The Handbook of Clinical Linguistics

Edited by

Martin J. Ball,
Michael R. Perkins,
Nicole Müller, and
Sara Howard

WILEY-BLACKWELL

A John Wiley & Sons, Inc., Publication

This paperback edition first published 2011
© 2011 Blackwell Publishing Ltd

Edition history: Blackwell Publishing Ltd (hardback, 2008)

Blackwell Publishing was acquired by John Wiley & Sons in February 2007. Blackwell's publishing program has been merged with Wiley's global Scientific, Technical, and Medical business to form Wiley-Blackwell.

Registered Office
John Wiley & Sons Ltd, The Atrium, Southern Gate, Chichester, West Sussex, PO19 8SQ, United Kingdom

Editorial Offices
350 Main Street, Malden, MA 02148-5020, USA
9600 Garsington Road, Oxford, OX4 2DQ, UK
The Atrium, Southern Gate, Chichester, West Sussex, PO19 8SQ, UK

For details of our global editorial offices, for customer services, and for information about how to apply for permission to reuse the copyright material in this book please see our website at www.wiley.com/wiley-blackwell.

The right of Martin J. Ball, Michael R. Perkins, Nicole Müller, and Sara Howard to be identified as the authors of the editorial material in this work has been asserted in accordance with the UK Copyright, Designs and Patents Act 1988.

Library of Congress Cataloging-in-Publication Data
The handbook of clinical linguistics / edited by Martin J. Ball . . . [et al.]
    p. ; cm. — (Blackwell handbooks in linguistics; 24)
    Includes bibliographical references and index.
    ISBN 978-1-4051-3522-1 (hardcover : alk. paper) ISBN 978-1-4443-3877-5 (paperback)
1. Language disorders. 2. Linguistics. I. Ball, Martin J. (Martin John) II. Series.
    [DNLM: 1. Language Disorders. 2. Linguistics. WL 340.2 H2354 2008]

    RC423.H3252 2008
    616.8525—dc22

                                                                            2007037584

A catalogue record for this book is available from the British Library.

Set in 10/12pt Palatino by Graphicraft
Printed and bound in Singapore by Fabulous Printers Pte Ltd

1 2011

Contents

Figures

Notes on Contributors

Elisabeth Ahlsén is Professor of Neurolinguistics at the Department of Linguistics and the SSKKII Center for Cognitive Science, Göteborg University. Her main areas of research are neurolinguistics, pragmatics, and communication disorders. She teaches neurolinguistics, psycholinguistics, cognitive science, communication analysis, and linguistic research methods. She coordinates a number of research projects on communication disorders in adults and children, focusing on pragmatics, semantics, gesture, and ICT support.

Shaheen N. Awan is Professor of Speech Pathology at Bloomsburg University of Pennsylvania. His research interests are in acoustic analysis of normal and disordered speech/voice and digital signal processing. His clinical work is focused on the administration and interpretation of stroboscopy, as well as other aspects of the assessment and treatment of voice disorders.

Martin J. Ball is Hawthorne Endowed Professor and Director of the Research Center in the Department of Communicative Disorders, at the University of Louisiana at Lafayette. He is co-editor of the journal *Clinical Linguistics and Phonetics* and of the book series Communication Disorders across Languages (Multilingual Matters). His main research interests include sociolinguistics, clinical phonetics and phonology, and the linguistics of Welsh. He is the immediate Past President of the International Clinical Phonetics and Linguistics Association. His most recent books are *Clinical Sociolinguistics* (Blackwell, 2005) and, co-authored with Nicole Müller, *Phonetics for Communication Disorders* (Erlbaum, 2005).

Tessa Bent is an Assistant Professor in the Department of Speech and Hearing Sciences at Indiana University. Her research has focused on speech intelligibility, perceptual learning and cross-language speech perception and production. Her research reports have appeared in the *Journal of the Acoustical Society of America*, the *Journal of Experimental Psychology: Human Perception and Performance, Linguistics, Cognition* and *Phonetica*.

(Barbara) May Bernhardt is Professor in the School of Audiology and Speech Sciences, University of British Columbia, specializing in child language acquisition, specifically on phonological development, assessment, and intervention.

Maria Black has taught linguistics and psycholinguistics at University College London from 1980 to 2009. Her research has focused on psycholinguistic approaches to language impairments in adults with aphasia. She has published studies on semantic, syntactic, and prosodic aspects of aphasia, and has co-authored with Shula Chiat *Linguistics for Clinicians* (Arnold, 2003), a textbook in clinical linguistics.

Joan L. Bybee is Distinguished Professor Emerita in Linguistics at the University of New Mexico. She has published books and articles on phonology, morphology, and language change. She is Past President and Fellow of the Linguistic Society of America.

Shula Chiat has taught linguistics and language development on speech and language therapy courses for many years, at City University and at University College London. Her research focuses on psycholinguistic approaches to language impairments in children. She is author of *Understanding Children with Language Problems* (Cambridge, 2000), and co-author with Maria Black of a textbook, *Linguistics for Clinicians* (Arnold, 2003).

Harald Clahsen's first degree was in German philology and sociology (1978). He went on to do research in first and second language acquisition, which led to his PhD in 1981. Over the following years his research focused on developmental language disorders, which led to his postdoctoral degree (Habilitation) in linguistics in 1987 at the University of Düsseldorf. Since then, he has also studied grammatical processing in native speakers and language learners using psycholinguistic experimentation. He has written seven books and over one hundred research articles on first and second language acquisition, language disorders, and language processing. He has received the Gerhard-Hess Award from the German Science Foundation for his work on language acquisition and an award for his book on child language disorders. He has coordinated several large research projects, and he co-edits Benjamins' book series on Language Development and Language Disorders. In addition to acquisition, disorders, and processing of language, his research interests include theories of morphology and syntax.

Martha Crago is a Professor and Vice-Rector at the University of Montréal. Her research and publications focus on language acquisition and socialization in monolingual and bilingual children who are typical and atypical learners and speakers of a variety of languages including English, French, Inuktitut, and Arabic languages.

Jack S. Damico is the Doris B. Hawthorne Eminent Scholar in Communication Disorders and Special Education at the University of Louisiana at Lafayette. He earned a master's degree in communicative disorders at the University of Oklahoma Health Sciences Center in 1976 and a doctorate in linguistics at the University of New Mexico in 1985. His research interests include language as a synergistic phenomenon and language as social action. His primary research focus is applications of qualitative research methodologies in communicative sciences and disorders including language and literacy, clinical aphasiology, language disorders in children, attention deficit hyperactivity disorder, and service delivery to multicultural populations. He has published over one hundred articles and chapters and has authored or edited several books including *Clinical Aphasiology: Future Directions* (with Martin Ball; Psychology Press, 2007), *Special Education Considerations for English Language Learners: Delivering a Continuum of Services* (with Else Hamayan, Barbara Marler and Cristina Sanchez-Lopez; Caslon, 2007), and *Childhood Language Disorders* (with Michael Smith; 1996, Thieme Medical).

Jan de Jong is an Assistant Professor and Senior Researcher at the University of Amsterdam (Amsterdam Center for Language and Communication). At present, he is involved in a research project on Specific Language Impairment (SLI) in Turkish-Dutch bilingual children with SLI. His previous research addressed the grammatical symptoms of SLI in Dutch (inflectional morphology and argument structure) and the linguistic precursors of dyslexia.

Daniel A. Dinnsen is Chancellor's Professor of Linguistics and Cognitive Science and Adjunct Professor of Speech and Hearing Sciences at Indiana University, Bloomington. His research draws on the latest developments in linguistic theory and is recognized for its theoretical and empirical discoveries about phonological acquisition and disorders.

Gerrard Docherty is Professor of Phonetics at Newcastle University, UK. His research is focused on investigating aspects of variability in speech production with a particular interest in determining how the phonetic performance of speakers is shaped by the various dimensions (physical, linguistic, cognitive, and social) of spoken communication, with a view to developing theories which account for the systematic properties of speech in its social context. While much of his recent work has focused on sociophonetic variability in normal adult speakers, he has also carried out research on the acquisition of speech sound patterning in children and on the nature of speech in populations of speakers with impaired speech production.

Alison Ferguson is Associate Professor and the Speech Pathology Discipline Convenor at the University of Newcastle, Australia, with over 20 years experience in the field of speech-language pathology. She has a strong track record of funded clinical research, mainly in the area of linguistic applications to aphasia (impaired language due to brain damage), and has published widely in international peer-reviewed journals.

Angela D. Friederici is Director of the Max Planck Institute for Human Cognitive and Brain Sciences, Leipzig, and Honorary Professor at the Universities of Leipzig, Potsdam, and Berlin. She studied linguistics and psychology. Dr. Friederici received her PhD from the University of Bonn and spent her postdoctoral period at the Massachusetts Institute of Technology. Her main field of research is neurocognition of language, particular language comprehension. She is a member of the International Neuropsychological Symposium and the German Academy of Natural Sciences Leopoldina, and Vice-President of the Berlin Brandenburg Academy of Sciences.

Stefan Frisch studied psychology, philosophy, and linguistics at the Universities of Heidelberg, Berlin, Leipzig, and Potsdam. He has been working as a research assistant at the Max Planck Institute of Human Cognitive and Brain Sciences in Leipzig and at the University of Potsdam. He is now in the neuropsychology department at the Day-Care Clinic of Cognitive Neurology, University of Leipzig. His research interests focus on electrophysiology and imaging of normal and impaired cognition, as well as on neuropsychological treatment.

Fiona E. Gibbon is a speech and language therapist and Professor and Head of Speech and Hearing Sciences at Queen Margaret University in Edinburgh. Her research focuses on the use of instrumentation to diagnose and treat speech disorders. She has published over seventy papers in professional and scientific journals and as book chapters, and has been awarded numerous research council- and charity-funded grants. Her research was awarded the Queen's Anniversary Prize for excellence in 2002. She is a Fellow of the Royal College of Speech and Language Therapists.

Judith A. Gierut is Professor of Speech & Hearing Sciences and Cognitive Science and Adjunct Professor of Linguistics at Indiana University, Bloomington. Her research draws upon linguistic and psycholinguistic theories in the process of language acquisition by children with typical and atypical speech sound development. Gierut is recognized for her innovative integration of linguistics, cognitive psychology, and speech pathology in assessment and experimental treatment of phonological disorders.

Louis M. Goldstein received his PhD in linguistics from the University of California at Los Angeles. He is Professor of Linguistics and Psychology at Yale University and a Senior Scientist at Haskins Laboratories. His research focuses on aspects of articulatory phonology, both experimental and modeling, and also on the emergence of phonological structure.

Jacqueline A. Guendouzi is an Associate Professor in the Communication Sciences and Disorders Department of Southeastern Louisiana University. Her research focuses on qualitative approaches to interactions involving clinical populations. She has recently published a book and several articles with Nicole Müller, examining discourse approaches to dementia. With the same author, she has published articles and chapters relating to the application of qualitative methods to clinical interactions. She has also published several articles examining socialized gender roles in women's interactions.

Bill Hardcastle is Professor of Speech Sciences and Director of the Speech Science Research Centre at Queen Margaret University, Edinburgh. From 1974 to 1993 he worked in the Department of Linguistic Science at Reading University, where he was Professor of Speech Science and Director of the Speech Research Laboratory. From 1993 to 2002 he was Head of the Department of Speech and Language Sciences then Dean of Health Sciences and Dean of Research at QMU. He has published numerous books and articles in areas such as the mechanisms of speech production, instrumental clinical phonetics and sensorimotor control in both normal and pathological speech. For his research on electropalatography he was recently honored by Queen Elizabeth as a Pioneer of the British Nation, and received the 2006 Lord Lloyd of Kilgerran award from the Foundation for Science and Technology. He is a Fellow of the British Academy and an Honorary Fellow of the Royal College of Speech and Language Therapists, and was President of the International Clinical Phonetics and Linguistics Association from 1991 till 2000.

Barry Heselwood is Senior Lecturer in the Department of Linguistics and Phonetics at the University of Leeds, where he specializes in phonetics and phonology. He has a research interest in disordered speech, having published several single- and joint-authored papers in this field. Along with Sara Howard he is co-convener of a recently formed Phonetic Transcription Group, its membership drawn from across the north of England.

Sara Howard is Reader in Clinical Phonetics and ESRC Research Fellow in the Department of Human Communication Sciences at the University of Sheffield. As well as her academic qualifications in phonetics and linguistics, she is professionally qualified as a speech-language therapist/pathologist. She has co-edited with Mick Perkins *Case Studies in Clinical Linguistics* (Whurr, 1995) and *New Directions in Language Development and Disorders* (Kluwer, 2000), and has published and presented widely in the area of clinical phonetics and phonology. Her research focuses on the interface between phonetics and phonology in normal and atypical speech production, with a particular emphasis on the perceptual and instrumental phonetic analysis of developmental speech impairment. She is currently President of the International Clinical Phonetics and Linguistics Association.

David Ingram is a Professor and Chair of the Department of Speech and Hearing Science at Arizona State University. His research interests are in language acquisition in typically developing children and children with language disorders, with a cross-linguistic focus. The language areas of interest are phonological, morphological, and syntactic acquisition.

Yves Joanette was trained in speech-language pathology and in neurosciences at the University of Montréal, and then completed postdoctoral training in clinical and cognitive neurosciences in Marseilles. In 1982, Dr. Joanette started his research career as a CIHR *Scholar* then *Scientist*. In 1990, he was awarded the Prix du jeune chercheur of the Club de recherches cliniques du Québec. In 1995, he was the recipient of the CASLPA Eve-Kassirer award for his outstanding achievements. Since 1997, he has been Research Director at the Institut universitaire de gériatrie de Montréal. His research work bears upon the age-influenced impact of right-hemisphere lesions on verbal communication as well as on the cognitive dimensions of dementia (e.g., Alzheimer's disease). Dr. Joanette is also very much involved in the international community. Formerly Chair of the Board of Governors of the prestigious Academy of Aphasia, he is now Chair of the Board of the Sociedad latinoamericana de neuropsicologia.

Karima Kahlaoui is Postdoctoral Fellow in Cognitive Neuroscience at the Centre de recherche de l'institut universitaire de gériatrie de Montréal. Her research interests include right hemisphere and processing of semantic relationships between isolated words, and functional neuroimaging of normal and pathological aging.

Ray D. Kent is Professor Emeritus of Communicative Disorders at the University of Wisconsin-Madison. His primary research interests are neurogenic speech disorders in children and adults, speech development in infants, speech intelligibility, and the acoustic analysis of speech. He currently serves as Vice-President for Research and Technology of the American Speech-Language-Hearing Association.

Ghada Khattab is a phonetics lecturer in the School of Education, Communication, and Language Sciences at the University of Newcastle upon Tyne. She is a native speaker of Lebanese Arabic and has a PhD in linguistics from the University of Leeds. Her research interests include monolingual and bilingual phonological development and sociolinguistics

Yunjung Kim recently completed a PhD in speech-language pathology at the University of Wisconsin-Madison after earning her undergraduate and master's degrees at the Korea University, Seoul. She is now an assistant professor at Louisiana State University in Baton Rouge. Her particular interests are in how type and severity of motor speech disorders influence acoustic and perceptual variability.

Sonja A. Kotz received her MS and PhD degrees in psychology at Tufts University, Medford, and also holds an MA degree in psycholinguistics from the University of Tübingen). She currently works as a senior research scientist in the departments of neuropsychology and neurology at the Max Planck Institute of Human Cognitive and Brain Sciences and the Day-Care Clinic of Cognitive Neurology at the University of Leipzig. Her main research interests focus on speech perception and language comprehension, in particular the representation and processing of language functions (prosody, semantics, and syntax; interaction of language functions). She is utilizing event-related brain potentials (ERPs), functional magnetic resonance imaging (fMRI), and behavioral measures to study these processes in both healthy and patient populations.

Alice S.-Y. Lee is a Lecturer in the Department of Speech and Hearing Sciences at University College Cork, Ireland. Her doctoral dissertation was on perceptual and instrumental investigations of hypernasality. Her research interests include perceptual and instrumental investigations of speech disorders in individuals with structural anomalies or neurological impairment.

Eeva Leinonen is a Professor in Clinical Linguistics and Vice Principal at King's College London and Privet Doscent in Clinical Linguistics at the University of Oulu, Finland. She has published two books and various articles, focusing particularly on clinical pragmatics and pragmatic language comprehension difficulties in children.

Li Wei is Professor of Applied Linguistics at Birkbeck, University of London. He was previously Head of the School of Education, Communication and Language Sciences at the University of Newcastle upon Tyne. His research interests are in bilingualism. He has researched code switching and bilingual interaction, language maintenance and language shift, bilingual and multilingual first language acquisition, and discursive practices in bilingual education. He is author of *Three Generations, Two Languages, One Family* (Multilingual Matters, 1997), and editor of *The Bilingualism Reader* (2nd edition, Routledge, 2007), *Opportunities and Challenges of Bilingualism*, with Jean-Marc Dewaele (Mouton de Gruyter, 2002), *Bilingualism: Beyond Basic Principles* (Multilingual Matters, 2003), *Handbook of Multilingualism and Multilingual Communication*, with Peter Auer (Mouton de Gruyter, 2007), and the *Blackwell Handbook of Research Methods in Bilingualism and Multilingualism*, with Melissa Moyer (Blackwell, 2007). He is also the editor of the *International Journal of Bilingualism*.

John Local is Professor of Phonetics and Linguistics at the University of York. His research over the past 30 years has engaged with non-segmental phonology and phonetic interpretation, speech synthesis, and, latterly, phonetics and talk-in-interaction. This work developed out of a close study of Firthian Prosodic Analysis (FPA) and an attempt to elaborate an impressionistic para-metric phonetics supported by instrumental findings. Some of the results of this research, conducted with his colleague John Kelly, are presented in their book, *Doing Phonology* (Manchester University Press, 1989). In recent years he has worked on phonetic variability in the 'liquid' system of English and the phonetic and interactional features of attitude in everyday conversation (supported by grants from the Economic and Social Research Council). He is currently writing a book, arising from research during a two-year British Academy Readership, on an interactionally grounded analysis of the phonetics of everyday talk.

Theodoros Marinis is Lecturer in Clinical Linguistics at the University of Reading. His research focuses on cross-linguistic first and second language acquisition and processing in adults, typically developing monolingual and bilingual children, and children with Specific Language Impairment. In 2003, he published the book *The Acquisition of the DP in Modern Greek* (John Benjamins).

Lise Menn is a Professor of Linguistics at the University of Colorado. She is a leading authority on the cross-linguistic nature of adult-acquired aphasia and author of numerous publications on the subject.

Adele Miccio (1952–2009) is the late Associate Professor of Communication Sciences and Disorders at the Pennsylvania State University, where she taught courses in phonetics and phonology. Her research interests included the assessment and treatment of disordered phonological systems and the relation of early phonological development to emerging literacy. Recent projects included the longitudinal study of bilingual Spanish-English phonological acquisition and the development of bilingual phonological assessment procedures.

Nicole Müller is Hawthorne-BoRSF Endowed Professor in Communicative Disorders, University of Louisiana at Lafayette. Dr. Müller has published widely in both books and journals in various areas of language disorders. Particular areas of interest include sociolinguistics and multilingualism, and clinical discourse studies and pragmatics, specifically as applied to dementia. She is co-editor of the journal *Clinical Linguistics and Phonetics*. Her most recent books include *Approaches to Discourse in Dementia*, co-authored with Jackie Guendouzi (Erlbaum, 2005), and *Multilayered Transcription* (Plural Publishing, 2006).

Johanne Paradis is an Associate Professor in the Linguistics Department at the University of Alberta. Her research and publications focus on typical and atypical learners who are monolingual, bilingual, and second language learners of French and English in majority and minority settings.

Martina Penke is working as Professor of German Linguistics at the University of Ghent, Belgium, and is a member of the Institut für Sprache und Information (Abt. Allgemeine Sprachwissenschaft) at the University of Düsseldorf. Her research interests center on language disorders (acquired and congenital), first language acquisition and the cognitive/neural representation of language capacities. The aim of her work in language disorders is to provide linguistically sound profiles of retained and impaired language capacities in the areas of syntax and morphology in different syndromes. She is involved in various research projects on morphological and syntactical deficits and the neural representation of morphology. She teaches courses in theoretical linguistics as well as in neuro- and psycholinguistics, language acquisition, language disorders, and the biology of language.

Michael R. Perkins is Emeritus Professor of Clinical Linguistics in the Department of Human Communication Sciences at the University of Sheffield. Dr. Perkins has published numerous articles and several books including *Modal Expressions in English* (Ablex, 1983), *Case Studies in Clinical Linguistics* (Whurr, 1995), *New Directions in Language Development and Disorders* (Kluwer, 2000), the last two co-edited with Sara Howard, and *Pragmatic Impairment* (Cambridge University Press, 2007). His research focuses on the relationship between semantics, pragmatics, and cognition in human communication, with a particular emphasis on pragmatic disability in a wide range of developmental and acquired communication disorders. He was a founder member of the International Clinical Phonetics and Linguistics Association (ICPLA) and was its Vice-President from 2000 to 2006.

David B. Pisoni carries out basic and clinical research on speech perception, spoken word recognition, language comprehension, and perceptual development. He has carried out numerous studies on the perception of synthetic speech produced by rule and was involved in the perceptual evaluation of the MITalk text-to-speech system at MIT in the late 1970s. For the last 12 years he has been working on several clinical problems associated with hearing and hearing impairment in deaf children and adults who use cochlear implants, at the IU School of Medicine. Dr. Pisoni has been the Program Director of the NIH-sponsored training program in Speech, Hearing and Sensory Communication, from NIDCD since 1978. Dr. Pisoni was awarded a Guggenheim Fellowship in 1978. He is a fellow of the AAAS, the ASA, and the APS.

Karen Pollock is Professor and Chair of the Department of Speech Pathology and Audiology at the University of Alberta. After receiving a master's degree in linguistics from the University of Oregon, Dr. Pollock pursued a clinical degree in speech-language pathology, also at the University of Oregon, and later received her PhD from Purdue University. Prior to taking her current position, she was an assistant professor at the University of Northern Iowa and an associate professor at the University of Memphis, where she conducted research and taught graduate courses in phonetics, phonological disorders, and multicultural issues in communication disorders. She has a broad range of research interests, including vowel errors in children with phonological disorders, phonological variation in regional and social dialects, and speech-language acquisition in children adopted internationally.

Nuala Ryder is a Research Fellow in the Psychology Department at the University of Hertfordshire. She has published articles on children's use of context in pragmatic interpretation and the assessment of pragmatic comprehension in normal and clinical populations.

Shelley E. Scarpino is a doctoral student of child language and phonology at the Pennsylvania State University. Her research interests are in the areas of phonological development and disorders, phonological awareness and early literacy, and the development of phonological precursors to literacy in bilingual children.

Anna Vogel Sosa is Assistant Professor of Communication Sciences and Disorders at Northern Arizona University, Flagstaff. She received her M.A. in linguistics from the University of New Mexico, and Ph.D. from the University of Washington. She recently conducted research in the area of early phonological development within a usage based framework, with Carol Stoel-Gammon.

Joseph P. Stemberger is a Professor in the Department of Linguistics, University of British Columbia, specializing in adult psycholinguistics (especially phonology and morphology in language production, and the interactions between them) and first language acquisition.

Brigitte Stemmer obtained her PhD in applied linguistics at the Ruhr-University of Bochum and completed her medical studies at the University of Essen. After completing her postdoctoral studies in neuropsychology and cognitive neuroscience at the University of Montréal and at McGill University, she worked as a physician and clinical researcher at a neurological acute care and rehabilitation hospital in Germany. She currently holds a position as a Canada Research Chair in Neuroscience and Neuropragmatics at the University of Montreal.

Carol Stoel-Gammon is Professor in the Department of Speech and Hearing Sciences at the University of Washington. She received her doctorate in linguistics from Stanford University. She has held teaching appointments at the University of Campinas in Brazil, the University of Colorado, the University of Washington, and Canterbury University in New Zealand. Her research interests include prelinguistic vocal development, cross-linguistic studies of phonological acquisition, speech development and disorders in early childhood, and early identification of speech and language disorders.

Julie Thomson is a speech pathologist with thirty years experience in the area of child language disorders. She is currently conjoint lecturer and clinical educator with the University of Newcastle, Australia and Hunter-New England Health. Her master's research thesis applied Systemic Functional Linguistics to children's discourse and she has also published on this topic in a number of refereed journals.

Kris Tjaden is an Associate Professor and Director of the Motor Speech Disorders Laboratory in the Department of Communicative Disorders and Sciences at the University at Buffalo. Dr. Tjaden's NIH-funded research focuses on the acoustic and perceptual consequences of vocal tract behavior in dysarthria. Her research has been published in a variety of scholarly journals, and a recent study published in the *Journal of Speech, Language and Hearing Research* was selected to receive the 2005 Speech Editor's Award. She has also authored or co-authored several book chapters. Dr. Tjaden is presently an associate editor for the *Journal of Speech, Language and Hearing Research*.

Pascal H. H. M. van Lieshout received his PhD in experimental psychology from the Radboud University, Nijmegen. He is Canada Research Chair in Oral Motor Function across the Lifespan, Associate Professor in Speech Science, and Director of the Oral Dynamics Lab in the Department of Speech-Language Pathology at the University of Toronto. His research is in the area of oral motor control in speech and swallowing.

Gary Weismer is a Professor in the Department of Communicative Disorders and Waisman Center at the University of Wisconsin-Madison. His research interests are in the areas of speech acoustics, speech physiology, and motor speech disorders.

Bill Wells is a full professor and currently Chair of the Department of Human Communication Sciences at the University of Sheffield. His principal research interests are: typical and atypical speech development in children, including linguistic, psycholinguistic, and interactional approaches; phonological aspects of children's connected speech; children's production and comprehension of intonation; children's processing of unfamiliar regional accents; and prosody in conversational interaction.

Tara L. Whitehill is Professor in the Division of Speech and Hearing Sciences and Director of the Motor Speech Laboratory at the University of Hong Kong. Her research focuses on the perceptual and instrumental evaluation of speech disorders in individuals with cleft palate, dysarthria, and other physiologically based disorders. She focuses on improving the validity and reliability of measures of disordered speech, and determining contributions to reduced speech intelligibility.

Sandra Whiteside is a Reader in Speech Sciences in the Department of Human Communication Sciences at the University of Sheffield. Her research interests include hormone-mediated developmental sex differences in speech across the human lifespan, and speech encoding in typical and atypical speech with a specific interest in acquired apraxia of speech, and related speech disorders.

Ray Wilkinson is a Reader in the Neuroscience and Aphasia Research Unit, School of Psychological Sciences at the University of Manchester. His research has predominantly focused on conversation analysis and communication disorders, particularly aphasia. Recent work has included the analysis of change over time in conversations of couples where one partner has aphasia, and the use of conversation analysis to guide and evaluate intervention programmes aimed at changing interactional behaviour.

Brent Wilson is an assistant professor at Radford University, Virginia. His major research interests include acquired and degenerative neurogenic communicative disorders, as well as qualitative research methodologies. He presented three papers at the 2006 International Clinical Linguistics and Phonetics Association conference, and three at the 2006 American Speech Language and Hearing Association conference. His dissertation was on discourse markers in Alzheimer's disease.

Alison Wray is a Professor of Language and Communication at Cardiff University. Her research has focused on modeling the forms and functions of formulaic sequences in normal and disordered language and in second language acquisition, with further applications to the evolution of language and to language profiling.

Zhu Hua is Reader in Applied Linguistics and Communication at Birkbeck, University of London. She was previously Sir James Knott Research Fellow, Lecturer and Senior Lecturer in Language and Communication at the University of Newcastle upon Tyne. Her research interests include cross-linguistic studies of children's speech and language development and disorders, and cross-cultural pragmatics. She is author of *Phonological Development in Specific Contexts* (Multilingual Matters, 2002), of *DEAP: Diagnostic Evaluation of Articulation and Phonology*, with Barbara Dodd, Sharon Crosbie, Alison Holm, and Ann Ozanne (Psycholocial Corporation, 2002), of *PAC: Phonological Assessment of Chinese (Mandarin)* (Speechmark, 2007), and of many articles in the *Journal of Child Language, Clinical Linguistics and Phonetics*, the *International Journal of Language and Communication Disorders*, the *Journal of Pragmatics, Multilingua*, and *Language and Intercultural Communication*. She is co-editor with Barbara Dodd of *Phonological Development and Disorders in Children: A Multilingual Perspective* (Multilingual Matters, 2006), and, with Paul Seedhouse, Li Wei, and Vivian Cook, of *Language Learning and Teaching as Social Inter-Action* (Palgrave Macmillan, 2007).

Wolfram Ziegler acquired his PhD in mathematics at the Technical University, Munich, and has worked as a research assistant at the Max Planck Institute for Psychiatry, Munich. He is Head of the Clinical Neuropsychology Research Group at the Department of Neuropsychology, City Hospital Bogenhausen, Munich, and lectures in neurophonetics at the University of Munich. The main topics of his research are dysarthria, apraxia of speech, and aphasia.

Introduction

MARTIN J. BALL, MICHAEL R.
PERKINS, NICOLE MÜLLER,
AND SARA HOWARD

Although the insights of the speech and language sciences have long been applied to the description and analysis of communication impairment, the widespread use of the term 'clinical linguistics' dates only from the publication of the book of that title by David Crystal (1981). Crystal defines clinical linguistics as "the application of linguistic science to the study of communication disability, as encountered in clinical situations" (Crystal, 1981, p. 1).Further, Crystal (1984, p. 31) adds to his definition: "clinical linguistics is the application of the theories, methods and findings of linguistics (including phonetics) to the study of those situations where language handicaps are diagnosed and treated."

Restricting the direction of application from linguistics to language disorder is deliberate: "the orientation . . . should be noted. It may be contrasted with the approach of neurolinguists, for example, who study clinical language data in order to gain insights into linguistic or neurological theory" (Crystal, 1984, pp. 30–1). However, it has since been recognized that the study of communication disorders can tell us a great deal about the nature of communication itself, and the scope of the term has subsequently been extended. For example, Ball and Kent (1987, p. 2) in the preface to the then newly launching journal *Clinical Linguistics and Phonetics*, state that they prefer a definition that covers "either applying linguistic/phonetic analytic techniques to clinical problems, or showing how clinical data contribute to theoretical issues in linguistics/ phonetics". This approach is the one we take in this handbook.

In the 1970s and 80s Crystal and his colleagues worked to develop linguistically based profiling techniques for the analysis of normal and disordered syntax (Crystal, Fletcher, & Garman, 1976; Crystal, 1979), and then phonology, prosody and semantics (Crystal, 1982). At about the same time a particular interest in the clinical application of phonology began to emerge, with work by Grunwell (1982), Ingram (1976, 1981), Edwards and Shriberg (1983), and Edwards and Gierut (1986) among many others. The founding of the journal *Clinical Linguistics and Phonetics* in 1987 provided an expanded forum for the development of clinical linguistics, and the lead article by Crystal pointed the way to the exploration of interactions between levels of analysis in clinical linguistics (Crystal, 1987). The 1990s saw a number of book-length treatments of specific areas of clinical linguistics such as syntax (Grodzinsky, 1990), pragmatics (Gallagher, 1991; Smith & Leinonen, 1992), psycholinguistics (Lesser & Milroy, 1993), new approaches to phonology (Ball & Kent, 1997), transcribing disordered speech (Ball, Rahilly, & Tench, 1996; revisited in Müller, 2006), instrumental aspects of clinical phonetics (Ball & Code, 1997), and the detailed application of these specific areas in the form of individual case studies (Perkins & Howard, 1995). The increasing momentum of research into clinical linguistics has continued into the current decade. Collections of research articles have been published which attest to the full scope of the discipline (e.g. Fava, 2002; Maassen & Groenen, 1999; Windsor, Hewlett, & Kelly, 2002). *Clinical Linguistics and Phonetics* now appears monthly with articles covering a range of linguistic areas and disorder types, and dealing with a variety of different languages. Recent books show the expansion of clinical linguistics into new areas: Ball (2007) describes a clinical sociolinguistics, Perkins (2007) provides a unified theory of pragmatic ability and disability, and Guendouzi and Müller (2006) investigate the nature of discourse in dementia. The discipline has clearly matured to a point where an up-to-date survey in the form of a handbook is warranted, if not overdue.

For this handbook we have commissioned state-of-the-art articles by leading clinical linguists and phoneticians with the aim of covering the main areas of research in the field. It is organized according to the different areas of linguistics – e.g. phonology, syntax, pragmatics – rather than to different types of communication disorder – e.g. aphasia, specific language impairment, dysarthria. The latter approach has been avoided partly because there are handbooks of communication disorders already in existence (e.g. Blanken, Dittmann, Grimm, Marshall, & Wallesch, 1993; Damico, Ball, & Müller, forthcoming; Kent, 2003), but also to reflect the status of clinical linguistics as a subdiscipline of linguistics rather than of speech and language pathology. The aim has been to include discussion of a range of pathologies, both developmental and acquired, in each chapter. In addition, we have invited authors to briefly consider the actual or potential influence of their particular specialist area on mainstream theories and descriptions of language, in line with our expanded definition of clinical linguistics above.

The handbook is divided into three parts: I: Discourse, Pragmatics and Sociolinguistics, II: Syntax and Semantics and III: Phonetics and Phonology.

Part I, Discourse, Pragmatics and Sociolinguistics, considers speech, language and communication impairment from the perspective of language *use*. In particular, it examines how the choices involved in language production and comprehension are influenced by underlying linguistic and cognitive abilities and also by the communicative context, including factors such as the age, sex and socio-cultural background of the interlocutors, their relationship, relative status and degree of shared knowledge, their interactional agendas, and the physical, social, cultural, institutional and political parameters of the interaction itself. The focus on use and context is a relatively recent development in clinical linguistics, which has been more traditionally concerned with the form and structure of speech and language. However, the vitality of this burgeoning area of the discipline is evident in the range of different theoretical approaches and methodological paradigms represented in the nine chapters of part I.

In the opening chapter, Müller, Guendouzi and Wilson review the application of Discourse Analysis (DA) in its various guises to the study of communication disorders. They focus in particular on Kintsch and Van Dijk's model of macrostructure and microstructure, on story grammars, and on socio-cultural approaches such as Critical Discourse Analysis, Discursive Psychology and Social Construction Theory. In addition, Speech Act Theory, which is also mentioned in several other chapters (e.g. chapters 4 and 5), receives its main treatment in this chapter. Two further theories of pragmatics – Conversational Implicature and Relevance Theory – are covered in chapters 2 and 3. Ahlsén examines how Grice's cooperative principle and conversational maxims can be used as a framework for elucidating communication impairment, and in particular focuses on ways in which the principle and maxims appear not to be adhered to for various reasons. Problems with world knowledge, cognition, language comprehension and language production can all affect the use of implicature, and she examines the impact of each on individual maxims. In chapter 3, Leinonen and Ryder review the clinical application of Relevance Theory (RT). The use of RT by clinicians has so far been fairly limited, though the authors argue that an account of pragmatic impairment in terms of cognitive processing, as proposed in RT, is of more explanatory value than description of behavioral symptoms alone. RT has proved to be particularly illuminating in the analysis of individuals with autism, and it is argued that RT itself is supported by studies of pragmatic impairment.

Rather than take pragmatic theory as its starting point as in chapters 2 and 3, Stemmer's chapter on 'neuropragmatics' – a recently coined term meaning the study of the neural substrates of pragmatic behavior – provides an overview of research which aims to identify links between a range of neurological impairments (e.g. right-hemisphere damage, traumatic brain injury, dementia and developmental disorders) and behaviors which have an impact on pragmatic competence, such as problems with inferential reasoning, interpretation of irony, sarcasm and jokes, and recognition of others' emotions and executive functions (e.g. attention, planning and problem solving). Perkins in chapter 5 likewise focuses on factors which underlie pragmatic impairment, but from a broader perspective. His 'emergentist' theory of pragmatics views pragmatic impairment not as a discrete phenomenon in its own right but as the complex outcome of interactions between semiotic, cognitive and sensorimotor systems during the process of communication. It extends the neuropragmatic account by (1) viewing phenomena such as cognitive processing and language use as inherently interpersonal, (2) seeing the relationship between underlying deficit and consequent behavior as being mediated via a process of compensatory adaptation, and (3) characterizing pragmatics as a multimodal rather than an exclusively linguistic phenomenon. The interpersonal dimension of language use is also highlighted by Wilkinson in chapter 6 from the perspective of conversation analysis (CA) – a variety of discourse analysis which focuses on the way in which conversation comes into being through a collaborative process of turn-by-turn construction in real time by both participants. Wilkinson examines how CA has been used to analyze interactions involving individuals with acquired and developmental communication disorders, and shows that such disorders are not the exclusive responsibility of individuals but are to a considerable degree the manifestation of jointly negotiated agendas.

In chapter 7, Damico and Ball examine the wider sociolinguistic context of communication disorder from the perspective of the variationist paradigm originally developed by Labov. They note, for example, the importance of being aware of the accent, dialect and socio-cultural features of the client's speech community which otherwise might be interpreted as evidence of impairment when compared to standard varieties/norms, and the necessity of setting ecologically valid remedial targets. They also discuss the way in which power relationships are negotiated between clinician and client, and the notion of literacy as a socio-political construct. Ferguson and Thomson (chapter 8) also take a sociolinguistically oriented view of communication impairment, but from the perspective of Systemic Functional Linguistics (SFL), a theory of language use developed by the British linguist Michael Halliday, in which syntax, semantics, phonology and pragmatics are all integral. They provide an outline of the theory, and of how it lends itself to clinical linguistic analysis, arguing that rather than simply providing a checklist of items for assessment or intervention, the value of SFL lies in its provision of a meaning-based conceptual and analytical paradigm which affords unique insight into the nature of communication impairment.

The final chapter in part I, by Hua and Wei, examines how cross-linguistic variation and bilingualism intersect with pragmatics, discourse and sociolinguistics in the context of clinical linguistics. There is still a relatively small literature on non-English speaking people with communication impairments, and within this literature discourse, pragmatics and sociolinguistics are the least researched topics. Hua and Wei point out that cross-linguistic and multilingual research in these areas is important not just in order to understand the nature of the impairments themselves and the extent to which they are influenced by the properties of specific languages and sociocultural factors, but also in order to provide effective assessment and treatment.

Part II is dedicated to syntax, morphology and semantics in the clinical domain. Whereas part I is concerned with language use in its various guises, the chapters in part II deal with formal aspects of language: sentence structure, word structure, and lexical meaning, traditionally considered core areas of both mainstream and clinical linguistics.

Chomsky's theory of generative grammar has been a dominant paradigm in theoretical syntax for roughly half a century. Clahsen's chapter (10) gives an overview of applications of generative grammar to issues in clinical linguistics.

Traditionally, favorite areas of application were aphasia and Specific Language Impairment (SLI), since, in these disorders, impairment appears to be specific to linguistic systems, while other cognitive domains remain more or less unimpaired. Clahsen outlines several approaches to the deficits observed in agrammatic aphasia: feature and trace deletion, Tree Pruning, and Underspecification of T/INFL, the former two being framed within Government and Binding Theory, the latter within the Minimalist Program. In the application of Chomskyan grammar to SLI, Clahsen discusses two types of approaches: those that identify quite broad syntactic impairments, and those that attempt to find specific linguistic markers for SLI. Chomskyan theory has thus far not been widely applied to broader developmental disorders that involve a broader range of cognitive and linguistic impairments, such as Down's syndrome. Clahsen discusses difficulties with pronoun comprehension, anaphoric binding and passivization that have been analyzed within this framework.

The topic of Wray's chapter (11) is formulaic language. Characteristics of formulaic sequences are that they appear to be stored and retrieved whole, rather than spontaneously created or analyzed at the point of use. Findings on the occurrence and nature of formulaic language in aphasia, Alzheimer's disease and autism are reviewed. Wray discusses dual systems models of language processing ('holistic' and 'analytic' processing), and contrasts them with a model of the lexicon as composed of different subunits on the basis of function.

Marinis (chapter 12) discusses syntactic processing in developmental and acquired language disorders, focusing on SLI and aphasia. He identifies as a major issue the question whether language disorder results from an incomplete language system (either incompletely developed, or affected by brain insult in acquired disorders), or from processing limitations. The chapter reviews literature investigating real-time syntactic processing, and compares differences in insights provided by on-line and off-line tasks.

In chapter 13, Penke surveys how inflectional systems are affected in language disorders. The factors identified as influencing errors with inflectional morphology are typology and complexity of inflectional systems, inflection type, regularity, frequency, and morphosyntactic specifications and markedness. Penke reviews theories that aim to account for deficits in inflectional systems, such as the role of mental lexicon versus that of mental grammar, and accounts based on problems with perception and production of inflectional affixes. Under the heading of the relevance of inflectional impairments for linguistic theory, the author discusses the implications of findings of selective deficits of regular and irregular inflections across a number of languages, differential impairment of different inflections with the same or similar surface forms, and the status of inflectional morphemes in the mental lexicon.

Kahlaoui and Joanette (chapter 14) give an overview of the neurological structures underlying word semantics, focusing on the specific contributions of the two cerebral hemispheres. The chapter surveys research on hemispheric asymmetries in semantic processing in normally functioning brains, as well as in studies of brain damage with a variety of etiologies (left-hemisphere lesions, right-hemisphere lesions, Alzheimer's disease). The authors conclude that semantic processing in the right cerebral hemisphere is unique, enriching and complementing processing by the left cerebral hemisphere.

Frisch, Kotz and Friederici (chapter 15) present research on the neural correlates of normal and pathological language processing at the sentence level. Their survey begins with the classical models of language as a neurological and psychological function, developed from the second half of the nineteenth century onwards. The chapter discusses the timing issue in language processing, as investigated via reaction-time experiments, event-related potentials (ERP), and neuroimaging methods that allow a high spatial resolution (positron emission tomography and functional magnetic resonance imaging – fMRI). The authors discuss ERP and fMRI research intro semantic integration and syntactic processes (word category integration, processing of morphosyntactic information, and syntactic repair analysis). They present a model of differential sequential phases of sentence processing, with the caveat that this is a very dynamic area of research and that therefore models are in a state of flux.

The main focus of de Jong's chapter (16) is on specific language impairment (SLI) in bilingual children. A brief discussion of aphasia in bilingual adults is included for comparative and contrastive purposes. Diagnostic concerns in bilingual SLI mirror major research questions, namely how to map the boundaries between language disorder and normally developing speakers of two or multiple languages with varying acquisition patterns (simultaneous or sequential, for example). The question of what constitutes bilingual SLI and how it differs from monolingual SLI is approached via a composite of group comparisons featuring bilingualism and/or SLI.

Crago, Paradis and Menn (chapter 17) offer cross-linguistic perspectives on impairments of syntax and semantics. The two populations focused upon are children with SLI, and adults with acquired aphasia. A key focus of cross-linguistic research in SLI has been the question of the extent to which clinical markers are language-specific or show tendencies across languages, with investigations of inflectional morphology dominating, while research on syntax or lexical semantics is thus far underrepresented. The authors conclude that while there are no universal cross-linguistic characteristics of SLI, there are characteristic tendencies, in particular within language families. The discussion of cross-linguistic research on aphasia begins with reviews of research on the comprehension of syntax and word-string interpretation studies, before moving on to production studies. The chapter concludes with a brief section on bilingual aphasia.

Black and Chiat's chapter (18) on interfaces between cognition, semantics and syntax focuses on verb argument structure, its impairments and linguistic analyses. A summary of deficits in verb argument structure in SLI and aphasia is followed by a review of thematic role analysis, in which each verb is categorized as having a specified thematic structure paired with a syntactic subcategorization frame. This permits an account of patterns of mapping between thematic and semantic roles shared by semantically diverse verbs. Given a number of shortcomings of thematic role analysis identified in the research literature, the authors conclude that thematic roles are insufficient to account for verb argument structures and their impairments. Rather, the authors argue that situations and their properties are crucial in the linguistic expression of situations, and that 'event structure' analysis should include the aspectual type of a situation, the causal structure of situations, and an indication of the properties of participants affecting their linguistic mapping.

Part III deals with phonetics and phonology. Because these related areas so often overlap in the clinical context (see Ball and Müller, 2002, for the difficulties in the use of the phonetics–phonology distinction with clinical data), we have combined these fields of study into the third part of the book.

Chapters 19 to 24, 'Phonetic Analysis', comprise a series of accounts of different methods for the phonetic analysis of clinical speech data, covering a range of instrumental, acoustic and perceptual approaches. In chapter 19, Gibbon describes a range of instrumental techniques used to capture aspects of articulatory activity during speech production, including electropalatography, X-ray, ultrasound, magnetic resonance imaging, electromagnetic articulography, optoelectronic systems and glossometry. As well as discussing the insights into the nature of impaired speech production which their use in research has supplied, Gibbon provides an assessment of the strengths and weaknesses of the techniques for use in the clinical context with children and adults with speech impairments, and also discusses the possible reasons why their clinical use is not as yet more widespread. In chapter 20, Whitehill and Lee continue the theme of instrumental analysis, describing a range of techniques which assess nasal resonance and airflow and velopharyngeal function, including direct visualization methods, such as nasendoscopy and videofluoroscopy, as well as acoustic and aerodynamic approaches including spectrography, nasometry, accelerometry and pressure-flow techniques. The authors note the care that is needed in the application of the techniques and in the interpretation of data gained from them, and discuss the relationship between instrumental and perceptual analyses in different clinical populations, including particularly speakers with cleft palate and speakers with a dysarthria.

Following on from the preceding accounts of articulation and resonance, in chapter 21 Awan considers the instrumental analysis of phonation and voice. Describing a range of direct and indirect techniques for investigating laryngeal structure and function, Awan points out the many challenges involved in voice analysis, given both the complex, multidimensional character of voice quality and phonatory activity, and also the additional consideration of inter- and intra-speaker variability and variation.

In chapter 22, Kent and Kim tackle the huge subject of acoustic analysis and its application in clinical phonetics. As they note, it is a particularly valuable technique in exploring the nature of speech impairments, as it can link the processes of speech production and speech perception. As well as providing a summary of the acoustic features of vowels and consonants, the authors use key areas of the research literature to discuss the ways in which acoustic analysis has contributed so extensively to our understanding of impaired speech production and perception. While acknowledging how much has already been achieved, Kent and Kim point the way forward to further work across a wide range of speech impairments.

Complementarily to the instrumental techniques already covered, in chapter 23 Heselwood and Howard explore the use of phonetic transcription in the analysis of atypical speech output. As well as a discussion of the motivation for carrying out narrow phonetic transcription, they describe its strengths and pitfalls. Issues considered by the authors include the content and layout of transcriptions, the various symbol systems and conventions available for capturing unusual aspects of speech production, and the different kinds and levels of detail which might be appropriate for different types of speech data.

Moving away from the approaches to clinical phonetic investigation addressed in the previous chapters, Bent and Pisoni (chapter 24) focus on the ways in which researchers have assessed speech perception and the extent to which different experimental paradigms support or undermine the claims made by competing theories of speech perception. Of particular interest is the degree to which the processes of speech perception are distinct from processes which human beings use to process other auditory events, as well as issues surrounding intelligibility and talker variability. The authors consider the implications of these issues for individuals with speech and language difficulties.

Chapters 25 to 30, 'Phonological Analysis', deals with clinical phonological concerns. A variety of phonological theories have been applied to the analysis of clinical data and recruited to aid in the planning of remediation for phonological errors, and these chapters explore the most dominant of these together with some innovations in the field. Miccio and Scarpino (chapter 25) critically evaluate the phonological processes approach to clinical phonology developed out of the theory of Natural Phonology, an approach that has been dominant among speech-language pathologists for some time. The authors note both the positive aspects of attention to patterns (rather than individual segments) and the frequent lack of phonetic grounding in some of the processes invented to deal with disordered speech.

The move to the nonlinear accounts of phonological patterning that have been part of the generative paradigm for many years came relatively late to clinical phonology. Developments such as autosegmental phonology, metrical phonology and feature geometry have all now been seen to have implications in the description and remediation of disordered speech. Bernhardt and Stemberger (chapter 26) describe these developments and move on to discuss how they operate within a constraints-based phonology. Dinnsen and Gierut (chapter 27) also take constraints as central, using the recently emerging approach of Optimality Theory to discuss phonological overgeneralization in children's speech. Optimality Theory accounts for phonological changes through the reordering of constraints, and the authors point out that a variety of disordered speech patterns could be described in this way. Government Phonology is in the same generative tradition as several of the preceding accounts. However, as Ball (chapter 28) explains, there are many important differences at both the segmental and the prosodic levels. One of the most important aspects of the theory is that feature values are unary and that governing relations may hold between features, and between segments. Often, the changes seen in disordered speech may be accounted for through changes in these governing relations.

An alternative to the generative paradigm is offered by Van Lieshout and Goldstein (chapter 29), who describe Articulatory Phonology and its application to speech impairment. As the name suggests, Articulatory Phonology is strongly phonetically based, with articulatory gestures acting as the primitive units of description. Changes in gestural coordination, gestural intrusion and decoupling are insightful ways of describing many aspects of disordered speech in both children and adults. The final chapter on phonological analysis (30) is by Sosa and Bybee; it describes the very recent work on phonology in use pioneered by the second author. This approach to phonology attempts psycholinguistic validity (rather than simply descriptive validity), and, in its modeling of phonological storage and emerging patterns influenced by frequency, may well have important implications for both the description and the treatment of disordered speech.

The remaining chapters of part III deal with other important topics in clinical phonetics and phonology. Ziegler, in chapter 31, deals with neurophonetics. He describes this area of study as a subdiscipline of neurolinguistics, and is concerned with those areas of neural functioning that deal with spoken language processing; he acknowledges the difficulty of disentangling phonetic from phonological concerns in neurolinguistics. The chapter concentrates on two main areas: motor disorders (including adult-acquired impairments and developmental problems in children), and perceptual neurophonetics. It concludes with the impact the study of neurophonetics has had on theory building in phonetics.

An issue which permeates many types of speech impairment, including those associated with aphasia, dysfluency, dysarthria, apraxia of speech and hearing impairment, is that of coarticulation, and specifically of impairments to coarticulation which disrupt the smooth and delicately timed overlapping of the different vocal organ movements for speech. In chapter 32 Hardcastle and Tjaden address this wide-ranging topic, examining different theoretical and methodological approaches to defining and measuring coarticulation, as well as discussing problems with coarticulation manifest across different clinical populations. They comment on the difficulties inherent in conducting clinical research in this area, but also note that further refinement and development of those analytic techniques currently available form a worthwhile endeavor.

Stoel-Gammon and Pollock's chapter (33) deals with vowels in normal acquisition and in disorder. The authors note the lack of research in this area in comparison to work with consonants. The chapter commences with a physiological description of vowel production, before examining the vowel system of American English in some detail. The literature on vowel acquisition in English and other languages is reviewed, and examples of vowel errors in normally developing and phonologically disordered children are given, including a discussion of childhood apraxia of speech. The chapter concludes with a discussion of assessment and treatment issues.

In chapter 34 Wells and Whiteside focus on prosody and on the ways in which atypical prosodic behavior may be investigated and assessed. As well as providing accounts of phonetic (perceptual and instrumental) and phonological/linguistic approaches to the analysis of prosody, the authors broaden their perspective to encompass both psycholinguistic and interactional approaches, the former focusing on the input and output processes involved in the perception and production of prosodic variables, and the latter exploring how various prosodic behaviors contribute to the negotiation of aspects of conversation such as turn-taking, topic control and repairs in real talk. They argue that the study of prosody in speech impairments is doubly valuable, both as a way of characterizing prosodic impairments, and also as a way of exploring how a speaker's comparative strengths in prosody might be employed to compensate for other speech production deficits.

Speech intelligibility is the focus of Gary Weismer's chapter 35. The author discusses the problem of defining what is meant by speech intelligibility, settling on the "relative measure of the degree to which a speaker's speech signal is understood". Weismer examines various approaches to the measuring of speech intelligibility, and then turns his attention to predicting intelligibility from error analyses, noting that feature-analytic measures prove better predictors than those based on transcription. Multiple regression models are also reviewed, the author concluding that a small number of the variables account for most of the variance in intelligibility scores.

Where clinical phonetic and phonological analysis has traditionally taken as its focus single words, in chapter 36 Howard, Wells, and Local adopt a different perspective, looking at how individuals with impaired speech produce words in sequence in multi-word utterances. As well as focusing in detail on word juncture behaviors and the ways in which speakers with speech difficulties negotiate word boundaries, they discuss the interplay between articulation and prosody in longer utterances, and the impact that connected speech difficulties can have on intelligibility. Insights from detailed phonetic analysis of clinical and developmental data lead the authors to call for analysis of connected speech to become a routine component of clinical assessment.

Another departure from traditional approaches to clinical phonetic and phonological analysis is made by Docherty and Khattab in chapter 37, where they present compelling reasons for researchers and clinicians to take account of sociophonetic factors in assessing and characterizing impaired speech. The authors explore issues associated with describing and interpreting sociophonetic variation and with seeking to understand how young children develop the ability to perceive and produce a repertoire of subtle and appropriate variants.

The implications of sociophonetic variation for clinical assessment and intervention as they relate to social and regional variation are explored, as well as the variation encountered in bilingual and second-language speakers.

The final contribution to the handbook deals with the cross-linguistic acquisition of phonology. Ingram (chapter 38) starts by considering the range of phonological differences between languages (from segmental inventories through prosody and phonotactics to morphophonology) and discussing theoretical aspects of phonology and phonological acquisition. He concentrates on consonant and word-complexity acquisition, in relation to theoretical concerns about the universal versus individual language nature of acquisition, and whether problems in acquisition have a phonological or articulatory basis. Ingram presents data from a range of different languages that lead to the conclusion that a considerable amount of cross-language variation is found in phonological acquisition, and that phonological disorders are not simply a reflex of articulatory limitations.

REFERENCES

Ball, M. J. (ed.) (2005). *Clinical Sociolinguistics*. Oxford: Blackwell.

Ball, M. J. and Code, C. (eds.) (1997). *Instrumental Clinical Phonetics*. London: Whurr.

Ball, M. J. and Kent, R. D. (1987). Editorial. *Clinical Linguistics and Phonetics*, 1, 1–5.

Ball, M. J. and Kent, R. D. (eds.) (1997). *The New Phonologies: Developments in Clinical Linguistics*. San Diego, CA: Singular Publishing.

Ball, M. J. and Müller, N. (2002). The use of the terms phonetics and phonology in the description of disordered speech. *Advances in Speech-Language Pathology*, 4, 95–108.

Ball, M. J., Rahilly, J., and Tench, P. (1996). *The Phonetic Transcription of Disordered Speech*. San Diego, CA: Singular Publishing.

Blanken, G., Dittmann, J., Grimm, H., Marshall, J. C., and Wallesch, C.–W. (eds.) (1993). *Linguistic Disorders and Pathologies: An International Handbook*. Berlin: Walter de Gruyter.

Crystal, D. (1979). *Working with LARSP*. London: Edward Arnold.

Crystal, D. (1981). *Clinical Linguistics*. Vienna: Springer Verlag.

Crystal, D. (1982). *Profiling Linguistic Disability*. London: Edward Arnold.

Crystal, D. (1984). *Linguistic Encounters with Language Handicap*. Oxford: Blackwell.

Crystal, D. (1987). Towards a 'bucket' theory of language disability: taking account of interaction between linguistic levels. *Clinical Linguistics and Phonetics*, 1, 7–22.

Crystal, D., Fletcher, P., and Garman, M. (1976). *The Grammatical Analysis of Language Disability*. London: Edward Arnold.

Damico, J., Ball, M. J., and Müller, N. (eds.) (forthcoming). *Handbook of Language and Speech Disorders*. Oxford: Blackwell.

Edwards, M. and Shriberg, L. (1983). *Phonology: Applications in Communicative Disorders*. San Diego, CA: College Hill.

Elbert, M. and Gierut, J. (1986). *Handbook of Clinical Phonology: Approaches to Assessment and Treatment*. Austin, TX: Pro-Ed.

Fava, E. (ed.) (2002). *Clinical Linguistics: Theory and Applications in Speech Pathology and Therapy*. Amsterdam: Benjamins.

Howard, S. and Heselwood, B. (2007). *Clinical Phonetics and Phonology: Analyzing Speech in a Clinical Context*. San Diego, CA: Academic Press.

Gallagher, T. M. (ed.) (1991). *Pragmatics of Language: Clinical Practice Issues*. London: Chapman Hall.

Grodzinsky, Y. (1990). *Theoretical Perspectives on Language Deficits*. Cambridge, MA: MIT Press.

Grunwell, P. (1982). *Clinical Phonology*. London: Croom Helm.

Guendouzi, J. A. and Müller, N. (2006). *Approaches to Discourse in Dementia*. Mahwah, NJ: Lawrence Erlbaum.

Ingram, D. (1976). *Phonological Disability in Children*. London: Edward Arnold.

Ingram, D. (1981). *Procedures for the Phonological Analysis of Children's Language*. Baltimore, MD: University Park Press.

Kent, R. (ed.) (2003). *MIT Encyclopedia of Communication Disorders*. Cambridge, MA: MIT Press.

Lesser, R. and Milroy, L. (1993). *Linguistics and Aphasia: Psycholinguistic and Pragmatic Aspects of Intervention*. London: Longman.

Maassen, B. and Groenen, P. (eds.) (1999). *Pathologies of Speech and Language: Advances in Clinical Phonetics and Linguistics*. London: Whurr.

Müller, N. (ed.) (2000). *Pragmatics in Speech and Language Pathology*. Studies in Speech Pathology and Clinical Linguistics, 7. Amsterdam: John Benjamins.

Müller, N. (ed.) (2006). *Multilayered Transcription*. San Diego, CA: Plural Publishers.

Perkins, M. R. (2007). *Pragmatic Impairment*. Cambridge: Cambridge University Press.

Perkins, M. and Howard, S. (eds.) (1995). *Case Studies in Clinical Linguistics*. London: Whurr.

Smith, B. R. and Leinonen, E. (1992). *Clinical Pragmatics: Unravelling the Complexities of Communicative Failure*. London: Chapman and Hall.

Windsor, F., Hewlett, N., and Kelly, L. (eds.) (2002). *Investigations in Clinical Phonetics and Linguistics*. New York: Lawrence Erlbaum.

Part I Pragmatics, Discourse, and Sociolinguistics

1 Discourse Analysis and Communication Impairment

NICOLE MÜLLER, JACQUELINE A. GUENDOUZI, AND BRENT WILSON

1.1 Introduction: Definitions and Conceptualizations of Discourse

1.1.1 What is discourse?

The applied clinical disciplines have a long history of borrowing theoretical constructs and methods of inquiry from, for example, theoretical linguistics, psycholinguistics, the philosophy of language, sociology, anthropology, and others. This means on the one hand that there is an impressive array of methodological resources and complementary (and sometimes contradictory) theoretical viewpoints that can inform our understanding of all manner of speech and language data. On the other hand, there is a danger of conceptual and terminological confusion, if the theoretical and philosophical heritage of terminologies is overlooked (see Guendouzi & Müller, 2006; Perkins, 2007, for more detailed discussion).

The terms *discourse* and *discourse analysis* are used in many different ways by different people, not only in clinical[1] linguistics (or, more broadly, clinical communication studies) and speech-language pathology, but also in non-clinical domains. The Latin word *discursus*, which became 'discourse' in English (Onions, 1966, p. 272), means 'running to and fro', from which derived the medieval Latin meaning 'argument'. Thus, within disciplines that deal with human language, speech and communication, 'discourse' can be understood, in the widest sense, as both the process of running to and fro, an exchange, between a human being and his or her environment, and the products arising from such exchanges.

Because of space limitations, we do not attempt to give a comprehensive overview of explicit and implicit definitions of the terms discourse and discourse analysis as they have been used in the non-clinical literature. Readers may find such overviews in the opening chapter of Jaworski and Coupland (1999) or Schiffrin (1994, ch. 2), and in the introduction to Schiffrin, Tannen, and Hamilton (2001). The latter volume groups the multitude of discourse-analytic approaches into three major strands: "(1) anything beyond the sentence, (2) language use, and (3) a broader range of social practice that includes non-linguistic and nonspecific instances of language" (p. 1). The conceptualization of discourse adopted, whether explicitly defined or left implicit to emerge from the data gathered and analyzed, depends of course on the research question asked, which in turn is constrained by the theoretical or analytical framework within which a researcher works.

Schiffrin (1994) distinguishes between formalist and functionalist traditions in discourse analysis. Formalist approaches aim at the discovery of structural properties pertaining between elements of discourse, (1) as defined in Schiffrin, Tannen, and Hamilton (2001). It would appear to follow that such approaches also implicitly focus on discourse as *product*, rather than as a *process*. In other words, while there are "producers and receivers of sentences, or extended texts, . . . the analysis concentrates solely on the product, that is, the words-on-the-page" (Brown & Yule, 1983, p. 23). Functionalist views of discourse, on the other hand, aim to capture patterns of language use, including the use of linguistic form (and other communicative devices) for interactive and communicative purposes, thus discourses (2) and (3). Brown and Yule, taking a *process* stance towards discourse, describe a discourse analyst as someone who is "interested in the function or purpose of a piece of linguistic data and also in how that data is processed, both by the producer and the receiver" (1983, p. 25), and who treats "data as the record (text) of a dynamic process in which language was used as an instrument of communication in a context by a speaker/writer to express meanings and achieve intentions (discourse)" (p. 26). Discourse (3) is the object of analysis in critical approaches, which examine language and its use within the context of social practices, and society and identities as constructed through discursive (linguistic and non-linguistic) practices. (Guendouzi & Müller, 2006, ch. 1, on which this section draws substantially, presents a more detailed overview of definitions and approaches to discourse, and additional references, with specific application to dementia studies.)

In reality, the distinction between discourse as process and discourse as product, and indeed between formalist and functionalist approaches, turns out to be less than straightforward to maintain. First of all, it has to be stressed that all analysis of discourse is an analysis of a product (with the possible exception of real-time neuroimaging studies; but even there we can argue that what is analyzed is an artifact of an analytical procedure, i.e. a pattern, or image). That is to say, the starting point of an analysis is always going to be a "piece of linguistic data", in Brown and Yule's phrase, or a *text*. In general, researchers in clinical contexts are primarily concerned with the mechanisms that underlie the processing of discourse and the production of text.

However, definitions of discourse in work that does not draw on the methods of conversation analysis (see Wilkinson, chapter 6 in this volume), particularly in experimental research, tend to fall squarely into Schiffrin, Tannen, and Hamilton's (2001) category (1), as for example Joanette, Goulet, and Hannequin's statement (1990, p. 163) that discourse "refers to a groups of sentences such as in a conversation or a story", or Cherney, Shadden, and Coelho's definition of discourse (1998, p. 2) as "continuous stretches of language or a series of connected sentences or related linguistic units that convey a message".

Research and assessment in clinical discourse analysis frequently targets specific discourse types, or genres. Table 1.1 summarizes a widely used taxonomy (based on Cherney, Shadden, & Coelho, 1998).

The distinction between discourse types and their characteristics is of course an oversimplification. A speaker's main purpose in telling a story may be instructional (a 'cautionary tale'), by way of entertainment. A business negotiation may have a conversational structure overall, but is likely to contain elements of expository and persuasive discourse, and possibly even narrative material (by way of illustrating elements of either expository or persuasive discourse). However, in terms of clinical applications the simplification inherent in the categorization is deliberate, since it limits the variables of analysis that have to be taken into account, and thus makes comparisons and generalizations easier. This is also the reason why in assessment or research contexts, 'naturalness' tends to be sacrificed for the sake of standardization in terms of the tasks and stimuli used. For example, one of the frequently used picture stimuli to elicit descriptive discourse is the well-known "Cookie Theft Picture" from the Boston Diagnostic Aphasia Examination (Goodglass & Kaplan, 1983). Narrative discourse is often elicited using action pictures, or picture sequences (see some of the references in sections 1.2 and 1.3 below. Thus a balance is attempted between achieving generalizability and, if not necessarily a discourse context that is entirely personally relevant and natural to the participant, one that is engaging enough to produce data that reflect the best of the participant's ability.

1.1.2   *Analyses of discourses in clinical domains, and the role and impact of disorder*

We believe it is safe to say that there is, in clinical domains, a common thread among the multiplicity of approaches to the analysis of discourse, namely the quest for mechanisms that permit humans the creation of meaning in context.[2] The chief instrument for meaning creation is of course language use. Within clinical linguistics and interaction studies, a focus of interaction is impairments that impede communicative language use. The object of analysis is always a text, and the properties of the said text may be formulated in a multitude of different ways; however, clinical discourse analysis in the end will always aim at a clinical purpose. The purpose may be the search for generalizable features, patterns or symptoms that characterize either disorders

Table 1.1 Discourse genres distinguished in clinical applications

Type	Characteristics	Purpose	Examples
Descriptive	Lists attributes and concepts; no chronological sequence	To translate a static visual image (real or imaginary) into language	Description of a picture or an object
Narrative	Presents events/ actions arranged in a chronological or temporal sequence	To entertain by relating real or fictitious event to an audience	Retelling a personal experience or a fictional event; retelling a story heard, read, or from a picture sequence or action picture
Procedural	Includes instructions and/or directions, in a specific order	To instruct as to how a procedure is carried out	Instructions how to make a cup of tea; how to change a wheel on a car
Persuasive	Expresses an opinion; gives reasons to support that opinion	That the addressee should come to share the opinion expressed by the speaker	Political canvassing (persuading voters to vote for a certain candidate)
Expository	Provides factual and interpretive information about a topic (compare and contrast; cause and effect; generalization, etc.)	To inform about a topic	Exposition of pros and cons of a certain therapy approach
Conversational	Interactive; participants switch roles (speaker–addressee)	To mutually communicate content	Chat between friends; interview

or populations with certain impairments, for strategies by which the impact of impairment is alleviated, or for the mechanisms by which societies construct images of impairment or disorder. Whatever the research question, the analysis of discourse in clinical domains is essentially *functional*, even though the measures employed may be borrowed from so-called formal approaches to discourse analysis.

As regards the enabling (or, depending on one's perspective, disabling) mechanisms in the creation of meaning in context, we can, at a minimum, distinguish the following:

1   Intra-individual or -personal: the cognitive, linguistic, but also organic (including neural) mechanisms that can be linked to the achievement of discourse. Michael Perkins (chapter 5 in this volume) lists a number of semiotic, cognitive and sensorimotor elements of pragmatics, which can be included here as part of the intra-individual discourse potential.
2   Inter-individual, or interactional: the mechanisms at work in an interaction that contribute to meaning creation. These mechanisms could be further subdivided into characteristics of interactants (which makes reference back to point 1), of an unfolding interaction, and of the context in which an interaction takes place.
3   Social: the mechanisms in the socio-cultural context beyond any given communicative situation that contribute to meaning creation.

This tripartite distinction is of course somewhat of a simplification: It is too gross-grained in that within each category, multiplicities of mechanisms and processes could be distinguished; and it is too rigid because meaning creation between communicating participants cannot happen without all three types of mechanisms. However, it may serve us as a simple structure to which to anchor some distinctions concerning the various approaches to clinical discourse analysis, and the presence and nature of *disorder*.

To say what it means for a skill, an anatomical or neurological mechanism, an interaction, or even a person (to name only a few possibilities) to be 'disordered' is not a trivial endeavor in clinical studies. The perspective on this question will determine how a researcher or clinician defines and approaches a research question or therapeutic activity. Our tripartite classification of contributing mechanisms, then, offers three different perspectives on the nature of texts, and on the role of disorder. We can look at texts as windows on cultural and social processes, and socially negotiated meanings of 'order' and 'disorder' (making reference to point 3). Another perspective is an interactional-emergent view of disorder that makes reference to point 2 above, and that looks at a text as a record of the joint, interactional negotiation of meaning. Furthermore, we can use texts, and in particular texts in which meaning construction is disrupted in some fashion, as reflections of certain configurations of impairments that are properties of a person (point 1).

Wilkinson (chapter 6 in this volume) discusses the application of conversation analysis (CA) to clinical data. Among the major methodological tenets of CA and clinical approaches based on CA is the principle that one's data must be approached with as few preconceptions as possible as to *how* mutual understanding (the joint negotiation of meaning within the interactional context) is or is not achieved. Further, the analyst's role is to discover, by way of detailed description of the 'local' (i.e. turn-by-turn, in conversational data) organiza-tion of a text (e.g. a transcript of a conversation), the mechanisms that inter-actants use to jointly negotiate meaning. Thus, there is no *a priori* 'ill-formed' or 'well-formed' structure; rather, what is or is not successful emerges out of the unfolding interaction (see also Atkinson & Heritage, 1984). Thus the search is for joint interactional mechanisms (including, for example, compensatory strategies, or even non-conventional uses of interactional tools; see also Perkins, chapter 5 in this volume), rather than primarily for indicators of communicative impairment.

In contrast to what could thus be termed a bottom-up approach to discourse as defined above, many investigators apply a top-down set of tools to the analysis of data from clinical contexts. These tools are then employed in the search for characteristics of discourse that can be considered typical for certain types of disorder; that is, discourse characteristics are analyzed as reflections of impairment. This perspective within clinical discourse analysis typically employs an experimental or quasi-experimental-reductionist approach to research, in which attempts are made to control for factors that may influence the production of texts and cloud the perspective on individual impairment. Top-down approaches to discourse typically employ, either implicitly or expli-citly, a notion of well-formedness. In other words, as well as applying a set of descriptive-analytic categories to a text, such approaches bring a set of assumptions as to appropriate or inappropriate realizations of categories.

Our presentation of approaches to the analysis of discourse is necessarily selective. In sections 1.2 and 1.3 below, we discuss perspectives on discourse that originated in research on language processing, namely the notion of micro- and macrostructures (1.2) and analyses of narrative, specifically story gram-mars (1.3). Section 1.4 deals with a perspective borrowed from the philosophy of language, speech act theory. While these perspectives emerge from very dif-ferent scientific and philosophical traditions, they have provided researchers in the clinical disciplines with analytical and descriptive frameworks that have been widely used (and at times widely criticized). Other influential work in the realm of clinical discourse analyses is discussed elsewhere in this volume: for example, cohesion analyses grounded in Systemic Functional Linguistics (Ferguson & Thomson, chapter 8 in this volume), and conversation analysis (Wilkinson, chapter 6 in this volume). Section 1.5 moves the discussion to the social construction of self and personhood in the presence of disorder, speci-fically dementia.

1.2   Perspectives from Discourse Processing: Micro- and Macrostructures

Theories that attempt to explain the processing of discourse, developed chiefly in the 1970s and 1980s, have had a considerable impact on the clinical domain. The research underlying the clinical application was deliberately and programmatically interdisciplinary, spanning psychology, linguistics, sociology and cognitive science (see e.g. Gordon, 1993; Kintsch, 1977; Mandler, 1984; Schank & Abelson, 1977; Van Dijk, 1977; Van Dijk & Kintsch, 1978, 1983). Attempts to model cognitive structures and processes underlying the comprehension (and by implication production)[3] of discourse were motivated by the view that "actual language use in social contexts" rather than "abstract or ideal language systems should be the empirical object of linguistic theories" (de Beaugrande, 1991, p. 265, excerpting from Van Dijk & Kintsch, 1983). This view is influenced by the traditions of European structuralism, literary scholarship and rhetoric, and sociolinguistics, and can also be seen in part as a reaction against the preoccupation of mainstream linguistics (in essence dominated by the transformational generative paradigm) and psycholinguistics with the syntax and semantics of isolated sentences. A central tenet of what Duchan (1994, pp. 2–3) briefly summarizes as the "thought behind the discourse" approach is that the comprehension and production of discourse involves a language user's establishing and subsequently drawing on mental representations (knowledge structures or schemas). Further, it is assumed that it is possible to formally model such representations. In the clinical literature, further assumptions that emerge are that such models can be used to describe and isolate deficits in processing (both linguistic and cognitive) associated with various diagnostic categories, such as aphasia, right-brain damage, and others, and that, in turn, the deficits associated with these diagnostic categories can shed light on normal, non-disordered language processing.

The categories micro- and macrostructure in particular, and by extension micro- and macrostructural deficits, are frequently employed in the clinical literature. Studies employing the notion of micro- and macrostructures frequently make reference to Kintsch and Van Dijk's (1978) model of discourse comprehension and production. Our brief summary of the model is based on Kintsch and Van Dijk (1978), Mross (1990), and Fayol and Lemaire (1993). One assumption in Kintsch and Van Dijk's model is that comprehension happens in real time. Processing the linguistic cues in a text and relating them to conceptual knowledge is constrained by the limitations of short-term memory. This circumstance forces cyclical, iterative processing. In Kintsch and Van Dijk's model, text is represented at three levels. The verbatim trace or surface of a text is the memory of specific words or phrases.[4] The text base represents the meaning of the text, and consists of a partially ordered list of connected propositions. Within the text base, Kintsch and Van Dijk distinguish between microstructure and macrostructure. The microstructure contains 'local' information, "corresponding to the individual words and their relationships in the text" (Mross, 1990, p. 55). Argument overlap, or co-reference, results in local coherence. The macrostructure of the text base represents global information; it represents the level of gist, topic, main ideas of the text. Correspondingly, global coherence operates at the level of the text as a whole. The macrostructure results from the operation of so-called macro-rules, which "relate sequences of propositions at the local level to higher-level sequences of propositions, in so doing yielding the global meaning of the discourse" (Mross, 1990, p. 59). The macro-rules (deletion, generalization and construction) operate recursively on the micropropositions, and thus produce a hierarchical, partially ordered list of propositions. Superstructures, in Kintsch and Van Dijk's (1978) terms, are abstract cognitive structures that correspond to conventionalized types of discourse (e.g. narrative). Superstructures are, as Mross points out (1990, p. 59), "more of a description of the overall form that a discourse *may take* and are *not* a representation of the semantic content of a particular discourse", in contrast to the macrostructure. Kintsch and Van Dijk further hypothesize that, in addition to the text base "readers construct a structure referred to as the situation model" (Mross, 1990, p. 62), in order to account for phenomena such as learning from texts, i.e. using information from texts, as opposed to remembering a text. Whereas Kintsch and Van Dijk's (1978) model proposes that the processing of micropropositions results in macrostructure (see above), other authors (e.g. Johnson-Laird, 1983; see also Van Dijk and Kintsch, 1983) stress the role of general world knowledge, and a heuristic model of processing.

The differentiation between micro-, macro- and superstructures, and between micro- and macroprocessing has been attractive to researchers in the area of memory (impaired or otherwise), and various impairments of linguistic and cognitive functioning. Mross (1990), as well as giving a detailed précis of the Kintsch and Van Dijk model in its philosophical and historical context, summarizes experimental studies on short-term and long-term memory and text processing. In the field of aphasia studies, Ulatowska and her colleagues in the 1980s investigated micro- and macrostructure availability in the production of procedural and narrative discourse (Ulatowska, Doyel, Freedman-Stern, Macaluso-Haynes, & North, 1983; Ulatowska, Freedman-Stern, Weiss-Doyel, Macaluso-Haynes, & North, 1983; Ulatowska, North, & Macaluso-Haynes, 1981). The superstructures of Kintsch and Van Dijk's model were here defined as "categories of story grammar", or "sets of instrumental scripts" (Huber, 1990, p. 171). The general conclusions are that even where significant language impairment at the syntactic and lexical level was present, the most essential elements were recognizably preserved. As Huber (1990, p. 172) points out, "methodologically, the discovery of macropropositions is difficult to achieve", given that macropropositions are abstractions and therefore not directly accessible. Ulatowska, Freedman-Stern, Weiss-Doyel, Macaluso-Haynes, and North (1983) chose to identify essential propositions empirically, as those most frequently used in the story summaries of their non-impaired control group. They found that none of the participants with aphasia produced the complete set of essential propositions, but that nonessential ones were omitted more often.

Huber (1990) contrasts heuristic macroprocessing and algorithmic microprocessing, the former relying significantly on world knowledge, the latter on linguistic knowledge. He summarizes experiments in text–picture matching, comprehension of metaphorical idioms, story arrangement (with cartoon stimuli), and verbal description of cartoon stories. Overall, the studies pointed towards knowledge based macroprocessing as "the preferred mode of text processing" in aphasia. However, they also found that macroprocessing was not completely spared in persons with aphasia, either in production or in comprehension.

In a review of aphasic discourse analysis, Armstrong (2000, p. 880) finds that investigations of micro- and macrostructural deficits in aphasia research have led to a separation of levels of processing "to the point where it has been suggested that a dissociation between the skills required for intact microstructure and macrostructure of text may exist". Glosser and Deser (1990) suggest that hemispheric specialization of micro- and macrolinguistic skills may underlie a dissociation. However, the existence of such a dissociation is not universally accepted (see e.g. Christiansen, 1995). Armstrong, who approaches micro- and macrostructure from the perspective of discourse coherence, calls for further research into the possible links between the two levels of processing, as well as investigations into their organization in speakers with aphasia.

The differentiation between micro- and macro-levels of processing has also been applied to populations with impairment other than aphasia. Coelho, Grela, Corso, Gamble, and Feinn (2005) summarize relevant research in the area of traumatic brain injury (TBI). They report on a study utilizing propositional density at the microstructural level, which finds that persons with TBI produce narratives with lower propositional density (number of propositions per sentence) than persons without brain injury. Myers (1993) summarizes findings on deficits in narrative production in persons with right-hemisphere damage, among them macrostructural deficits.

Research involving persons with various types of brain damage assumes, in general, that neural correlates of characteristics of texts (e.g. propositional density) can be identified; in other words, a departure from well-formedness reflects patterns of processing deficits. At times, however, the terms micro-, macro- and superstructure are used in a more or less theory-neutral fashion in the clinical literature. Cherney, Shadden, and Coelho (1998, p. 5), for example, refer to micro-, macro- and superstructural *analyses*, the first being defined as a focus on the word or sentence level, investigating the "small elements" in a text and the relationships between them. Macrostructural analyses operate at the level of the text, looking at "gist, theme, or main ideas". Superstructural analysis "overlies the text"; the term is essentially used in the sense of genre or discourse type. Thus terms that were originally conceived of as distinguishing between levels of processing become analytic, or assessment, categories, that do not necessarily make an *a priori* claim to psychological, or neural, reality.

1.3   Perspectives from Discourse Processing: Story Grammars

Narratives have been an object of analysis for many disciplines within the humanities, sciences and cognitive sciences (see Johnstone, 2001, for an overview). While there is great potential for the use of narratives (especially

personal autobiographical narratives) as a tool to explore the social construction of disease and disorder, the analysis of narrative structure has also been
frequently used to investigate patterns of cognitive and linguistic deficit in the
context of various types of impairment.

Story grammars were developed, in the 1970s, within a generative perspective on language and language processing which, however, aspired to provide
formal models of language beyond the level of isolated sentences (see above).
Story grammars are, in essence, "systems of rules defining the regularities
found in narrative texts" (Fayol & Lemaire, 1993, p. 4).

Stein and Glenn's (1979) story schema is an example of such a grammar.
Initially drawing on, and then departing from, earlier work by Rumelhart
(1975), they propose to set out a grammar that represents the internal representation involved in comprehending (and, by implication, producing) stories.
The story grammar has a set of ordered generative (or 'rewrite') rules that
specify category structures and intercategory relations; further, a "story consists of a setting category plus an episode system" (Stein & Glenn, 1979, p. 59).
The internal structure of a simple episode comprises (1) an initiating event,
(2) the protagonist's internal response to (1), (3) her or his internal plan to achieve
a goal, (4) an attempt to carry out the plan and attain the goal, (5) the consequence of (4), and (6) the protagonist's reaction to (5). A story's episode system consists of one or more episodes linked by the connectors AND (includes
simultaneous or a temporal relation), THEN (includes temporal but not direct
causal relations), or CAUSE (includes temporal relations which are causal in
nature) (Stein & Glenn, 1979, pp. 60–2; see also e.g. Mandler, 1984; Mandler &
Johnson, 1977). Story grammars have not been universally accepted as adequate models of story processing; however, as Fayol and Lemaire (1993) point
out, canonical story structure has widely been considered a relevant factor.

The notion of story grammar has experienced considerable popularity as an
analytical tool in the investigation of narratives produced by persons with a
variety of linguistic and cognitive impairments. For example, Roth and Spekman
(1986) used Stein and Glenn's (1979) structure, with slight modifications, to
analyze oral narratives by children with learning disabilities, who produced
stories containing fewer propositions overall, fewer complete episodes and
fewer Minor Setting statements than normally developing controls. Jordan,
Murdoch, and Buttsworth (1991) replicated Roth and Spekman's procedure
with groups of children with closed head injury (CHI). In contrast to other
studies discussed in the paper, story grammar analysis did not result in significant differences between narratives by children with either mild or severe
CHI and those by normally developing peers. Ska and Guénard (1993) analyzed
narratives produced by persons with dementia of the Alzheimer's type (DAT)
using Stein and Glenn's (1979) categories. They found that persons with
DAT produced fewer story components than normally aging controls, made
sequential-order errors, and produced more irrelevant propositions. In addition, for both participants with DAT and controls, the nature of the task
(narratives produced with no visual stimulus, with a single picture stimulus,

or an ordered series of pictures) significantly affected performance. Pearce, McCormack, and James (2003) used picture stimuli (a wordless picture book, and an isolated picture) to elicit oral narratives from children with specific language impairment (SLI), normally developing (ND) age-matched peers, and children with language impairment and low non-verbal ability (LNVA). Children with SLI produced more complex stories than children with LNVA, but only with the wordless picture book. The authors interpret their findings as challenging notions about SLI as "a unique classification that may be defined by morphosyntactic characteristics" (p. 331). McDonald and Turkstra (1998) review literature on assessing pragmatic language function, including story grammar analyses of narratives, in adolescents with traumatic brain injury (TBI). Coelho, Youse, Le, and Feinn (2003) included elements of story grammar analyses (number of complete and incomplete episodes, and the completion of T-units contained within episode structure) in a discriminant analysis of narrative and conversational discourse produced by adults with CHI and non-brain injured adults.

In terms of story grammar, a well-formed story is one that contains the elements specified in the story grammar, and no (or little) extraneous information that would distract from the well-formed story structure. McCabe and Bliss (2003, pp. 12–14) urge caution in the use of story grammar analysis as an assessment tool for children's narrative production. Story grammar analysis does not necessarily discriminate between children with and without language impairment, particularly on story-retelling tasks. Furthermore, a prescriptive use of story grammar in the sense of an assessment template produces a bias against narratives which are not produced in the European tradition.

1.4 A Perspective from the Philosophy of Language: Speech Acts in Theory and Practice

Communicative intent, its expression and comprehension – in other words, what people do with language – is of course a fundamental concern in clinical contexts. Austin's (1962) tripartite division of a speech act into *locutionary act*, *illocutionary act*, and *perlocution* looks simple and straightforward. A locutionary act, or locution, is a speaker's use of words with determinate sense or, in other words, unambiguous meaning, and reference. The *illocutionary act* or *illocution* is the act carried out by the speaker uttering the locution; in other words, the illocution embodies the speaker's intention in making an utterance. The *illocutionary effect* is the addressee's (or listener's) recognition of the speaker's intention (Searle, 1969). The listener's acting upon the speaker's expressed intention is the *perlocution*, or *perlocutionary act*. The effect, or force, of an utterance is a source of meaning that can be distinguished from the truth or falsity of a sentence, another source of meaning. To illustrate, the proposition expressed by means of the sentence *It's raining* will be true if at the time specified (the present) watery precipitation is indeed happening. However, the sentence can be used in an utterance to express, for example, a reminder by the speaker to the listener to pick up an umbrella before stepping outside, or as an excuse by the speaker when asked why she hasn't cut the grass yet. Certain conditions, often referred to as *felicity conditions* (see e.g. Austin, 1962; Searle, 1969, 1975) have to be met for illocutionary acts to be successful, i.e. lead to the desired perlocutions. For example, a promise can only 'count as' a promise if the action to which a speaker is committing represents something that is desirable to the addressee.

Searle (1975) classifies illocutionary acts into five major categories, using their *illocutionary point* as a criterion. The illocutionary point can be described as the main source of meaning of the illocutionary act. As an illustration, an order has the same illocutionary point as a request: the speaker's intent is that the addressee will carry out an action. However, the former has an element of compulsion or obligation on the part of the addressee and an element of authority on the part of the speaker; the latter does not. Searle's classification has been modified by various authors both in terms of terminology and defini- tions (see e.g. Bach & Harnisch, 1979; Hancher, 1979; Clark, 1996; Levinson, 1983); the following is based on Searle (1979, pp. 12–20).

Illocutionary acts	Illocutionary points
Assertives	"commit the speaker . . . to something's being the case, to the truth of the expressed proposition" (p. 12).
Directives	"are attempts by the speaker to get the hearer to do something" (p. 13).
Commissives	"commit the speaker to some future course of action" (p. 14).
Expressives	"express the psychological state specified in the sincerity condition about a state of affairs specified in the propositional content" (p. 15); "express a feeling toward the addressee" (Clark, 1996, p. 135).
Declaration:	"bring about some alteration in the status or condition of the referred to object . . . solely in virtue of the fact that the declaration has been successfully performed" (p. 17).

Subclassifications of these basic categories can be found in various treatments and applications of speech act theory; we shall return below to potential prob- lems of taxonomies and their applicability to texts.

As mentioned above, the success or failure of a speech act depends on the addressee's 'uptake', which presupposes that the addressee recognizes the illocutionary force and acts accordingly. In day-to-day language use, speakers typically do not have any problems with decoding a declarative sentence form that could in some context express the illocutionary point of an assertive ('I'm cold') as a directive (the point of which is to get the hearer to achieve a rise in the ambient temperature, e.g. by turning the heating up). Speech act theory (SAT) distinguishes between *direct* and *indirect* speech acts. In the former category, there is a direct mapping between sentence form and illocutionary force, or, to put it differently, the illocutionary force is derived from grammatical structure and semantic meaning (e.g. 'I'm cold' used as an assertive). With indirect speech acts, a distinction is made between primary and secondary illocutionary acts, where the primary act consists of the 'literal' act, whereas the secondary (and dominant) illocutionary act is inferable (e.g. the use of a 'literal' assertive to perform a directive). Various mechanisms have been proposed to account for how a listener arrives at a speaker's intended interpretation of an illocutionary act, including reference to felicity conditions, Gricean implicature (Grice, 1975; Searle, 1975), idiom theory and convention, and so-called *ifids*, or 'illocutionary force identifying devices' (Levinson, 1983) (see e.g. Geis, 1995; Grundy, 1995, for summaries and discussions).

1.4.1   Critiques of SAT and its application to contextualized data

Speech act theory as developed in the 1960s and 1970s was not intended as a framework for the analysis of naturally occurring conversational language, nor indeed as a taxonomy to capture the cognitive (even less the neurological) processes underlying the expression of communicative intent in authentic communicative situations (see e.g. Searle, 1986). Indeed, the limitations of SAT in terms of its applicability to contextualized, interactive language use have drawn much comment. For example, H. H. Clark (1996, pp. 136–9) points out that Searle's basic five categories are too general to generate all possible illocutionary acts. Further, he notes that there is an assumption that an illocutionary act belongs to only one category; however, utterances, in practice, can and do fulfill multiple functions simultaneously. In Clark's discussion, the greatest drawback of Searle's approach is the almost exclusive focus in SAT on the speaker's actions, all but ignoring the listener's contribution (but see Austin, 1962). According to Clark, "illocutionary acts . . . can be accomplished only as parts of joint actions, and the same is true for perlocutionary acts" (1996, p. 139). Clark makes reference to Streeck's (1980) critique of SAT and subsequent attempt to extend and modify the theory into a framework that lends itself to the analysis of naturally occurring interactive language. Streeck identifies several principles which a theory of communicative interaction needs to accommodate: Interaction cannot be reduced to intentional action on the part of the speaker (pp. 146–7). Meaning is constituted interactively, rather than predetermined (pp. 147–9), so that "[i]llocutionary forces are created and can only be identified within the context of prior and subsequent speech acts" (p. 149). Further, SAT's insistence on the complete sentence as the typical grammatical form of an illocutionary act is problematic, since what functions as a communicative unit is constructed interactively (pp. 149–50). A further principle is the indefiniteness of shared understandings (pp. 150–1). According to Streeck, an analysis of speech acts only makes sense within a framework for the analysis of interaction, which aims to discover the participants' "methodic *procedures* for accomplishing shared understanding and coordinated behavior" (p. 151). This call for procedural, as it were, analysis of situated talk of course brings us into the neighborhood of conversation analysis (see further below, and Wilkinson, chapter 6 in this volume).

Lesser and Milroy (1993, p. 149) point out that "indeterminacy and multiplicity of meaning have plagued attempts to apply a speech-act framework to *situated* speech . . . But from the point of view of the practical analyst, perhaps the most serious problem is that meanings seem to be jointly negotiated as conversation proceeds, interpretation cosequently changing as the discourse unfolds." They also stress the problematicity of using top-down analyses that attempt to specify sets of rules for the production and interpretation of utterances, and the need for more bottom-up "empirical analysis" that approaches contextualized data with a "minimum of prior theoretical constraint" (p. 151).

1.4.2 Applications of concepts from SAT in clinical domains

Lesser and Milroy (1993, p. 147) comment on SAT that while "it hardly holds water as a theoretical model [to be applied to authentic communication], some of its basic distinctions and concepts are quite fundamentally relevant to clinical practice", which would explain why, for several decades, many researchers have sought to apply concepts from SAT to clinical data, in a variety of contexts. As elsewhere in this chapter, the examples given below are intended to be illustrative, rather than exhaustive. Our focus will be on taxonomies, categories and classifications, rather than on the results of individual studies.

Classifications from SAT have been used in the construction of communication assessments. The earlier version of Prutting and Kirchner's (1983) Pragmatic Protocol includes a taxonomy of behaviors based on SAT, distinguishing between utterance acts (how a speaker presents a message), propositional acts (linguistic meaning), illocutionary acts and perlocutionary acts. In the later (1987) version of the Pragmatic Protocol, this classification was abandoned; the notion of speech acts (*speech act pair analysis* and *variety of speech acts* are to be rated as either 'appropriate' or 'inappropriate', or 'no opportunity to observe') was, however, maintained. The Profile of Communicative Appropriateness (Penn, 1988) includes the management of indirect speech acts (without further subclassification) as one aspect under the metacategory of sociolinguistic sensitivity. Damico's Systematic Observation of Communicative Interaction (see e.g. Damico, 1991) is a tool for 'real-time' observation of communicative interaction which uses Bach and Harnisch's (1979) modification of Searle's original classification of illocutionary acts as a framework. Inappropriate execution of illocutionary acts is classified by means of 16 types of problematic verbal that are categorized according to Grice's maxims of conversational cooperation

(Grice, 1975; also Ahlsén, chapter 2 in this volume), as well as four types of problematic non-verbal behaviors. (See Adams, 2002, for a review of other assessment methods and analytic procedures that employ concepts from SAT, among other aspects of interaction and pragmatics.)

Attempts to use concepts and taxonomies from SAT have frequently led to extensions and modifications of the original classification, both on the level of *what* is categorized (speaker's intent, as in 'classical' SAT, or other levels of interaction as well as speaker's intent, or comprehension of speaker's intent), and *how* the taxonomies are structured. Given that the development of intentions and their expression is a cornerstone of cognitive and linguistic maturation, it is not surprising that the area of child language development (both normal and disordered) represents a particularly rich, and sometimes bewildering, array of classification schemes. Bates, Camaioni, and Volterra (1975) applied the tripartite conceptualization of the speech act into perlocution(ary act), illocution(ary act) and locution(ary act) to the communicative development of children, drawing on Piaget's developmental model, and used them as labels in a chronological stage model: The first stage is the *perlocutionary* stage (birth to approximately 8 months, by the end of which the child produces goal-directed behaviors. During the second stage, labeled the *illocutionary stage* (approximately 8–12 months), the child conveys a range of intentions, by gesturing and the use of phonetically increasingly consistent vocalizations. The *locutionary* stage (from approximately 12 months) begins with the production of the first meaningful words.

Halliday's longitudinal observations of his son (Halliday, 1975) resulted in seven categories of the expression of communicative intentions with the introduction of the first words (Instrumental, Regulatory, Interactional, Personal, Heuristic, Imaginative, Informative). Dore's (1974, 1975) classification of the communicative intentions of children at the one-word stage distinguishes nine major categories of so-called 'primitive speech acts' (Labeling, Answering, Requesting action, Requesting an answer, Calling/addressing, Greeting, Protesting, Repeating/imitating, Practicing (language). In the language of preschool children, Dore (1978, 1979) makes 38 distinctions in total, in six major categories (Requestives, Assertives, Responsives, Regulatives, Expressives, and Performatives). Fey's (1986) coding system of speech acts distinguishes the major categories of requestives, assertive acts, and performatives, all with several subcategories.

Ninio, Snow, Pan, and Rollins (1994) review several taxonomies of speech acts, as well as a number of studies that apply speech act classifications to the spoken language output of children with a variety of communicative disorders. They come to the conclusion that "there is rather little comparability of analysis across the various studies" (p. 161) and, further, that it is not sufficient to classify communicative intent in terms of an illocutionary act. Their classification scheme distinguishes between the propositional or semantic level, the performance or speech act level, the interactive level, and the conversational level, with the caveat that these levels are easily distinguishable, but that "there are undoubtedly more" (p. 157). The authors offer the "Inventory of

Communicative Acts-Abridged (INCA-A)", which distinguishes between 22 interchange types and 66 speech acts. Rollins, Pan, Conti-Ramsden, and Snow (1994) distinguish three levels of communicative act, namely the social interchange, speech act and conversational levels. Their major speech act categories (with subcategories of "openers" and "responses" for each with the exception of the category "other") are: directives, statements/declarations, questions, commitments, and other (p. 199).

Research employing various taxonomies of speech acts is not restricted to the investigation of child language development and disorders. For example, Ripich, Vertes, Whitehouse, Fulton, and Ekelman (1991) adapt their classification of speech acts from Dore (1979). Causino Lamar, Obler, Knoefel, and Albert (1994) include the categories "directives" (and responses to directives), comments and representatives, and expressives and commissives in a series of 13 pragmatic parameters (derived from Prutting & Kirchner, 1983) in their investigation of conversations between persons with late-stage Alzheimer's disease and hospital care staff.

The distinction between direct and indirect speech acts has also received considerable attention in clinical contexts. Stemmer (chapter 4 in this volume) outlines research in this area as involving persons with right-hemisphere damage and other acquired neurological impairment, and the reader is referred to that chapter for more detailed discussion. Earlier experimental literature relating to how listeners use contextual information in identifying the intended meaning of an utterance (e.g. whether an interrogative serves as a request for information or as an order) is summarized in Abbeduto, Furman, and Davis (1989) (see also Lesser & Milroy, 1993, with specific reference to aphasia).

That the existence of multiple taxonomies and categorizations makes it difficult to make comparisons between studies has been remarked upon by many researchers (see e.g. Lesser & Milroy, 1993; McTear, 1985; Ninio, Snow, Pan, & Rollins, 1994; Rollins, Pan, Conti-Ramsden, & Snow, 1994; also Perkins, chapter 5 in this volume, and 2007). This *embarras de richesses* of course also represents the continued search for methods to systematically, reliably and categorically capture the logical, syntactic, and interactive relationships between communicative intent and linguistic expression over several decades (see e.g. Geis, 1995 for a comparatively recent attempt to synthesize principles from speech act theory, conversation analysis, and artificial intelligence in natural language processing). However, it also points towards the inherent problematicity of top-down approaches in the analysis of human communicative activity.

1.5   Social and Cultural Discourses of Disorder and Impairment: Critical Approaches

Critical approaches to discourse investigate the linguistic and non-linguistic social practices that contribute to and express the world views and sense of self of individuals within a society, and that both reflect and give rise to value systems and ideologies. Our discussion of the investigation of discourse as a social-cultural process draws its illustrations mainly from the field of dementia studies, and is based in part on the more detailed discussion in Guendouzi and Müller (2006). In the areas of gerontology, investigations of normal and pathological aging, and dementia studies, critical analyses have gained much prominence over the past two decades, in particular in the so-called 'caregiving' or 'caring' professions, such as nursing, elder care, and geriatric medicine (see e.g. Golander & Raz, 1996; Kitwood, 1990, 1997; Sabat, 2001).

1.5.1   Critical Discourse Analysis and Discursive Psychology: Philosophical and political roots

Two influential approaches in the critical tradition are Critical Discourse Analysis (CDA) and Discursive Psychology (DP), both seeking to investigate the values and constructs underlying, and giving rise to, discourses of various types. Critical approaches allow researchers to describe, interpret and explain how language is used to accomplish clinical interactions and interventions (Candlin, 1995).

CDA "primarily studies the way social power abuse, dominance, and inequality are enacted, reproduced, and resisted by text and talk in the social and political contexts" (Van Dijk, 2001, p. 35). Texts are viewed as the products of social and historical traditions, and it is the analyst's task to situate current discourses within those traditions. CDA looks for patterns within texts that may reveal the interests and influences of particular groups within society. An important contributing tradition to CDA is critical linguistics (e.g. Fowler, Hodge, Kress, & Trew, 1979; Kress, 1988; Mey, 1985), a major objective the examination of power and ideology (Fairclough, 1989; Hodge & Kress, 1992). CDA analysis, however, is more than just a commentary on texts, but calls for a systematic analysis of the form and organization of texts. CDA has also drawn on traditions that are not primarily linguistically oriented, for example work in media studies by the Glasgow University Media Group (1976) and by Stuart Hall and colleagues (1980), and studies by Anthony Giddens in sociology (1976, 1991). Unlike conversation analysis, CDA does not regard conversational interaction as the prime site of analysis. Rather, it takes a broader perspective to include non-conversational spoken, written, and non-linguistic texts, for example images (e.g. Kress & van Leeuwen, 1996). Critical approaches are multi-layered and situate their data samples within broader social and institutional discourses. For example, work in gender studies has looked at how women's talk is embedded within the patriarchal texts of Western cultural and historical traditions (see e.g. Cameron, 1992; Coates, 1996).

CDA is not a philosophically or politically neutral form of analysis (see e.g. Verschueren, 2001). It draws on a long line of philosophical traditions, and often makes reference to prominent social philosophers and social scientists (e.g. Bakhtin, 1981, 1986; Bourdieu, 1991; Foucault, 1984; Habermas, 1989). Fairclough (1995) suggests that CDA is a successor to the tradition of European philosophy and critical theory, and much of the early work in CDA has been grounded in the Marxist tradition (e.g. Althusser, 1971) and the notion of power struggles. Drawing on Gramsci's work (1971), "which foregrounds the winning of consent in the exercise of power" (Fairclough, 1995, p. 27), CDA suggests that ideological perspectives are embedded within our everyday discourse practices, and institutions are held together as much by discourse practices as by constitutional power. Therefore if we study the organization of those discourses we can examine how ideologies affect our everyday inter-actions. Thus, CDA starts from the premise that discourse practices represent the "social power of groups and institutions" (van Dijk, 2001, p. 354).

Discursive Pyschology (DP) is a critical approach that draws on the tradition of ethnomethodology in seeking to understand the individual's own perspec-tive of the world. Potter (2003, p. 6), drawing on Edwards (1997), suggests that one of the "central themes in discursive psychology is the way that versions of the world and versions of psychological states are linked together in talk for the purposes of action". DP, like conversation analysis, calls for researchers to approach their data with an open mind, and to avoid bringing preconceptions of power to the analysis. DP does, however, examine how ideologies are linked to the psychological constructs of the individual, and utilizes "the analytical resources of both discourse analysis and conversation analysis" (Potter, 2003; see also Potter & Wetherell, 1987). Thus, although DP may seek to make links to ideologies it does not posit *a priori* viewpoints.

1.5.2   Critical approaches to discourses of Alzheimer's disease and dementia

1.5.2.1   Media discourses

A powerful mediator of public awareness of health issues is the institutional, political and economic perspective of the news media. Negativity is a strong news value (Galtung & Ruge, 1973); 'bad news is good news' (Fowler, 1991; Bell, 1991). Stories involving death, disease or crime gain wide media cover-age, they attract a large audience and are therefore profitable for the owners or shareholders of media companies.

Alzheimer's disease, along with its accompanying deterioration of cognition and communication, has received a great deal of media attention in recent years. The most dominant themes emerging from the media relating to dementia are that of a horrific loss of self, and the rapidly growing number of people diagnosed with dementia. Televised documentaries of people living with dementia tend to focus on the negative aspects of dementia, on progressive and irreversible loss of independence and functioning. The public is made very aware, and indeed potentially very fearful, of the growing 'threat of dementia', and of increasing numbers of persons diagnosed with a dement-ing disease (such as Alzheimer's disease); the latter circumstance is at times referred to as an "Alzheimer's epidemic". An example from a newspaper (see

below) reveals themes of hopelessness and negativity in current public discourses that dehumanize people with dementia:

> Alzheimer's disease [is] a progressive and frightening neurological disorder . . .
> it begins as forgetfulness. As time passes the brain increasingly malfunctions,
> resulting in profound deficiencies in cognitive thought. This eventually ends in a
> catastrophe: extreme confusion, loss of judgment, inability to recognize loved
> ones, belligerency . . . in the truest sense of the word the advanced Alzheimer's
> patient has lost all of the qualities that make him or her human. (Gott, 2004)

Negative images may raise public awareness and therefore result in more
public pressure for funding for research and treatment. However, research has
shown that repeated, continuous exposure to negative images may result in a
general acceptance of these socially constructed stereotypes (e.g. Fowler, 1991;
Hodge & Kress, 1992). Continuous dwelling on negative images of the threat
of terminal cognitive deterioration and loss of self may thus lead to an acceptance of this stereotype as 'inevitable', or even 'inescapable', and therefore be
counterproductive in terms of mobilizing public pressure.

1.5.2.2   *Discourses of 'selfhood' and 'personhood': the social construction of self and dementia*

Debates surrounding the concept of 'self' stretch (at least) as far back as Socrates,
and are still with us in recent and current critical thinking (e.g. Dennett, 1990),
neuroscience (e.g. Damasio, 1999), genetic research (e.g. in the area of research
involving embryonic stem cells) and artificial intelligence (Clark, 2003; Kurzweil,
1999). Whether the self should be conceptualized as a product of evolution
(Barkow, Cosmides, & Tooby, 1992), of physiology (LeDoux, 2002), or as an
emergent phenomenon of social interaction, we appear no closer to a defini-
tive answer than earlier philosophers and researchers. Indeed, much depends
on how 'self' is defined (a thorough discussion of which would lead us beyond
the scope of this chapter; see also Gergen, 1991; Goffman, 1964).

The self as a socially constructed entity may at first sight be a philosophical
concern of limited relevance to the clinical professions and research communities. However, perspectives on selfhood and personhood, and the possible
or probable links between a person's self or sense of self, and the functioning
of the brain (both 'higher' and 'lower' neurological functions) present medical
and moral dilemmas. For example, at what point in a progressive degeneration of the brain does 'loss of self' occur? Of what benefit are social contacts
to a person with dementia (e.g. in nursing homes); conversely, what harm
does social isolation cause to a dementing brain, and the person that this
brain inhabits? Can intervention geared towards maintaining a sense of self,
or personhood, be effective (and how would such effectiveness be assessed, or
measured)? Following on from this, should such intervention be considered a
right, and therefore be available to all? Questions of what constitutes 'selfhood'
or 'personhood' are highly relevant to how we treat persons with dementia

(especially progressive dementias, such as dementia of the Alzheimer's type), both in the medical sense, and in terms of according them the status of social human beings.

Experimental reductionist science centers on the "psychometric person" (Sabat, 2001, p. 263), a context-free personification of measures and norms used to assess impairment. This of course cannot capture the real-life variations and context-dependent fluctuations in functioning we see in the daily life experiences of persons with dementia. Therefore, Sabat (2001, p. 171) proposes to view persons with dementia as "semiotic or meaning-driven subjects", to consider whether they are capable of forming and retaining (1) intact goals, (2) intentions, and (3) long-standing dispositions, and how their life-contexts are facilitative or counterproductive in these terms. For example, institutional settings, such as long-term residential facilities, may overregiment the residents' lives to the point where they become overly dependent, lacking the power to influence even minor day-to-day life events or make decisions for themselves. Sabat (2001, p. 97), drawing on work by Kitwood and Bredin (1992), and Kitwood (1997), lists a host of "malignant" social behaviors that people in institutions encounter that impact on the "afflicted person's feelings of self-worth and personhood".

Social construction theory (Coulter, 1979; Harré, 1983, 1991; Sabat & Harré, 1992) provides ways of analyzing projections of self within daily interactions. For example, one way to construct self within discourse is through the use of linguistic tokens, such as the pronouns 'I', 'me' or 'you'. These pronouns index the individual's awareness of self as a singularity, separate from their surroundings and identifiable as such. Whether the 'I' is indexical of the individual we have always known or some new 'I' is not always clear to the caregiver or family member. This expectation of unpredictability makes it difficult for others to adjust their orientation to the person with dementia.

Sabat (2001) differentiates between three constructions of 'self'. "Self 1" is the "self of personal identity" a person's experience of personal, individual identity (p. 276). The "self of mental and physical attributes" is referred to as "Self 2" (p. 190). This concept of self includes factors such as the individual's beliefs and cognitive and physical attributes (e.g. being a gifted mathematician, short, thin or blonde). Some of these attributes remain largely unchanged over the course of the lifespan, and are not affected by disease processes (for example dementia), whereas other are (e.g. losing the ability to play chess, or to balance a check book), and these have to be accommodated into a new concept of self. The term "Self 3" (p. 294) refers to the multiple social personae, roles and role-specific patterns of behavior that an individual adopts throughout the lifespan, many of them coexisting with each other, for example those of being someone's child, a parent, a spouse, a co-worker. In order to fulfill their roles, social actors need to be aware of the context, the social status and identity of interlocutors, and their own role in relation to the other persons (e.g. mother, spouse, friend). They also need to discursively position themselves within a specific temporal framework, that is, which aspect of self needs to be foregrounded in a given situation. A person with dementia may confuse or misinterpret any, or all, of these variables, therefore enacting the 'wrong' role for the particular context or audience, and creating a mismatch between actions and expectations.

Such a mismatch may result in attempts of persons without dementia (e.g. family or professional caregivers) to compensate, which in turn may lead to either overaccommodation (e.g. oversimplification of a communicative situation) or underaccommodation (e.g. preventing further contributions from happening). The dynamics of social interaction require that interactional partners recognize each other's social role(s), intentions and states of mind. Thus, three variables that have an important effect on the dynamics of dementia interactions are (1) the internal concept of selfhood on the part of the person with dementia, (2) the socially negotiated self accorded them by interactional partners, and (3) mismatches between the two. Such mismatches may be difficult or even impossible to resolve, depending on the levels of communicative impairment and the expectations of communication partners.

1.5.2.3   *Critical approaches to discourse and clinical research*

Critical approaches to discourse can shed light on the socially constructed values and ideologies that impact the lives of persons with communicative (or other) impairments within their social contexts. Therefore, they can help to raise public awareness, and to identify ideologies that are inimical to the equitable treatment of persons with impairments. However, we need to be aware that there is never only one 'correct' or 'possible' interpretation of texts (see Verschueren, 2001). A further issue arising out of the critical enterprise is that it creates responsibilities: Identification of counterproductive ideologies should be accompanied by attempts to adjust public discourses in order to introduce alternative ways of conceptualizing, for example, dementia or other communicative or cognitive impairment. Researchers in the clinical disciplines can play a role in this process, by carrying out detailed critical analyses of communicative patterns in institutional, medical and media discourses to overcome negative stereotypes, and expectations of failure. Critical approaches to analysis of discourse serve two very important roles in clinical research: CDA can reveal how institutional discourses frame disorder (in relation to, for example, measurable impairment), often identifying impairment with an identity of helplessness, lack of choice, negativity and fear. DP attempts to examine the experience of impairment from the perspective of the person affected. In the case of dementia, for example, it would be overoptimistic to state that any analysis can truly recreate the experience of a person with a progressive deterioration of cognitive and communicative ability. However, work grounded in DP does attempt to let dominant themes (and therefore the priorities and concerns of the person with dementia) arise out of the texts examined, rather than use preconceived expectations of disorder.

Critical perspectives on discourse have not only been applied to dementia. A further context that is experiencing a discussion of the social construction of disorder is autism and its ramifications. For example, Avdi, Griffin, and Brough (2000) analyze how parents of children with autism represent the 'problem' during the diagnostic assessment process, and identify three discourses employed by families in the construction of medical diagnoses, namely the discourses of normal development, the medical discourse, and the discourse of disability. O'Dell and Brownlow (2005) investigate media reports on purported links between the MMR vaccination and the development of autism. They find that a prominent theme in news reports is parental fear of 'damage' to affected children (i.e. onset of autism), noting that "[i]mplicit within the debate is the notion that an autistic child/adult is less acceptable than a (supposedly) 'normal' child" (p. 194). Thus the emergence of an "autistic identity" (p. 194) is constructed as negative, which, according to the authors, contrasts with the fact that "such identities can be highly valued by those so labelled" (p. 194). Avdi (2005) focuses on the negotiation of a pathological identity in family therapy involving a family with an autistic child. She concludes that dominant medical, pathology-maintaining accounts need to be deconstructed in order to allow for less disorder-centered, less problematic discourses to emerge.

1.6   Whither Clinical Discourse Analysis?

As mentioned in our introductory paragraphs, and illustrated in our discussion, there is a multitude of approaches to discourse (however defined) in the clinical disciplines, using a wide variety of data. Approaches range from the use of top-down frameworks with predetermined categories (e.g. story grammars in their original conception, or speech acts), to bottom-up, essentially emergentist methods such as conversation analysis. In addition, terminologies and concepts have been borrowed from a number of different disciplines, and in this process of adoption their meanings have adapted to a new context of use. Further, a tension can be perceived between 'naturalness' of data, and generalizability of findings: On the one hand, the quest for generalizable characteristics of certain types of impairments, typically cast in a traditional reductionist-experimental framework, carries with it the requirement for not only replicability, but also the control of potentially confounding extraneous variables. On the other hand, discourse by its very nature (whether discourse as text, or as an interactional process) is context-shaped, and indeed context-creating.

A potential terminological landmine which thus far we have studiously avoided is the delimitation of discourse and pragmatics. Perkins (2007) discusses this question in some detail. As he points out, whether pragmatics is considered a component of discourse or discourse a component of pragmatics depends on the theoretical tradition framing the inquiry, and the object under investigation. Other chapters in part I of this volume may serve as an illustration of this point: Conversational Implicature (Ahlsén, chapter 2), Relevance Theory (Leinonen & Ryder, chapter 3), Neuropragmatics (Stemmer, chapter 4), conversation analysis (Wilkinson, chapter 6), Systemic Functional Linguistics

(Ferguson & Thomson, chapter 8) and all deal, in various ways and with various types of data, with phenomena of discourse.

Rather than viewing this diverse universe of approaches to clinical discourse as disorderly and in need of unification, we see it as the reflection of a rich tradition of inquiry into human communicative action and interaction, its contributing processes, and indeed impairments. As the sciences contributing to the understanding of human communication continue to progress and interact (see, for example, Perkins in chapter 5 on pragmatic impairment as an emergent phenomenon), so the analysis of clinical discourse will adopt and adapt new frameworks, and in turn contribute to the non-clinical sciences.

NOTES

1 For the purposes of this chapter, the term 'clinical' is used as a shorthand to summarize contexts of communication impairment, and data arising out of such contexts, following the convention in use in, e.g., 'clinical linguistics' or 'clinical phonetics'.
2 See also Jaworski and Coupland (1999, p. xi) on the multiplicity of definitions of 'discourse' in non-clinical domains: "Whatever discourse is, and however concretely or abstractly the term is used, there will at least be agreement that it has focally to do with language, meaning and context."
3 Huber (1990) discusses the problematicity of regarding comprehension and production essentially as reverses of each other.
4 Note that Kintsch and Van Dijk's (1978) discussion centers on the reading and recall of texts.

REFERENCES

Abbeduto, L., Furman, L., and Davis, B. (1989). Identifying speech acts from contextual and linguistic information. *Language and Speech*, 32, 189–203.

Adams, C. (2002). Practitioner review: The assessment of language pragmatics. *Journal of Child Psychology and Child Psychiatry*, 48, 973–87.

Althusser, L. (1971). *Lenin, Philosophy and Other Essays*. London: New Left Books.

Armstrong, E. (2000). Aphasic discourse analysis: The story so far. *Aphasiology*, 14, 875–92.

Atkinson, J. M. and Heritage, J. (1984). *Structures of Social Action*. Cambridge: Cambridge University Press.

Austin, J. L. (1962). *How to Do Things with Words*. Oxford: Oxford University Press.

Avdi, E. (2005). Negotiating a pathological identity in the clinical dialogue: Discourse analysis of family therapy. *Psychology and Psychotherapy: Theory, Research and Practice*, 78, 493–511.

Avdi, E., Griffin, C., and Brough, S. (2000). Parents' constructions of the 'problem' during assessment and diagnosis of their child for an autistic spectrum disorder. *Journal of Health Psychology*, 5, 241–54.

Bach, K. and Harnisch, R. M. (1979). *Linguistic Communication and Speech Acts*. Cambridge, MA: MIT Press.

Bakhtin, M. (1981). *The Dialogical Imagination*. Austin: University of Texas Press.

Bakhtin, M. (1986). *Speech Genres and Other Late Essays*. Austin: University of Texas Press.

Barkow, J. H., Cosmides, L., and Tooby, J. (1992). *The Adapted Mind: Evolutionary Psychology and the Generation of Culture*. Oxford: Oxford University Press.

Bates, E., Camaioni, L., and Volterra, V. (1975). The acquisition of performatives prior to speech. *Merrill-Palmer Quarterly*, 21, 205–16.

Bell, A. (1991). *The Language of News Media*. Oxford: Blackwell.

Bourdieu, P. (1991). *Language and Symbolic Power*. Cambridge: Polity Press.

Brown, G. and Yule, G. (1983). *Discourse Analysis*. Cambridge: Cambridge University Press.

Cameron, D. (1992). *Feminism and Linguistic Theory*. 2nd ed. London: Macmillan.

Candlin, C. (1995). General introduction. In N. Fairclough (ed.), *Critical Discourse Analysis* (pp. vii–xi). London: Longman.

Causino Lamar, M. A., Obler, L. K., Knoefel, J. A., and Albert, M. L. (1994). Cohesive devices and conversational discourse in Alzheimer's disease. In R. L. Bloom, L. K. Obler, S. De Santi, and J. S. Ehrlich (eds.), *Discourse Analysis and Applications: Studies in Adult Clinical Populations* (pp. 201–16). Hillsdale, NJ: Lawrence Erlbaum Associates.

Cherney, L. R., Shadden, B. B., and Coelho, C. A. (1998). *Analyzing Discourse in Communicatively Impaired Adults*. Gaithersburg, MD: Aspen Publishers.

Christiansen, J. A. (1995). Coherence violations and propositional usage in the narratives of fluent aphasics. *Brain and Language*, 51, 291–317.

Clark, A. (2003). *Natural-born Cyborgs*. Oxford: Oxford University Press.

Clark, H. H. (1996). *Using Language*. Cambridge: Cambridge University Press.

Coates, J. (1996). *Women Talk*. Oxford: Blackwell.

Coelho, C. A., Grela, B., Corso, M., Gamble, A., and Feinn, R. (2005). Microlinguistic deficits in the narrative discourse of adults with traumatic brain injury. *Brain and Language*, 19, 1139–45.

Coelho, C. A., Youse, K. M., Le, K. N., and Feinn, R. (2003). Narrative and conversational discourse of adults with closed head injuries and non-brain-injured adults: A discriminant analysis. *Aphasiology*, 17, 499–510.

Coulter, J. (1979). *The Social Construction of Mind: Studies in Ethnomethodology and Linguistic Philosophy*. London: Macmillan.

Damico, J. S. (1991). Systematic observation of communicative interaction: A valid and practical descriptive assessment technique. *Best Practices in School Speech-Language Pathology*, 2, 133–42.

Damasio, A. (1999). *The Feeling of What Happens: Body and Emotion in the Making of Consciousness*. Orlando, FL: Harcourt.

De Beaugrande, R. (1991). *Linguistic Theory: The Discourse of Fundamental Works*. London: Longman.

Dennett, D. C. (1990). True believers: The intentional strategy and why it works. In W. G. Lycan (ed.), *Mind and Cognition* (pp. 75–86). Oxford: Blackwell.

Dore, J. (1974). A pragmatic description of early language development. *Journal of Psycholinguistic Research*, 3, 343–50.

Dore, J. (1975). Holophrases, speech acts and language universals. *Journal of Child Language*, 2, 21–40.

Dore, J. (1978). Variation in preschool children's conversational performances. In K. Nelson (ed.), *Children's Language*, vol. 1 (pp. 397–444). New York: Gardner Press.

Dore, J. (1979). Conversation and preschool language development. In P. Fletcher and M. Garman (eds.), *Language Acquisition*. New York: Cambridge University Press.

Duchan, J. (1994). Approaches to the study of discourse in the social sciences. In R. L. Bloom, L. K. Obler, S. De Santi, and J. S. Ehrlich (eds.), *Discourse Analysis and Applications: Studies in Adult Clinical Populations* (pp. 1–14). Hillsdale, NJ: Lawrence Erlbaum.

Edwards, D. (1997). *Discourse and Cognition*. London: Sage.

Edwards, D. and Potter, J. (2001). Discursive Psychology. In A. W. McHoul and M. Rapley (eds.), *How to Analyze Talk in Institutional Settings: A Casebook of Methods*. London: Continuum International.

Fairclough, N. (1989). *Language and Power*. London: Longman.

Fairclough, N. (1995). *Critical Discourse Analysis*. London: Longman.

Fayol, M. and Lemaire, P. (1993). Levels of approach to discourse. In H. H. Brownell and Y. Joanette (eds.), *Narrative Discourse in Neurologically Impaired and Normally Aging Adults* (pp. 3–22). San Diego: Singular.

Fey, M. E. (1986). *Language Intervention with Young Children*. San Diego: College Hill.

Foucault, M. (1984). The order of discourse. In M. Shapiro (ed.), *Language and Politics*. Oxford: Blackwell.

Fowler, R. (1991). *Language in the News: Discourse and Ideology in the Press*. London: Routledge.

Fowler, R., Hodge, B., Kress, G., and Trew, T. (1979). *Language and Control*. London: Routledge and Kegan Paul.

Galtung, J. and Ruge, M. (1973). Structuring and selecting news. In S. Cohen and J. Young (eds.), *The Manufacture of News: Social Problems, Deviance and the Mass Media* (pp. 62–72). London: Constable.

Geis, M. L. (1995). *Speech Acts and Conversational Interaction*. Cambridge: Cambridge University Press.

Gergen K. J. (1991). *The Saturated Self: Dilemmas of Identity in Everyday Life*. New York: Greenwood Press.

Giddens, A. (1976). *New Rules of Sociological Method: A Positive Critique of Interpretive Sociologies*. London: Hutchinson.

Giddens, A. (1991). *Modernity and Self-identity*. Cambridge: Polity Press.

Glasgow University Media Group (1976). *Bad News*. London: Routledge and Kegan Paul.

Glosser, G. and Deser, T. (1990). Patterns of discourse production among neurological patients with fluent language disorders. *Brain and Language*, 40, 67–88.

Goffman, E. (1964). *Asylums: Essays on the Social Situation of Mental Patients and Other Inmates*. New York: Doubleday.

Golander, H. and Raz, A. E. (1996). The mask of dementia: Images of 'demented residents' in a nursing ward. *Ageing and Society*, 16, 269–85.

Goodglass, H. and Kaplan, E. (1983). *The Boston Diagnostic Aphasia Examination*. 2nd ed. Boston: Lea and Febiger.

Gordon, P. (1993). Computational and psychological models of discourse. In H. H. Brownell and Y. Joanette (eds.), *Narrative Discourse in Neurologically Impaired and Normally Aging Adults* (pp. 23–46). San Diego: Singular.

Gott, P. (2004). Ask Dr Gott: Alzheimer's devastates lives of patient, family. *Hammond Daily Star*, March 28, section G, p. 4.

Gramsci, A. (1971). *Prison Notebooks*. New York: International Publishers.

Grice, H. P. (1975). Logic and conversation. In P. Cole and J. L. Morgan (eds.), *Syntax and Semantics. Volume 3: Speech Acts* (pp. 41–58). New York: Academic Press.

Grundy, P. (1995). *Doing Pragmatics*. London: Edward Arnold.

Guendouzi, J. A. and Müller, N. (2006). *Approaches to Discourse in Dementia*. Mahwah, NJ: Lawrence Erlbaum Associates.

Habermas, J. (1989). *The Structural Transformation of the Public Sphere*. Cambridge: Polity Press.

Hall, S., Hobson, D., Lowe, A., and Willis, P. (1980). *Culture, Media, Language*. London: Hutchinson.

Halliday, M. A. K. (1975). *Learning How to Mean: Explorations in the Development of Language*. New York: Arnold.

Hancher, M. (1979). The classification of cooperative illocutionary acts. *Language in Society*, 8, 1–14.

Harré, R. (1983). *Personal Being*. Oxford: Blackwell.

Harré, R. (1991). The discursive production of selves. *Theory and Psychology*, 1, 51–63.

Harré, R. and van Langenhove, L. (eds.) (1999). *Positioning Theoryy: Moral Contexts of Intentional Action*. Oxford: Blackwell.

Hodge, R. and Kress, G. (1992). *Language as Ideology*. 2nd ed. London: Routledge.

Huber, W. (1990). Text comprehension and production in aphasia: Analysis in terms of micro- and macrostructure. In Y. Joanette and H. Brownell, *Discourse Ability and Brain Damage: Theoretical and Empirical Perspectives* (pp. 154–77). New York: Springer.

Jaworski, A. and Coupland, N. (1999). *The Discourse Reader*. London: Routledge.

Joanette, Y., Goulet, P., and Hannequin, D. (1990). *Right Hemisphere and Verbal Communication*. New York: Springer.

Johnson-Laird, P. N. (1983). *Mental Models*. Cambridge: Cambridge University Press.

Johnstone, B. (2001). Discourse analysis and narrative. In D. Schiffrin, D. Tannen, and H. E. Hamilton (eds.), *The Handbook of Discourse Analysis*. Oxford: Blackwell.

Jordan, F. M., Murdoch, B. E., and Buttsworth, D. L. (1991). Closed-head-injured children's performance on narrative tasks. *Journal of Speech and Hearing Research*, 34, 572–82.

Kintsch, W. (1977). On comprehending stories. In M. A. Just and P. A. Carpenter (eds.), *Cognitive Processes in Comprehension* (pp. 33–62). New York: Wiley.

Kintsch, W. and Van Dijk, T. (1978). Towards a model of text comprehension and production. *Psychological Review*, 85, 363–94.

Kitwood, T. (1988). The technical, the personal, and the framing of dementia. *Social Behaviour*, 3, 161–79.

Kitwood, T. (1990). The dialectics of dementia: with particular reference to Alzheimer's disease. *Ageing and Society*, 10, 177–96.

Kitwood, T. (1997). *Dementia Reconsidered: The Person Comes First*. Philadelphia, PA: Open University Press.

Kitwood, T. and Bredin, K. (1992). Towards a theory of dementia care: Personhood and well-being. *Ageing and Society*, 10, 177–96.

Kress, G. (1988). *Linguistic Processes in Sociocultural Practice*. Oxford: Oxford University Press.

Kress, G. and van Leeuwen, T. (1996). *Reading Images: The Grammar of Visual Design*. London: Routledge.

Kurzweil, R. (1999). *The Age of Spiritual Machines*. New York: Penguin.

LeDoux, J. (2002). *Synaptic Self: How Our Brains Become Who We Are*. Harmondsworth: Penguin.

Lesser, R. and Milroy, L. (1993). *Linguistics and Aphasia: Psycholinguistic and Pragmatic Aspects of Intervention*. Harlow, Essex: Longman.

Levinson, S. (1983). *Pragmatics*. Cambridge: Cambridge University Press.

Mandler, J. (1984). *Stories, Scripts and Scenes: Aspects of a Schema Theory*. Hillsdale, NJ: Lawrence Erlbaum.

Mandler, J. and Johnson, N. S. (1977). Remembrance of things parsed: Story structure and recall. *Cognitive Psychology*, 9, 111–51.

McCabe, A. and Bliss, L. S. (2003). *Patterns of Narrative Discourse: A Multicultural, Lifespan Approach*. Boston: Allyn and Bacon.

McDonald, S. and Turkstra, L. (1998). Adolescents with traumatic brain injury: Issues in the assessment of pragmatic language. *Clinical Linguistics and Phonetics*, 12, 237–48.

McTear, M. (1985). Pragmatic disorders: A question of direction. *British Journal of Disorders of Communication*, 20, 119–27.

Mey, J. L. (1985). *Whose Language: A Study in Linguistic Pragmatics*. Amsterdam: Benjamins.

Mross, E. F. (1990). Text analysis: Macro- and microstructural aspects of discourse processing. In Y. Joanette and H. Brownell (1990), *Discourse Ability and Brain Damage: Theoretical and Empirical Perspectives* (pp. 50–69). New York: Springer.

Myers, P. S. (1993). Narrative expressive deficits associated with right hemisphere damage. In H. H. Brownell and Y. Joanette (eds.), *Narrative Discourse in Neurologically Impaired and Normally Aging Adults* (pp. 279–98). San Diego: Singular.

Ninio, A., Snow, C. E., Pan, B. A., and Rollins, P. R. (1994). Classifying communicative acts in children's interactions. *Journal of Communication Disorders*, 27, 157–87.

O'Dell, L. and Brownlow, C. (2005). Media reports of links between MMR and autism: A discourse analysis. *British Journal of Learning Disabilities*, 33, 194–9.

Onions, C. T. (1966). *The Oxford Dictionary of English Etymology*. Oxford: Oxford University Press.

Pearce, W. M., McCormack, P. F., and James, D. (2003). Exploring the boundaries of SLI: Findings from morphosyntactic and story grammar analyses. *Clinical Linguistics and Phonetics*, 17, 325–34.

Penn, C. (1988). The profiling of syntax and pragmatics in aphasia. *Clinical Linguistics and Phonetics*, 2, 179–207.

Perkins, M. (2007) *Pragmatic Impairment*. Cambridge: Cambridge University Press.

Potter, J. (2003). A discursive psychology of institutions. Paper presented at the BPS Social Psychology Section Annual Conference, London School of Economics.

Potter, J. and Wetherell, M. (1987). *Discourse and Social Psychology*. London: Sage.

Prutting, C. and Kirchner, D. (1983). Applied pragmatics. In T. Gallagher and C. Prutting (eds.), *Pragmatic Assessment and Intervention Issues in Language*. San Diego: College Hill.

Prutting, C. and Kirchner, D. (1987). A clinical appraisal of the pragmatic aspects of language. *Journal of Speech and Hearing Disorders*, 52, 105–19.

Ripich, D. N., Vertes, D., Whitehouse, P., Fulton, S., and Ekelman, B. (1991). Turn-taking and speech act patterns in the discourse of senile dementia of the Alzheimer's type patients. *Brain and Language*, 40, 330–43.

Rollins, P. R., Pan, B. A., Conti-Ramsden, G., and Snow, C. E. (1994). Communicative skills in children with Specific Language Impairments: A comparison with their language-matched siblings. *Journal of Communication Disorders*, 27, 188–201.

Roth, F. P. and N. J. Spekman (1986). Narrative discourse: Spontaneously-generated stories of learning-disabled and normally achieving students. *Journal of Speech and Hearing Disorders*, 51, 8–23.

Roth, F. P. and N. J. Spekman (1994). Oral story production in adults with learning disabilities. In R. L. Bloom, L. K. Obler, S. De Santi, and J. S. Ehrlich (eds.), *Discourse Analysis and Applications: Studies in Adult Clinical Populations* (pp. 131–48). Hillsdale, NJ: Lawrence Erlbaum.

Rumelhart, D. E. (1975). Notes on a schema for stories. In D. Bobrow and A. Collins (eds.), *Representation and Understanding: Studies in Cognitive Science* (pp. 185–210). New York: Academic Press.

Sabat, S. R. (1991). Turn-taking and turn-giving, and Alzheimer's disease: A case study in conversation. *Georgetown Journal of Languages and Linguistics*, 2, 161–75.

Sabat, S. R. (2001). *The Experience of Alzheimer's Disease: Life through a Tangled Veil.* Oxford: Blackwell.

Sabat, S. and Harré, R. (1992). The construction and deconstruction of self in Alzheimer's disease. *Ageing and Society*, 12, 443–61.

Schank, R. and Abelson, R. (1977). *Scripts, Plans, Goals and Understanding.* Hillsdale, NJ: Lawrence Erlbaum.

Schiffrin, D. (1994). *Approaches to Discourse.* Oxford: Blackwell.

Schiffrin, D., Tannen, D., and Hamilton, H. E. (eds.) (2001). *The Handbook of Discourse Analysis.* Oxford: Blackwell.

Searle, J. (1969). *Speech Acts.* Cambridge: Cambridge University Press.

Searle, J. (1975). A taxonomy of illocutionary acts. In K. Gunderson (ed.), *Language, Mind and Knowledge*. Minnesota Studies in the Philosophy of Science (pp. 344–69). Minneapolis: University of Minnesota Press. Reprinted in Searle (1979), pp. 1–29.

Searle, J. (1979). *Expression and Meaning.* Cambridge: Cambridge University Press.

Searle, J. (1986). Introductory essay: Notes on conversation. In D. G. Ellis and W. A. Donahue (eds.), *Contemporary Issues in Language and Discourse Processes* (pp. 7–19). Hillsdale, NJ: Lawrence Erlbaum.

Ska, B. and Guénard, D. (1993). Narrative schema in dementia of the Alzheimer's type. In H. H. Brownell and Y. Joanette (eds.), *Narrative Discourse in Neurologically Impaired and Normally Aging Adults* (pp. 299–316). San Diego: Singular.

Stein, N. L. and Glenn, C. G. (1979). An analysis of story comprehension in elementary school children. In R. O. Freedle (ed.), *New Directions in Discourse Processing* (pp. 53–120). Norwood, NJ: Ablex.

Streeck, J. (1980). Speech acts in interaction: A critique of Searle. *Discourse Processes*, 3, 133–54.

Ulatowska, H. K., Doyel, A. W., Freedman-Stern, R. F., Macaluso-Haynes, S. M., and North, A. J. (1983). Production of procedural discourse in aphasia. *Brain and Language*, 18, 315–41.

Ulatowska, H. K., Freedman-Stern, R., Weiss-Doyel, A., Macaluso-Haynes, S., and North, A. J. (1983). Production of narrative discourse in aphasia. *Brain and Language*, 19, 317–34.

Ulatowska, H. K., North, A. J., and Macaluso-Haynes, S. (1981). Production of narrative and procedural discourse in aphasia. *Brain and Language*, 13, 345–71.

Van Dijk, T. (1977). *Text and Context: Explorations of the Semantics and Pragmatics of Discourse.* London: Longman.

Van Dijk, T. (2001). Critical discourse analysis. In Schiffrin, Tannen, and Hamilton (2001) (pp. 352–71).

Van Dijk, T. and Kintsch, W. (1978). Cognitive psychology and discourse: Recalling and summarizing stories. In W. Dressler (ed.), *Current Trends in Text Linguistics*. New York: de Gruyter.

Van Dijk, T. and Kintsch, W. (1983). *Structures of Discourse Comprehension*. New York: Academic Press.

Verschueren, J. (2001). Predicaments of criticism. *Critique of Anthropology*, 21(1), 59–81.

2 Conversational Implicature and Communication Impairment

ELISABETH AHLSÉN

2.1 What is Conversational Implicature?

The notion of conversational implicature stems from H. P. Grice's 1975 paper 'Logic in Conversation'. That paper set out an overriding principle of cooperation and a series of subordinate conversational maxims, which make human communication possible and 'smooth'. Before looking more closely at conversational implicature, it is important to situate the framework as one of the main ways in which the pragmatic functions of language comprehension and production in context can be studied and understood. As Stephen Levinson stated in his 1983 book *Pragmatics*, "given a linguistic form uttered in a context, a pragmatic theory must account for the inference of presuppositions, implicatures, illocutionary force and other pragmatic implications" (p. 21).

Implicatures are, thus, one of the sets of phenomena that constitute pragmatics; they are related to others, especially to inference. Inference is described by Levinson as follows: "Understanding an utterance involves the making of *inferences* that will connect what is said to what is mutually assumed or what has been said before" (Levinson, 1983, p. 21). In light of this description, presuppositions (what is mutually assumed), implicatures (what has to be inferred from context and convention or from conversational principles), and illocutionary force (the function that a speaker intends an utterance to have) all serve to make the relevant connections.

Implicature, according to Grice (1975), is what a speaker may imply, suggest or mean, as distinct from what the speaker literally says. *Conventional* implicatures are determined by the conventional meanings of the words used. We will not dwell on conventional implicatures here, but simply note that Grice assumes some kind of 'literal meaning'. It is not clear that a specific 'literal meaning' really exists when the semantics and pragmatics of utterances in context are the focus; one might instead think of the conventional or typical meanings of words.

The general principle behind *conversational* implicature is the *cooperative principle*.

> Make your conversational contribution such as is required, at the stage at which it occurs, by the accepted purpose or direction of the talk exchange in which you are engaged (Grice, 1975, p. 45).

In order to adhere to the cooperative principle, which is necessary for communication to work, language users employ a set of *conversational maxims*, which present the principle in more detail. These are the maxims of quantity, quality, relation, and manner, as described below.

Quantity: Make your contributions as informative as is required (for the current purposes of the exchange). Do not make your contributions more informative than is required.

Quality: Do not say what you believe to be false. Do not say that for which you lack adequate evidence.

Relation: Be relevant.

Manner: Be perspicuous. Avoid obscurity of expression. Avoid ambiguity. Be brief (avoid unnecessary prolixity). Be orderly.

These are the four most important conversational maxims mentioned by Grice. This list should not, however, be seen as exhaustive. Other maxims may also apply, for example politeness (Be polite). Allwood (1976) made use of Grice's principle and maxims, but also criticized them. According to Allwood, it is not enough to have the cooperative principle, which means that people take each other into *cognitive* consideration. We also need a principle of *ethical* consideration. In other words, we should not only care about how other persons cognitively understand or share the content of what we say, but we must also care about their feelings. Conversational implicatures are, thus, not straightforward semantic interpretations or semantic inferences, in a logical, deductive sense, about the relations between utterances. Instead, they are inferences about what is said, made on the basis of assumptions about how we cooperate in spoken interaction. Since they emanate from general considerations of rationality, the claim is that they can be universally applied to *all* kinds of cooperative exchanges.

How are conversational principles and maxims used in speech and how can linguists use them in describing and explaining communication?

It has been suggested that the conversational maxims can be:

1   observed directly (by standard implicature, or so-called generalized
    implicature, if no particular contextual conditions are needed);
2   flouted (deliberately breached).

Maxims are flouted through the use of irony, sarcasm, jokes, etc., which function
by breaking one of the maxims in a particular way. This mechanism would
not work if the maxims were not assumed to be adhered to by persons who
communicate. In other words, when we observe successful flouting, we know
that the maxims work. We cannot directly observe what goes on in speakers'
minds, so only in their output can we find flouting and other signs that allow
us to study conversational implicature.

2.2   Conversational Implicature and Clinical Linguistics

Some of the advantages of studying conversational implicature in pragmatics,
according to Levinson (1983), are as follows:

- that the general principles originate outside the organization of language
  but profoundly affect the structure of language and therefore offer significant functional explanations of linguistic facts;
- that they make it possible to explicitly account for how one can mean more
  than what one actually says;
- that they are likely to simplify semantic descriptions;
- that they are essential for understanding various basic facts about language;
- that they have very general explanatory power.

This also makes them useful and interesting for clinical linguists (cf. Ahlsén,
1993).

Conversational implicature makes conversation maximally efficient, rational
and cooperative. It is quite fundamental to most of human communication
and fulfills a number of functions, as we have seen above. It affects our co-
construction of meaning in spoken interaction, since it determines what we
say and how we organize our contributions, as well as how we perceive and
understand the contributions of others. In clinical linguistics, this becomes
relevant in several ways. We are interested in the causes and effects of what
we can describe in terms of conversational implicature. For some communication disorders, conversational principles and maxims can provide an important framework for their description and explanation, where perhaps no other
available framework can capture the same phenomena. In other cases, they
provide additional information that can help us understand the disorder and
assist patients in developing communicative strategies. We can study how

conversational implicature helps communication and we can also study how it goes wrong. In this way, we can study how the maxims are observed either more or less successfully, or possibly how they are not fully observed at all. We can study:

1   Cases when conversational principles and maxims appear not to be adhered to. Either they cannot be used in the usual way as a basis for interpretation, although they can be used with addition/qualification, or they are put out of play, perhaps by a disorder that affects them more directly. We can study how the participants in a conversation handle this situation.
2   Cases when flouting is attempted but is not successful, or possibly is not attempted. Since the maxims cannot be assumed in the same way by the two participants, the possibility of flouting as a 'device' in the conversation vanishes. Since this is a negative identification, it is hard to study, but it is still important. Many persons with communication disorders have subjective problems that can be explained in terms of problems with flouting. The focus in our examples will, however, be instances of the first kind of case.

The Gricean maxims rely on (1) the participants' cognitive ability to use the principles and maxims as such, and (2) the ability of all participants to control and execute their own linguistic processing. We can therefore assume that they will be affected in some way by all communication disorders. Thus, we have to consider the role of underlying cognitive processing in communication, such as memory processes, for example working memory and the availability of long-term memory, central executive functions and attention. We also have to consider all possible disturbances of language processing, on the input as well as the output side. Thirdly, we have to consider the communicative interaction between participants, their co-construction of meaning and their general alignment and coordination. In some cases, it might be possible to see that – and how – conversational implicature is specifically affected by one factor, but in most cases it will depend on the complex interaction between several factors. Conversational implicature is always at work and it is likely to adapt to the circumstances, for example, to the effects of communication disorders, in particular ways. It is therefore important to try to find out how this comes about and what the consequences are.

A prerequisite for the successful use of conversational implicature is that the participants must have sufficient experience and background knowledge, in a general sense, to 'anchor' the application of conversational maxims, and, specifically, knowledge of how people interact in communication. We will therefore consider this factor in more detail below.

We will take a closer look at the principles and maxims at work in relation to a number of types of communication disorders. Let us first briefly consider cooperation, ethical consideration, strategies and context.

2.2.1   The principles of cognitive cooperation and ethical consideration

We have seen and will see that the full-fledged use of the conversational maxims can be affected in many ways by communication disorders. Since the maxims specify how we use the *cooperative principle*, the actual outcome of this principle is usually affected, although we can assume that in most cases, the cooperative and *ethical principles* are at work as much as, or perhaps more than, in typical communication.

Strategies play a central role in communication involving persons with communication disorders. Strategies may be more or less conscious manipulations of how we use conversational implicature to make sense of communicative contributions. They also affect how persons communicate in many ways that go beyond the direct effects of the communication problem in itself and thereby affect the basis for conversational implicature. Consequently, we need to be aware of strategies at work.

Context is another factor that continuously affects how we communicate and how we use conversational implicature. This means that the situation makes it easier or harder to communicate linguistically, depending on the available objects, the persons involved, what has been said before, the communicative requirements for taking part in an activity, etc.

2.3   Communication Impairment and Conversational Implicature: Types and Examples

In addition to background experience, there are three basic types of disorders that can affect the use of conversational implicature: (1) cognitive disorders of different types, (2) disorders affecting language comprehension, and (3) disorders affecting language production. (These three types are by no means mutually exclusive – in fact, they are rather interdependent – they are simply three main aspects of how we usually look at these types of disorders.) We will use them to illustrate how the maxims are used by and affected in persons with communication impairments.

2.3.1   Background experiences: A prerequisite

As a general background for being able to participate fully in communicative interaction, we need the necessary 'knowledge of the world' and awareness of the situation at hand. This store of knowledge develops over time and we do not expect small children to have very much of this knowledge and awareness, since they have not yet had many life experiences. As communicators we usually expect children to be less experienced, and adapt to it, so this does not become a problem. When the development is not appropriate to the person's age, problems in everyday interaction arise. This may depend on an inadequate social environment and experiences. It may also be caused by late or atypical cognitive and/or linguistic development (see below). The result can be, for example, a lack of vocabulary and knowledge about different topics, but also a lack of experience with how people interact in communication and what one can expect from others. That is, parts of the basis for using conversational implicature may be lacking. For adults, dementia, amnesia or other types of problems affecting long-term memory and attention can lead to this kind of problem (see below).

2.3.1.1 Resulting problems with maxims

Quantity: It becomes impossible to correctly judge what is the right amount and type of information to produce in a given situation, if there is a lack of experience (or memory problems causing a lack of access to experience). This can lead to giving too much or too little information and to problems interpreting and understanding what other people say.

Manner: Lack of available experience with the manner of presentation of information leads to comprehension problems and to seemingly disorganized presentation, which requires the interlocutor to make an extra effort.

Relation: It is impossible to correctly assess what information is relevant at a given point in an interaction, if there is a lack of available background information.

Quality: Quality can sometimes be affected by deficient world knowledge.

Concrete examples of the effects include vocabulary errors: deviant use of words such as overgeneralization (calling all animals *dog* or all colors *red*), speech output that appears to lack precise content words, and dispreferred answers and comments to the interlocutor's utterances, due to comprehension problems caused by the lack of available background knowledge.

2.3.2 Cognitive disorders of memory, attention, central executive functions and 'Theory of Mind' (ToM)

Cognitive disorders affect how we can acquire and use knowledge of the world and life experiences. They are also closely related and integrated into linguistic processing on both the input and output sides and this is very important for conversational implicature, which involves the ability to make inferences. One of the most important abilities needed is the ability to select among alternatives in a given situation, which involves cognitive flexibility and sensitivity to context. Related to this ability, but focusing specifically on the interlocutor, some form of ToM-like ability is required. Memory, central executive functions and sustained attention (the ability to focus and remain focused) are also very important.

2.3.2.1   Children
Many children who have cognitive problems are characterized by a slow or atypical cognitive development in general, which affects attention, focus, central executive function, etc. Another group is made up of children with a diagnosis of ADHD, who have problems with sustained attention and focusing. A third group comprises children with autism spectrum disorder or Asperger syndrome, where ToM and experiences with alignment, coordination and fine-tuned interpersonal interaction can be deficient (Happé & Loth, 2002). Children with acquired brain damage are also likely to have cognitive problems affecting memory and attention, as well as so-called 'subtle' or 'high-level' language (HLL) disorders, which are closely linked to cognitive processing.

2.3.2.2   Adults
Cognitive disorders have been studied in people with acquired cortical and subcortical lesions in the left and right hemispheres after a stroke or traumatic brain injury (TBI) and in people with dementia. Since these groups show some interesting phenomena that are directly and indirectly of importance for conversational implicature, we will consider some of the specific findings. In this category, which borders on (and intersects with) language comprehension problems, a number of symptoms have been described that directly relate to inference and more specifically to conversational implicature.

Many possible causal factors have been suggested, both more direct ones that are often described in terms of some type of pragmatic impairment and more indirect ones that refer to an underlying cognitive deficit of a more basic ability. Some of the factors suggested include:

- reduced sensitivity to conversational conventions,
- reduced sensitivity to context,
- reduced sensitivity to others' intentions, beliefs and motivations (ToM),
- reduced ability to generate the holistic theme or topic of a conversation (topic drift),
- reduced ability to make fine semantic distinctions,
- reduced sensitivity to facial expressions and prosody,
- disorders of attention,
- disorders of working memory,
- cognitive rigidity, for instance, difficulties in making revised inference,
- impaired selective ability (reduced specificity).

(Martin & McDonald, 2003; McDonald, 1993; McDonald & Pearce, 1996; McDonald, Togher, & Code, 1999; Myers, 1999; Perkins, Body, & Parker, 1995; Rehak, Kaplan, & Gardner, 1992; Saldert, 2006)

2.3.2.3   *Resulting problems with maxims*

Quantity: Memory disorders will cause the same problems as the problems with lack of available background knowledge that we noted above, since general world knowledge/experience is not totally available and therefore quantity demands cannot be assessed. Disorders affecting attention and short-term memory make it impossible to keep items and sequences in focus long enough to maintain an overview of single utterances and/or the interaction sequence, which directly affects the ability to apply the maxim of quantity, since it is impossible to know what has been said in the conversation. These kinds of disorders, for instance HLL disorders, are especially sensitive to conversational maxims. If the disorder affects ToM abilities, there will be an even more direct relationship to deficient use of the quantity maxim, since the lack of an ability to judge what information the interlocutor might need is the core of this disability. The same factors make it difficult to judge whether the interlocutor has provided enough information or not.

Manner: Many of the elements affecting the maxim of quantity also affect the different aspects of the maxim of manner. If one cannot keep attention and working memory focused long enough, it is hard to organize one's own contributions, and it might also be hard to make sense of the organization of the interlocutor's contributions. Central executive function disorders can have a considerable impact in this regard.

Relation: To judge what is relevant in interpreting the interlocutor's output and planning one's own utterances also requires an overview that is dependent on the cognitive functions of memory and sustained attention. It is also dependent on ToM-like abilities.

Quality: Quality is only secondarily affected, for example by memory disorders.

Examples 1 and 2 below illustrate how the output of a person with right-hemisphere damage does not facilitate the application of the maxims of manner and relevance by the listener.

Example 1. Man with right-hemisphere lesion (R) in conversation with a speech and language therapist (SLT) (S) about having been to a clinic at the 'social house' (from Saldert, 2006).

(/ = pause of up to 3 seconds; // = pause of 3 seconds or more)

R: and then / oh yes then I met // a warder /
S: uhum

R: from 'name of prison' / he had a lot of pa- / that one I met later because he
worked at 'name of amusement park' as a guard /because I met . . . had a
gang with him there then see / from 'name of prison'

S: at 'name of amusement park'

R: /n- / no [no at there]

S: [where did you meet him]

R: at / at this social house

Example 2. Man with right-hemisphere lesion in conversation with an SLT about what happened in a shop (from Saldert, 2006).

R: but I was there in half a tick I ran forward / then said you have to watch out
the said // and was pretty much a boy in the same age / same length / that
opened a door in another place that was a young mother too / and I said
thank you and she got so very surprised because of that

Examples 1 and 2 both relate fairly directly to the use of conversational maxims and how problems can arise when speakers do not present their output in the best possible way, making it hard for the interlocutor to assess the relevance of what is said. Fast-changing associations, word-finding problems and topic drift make the contributions hard to interpret. It is especially hard to know what situation, place or person is being referred to, and the interlocutor has to ask clarification questions, as in Example 1.

2.3.3   Language comprehension

In order to use conversational implicature optimally, one has to be able to follow the conversation, which requires good language comprehension. All aspects of language processing, including sensitivity to prosodic or body communication cues to information structure, emotion, etc., are used. The successful use of conversational implicature requires attention to individual cues, selection of relevant cues, integration of relevant cues, and association of cues with prior experiences or world knowledge (Myers, 1999, p. 105). We can see that this requires language comprehension, cognitive abilities, and access to and ability to use background knowledge/experiences. Conversational implicature is likely to play an important role in interactions involving persons with language comprehension disorders, but since parts of the basis for its use are damaged or missing, the results can be 'deviant.'

2.3.3.1   Children

In children with delayed or atypical language development, this is an area of some controversy, since it is not easy to distinguish more specific language disorders from more general (or specific) cognitive disorders. There may also be difficulties in distinguishing between language comprehension problems and problems caused by deficient background knowledge and experience. Finally, different alternatives have been suggested with regard to labeling some of these children as having a semantic-pragmatic, semantic or pragmatic disorder. In either case, this brings us to problems with conversational implicature, which can be secondary to or part of language comprehension problems (cf. Letts & Leinonen, 2001; McTear & Conti-Ramsden, 1992).

2.3.3.2 Adults
Language comprehension problems in adults are mainly found in persons with acquired left- and right-hemisphere cortical and subcortical lesions after a stroke or TBI and in persons with dementia.

2.3.3.3 Resulting problems with maxims
Language comprehension problems limit the accessibility of what is being said and therefore also limit the use of the maxims of quantity, manner and relation.

Quantity: Since what is said is not properly understood, it is hard to know whether (1) the interlocutor has provided the right amount of information, and (2) one's own contributions are providing the right quantity of information. It is also hard for the interlocutor to know (1) how much needs to be said so that the person with the communication disorder will understand, and (2) how well the language production of the person with a communication disorder matches their intended amount of information and how to interpret what is said. Neither participant can assume that the right quantity is being produced. One of the prominent features identifying persons with comprehension disorders is the production of 'too much' speech.

Manner: Not only the quantity but also the manner in which language is produced is affected, since semantic-pragmatic problems, such as word-finding problems, increased fluency of speech, and circumlocutions and neologisms, make the patient produce information in suboptimal ways. It is also hard for the interlocutor to know how to best organize his or her own speech, in order to be understood.

Relation: The features mentioned under quantity and manner also affect relation. It is not clear to either participant that what is produced by the patient is relevant, or how it should be interpreted as relevant.

Quality: Since comprehension of one's own speech is often affected, the quality maxim can also be affected on the output side, so that the interlocutor cannot assume that what is said is always correct. Children's language comprehension problems affect their acquisition of knowledge of the world and experience of how people communicate and consequently affect their use of conversational implicature (Beeman, 1993; Letts & Leinonen, 2001; McDonald, 1993; McTear & Conti-Ramsden, 1992; Rehak, Kaplan, & Gardner, 1992).

Examples 3 and 4 below illustrate some typical effects of language comprehension problems on spoken interaction.

Example 3. Conversation between a woman with aphasia (A) and an SLT (S) (from Ahlsén, 1993).

Context: The SLT is interviewing A about her family and asks her the ages of her two children.

> S: both are older than ten
>   (shows ten fingers)
> A: what did you say
> S.   are they OLDER than ten years they are bigger than ten
>   (shows ten fingers, then shows height of ten-year-old with hand)
> A: so hard what's it called
>   (looks at her fingers, shows three fingers)
> S: three
>   (shows three fingers)
> A: yes
> S: is one of them so small
> A: yes
> S: oh
> A: what did you say
> S: three
> A: no that must be wrong mustn't it

Example 4. Interaction in a confrontation naming test between a child with specific language impairment (SLI) who has language comprehension difficulties (C) and an SLT (S) (from Månsson, 2004).

Context: Confrontation naming task – the SLT mishears the child's contribution and reformulates her question.

> C: tongs
> S: what was the NAME for it
>   (C shrugs shoulders, looks down, tilts head to one side and smiles)
> S: It was correct what you said
> C: TONGS
>   (looks at S)
> S: yes TONGS

Both of the above examples reveal an increased insecurity in the use of conversational maxims on the part of both participants. They involve both comprehension and production difficulties, making it hard for participants to know exactly how to use conversational implicature.

In Example 3, the woman with aphasia does not at first understand the question; when she asks for a repetition, the SLT does not know what aspects of her question were not understood or why. This is reflected in the changed formulation of her second question. She makes a number of changes:

1 emphatic stress on the adjective *older* (*older* → *OLDER*),
2 the addition of the noun *years* (*ten* → *ten years*),
3 the reformulation of a declarative question as an interrogative question (SVO → VSO word order),
4 the addition of a repetition of the declarative question while changing the adjective to *bigger* (*older* → *bigger*),
5 the addition of the gesture illustrating the height of a ten-year-old.

This reflects the fact that she does not know whether she has to deal with problems related to quantity or manner, and thus she is not sure which specific aspects – vocabulary, word order, or more redundancy in presentation (verbal-vocal and body communication) – to change.

In the subsequent attempts to establish the age of the children, each participant has problems establishing whether the number suggested by the other participant is correct or not. A's comprehension and production problems make her unsure about the correctness of her own contributions and the SLT's interpretation. They also cause the SLT to be insecure about whether A's expression is correct. Questions concerning how much redundancy should be used and how mutual agreement should be established are typically directly related to conversational inference.

Example 4 illustrates how the child's comprehension and production problems result in insecurity in the use of conversational maxims. The fact that the SLT did not initially understand C's first contribution, which was correct, can probably be traced back to her expectations, that is, she cannot assume that C will understand and produce utterances correctly. But, more importantly, the fact that she then reformulates her question (in a way that is reminiscent of the strategy used in Example 3) makes C unsure. The child may doubt whether he contributed the correct information (that is, he doubts the quality and relevance of his own output) and, since he is aware that he does not know the name of everything that is asked for in the test, he is likely to do just that, given the SLT's new question. This is also indicated by his body communication.

2.3.4 Language production problems

In language production, the ability to make choices of pragmatic (for example, communication act), semantic, lexical, syntactic, morphological and phonological structures and units, as well as prosody and body communication, has to be intact, if one is to produce contributions that will facilitate the use of conversational implicature. This ability is, of course, also secondarily affected by cognitive and world knowledge prerequisites for making the appropriate choices.

2.3.4.1   Children

We find it natural that small children can only use a subset of language, and that not always correctly, and so we adapt to their abilities. But children with delayed or atypical language development, such as SLI, have more difficulties observing conversational maxims in their production and this will cause difficulties for their interlocutors. There are qualitatively different kinds of production problems. Grammar and phonology problems result in more direct production difficulties, even when semantic-pragmatic and cognitive abilities function properly. Problems with semantics and pragmatics may also be related to different linguistic and cognitive factors as well as background knowledge and are more challenging with respect to conversational implicature.

2.3.4.2   Adults

Language production problems are found in the same groups of adults as language comprehension problems and in many cases in those with other types of cognitive problems as well, that is, in persons with acquired left- and right-hemisphere cortical and subcortical lesions after stroke or TBI and in persons with dementia. In addition, they occur in persons with more specific speech production problems, such as speech apraxia and dysarthria.

2.3.4.3   Augmentative and alternative communication (AAC)

A special case for both children and adults concerns persons who have reduced mobility, caused by cerebral palsy, hemiplegia after a stroke, apraxia or dysarthria, where production problems can be severe and have a huge impact on the use of conversational implicature. The use of communication aids often also imposes specific demands on the interaction.

2.3.4.4   Resulting problems with maxims

What are described here are problems that primarily result from production difficulties. In reality, comprehension and production problems very often co-exist in the same patient, so section 2.3.3 above, 'Language comprehension', is also relevant in these cases. Examples 3 and 4 above are also relevant with respect to language production problems.

Quantity: Many production problems affect the amount of speech that is produced so that it becomes either too sparse or (less frequently) too verbose.

Manner: If you cannot produce speech in the best-ordered manner, you have to do it in some other way, by applying a strategy; alternatively, you might not be able to control the manner at all.

Relation: Production problems and strategies can make it a bit harder for the listener to interpret relevance in a straightforward way, but in principle relation is not affected so much.

Quality: The quality maxim is not affected much, except in cases where, for example, the patient cannot voluntarily choose between producing a 'yes' and a 'no' answer.

The maxim of quantity is maybe best exemplified by the typical speech production of persons with so-called fluent and nonfluent aphasia. We can see in examples 5 and 6 how not only quantity but also manner and, to some extent, relevance are affected. In both examples, the context is a task where the subject is asked to narrate what happens in an ordered sequence of four pictures. The pictures show: (1) a man sweeping up leaves with two children and a dog watching him in the background, (2) the man putting the leaves into a basket, (3) the wind blowing all the leaves out of the basket, and (4) the man angrily swinging the basket over his head, while the children and dog in the background walk away laughing.

Example 5. Nonfluent aphasia: narration of picture story (from Ahlsén, 1993).

a basket and one sweeps a leaf // takes // basket // takes up // takes up the leaf // leaf leaves fly // he gets angry

Example 6. Fluent aphasia: narration of picture story.

it is a man who eh // he // yes when s when is is a little colder outside then then comes k- a- on the snow or on that the // next to // eh he picks in in what's that called // what's it called // he he lies iiin bag not bag // yes almost bag and then it blows too much then it it fla- flo- floats away and then it lies on the ground and then he must // and he must then do again once more you see

Whereas control subjects normally tell the story in about 50 words, Example 5 contains 21 words and Example 6 contains 82.

The 'nonfluent' story is fairly well organized in terms of manner, although the sparse grammar and grammatical insecurity make it far from optimal. In terms of reference, the speaker does not include enough of the relevant information. The story does not specify who the main character is or what roles the wind, the children and the dog play. There is, thus, too little output.

The 'fluent' story, on the other hand, although it is fairly verbose, also lacks some referential information (to the children and the dog), while word-finding problems and substitutions (*lies* for *puts*, *bag* for *basket*), as well as circumlocutions, create problems of manner and relevance. In sum, there is too much quantity in terms of words and phrases produced, whereas manner, relevance and quality of content are not optimal. The word substitutions could also affect quality.

2.4 Cooperation: Cognitive and Ethical Consideration

Conversational implicature is a complex phenomenon, as we have seen, with a set of maxims specifying the assumptions that, if there are no indications to the contrary, are made by participants in a communicative situation about the contributions they make. In addition to being complex, it is also not explicit or directly observable in most cases. The examples above represent attempts to show how the usually quite automatized use of the maxims can become less reliable in different types of communication disorders and how this, in its turn, affects communication. The conversational maxims can be helpful tools for analyzing communication disorders and their consequences and they can also help to identify successful and less successful communication strategies.

The cases discussed above are, thus, not really cases where the maxims are not observed at all or where they are flouted, but cases where their use is restricted or less reliable because of the communication disorder. One can interpret these subjects' output as showing that the maxims are not adhered to, but this probably applies above all to the surface symptoms and may not necessarily mean that the subjects are not, in some sense, adhering to them internally. Instead, we might say that the participants in these interactions automatically and sometimes, when necessary, consciously try to use the maxims as much as possible and that this is one reason why the conversations work as well as they do, given the communication disorder. So conversational implicature can be a helpful, as well as a somewhat misleading, strategy in this context.

Flouting of the conversational maxims is often reported as a major subjective problem by persons with communication disorders, especially acquired disorders. We can see why this is so, in the above examples. Since the maxims cannot be effectively used and trusted in the usual way, the participants adapt their conversational inferences. Every deviation from the preferred use of maxims must be interpreted as being potentially *not* an intended deviation but a problem of production, comprehension, cognition or experience/world knowledge. Therefore, an intentional flouting is not only (because of these problems) difficult to produce, but nearly always fails to be interpreted as intentional by the interlocutor. This can be extremely frustrating for the person with the communication disorder, who can no longer make jokes or use irony successfully.

The overriding principles of cognitive and ethical consideration are always at work. In spite of, or possibly because of, the problems affecting production, comprehension, cognition and experience/world knowledge and the resulting insecurity in using the specific conversational maxims, there seems to be an 'overconsideration' of the interlocutor. This may lead to the unimpaired participant's engaging in overinterpretation and often leads to an almost extreme use of politeness strategies, failure to mention communication problems and explicitly taking on the 'guilt' when the other participant fails to communicate fully.

2.5 Influence of Clinical Linguistics on General Linguistics

As in many other cases, clinical linguistics can provide valuable insights for the study of conversational implicature in general linguistics. It is sometimes claimed that the conversational maxims can really only be studied when they are being flouted. However, as we have seen above, communication disorders provide a broad spectrum of ways in which we can at least attempt to study how conversational maxims and principles are adhered to more or less successfully in communication. We can use them to explain other linguistic phenomena and we can study how they are affected by cognitive and linguistic constraints. This can help us in further developing linguistic theory and applications concerning conversational implicature.

REFERENCES

Ahlsén, E. (1993). Conversational principles and aphasic communication. *Journal of Pragmatics*, 19, 57–70.

Allwood, J. (1976). *Linguistic Communication as Action and Cooperation*. Gothenburg Monographs in Linguistics, 2. Göteborg University, Department of Linguistics.

Beeman, M. (1993). Semantic processing in the right hemisphere may contribute to drawing inferences from discourse. *Brain and Language*, 44, 80–120.

Grice, H. P. (1975). Logic and conversation. In P. Cole and J. L. Morgan (eds.), *Syntax and Semantics. Volume 3: Speech Acts* (pp. 41–58). New York: Academic Press.

Happé, F. and Loth, E. (2002). 'Theory of mind' and tracking speakers' intentions. *Mind and Language,* 17, 24–36.

Letts, C. and Leinonen, E. (2001). Comprehension of inferential meaning in language-impaired and language normal children. *International Journal of Language and Communication Disorders*, 36(3), 307–28.

Levinson, S. (1983). *Pragmatics*. Cambridge: Cambridge University Press.

Månsson, A.-C. (2003). *The Relation Between Gestures and Semantic Processes: A Study of Normal Language Development and Specific Language Impairment in Children*. Gothenburg Monographs in Linguistics, 23. Göteborg University, Department of Linguistics.

Martin, I. and McDonald, S. (2003). Weak coherence, no theory of mind, or executive dysfunction? Solving the puzzle of pragmatic language disorders. *Brain and Language*, 85, 452–66.

McDonald, S. (1993). Viewing the brain sideways? Frontal versus right hemisphere: Explanations of non-aphasic language disorders. *Aphasiology*, 7, 535–9.

McDonald, S. and Pearce, S. (1996). Clinical insights into pragmatic theory: Frontal lobe deficits and sarcasm. *Brain and Language*, 52, 81–104.

McDonald, S., Togher, L., and Code, C. (1999). The nature of traumatic brain injury: Basic features and neuropsychological consequences. In S. McDonald, L. Togher, and C. Code (eds.), *Communication Disorders Following Traumatic Brain Injury* (pp. 19–54). Hove, Sussex: Psychology Press.

McTear, M. F. and Conti-Ramsden, G. (1992). *Pragmatic Disability in Children*. London: Whurr.

Myers, P. S. (1999). *Right Hemisphere Damage*. London: Singular Publishing Group.

Perkins, M. R., Body, R., and Parker, M. (1995). Closed head injury: Assessment and remediation of topic bias and repetitiveness. In M. R. Perkins and S. J. Howard (eds.), *Case Studies in Clinical Linguistics* (pp. 293–320). London: Whurr.

Rehak, A., Kaplan, J. A., and Gardner, H. (1992). Sensitivity to conversational deviance in right-hemisphere-damaged patients. *Brain and Language*, 42, 203–17.

Saldert, C. (2006). *Inference and Conversational Interaction*. Gothenburg Monographs in Linguistics, 30. Göteborg University, Department of Linguistics.

3 Relevance Theory and Communication Disorders

EEVA LEINONEN AND NUALA RYDER

3.1 Introduction

Clinical Pragmatics is a term coined in the early 1990s to reflect an emerging awareness that some communication difficulties could not be attributed to 'purely' linguistic problems. For a long time before that, practicing speech and language therapists had worked with children and adults whose primary difficulties seemed to lie with the understanding and/or production of connected discourse. The language produced seemed to be grammatically and semantically well-formed but not appropriate to the particular context in which it was produced. Conversational contributions produced by these individuals appeared not always to be connected and relevant to those of others, suggesting difficulty with contextual or pragmatic comprehension.

Smith and Leinonen (1992) reviewed much of the early work in clinical pragmatics. Many different linguistically based methodologies were used to investigate these difficulties. One methodology was the analysis of conversations for unacceptable and irrelevant contributions leading to categorizations of different types of 'semantic-pragmatic disorder'. This led to discussion of whether descriptions of surface manifestations of underlying difficulties are sufficient for an understanding of pragmatic impairment. There was a need for a theoretical framework that would have psycholinguistic validity.

In the mid-1990s, Happé found Relevance Theory to be a useful theoretical framework for investigating theory-of-mind abilities in autistic children. Leinonen and Kerbel (1999) also used Relevance Theory to explore pragmatic failure in conversations involving children with comprehension difficulties. More recently, Ryder and Leinonen (2003) and Leinonen, Ryder, Ellis, and Hammond (2003) have used this framework successfully to study the development of language comprehension and comprehension difficulties in children. The methodology developed for these studies has subsequently been used by Loukusa, Leinonen, Kuusikko, et al. (2007) to explore the pragmatic performance of normally developing Finnish-speaking children and those with a diagnosis of Asperger syndrome. Relevance Theory has been used to a lesser extent in the study of acquired language disorders in adults. Dipper, Bryan, and Tyson (1997) found the framework useful in exploring why patients with right-hemisphere damage had impaired semantic and pragmatic knowledge.

In this chapter, we first give a brief introduction to Relevance Theory. This is an oversimplification of this very complex and rapidly evolving theory, but we have striven for succinctness rather than completeness in our exposition. We will then review studies on developmental and acquired disorders using the Relevance Theory framework. One advantage of using a rigorous theoretical framework in studying language disorders is the information we gain about the theory itself. In the final section we will comment on the impact that these studies have had on Relevance Theory.

3.2   Introducing Relevance Theory

Relevance Theory (Sperber & Wilson, 1995) is a theory of communication which aims to elucidate in detail the claim that an essential feature of most human communication (verbal and non-verbal) is the expression and recognition of intentions (Wilson & Sperber, 2004). The theory attempts to explain how meaning is stored in memory (concepts) and how information is processed to successfully understand an intended meaning. This inferential model of communication suggests that an utterance is a linguistically coded piece of information which is only a starting point for the comprehension of intended meaning. Relevance Theory (RT) explains how the hearer infers the speaker's meaning on the basis of the evidence provided, i.e. the linguistic expression and the context. The context may include any relevant information (including gestures, intonation and so on), whether stored in the memory or directly obtained from the encyclopedic entries (see below) of the concepts which may be accessed during interpretation.

The comprehension of language in communication requires the ability to interpret meaning in context. As children develop toward becoming more competent comprehenders of language, they need to become increasingly skilled at interpreting meaning that arises in context (Bishop, 1997; Milosky, 1992; Oakhill & Yuill, 1986). RT provides a model of the processes that facilitate the understanding of implicated meaning (implicatures), and it lends itself to the empirical investigation of language interpretation in both normal and clinical populations.

Sperber and Wilson (1995) argue that inferential comprehension involves central cognitive processes rather than specialized mechanisms. Hence, comprehension and production of pragmatic meaning and cognition are intrinsically linked. They further propose that in any given communicative situation, our cognitive systems are equipped to process the most relevant information. Language interpretation is guided by a principle of relevance, which ensures that only the most relevant information is processed. The principle of relevance states that every communication intended to be communicative guarantees to the listener that it is optimally relevant. For information to be optimally relevant to the hearer, it has to interact in certain ways with previous knowledge and/or contextual information to produce an outcome with the least possible processing effort. For example, indirect answers to questions are intended to be relevant and are intended to produce a particular interpretation by the speaker. The hearer interprets the intended meaning with minimum processing effort. So in the following example (from Leinonen & Kerbel, 1999), B's utterance is indirect.

Example 1

    A: Is Mary a good friend?
    B: I know her.

Minimum processing effort in this context means that B's intended meaning is the first interpretation available for the listener in this context. There are many possible meanings of 'I know her' depending on the context in which it is uttered. In uttering 'I know her' in this context, B intends this to mean 'Mary is not a good friend' and expects that A will recover this meaning.

According to the principle of relevance, the hearer recovers the meanings 'I only know Mary slightly' and 'one knows a good friend more than slightly' in this context. The former is arrived at on the basis of the context in which the utterance occurs and the latter on the basis of one's world knowledge. Both meanings are integrated (interact) to produce the meaning intended by B (Mary is not a good friend of mine). The interaction process results in a probable conclusion (implicature); for example, if B says he only knows Mary slightly, and a good friend is someone you know well, then Mary is not a good friend of B. RT suggests that "the more worthwhile the conclusions achieved by processing an input, the more relevant it will be" (Wilson & Sperber, 2004, p. 4). A conclusion is worthwhile if it answers a question that the speaker had in mind (as in the example above), strengthens an assumption already held, or contradicts an assumption held. The example given here shows how the intended meaning of an utterance is arrived at through the interaction of incoming information (i.e. the linguistic expression) with the listener's existing knowledge or other contextually available information, and via this interaction the relevance of the utterance is arrived at and understood as intended.

Understanding indirect meaning in this way is cognitively effortful. RT suggests that recovering an implicature (the probable conclusion resulting from the processing of contextual information) is a more sophisticated ability than inferring semantic meaning or inferring a referent. Although understanding semantic meaning requires inferencing within context, it does not require the generation of implicatures.

The meaning of 'worked' in Example 2 depends on the context in which it is uttered and has to be inferred from the context.

Example 2

   Teacher: Well done everybody, you worked hard today.

If uttered by an aerobics teacher at the end of a class, 'worked' is correctly interpreted as 'exercised,' whereas in other contexts, for example when spoken by a school teacher, it would be intended to mean school work of some kind. Language is often underdetermined and context can be said to determine successful interpretation. Sperber (1994) suggests that all typically developing children are able to infer meaning and that language development is characterized by children's increasing ability to use context and integrate relevant information in the interpretation of intended meaning. RT's model of pragmatic processing can provide a way of investigating how context is utilized in interpretation and lends itself to studying the development of children's ability to comprehend contextual meaning.

   In clinical populations, research focuses on the impairment of language skills, which can include reduced ability to draw correct inferences or correctly integrate information in order to understand meaning. RT argues that meaning is dependent on context. Meanings of words may be enriched on the basis of context and constrained by the principle of relevance. RT suggests that concepts (the meaning of words) include encyclopedic, logical and lexical addresses which are accessed on attending to the utterance. The conceptual address of a word such as 'work' is treated merely as a point of access to an ordered array of encyclopedic information from which the hearer selects in order to construct a satisfactory interpretation. The hearer follows a path of least effort in selecting the relevant meaning and stops when their expectations of relevance are satisfied. That is, the principle of relevance prevents all possible meanings being considered (as in Example 2 above), but rather the context triggers expectations and the first interpretation meeting those expectations is selected.

   Sperber and Wilson (1995) suggest that the ability to successfully engage in communicative dialogue requires levels of 'mind-reading' ability (first-order, second-order, third-order, and so on). First-order mind reading ability is a metarepresentational ability facilitating recognition of the speaker's informative intention (awareness that she or he intends to inform you of something). Second-order mind-reading ability, the ability to represent the mental states of others, is necessary for successful interpretation of metaphor, irony, sarcasm, and some humor. That is, the hearer is aware of the speaker's intent to communicate something and of the speaker's intention that the hearer will believe what she or he intends her or him to believe. It is suggested that irony and sarcasm require third- and fourth-order abilities (Langdon, Davies, & Coltheart, 2002), whereby the hearer attributes thoughts to the speaker and the speaker's attitude towards them (Papp, 2006).

   Like indirect questions, metaphor, sarcasm and irony cannot be understood from the linguistic form alone, and the intended meaning is not gleaned from interpretation of enriched semantic meaning of the words used. The meaning is interpreted by metarepresentation and by attributing the speaker's attitude to the utterance. For example, a sarcastic comment such as 'Barbecue weather indeed!' is interpreted as relevant because the hearer interprets the speaker's intention to communicate a thought (that the weather is not suitable for cooking outside) and an attitude (derogatory) towards it. Interpreting metaphors is similarly explained. For example, in the utterance below, speaker A refers to a friend known also by the hearer (B).

> A: 'John is an animal.'

Speaker A intends the hearer to interpret this as 'John's behavior is like that of an animal (rather than a human)' in the situation being discussed. The hearer uses the context to interpret the meaning and the utterance achieves most of its relevance by expressing the speaker's attitude towards John's behavior. Metaphor and sarcasm necessitate understanding both what the metaphor is referring to (the behavior of John) and the speaker's intention in using it (to state that John's behavior is like that of an animal rather than human). The attribution of the speaker's attitude towards something is thought to increase processing costs. RT therefore lends itself to providing a framework for investigating the ability of clinical populations to process language expressions which differ in terms of their processing cost.

3.3   Developmental Disorders

Relevance theory has been used to empirically investigate the development of language understanding in normal children (Foster-Cohen, 1994, 1999) including the cognitive processes of pragmatic comprehension (Ryder & Leinonen, 2003), in children with SLI (Leinonen, Ryder, Ellis, & Hammond, 2003), with Asperger syndrome and autism (Loukusa, Leinonen, Kuusikko, et al., 2007) and in investigating the features of autistic communication, including the ability to understand communicative attention and attribute mental states (Happé, 1993, 1995).

Studies of children's language development suggest that early language development (before the age of three years) is centered on concrete events in their world (things they can see, touch or do), after which children develop the ability to understand more abstract events and to think about the intentions of the hearer (pragmatic understanding) and are able to understand meaning in context (Bishop, 1997). Young children utilize contextual cues such as nonverbal signals, facial expressions and the environment in interpreting expressions that are addressed to them. Children's early comprehension is contextually driven, and the developmental process can be seen to involve an increasing ability to utilize language in the comprehension process (pragmatic understanding). Children with developmental language disorders often have difficulties in understanding and/or using words in context, whether written or spoken. Other characteristics may also be present, such as using words (and their meanings) inappropriately and difficulty in comprehension (they may hear a word and not understand its meaning), and an inability to express ideas. These children are developing typically with the exception of their language abilities, which results in difficulties in communicating. The grammatical difficulties of children with language impairment have been researched extensively, but less is known about their difficulties in understanding intended meaning.

RT suggests that the development of pragmatic comprehension includes the ability to utilize relevant context in assigning referents, enriching semantic meaning and integrating contextual information to recover implicature(s). The recovery of implicatures is argued to involve reasoning whereby the contextual information is integrated to yield a probable conclusion or assumption based on the context. This conclusion is called an implicature. As children become more sophisticated in their use of language, they develop the ability to utilize context and combine information from different sources to interpret intended meaning. In a study of three- to five-year-old children, Ryder and Leinonen (2003) found a developmental trend in the use of context in typically developing children. The three-year-olds were unable to answer questions targeting the recovery of implicatures and the five-year-olds were still developing this ability, but all the children were able to infer referents successfully and enrich semantic meaning. In a further study, age-matched SLI children (mean age eight years) performed similarly to the four-year-olds, suggesting a delayed developmental pattern (Leinonen & Ryder 2003). These findings supported the view of RT that assigning referents and enriching semantic meaning, while they involve inferencing, are less pragmatically complex than generating implicatures which require the integration of context (such as world knowledge and previously constructed meaning from prior context). The questions targeting implicatures were particularly problematic for the SLI children compared to their age-matched peers. That is, the pragmatic demands of the question (based on a storybook methodology) affected the ability of the SLI children to answer correctly, and these children appear delayed in pragmatic language development. Ryder, Leinonen, and Schulz (in press) investigated the effect of context (verbal and pictorial) on the ability of children with SLI and children with pragmatic difficulties to answer pragmatically demanding questions. Children with SLI were found to perform similarly to typically developing five- and six-year-olds when only verbal context was available, but where strong pictorial support was given, the children performed similarly to their age-matched peers (seven-year-olds). As predicted by RT, the performance on questions targeting implicature(s) was found to be significantly poorer in SLI children.

Children with Asperger syndrome (AS) and high-functioning autism (HFA) have also been found to have difficulty with pragmatically demanding questions (requiring implicature(s) to be generated). In a study using a similar methodology to Ryder and Leinonen (2003), Loukusa, Leinonen, Kuusikko, et al. (2007) used questions to target the processes of reference assignment, enrichment and implicature (based on short scenarios) in monolingual Finnish-speaking children with normal language abilities and AS/HFA. The children were found to have difficulties with the most pragmatically demanding questions. In line with developmental trends found in English-speaking typically developing children and children with SLI, the older Finnish-speaking children with AS/HFA in this study (10- to 12-year-olds) performed better than the younger AS/HFA group (seven- to nine-year-olds) when answering the more pragmatically complex questions. The younger group were able to answer some of the questions targeting implicatures, though they were less successful overall than the typically developing seven- to nine-year-old Finnish-speaking children. Results of this study (and the Ryder and Leinonen studies with English-speaking children) suggest that in typically developing children, pragmatic abilities have developed by the age of seven years. In children with SLI and AS/HFA this development appears delayed.

RT makes it possible to derive predictions about the levels of communicative competence in children and adults with either (1) no theory of mind, (2) first-order theory of mind only, or (3) second-order theory of mind abilities (Happé, 1993). These 'mentalizing' abilities (i.e. being able to think about thoughts and attribute mental states) were investigated in individuals with autism and with mild learning disabilities (Happé, 1995). The ability to understand figurative language (sarcasm, metaphor, irony) develops gradually in typically developing children from around the age of five upwards (Laval & Bert-Erboul, 2005). Three-year-old children (English and French) were found to be unable to understand sarcasm or metaphors as were children and adults with autism. This difficulty in individuals with autism is linked to their inability to understand the intentions of others in communicative situations. As RT predicts that figurative language such as similes requires less processing than metaphor, and metaphor less than irony (because of the attribution of mental states), Happé (1993, 1995) investigated figurative language in individuals with autism. The participants with autism (aged 9–28 years) were grouped according to their ability on theory-of-mind tasks and then answered questions targeting similes, metaphors, and irony. The control subjects (aged 12–38 years) had mild learning disabilities. Findings supported RT's predictions about the increasing levels of representation necessary for understanding simile, metaphor, and irony, and suggested that the ability to understand the intentions of others (i.e. theory of mind) was directly associated with the comprehension of pragmatically demanding figurative language (Happé, 1993). There were also underlying differences in the mentalizing abilities of the groups with autism, which mediated false-belief performance and utterance comprehension (Happé, 1995).

3.4   Acquired Disorders

There have been many studies suggesting that damage to the right hemisphere results in pragmatic language difficulties. These difficulties include an inability to understand non-literal language (e.g. metaphor, sarcasm, and humor), an inability to utilize context effectively (including an inability to judge whether facts are plausible given a specific context), and an inability to make inferences (Bihrle, Brownell, Powelson, & Gardner, 1986; Brownell, Michel, Powelson, & Gardner, 1983; Gardner, Brownell, Wapner, & Michelow, 1983; Roman, Brownell, Potter, Seibold, & Gardner, 1987; Wapner, Hamby, & Gardner, 1981; Winner & Gardner, 1977).

Dipper, Bryan, and Tyson (1997) investigated the pragmatic difficulties of individuals with right hemisphere damage (RHD) using RT. The participants were six stroke patients aged 31–74 years with unilateral right-hemisphere damage following a single neurological episode, and twelve age-matched controls. They noted that when answering questions based on a story, the patients with RHD did not use the context of the story in their answers, but were able to justify their answers. The justifications revealed that the RHD participants did not appear to be aware of the contextual information but were relying on world knowledge to generate semantically related inferences rather than utilizing the context given in the story. Dipper et al. proposed RT as a way of investigating the reasons for their answers.

RT's model of language comprehension suggests that a deductive system operates on linguistic input, and concepts consist of addresses in memory which give rise to logical, encyclopedic and lexical information. Participants in Dipper et al.'s study listened and read two sentence scenarios and answered three question types targeting three types of bridging inference. The first (textual inference) required utilizing linguistic input in order to answer correctly. The second (textually reinforced inference) targeted information derived from discourse connectives which generate the context and inference, without accessing encyclopedic information (RT suggests discourse connectives are procedural and do not have encyclopedic entries). The third inference was encyclopedic, that is, where a correct answer required access to knowledge, for example that peeling onions can make your eyes water.

Dipper et al. (1997, p. 227) found that RHD participants performed less well than controls on all inference types and that there was not one inference type which was 'easier' for both groups. The clinical group was found to rely on encyclopedic information; questions targeting linguistic deduction were problematic for this group, particularly discourse connectives. If RT's account of the procedural and non-encyclopedic nature of discourse connective concepts is correct, then, as Dipper et al. suggest, the brain damage suffered by RHD patients affects the logical deductive device, and the use of linguistic context to infer intended meaning is therefore affected.

RT has also been used to investigate the process of inferencing when interpreting sarcasm in clinical populations (McDonald, 1999). RT suggests that the most relevant and least effortful interpretation possible in a given context is inferred along with recognition of the speaker's attitude. The comprehension of sarcasm draws on linguistic and contextual features in the same way as other linguistic expression but, additionally, sarcastic comments echo a prior proposition (shared knowledge), and this echoing communicates the speaker's derogatory attitude. The contextual information relevant to the interpretation of sarcasm often includes tone of voice, facial expression, and in some studies recognising the relationship between speakers (McDonald 2000). McDonald's (1999) review of studies of sarcasm comprehension (in normal and clinical populations) suggests that patients with traumatic brain injury (TBI) generally had difficulty in inferential reasoning, and the differences in successful interpretation of sarcasm were found to be related to the different types of contextual information which had to be processed. McDonald (2000) notes that TBI populations are heterogeneous and that there is evidence that some TBI patients have difficulties with non-verbal context (intonation, gesture) and in recognizing the relationship between speakers, which impedes their ability to understand sarcasm.

Patients with RH brain damage were also found to have difficulties in interpreting counterfactual comments (sarcastic) when the contradiction was verbal rather than physical contextual information (i.e., recognizing the contradiction depended on interpreting the verbal contradiction rather than an action). McDonald (1999) argues that these patients understand the literal meaning of the comment and are therefore able to recognise the scornful echo (as proposed by RT), but this is not sufficient to understand the sarcastic intent. RH patients appeared to attribute a perception of the literal interpretation to the listener. Therefore McDonald suggests that the conversational inferences are essential for the understanding of sarcasm.

McDonald (1999) notes that the way in which questions target the understanding of sarcasm differs in research in this area. Some target the speaker's intention or attitude when replying to a sarcastic remark, others target whether the speaker intended the meaning of his utterance to be understood literally, and some target counterfactual meaning (i.e. they ask if the speaker meant the opposite of what was uttered). TBI patients improved their success rate when the number of inferences made about the speakers was reduced. That is, questions asking whether the speaker uttering a sarcastic remark intended the utterance to be taken literally were answered correctly more often than questions asking if the speaker responding to the sarcasm meant the opposite to what was said (e.g. whether the speaker of 'Sorry I made you come' was pleased that he made his addressee come). This suggests that inferences about both the facts of the situation and the mental state of the speaker (attitudes, knowledge, and intentions) are important for comprehending sarcasm. RT's notion of attitudinal cues in sarcasm was considered to be well founded, though McDonald questions the suggestion that the echoic interpretation is involved. The generation of inferences regarding mental state may be crucial for some interpretations of sarcasm and this appears to be a difficulty in individuals with TBI. There is also the possibility that the number of inferences necessary (or the integration of information) is implicated.

3.5   Conclusions

Studies of language disorders using Relevance Theory have validated the predictions of pragmatic complexity made by RT. They have shown, for instance, that predicted level of complexity of pragmatic processing is related to order of development. Furthermore, it has been shown that instances of pragmatic breakdown can be predicted and explained by the theory. These support the psychological validity of the theory itself and its consequent usefulness for exploring and understanding both development and disorders.

The theory also places responsibility for conversational success and failure squarely on the shoulders of all parties involved. Studies using this framework have demonstrated this in contexts where one of the participants has difficulty with pragmatic processing and how others can compensate for or, unfortunately, compound the ensuing conversational difficulties. These observations have important implications for the type of therapy that is used with individuals with pragmatic difficulties. Therapy which encourages the understanding of how context is utilized in comprehension may be valuable.

Working within a theoretical framework enables one to make testable predictions about the nature of language disorders and the kinds of behaviors that children and adults with impaired language production and comprehension are likely to exhibit. We have found that working with RT has enabled us to move from description of surface behaviors to a deeper understanding of why pragmatic language difficulties may come about and why they have the impact that they do on the quality of conversational interactions. We have also been able to make progress in suggesting useful ways of facilitating interactions with pragmatically impaired individuals both within and outside therapeutic contexts.

REFERENCES

Bihrle, A. M., Brownell, H. H., Powelson, J. A., and Gardner, H. (1986). Comprehension of humorous and nonhumorous materials by left and right brain-damaged patients. *Brain and Cognition*, 5, 399–411.

Bishop, D. V. M. (1997). *Uncommon Understanding: Development and Disorders of Language Comprehension in Children*. Hove, Sussex: Psychology Press.

Brownell, H. H., Michel, D., Powelson, J., and Gardner, H. (1983). Surprise but no coherence: Sensitivity to verbal humor in right-hemisphere patients. *Brain and Language*, 18, 20–7.

Dipper, L. T., Bryan, K. L., and Tyson, J. (1997). Bridging inference and relevance theory: An account of right hemisphere inference. *Clinical Linguistics and Phonetics*, 11(3), 213–28.

Foster-Cohen, S. (1994). Exploring the boundary between syntax and pragmatics: relevance and the binding of pronouns. *Journal of Child Language*, 21, 237–55.

Foster-Cohen, S. (1999). A relevance-theoretic account of children's referential communi-
nication skills: Arguments for continuity of pragmatic processing. Paper presented
to the Child Language Seminar, City University, London, September.

Gardner, H., Brownell, H. H., Wapner, W., and Michelow, D. (1983). Missing the
point: The role of the right hemisphere in the processing of complex linguistic
materials. In E. Perecman (ed.), *Cognitive Processing in the Right Hemisphere*. New
York: Academic Press.

Happé, F. G. E. (1993). Communicative competence and theory of mind in autism: A
test of relevance theory. *Cognition*, 48(2), 101–19.

Happé, F. G. E. (1995). Understanding minds and metaphors: Insights from the study
of figurative language in autism. *Metaphor and Symbol*, 10(4), 275–95.

Langdon, R., Davies, M., and Coltheart, M. (2002). Understanding minds and understanding communicated meanings in schizophrenia. *Mind and Language*, 17(1), 68–104.

Laval, V. and Bert-Erboul, A. (2005). French-speaking children's understanding of
sarcasm: The role of intonation and context. *Journal of Speech, Language, and Hearing
Research*, 48, 610–20.

Leinonen, E. and Kerbel, D. (1999). Relevance theory and pragmatic impairment. *International Journal of Language and Communication Disorder*, 34(4), 367–90.

Leinonen, E., Ryder, N., Ellis, M., and Hammond, C. (2003). The use of context in
pragmatic comprehension by specifically language impaired and control children.
Linguistics, 41(2), 407–23.

Loukusa, S., Leinonen, E., Kuusikko, S., Jussila, K., Mattila, L., Ryder, N., Ebeling, H.,
and Moilanen, I. (2007). Use of context in pragmatic language comprehension by
children with Asperger syndrome or high-functioning autism. *Journal of Autism
and Developmental Disorders*, 37(6), 1049–59.

McDonald, S. (1999). Exploring the process of inference generation in sarcasm: A
review of normal and clinical studies. *Brain and Language*, 68, 486–506.

McDonald, S. (2000). Putting communication disorders in context after traumatic brain
injury. *Aphasiology*, 14(4), 339–47.

Milosky, L. M. (1992). Children listening: the role of world knowledge in comprehension. In R. Chapman (ed.), *Processes in Language Acquisition and Disorders*. St. Louis,
MO: Mosby.

Oakhill, J. and Yuill, N. (1986). Pronoun resolution in skilled and less skilled comprehenders: effects of memory load and inferential complexity. *Language and Speech*,
29, 25–36.

Papp, S. (2006). A relevance-theoretic account of the development and deficits of theory
or mind in normally developing children and individuals with autism. *Theory and
Psychology*, 16(2), 141–61.

Roman, M., Brownell, H. H., Potter, H. H., Seibold, M. S., and Gardner, H. (1987). Script
knowledge in right hemisphere-damaged and in normal elderly adults. *Brain and
Language*, 31(1), 151–70.

Ryder, N. and Leinonen, E. (2003). Use of context in question answering by 3, 4 and 5
year old children. *Journal of Psycholinguistic Research*, 32(4), 397–415.

Ryder, N., Leinonen, E., and Schulz, J. (in press). A cognitive approach to assessing
pragmatic language comprehension in children with Specific Language Impairment. *International Journal of Language and Communication Disorders*.

Smith, B. and Leinonen, E. (1992). *Clinical Pragmatics*. London: Chapman and Hall.

Sperber, D. (1994). Understanding verbal understanding. In J. Khalfa (ed.), *What is
Intelligence?* (pp. 179–98). Cambridge: Cambridge University Press.

Sperber, D. and Wilson, D. (1995). *Relevance: Communication and Cognition.* Oxford: Blackwell.

Wapner, W., Hamby, S., and Gardner, H. (1981). The role of the right hemisphere in the apprehension of complex linguistic materials. *Brain and Language,* 14, 15–33.

Winner, E. and Gardner, H. (1977). The comprehension of metaphor in brain-damaged patients. *Brain,* 100, 717–29.

Wilson, D. and Sperber, D. (2004). Relevance theory. In G. Ward and L. Horn (eds.), *Handbook of Pragmatics* (pp. 607–32). Oxford: Blackwell

4 Neuropragmatics

BRIGITTE STEMMER

4.1 Introduction

While the study of pragmatics has a long tradition in philosophy and linguistics, its incorporation into the neuroscience of language is relatively recent. The observation that some patients with damage to the right hemisphere (RHD) do not show any obvious impairments in producing or comprehending words or sentences, but nevertheless exhibit communication problems, led to the incorporation of pragmatic theories into neurolinguistic research (for a summary see Paradis, 1998; Stemmer, 1999b). This research has mainly been concerned with providing detailed descriptive accounts of communicative difficulties, first in patients with RHD, and subsequently in other clinical populations such as in patients with autistic, schizophrenic, or developmental disorders and with dementia. Attempts have been made to investigate and explain the processes leading to such impairments. In doing so, questions naturally evolved regarding the role of the brain in the comprehension and production of pragmatic behavior, along with an interest in the neural substrates of cerebral involvement. This research has become known as neuropragmatics. Traditionally, insights have been gained from studies with patients who have sustained some sort of brain damage and, more recently, from studies of both healthy individuals and patients with brain lesions that use such neuroimaging techniques as PET, fMRI or EEG/ERP.

The studies usually subsumed under neuropragmatics deal with how aspects of communication such as discourse, conversation and figurative language are comprehended and/or produced by individuals with and without brain pathologies. While pragmatic theories are frequently used to provide a description and explanation of communicative behavior, knowledge from neuroscience or other 'neuro' disciplines is drawn upon to explain how aspects of pragmatics are represented or processed in the brain and to gain insights about the neural substrates and networks involved. Although neuropragmatics research involves both healthy and clinical populations, this contribution will focus on the various patterns of neural dysfunction that lead to pragmatic impairment.

4.2   Neuropragmatics and Clinical Populations

Early observations of a dissociation between *language* problems occurring after left-hemisphere damage and *communication* problems after right-hemisphere damage probably contributed strongly to a situation in which the most frequently studied patient population in neuropragmatics is patients with focal lesions in the right hemisphere. We thus discuss this research first and then continue with examples of neuropragmatic impairment in other clinical populations.

4.2.1   *Pragmatic impairment in right-hemisphere damaged (RHD) individuals*

Ample evidence has accumulated that in right handed people damage in the left (and not right) hemisphere may lead to various forms of aphasia, and it is usually assumed that damage to the right hemisphere can lead to pragmatic impairment. RHD patients are often described as behaving conversationally oddly or inappropriately in social situations despite intact linguistic abilities. Their conversational style has been described as embellishing, rambling, tangential, non-informative, irrelevant, repetitive, confabulatory, and literal. They jump from topic to topic and leave the listener with gaps of information; they miss the overall point of a conversation and have difficulties maintaining the theme of a conversation. There is a large literature describing the effects of RHD on the comprehension and production of discourse. One aspect of this literature is concerned with the difficulties RHD patients have in producing, comprehending, or interpreting appropriately 'non-literal', 'indirect' or figurative language such as indirect requests, metaphor, proverbs, sarcasm and irony, idioms, or some types of humor (for reviews see Brownell, Carroll, Rehak, & Wingfield, 1992; Brownell & Stringfellow, 1999; Joanette & Brownell, 1990; Shammi & Stuss, 1999; Stemmer, 1994; Stemmer, Giroux, & Joanette, 1994; Tompkins, 1990).

4.2.1.1   *Indirect speech acts*
The difficulties that RHD patients have with indirectness and non-literalness have been key features in many neuropsychological studies. The underlying assumption usually is that 'indirect' and 'non-literal' language is more 'abstract' and requires more complex or different inferencing processes, and more processing efforts, than 'literal' or 'direct' language. For example, uttering or comprehending a request such as 'Are you here by car?' (meaning 'Give me a lift home') underlies a complex interplay between social, situational, interpersonal and

cognitive variables – although such a request is part of our daily routine. We usually do not spend much time thinking about how to phrase the request or interpret it. Consider the request 'Could you please pass the bread?' Although the wording of this utterance might be interpreted as a question as to whether or not you are indeed able to physically pass the bread, primary pragmatic knowledge (Gibbs, 1999) or high saliency (Giora, 2003) leads us to interpret the utterance as a request to pass the bread. In early studies, it was claimed that RHD patients had problems understanding such indirect requests (Foldi, 1987; Hirst, LeDoux, & Stein, 1984; Weylman, Brownell, Roman, & Gardner, 1989). There is, however, nothing either particularly indirect or abstract about this utterance; there are likewise no reasons to believe that its comprehension demands complex processes of inference or particular processing efforts. Also utterances such as, 'I have no idea how to get home', where the wording of the utterance may suggest several meanings, are readily understood as 'Please give me a lift home' as secondary pragmatic knowledge leads to the intended meaning (Gibbs, 1999). Later studies on requests, using other designs and better-defined theoretical frameworks, only partially supported the findings of earlier studies. In particular, it was shown that RHD patients were quite able to understand and produce a whole range of types of direct and indirect requests. However, a rather reduced and, at times, inappropriate use and evaluation of explanatory material was observed. Pragmatic knowledge *per se* seemed to be preserved but there was a lack of ability to establish a relationship between request types (non-conventional indirect requests) involving primarily secondary pragmatic knowledge and the supporting material (Brownell & Stringfellow, 1999; Stemmer, Giroux, & Joanette, 1994). Another study investigating basic speech acts (among them requests) reported left-hemisphere damaged (LHD) patients and RHD patients to be impaired compared to healthy controls, with LHD showing poorer performance than the RHD patients (Soroker, Kasher, Giora, Batori, Corn, Gil, & Zaidel, 2005). These findings are difficult to reconcile with previous research. One explanation is that structural and functional aspects of language seem to have been confounded in the stimuli used. It cannot be excluded that the LHD patients performed more poorly because of more demanding structural language aspects and that the RHD patients did not show problems because the speech acts were of the conventional or salient type. The authors also tried to assign each basic speech act to a distinct pattern of localization. Such assignments seem somewhat premature, however, considering the heterogeneity of both the patient population and the details of the lesions shown in the CT scans.

Indirect requests have also been investigated in traumatic brain injury (TBI) patients who showed preserved sensitivity to various social factors but had difficulties in formulating non-conventional indirect requests (McDonald & van Sommers, 1993), or in producing non-conventional requests that would overcome listener reluctance (McDonald & Pearce, 1998). The TBI patients investigated in these studies were extremely heterogeneous with respect to the nature of their brain damage and thus no claims were made concerning underlying neural substrates possibly implicated in the pragmatic impairments described. In one study, all patients were impaired in their ability to perform executive functions. There is thus some indication that impaired reasoning abilities may have influenced pragmatic performance.

4.2.1.2   *Irony, sarcasm, lies and jokes*

Other types of figurative language such as irony, sarcasm, lies or jokes have also been investigated in RHD patients. Similar to non-conventional indirect requests, these types of figurative language imply complex metarepresentational abilities (Gibbs, 1999; Sperber, 2000). RHD patients have been found to be impaired in their ability to reply to inferential questions concerning sarcastic final comments with regard to a narrative, despite an intact ability to infer attitudinal and emotional information about the speakers. Difficulties have also been observed with the interpretation of counterfactual comments at the end of a story (Kaplan, Brownell, Jacobs, & Gardner, 1990; Tompkins & Mateer, 1985). RHD patients have also demonstrated problems using contextual information to guide interpretations of sarcastic, humorous or deceitful utterances. Similar difficulties have been observed in autistic children, however, and thus these observations in RHD patients were not taken as evidence that the deficits were specific to right-hemisphere pathology (Kaplan, Brownell, Jacobs, & Gardner, 1990).

Some RHD patients have been observed to be impaired in tasks involving second-order metarepresentational judgments involving lies and ironic joke stories (Winner, Brownell, Happé, Blum, & Pincus, 1998). Although it seemed that the right hemisphere might be involved in second-order metarepresentational processes, as expressed in the theory of mind, inasmuch as not all RHD subjects showed a poor performance and a few control subjects performed poorly on this task, it was suggested that the underlying impairment may not be restricted to right-hemisphere pathology. Aside from RHD patients, TBI patients and autistic children have also demonstrated difficulties interpreting sarcastic remarks (for a summary see McDonald, 1999).

Arriving at metarepresentational judgments involves making inferences at various levels of complexity, just as does interpreting various types of figurative language, such as sarcasm. It is thus not surprising that a relationship between impaired executive functions and a diminished ability to interpret sarcasm in patients with frontal lobe lesions has been observed by McDonald and Pearce (1996). Executive functions are often conceptualized as the central executive of the information-processing system and encompass the control of attention, goal setting (initiating, planning, problem solving, strategic behavior) and cognitive flexibility (attention shifting, working memory, self-monitoring, self-regulation) (Fuster, 2002; Stuss & Alexander, 2000). It can easily be seen that some, if not all, of these components are necessary for drawing complex inferences and for tasks involving integration.

RHD and LHD patients have been compared with respect to their abilities to comprehend jokes and cartoons. Similarly to the comprehension of non-conventional indirect requests or ironic and sarcastic remarks, context, knowledge and experience guide joke and cartoon comprehension, and the listener must be able to revise or update his or her assumptions made during the comprehension process. Apprehension, unexpectedness, surprise and appreciation are all elements involved in cartoon and joke comprehension. Compared to LHD, RHD patients were unable to use new information to arrive at a revised interpretation of the humorous discourse (Bihrle, Brownell, Powelson, & Gardner, 1986; Brownell & Gardner, 1988; Brownell, Michel, Powelson, & Gardner, 1983). While they were sensitive to the surprise element of the joke or cartoon, they were unable to establish appropriate coherence with the previous discourse. LHD patients also did not arrive at the correct joke or cartoon interpretation but, unlike RHD patients, they were able to maintain coherence between the critical utterance and the opening text body. Another study investigated the role of specific cognitive processes in humor appreciation and the underlying neural networks (Shammi & Stuss, 1999). Impairment of aspects in the humor task was found in two patients with right frontal damage, and in one patient with left frontal and three patients with bilateral frontal lesions (Shammi & Stuss, 1999, p. 659). The authors' conclusion that the ability to appreciate humor was related to the anterior portion of the right frontal lobe needs to be viewed with caution considering the few subjects who showed the impairment pattern. Similarly to McDonald and colleagues in their studies of sarcasm, Shammi and Stuss reported a relationship between executive functions (working memory, mental shifting, verbal abstraction) and humor appreciation for all frontal-lobe-damaged patients.

4.2.1.3 *Emotions and verbal communication*

Studies investigating the impact of emotional content on verbal communication have suggested that emotional context may suppress pragmatic performance in RHD but facilitate pragmatic performance in LHD (Bloom, Borod, Obler, & Gerstman, 1993). In a comparison of RHD, LHD and healthy controls in a picture story test that elicited emotional, visuospatial or procedural/ neutral content, LHD patients were found to be more impaired than RHD on a total pragmatic feature score and RHD more impaired with respect to the emotional content story. Another study found that positive emotional content induced poorer performance in RHD patients while negative emotional content influenced the processing of information in LHD patients (Borod, Rorie, Pick, et al., 2000).

Generally, lesion studies have thus shown that some aspects of figurative language comprehension and/or production are impaired in RHD and TBI patients. It remains unclear to what extent the right hemisphere is involved in the pragmatics-associated difficulties of the TBI patients. Lesion studies indicate that the right hemisphere, and possibly the right frontal lobe, are involved in humor processing. However, some studies also indicate an involvement of the left hemisphere. It is conceivable that each hemisphere contributes different aspects to specific facets of figurative language and humor processing, and to various degrees.

4.2.2   *Pragmatic abilities in other patient populations*

Although pragmatic abilities have been investigated most often in RHD patients, pragmatic impairments have also been observed in other patient populations. It should be noted that the observation of similar pragmatic impairments in different patient populations does not necessarily mean that the reasons for the impairment are the same: nor do identical lesions always lead to the same pragmatic impairments.

4.2.2.1   *Aphasia*

Aphasia is most frequently provoked by a lesion to the left hemisphere. Studying pragmatic abilities in these patients can be challenging due to their language impairment, and frequently no clear conclusion can be drawn as to whether the impairment is linguistically based or of a pragmatic nature. Good command of pragmatic abilities and functions has been described in a patient with severe Broca's aphasia. Frequent discourse initiation and topic change and a reduced query production were ascribed to the linguistic impairment in this patient (Dronkers, Ludy, & Redfern, 1998). Similarly, linguistic impairment seems to have influenced the performance of patients with fluent aphasia whose discourse was less informative than that of non-brain-damaged adults (Chapman, Highley, & Thompson, 1998). However, these patients' ability to draw inferences between textual content and real-world knowledge was intact. Other problems that have been described include inappropriate pause times during turn-taking in discourse, a reduced variety in the use of types of speech acts, and less specificity and accuracy of the message (Borod, Rorie, Pick, et al., 2000; Kasher, Batori, Soroker, Graves, & Zaidel, 1999; Kee, Green, Gizer, Laack, & Zaidel, 2000; Prutting & Kirchner, 1987; for a summary see Wright & Newhoff, 2005).

Generally, some pragmatic abilities seem to be intact in aphasic patients, and those abilities that have been found to be impaired may be related to the linguistic impairments. There is, however, the possibility that cognitive impairment – for instance in working memory – is implicated (Caplan & Waters, 2002). This possibility has rarely been investigated in these patients. Research further suggests that the type of aphasia influences pragmatic abilities. There is currently no clear evidence to suggest that the pragmatic weaknesses described in aphasic patients are independent of their language problem or other cognitive problems.

4.2.2.2   *Dementia*

Comparing linguistic and pragmatic abilities in fluent aphasics of mild severity with patients with Alzheimer's disease (AD) in the early stages showed that the AD patients as a group (but not every individual patient) exhibited prominent difficulties in drawing inferences in a fable retell task, a picture generation story task, a task in which the central meaning had to be abstracted, and a task in which the didactic meaning had to be derived in the form of a lesson

(Chapman, Highley, & Thompson, 1998). These disturbances were independent of linguistic formulation difficulties in these patients. As possible causes for the impairments, the authors discuss memory problems, not attending to the most salient aspects of the task, and affliction of the right hemisphere in the disease process.

Traumatic brain injury (TBI). TBI patients have been shown to be impaired in formulating non-conventional requests despite appropriate sensitivity to various social factors, and in the appropriate use of politeness markers in telephone conversations (McDonald & van Sommers, 1993; Togher & Hand, 1998). A detailed single case study with a TBI patient demonstrated that a range of cognitive deficits (attention, executive functions, impulse control) can lead to inappropriate pragmatic language use (Body, Perkins, & McDonald, 1999).

4.2.2.3   Williams syndrome
This genetic syndrome is characterized by relatively spared language in the context of general cognitive impairment and hyper-sociability. A comparison of children and adolescents with Williams syndrome (WS) with those with Down syndrome (DS) patients and healthy controls while telling a story based on pictures found that the WS patients produced more social evaluations during story telling than the control and DS individuals. Compared to healthy controls, both WS and DS demonstrated difficulties with the story structure (canonic schema) and with maintaining the theme of a story (Bernicot, Lacrois, & Reilly, 2003).

4.2.2.4   Schizophrenia
A number of researchers have ascribed the communicational oddities in patients with schizophrenia to the area of pragmatics. The described abnormalities include a failure to structure discourse at higher levels, to adhere to a topic, and to distinguish relevant from non-relevant content topic maintenance, and those abilities evaluated by the pragmatic protocol (Prutting & Kirchner, 1987) (for a summary see Meilijson, Kasher, & Elizur, 2004). Schizophrenic patients have also shown problems with understanding false-belief stories and non-literal language (metaphors and irony) (Langdon, Coltheart, Ward, & Catts, 2002). There is some indication that schizophrenic patients may be grouped according to their patterns of pragmatic impairments. Meilijson, Kasher, and Elizur (2004) identified two schizophrenic patient groups who demonstrated problems in speech act, turn-taking and lexical and non-verbal performance, and one group that was mostly impaired in lexical performance.

4.3   Explaining Pragmatic Impairments in RHD Patients

Numerous explanations have been advanced to explain the pragmatic difficulties identified in RHD patients. Most generally, they can be summarized as the inferencing hypothesis, the theory of mind hypothesis, and the mental model hypothesis (for a summary and discussion see Martin & McDonald, 2003; Stemmer & Cohen, 2002; note that these authors use a different terminology). The inferencing hypothesis suggests that the communicative impairments observed are due to difficulties generating inferences (Beeman, 1993; Bisset & Novak, 1995; Brownell & Martino, 1998; Brownell, Potter, Bihrle, & Gardner, 1986; McDonald & Wales, 1986; Moya, Benowitz, Levine, & Finkelstein, 1986; Read, 1981; Rehak, Kaplan, Weylman, et al., 1992; Tompkins, Lehman, & Baumgaertner, 1999; Wapner, Hamby, & Gardner, 1981). Controversies in the interpretation of research findings concerning the ability to comprehend or generate inferences have been explained by the lack of a proper definition of inferencing, a neglect in distinguishing between different types of inferencing and a lack of consideration of inference generation models (Frederiksen & Stemmer, 1993; Lehman & Tompkins, 2000; Stemmer & Joanette, 1998).

The theory of mind hypothesis refers to the ability of a person to form representations of other people's mental states (such as hopes, beliefs, beliefs about beliefs, moods, desires, intentions) and to employ such representations to interpret, predict, and judge utterances and behavior. The theory of mind hypothesis is thus closely related to the inferencing hypothesis in that it refers to the ability to make inferences about other people's mental states. It is typically tested with tasks that assess the subject's ability to infer that someone can have a mistaken belief that is different from her or his own true belief (first-order false beliefs). It is assumed that this situation requires an understanding of the other's mental state. Second-order false belief tasks assess the ability to understand what someone else thinks about what another person thinks.

Several authors have investigated whether the communicative difficulties of RHD patients are due to a compromised theory of mind. Compared to LHD, RHD patients made more errors in responses to false belief questions if the false belief question was ambiguous (Siegal, Carrington, & Radel, 1996). No difference between the patient groups were found when the false belief question was unambiguous. Interpretation of the study is compromised by the small amount of information provided on the functional abilities of the patients investigated. Further, both patient groups were extremely heterogeneous in terms of lesion site, time post-onset and education. It has also been suggested that RHD patients' difficulties with distinguishing lies from jokes was related to difficulties in inferring second-order mental states (Winner, Brownell, Happé, Blum, & Pincus, 1998). The authors concluded that although the right hemisphere clearly seems to be implicated in the theory of mind, the frontal lobes and possibly the prefrontal region may also be involved in the conceptualization of mental events. This is further supported by the observation that some of the non-brain-damaged control subjects also performed poorly on the second-order belief tasks.

The assumption that successful performance on theory of mind tasks is non-specific in relation to right-hemisphere involvement is supported by Stone, Baron-Cohen, and Knight's (1998) study on frontal lobe contributions to the theory of mind. These authors investigated the ability of patients with bilateral orbito-frontal lesions and patients with left dorsolateral frontal lesions using first- and second-order theory of mind tasks and a *faux pas* task. No theory of mind effect as tested with the first- and second-order belief tasks was found in the bilateral orbito-frontal lesioned patients or in the left dorsolateral frontal lesioned patients. The latter group showed a working memory effect. In the *faux pas* task, most of the bilateral orbito-frontal lesioned patients (but not the dorsolateral frontal patients) failed to recognize the *faux pas* although they were quite able to make appropriate empathic inferences about what the characters in the stories would have felt. The authors concluded that the empathic understanding of what another person would find upsetting was intact in the orbito-frontal lesioned patients, and they ascribed the *faux pas* errors to problems connecting the theory of mind inferences with an understanding of emotion. They further concluded that the orbito-frontal cortex is part of the circuit involved in theory of mind tasks. As these authors tested bilateral orbito-frontal and left dorsolateral frontal lesioned patients the involvement of the right hemisphere remains unclear. In an attempt to elucidate the contribution of various prefrontal regions to theory of mind tasks, Stuss and colleagues (Stuss, Gallup, & Alexander, 2001) investigated patients with frontal (right, left, bilateral) lesions and compared them with non-frontal lesion patients and healthy controls. They used a simple 'direct inference' task, a more complex 'transfer inference' task and a deception task in which the subject had to infer that someone was trying to deceive them. For the deception task bifrontal lesions were related to impaired performance on the deception task. There was less specificity of lesion location within the frontal lobe for the transfer inference task with some tentative suggestion for a greater involvement of the right frontal region.

The mental model hypothesis (Frederiksen & Stemmer, 1993; Stemmer, Giroux, & Joanette, 1994; Stemmer & Joanette, 1998) is based on Johnson-Laird's (1983, 1989) concept of a mental model. Mental models are dynamic symbolic representations of how we perceive and represent the world. From external events and internal experiences people construct and employ mental models in order to understand, explain, and predict phenomena of the environment, and to act accordingly (for a summary see Stemmer & Cohen, 2002). Note that aspects of the theory of mind are encompassed in the mental model approach. A main concern of the theory of mental model is to explain higher cognitive processes such as comprehension, drawing inferences, and intention in communication and action. Investigating single cases and using a mental model approach, it was suggested that RHD patients had no problems drawing inferences *per se* and no problems with manipulating mental representations that involved only one mental model. Instead, those processes seemed to be impaired that constructed mental representations which required the manipulation of more than one conceptual model to arrive at a new conceptual model (Frederiksen & Stemmer, 1993; Stemmer & Joanette, 1998; Stemmer, Giroux, & Joanette, 1994). LHD patients did not show these problems.

4.4   Cognitive Functions and Aspects of Pragmatics

Previously, we have discussed various pathologies that affect pragmatic performance. With these pathologies it is more the rule than the exception that they are accompanied by (not always obvious or easily measured) cognitive impairments, and the question is to what extent these impairments influence pragmatic performance (for a discussion see Body, Perkins & McDonald, 1999; Brownell & Friedman, 2001; McDonald, 1999; McDonald, 2000; Stemmer, 1999a; Stemmer & Cohen, 2002). Many studies have not addressed these issues and those that did have not always been conclusive. The relationship between working memory (WM) (using a sentence span task) and discourse comprehension was studied in RHD, LHD patients and healthy controls by Tompkins, Bloise, Timko, and Baumgaertner (1994). A strong correlation was reported between WM and one aspect of inferencing that required the subject to interpret a final utterance in a discourse that contradicted the speaker's attitude. The LHD patients performed worse than controls on this inference task but no reliable correlation between WM and performance on the tasks were found. Another study found a correlation between working memory (using the reading span task) and reading comprehension performance in LHD aphasic patients (Caspari, Parkinson, LaPointe, & Katz, 1998). A reason for these controversial findings may be subtle differences in the implicated lesioned network(s) (see section 4.5 below for a discussion).

More studies have investigated the relationship between executive functions and pragmatic performance. There is some indication that a loss of inhibition may influence request performance in TBI patients, and impaired executive functions and poor sarcasm interpretation were found to be correlated in patients with frontal lobe lesions (McDonald & Pearce, 1996, 1998). A relationship between facets of executive functions (perseveration errors) as measured by the Wisconsin Card Sorting Test (WCST) and incomplete story episode description in TBI patients was also reported by Coelho, Liles, and Duffy (1995). In a single case study of a TBI patient, Body, Perkins, and McDonald (1999) reported impairment in verbal abilities, all facets of attention, verbal learning and memory, perception, problem solving, impulsiveness and perseveration – that is, impairments frequently observed in patients with frontal lobe lesions. From a pragmatic perspective, the patient demonstrated impaired conversational interaction by not taking sufficient account of the interlocutor's perspective. No detailed lesion analysis is provided but the left temporoparietal region seemed to have been involved.

It is reasonable to assume that the neural substrates underlying arousal, attention, perception, emotion, memory, learning, or cognitive control directly or indirectly influence aspects of pragmatic processing. Many studies investigating RHD patients and patients with other brain pathologies did not include extensive or subtle neuropsychological testing, and the findings reported by

those who did vary widely or are inconclusive. Investigating request performance in TBI patients, McDonald and Pearce (1998) did not find a relationship
to facets of executive dysfunction. They did, however, demonstrate that a loss
of inhibition influenced the capacity to take mental states into account when
producing requests. It may be that the tests used to explore facets of executive
functions either were not sensitive enough, involved facets of executive functions different from those tested in other studies, or used the notions of executive functions and control mechanisms in a somewhat unusual way. In another
study McDonald (2000) examined the influence of an impaired executive system
or an impaired system for visuospatial mental constructions and synthesis on
pragmatic performance in RHD patients. The author reported that visuospatial
but not executive function was related to pragmatic performance. Unfortunately,
the interpretation of the results is rather limited in this study due to the
heterogeneous patient group (four right subcortical lesions, two right parietal/
occipital lesions, two bilateral lesions, five mixed right fronto/temporal/pari-
etal lesions, one no imaging available and one without CT pathology), a failure
to account statistically for this diverse patient group and the rather limited
testing for executive impairment. With regard to the relationship between
facets of attention or memory and pragmatic performance, there are only a few
studies that allude to a possible relationship and there are no studies primarily
investigating these issues. The situation is aggravated by the fact that standard
neuropsychological testing may not reveal impairments although most brain-
damaged individuals are impaired to some degree in their mental capacities
(see e.g. Stuss, Alexander, Floden, et al., 2002; Stuss & Levine, 2002).

4.5   Pragmatic Behavior and the Brain

Despite numerous studies aimed at investigating pragmatic abilities in various
pathological populations, no clear picture has emerged concerning the neural
substrates and networks involved. The researcher investigating pragmatic
abilities in brain-damaged populations is faced with several non-trivial challenges. First, there is the heterogeneity of the patients; age, level of education,
severity of functional impairment (at all kinds of levels), extent of structural
impairment, and time of testing post-onset should all be considered. Second,
a choice has to be made concerning the theoretical framework and model of
analysis the research is based on. Third, the construction of the stimuli needs
to satisfy the theoretical framework, and, at the same time, be applicable to the
patients with or despite their individual functional impairments. These constraints certainly add to the frequently found discrepancy of findings among
various studies. In addition, many studies lack a precise lesion analysis with
neuroimaging techniques, which, naturally, was not available for early studies.
With today's advanced technology, we are now in a position to provide better
lesion descriptions, base our research on more advanced pragmatic theories
and models and integrate a variety of cognitive measures that have been

related to specific brain functions. Another consideration has to do with the perspective one has of pragmatic performance and with the elements of which such performance consists. It seems unlikely that these diverse elements comprise a cohesive entity with a specific localized topological representation in the brain. Pragmatically appropriate communicative behavior depends on complex interplays of linguistic, emotional, cognitive, and regulatory mechanisms (see, for example, Perkins, chapter 5 in this volume). Just as different organic disease processes can produce similar symptoms and similar symptoms can reflect different organic etiologies, different cognitive disease processes can also produce similar pragmatic impairments and vice versa. It thus seems that knowledge about the ways these various mechanisms work and interact – and the neural substrates and networks involved in these interactions – will help us to understand what the individual facets of pragmatic performance and impairment actually are. This will involve looking beyond the confines of linguistics and pragmatics as has been done, for example, by some researchers who have related research of frontal lobe functions to pragmatic impairments.

There is extensive research on the neuroanatomy, physiology and neuropsychology of frontal lobe functions that suggests links to the pragmatic communicative behavior that has been described. The dorsal frontal lobes have been related to cognitive and the ventral frontal lobes to affective functions (for summaries see Knight & Stuss, 2002; Mesulam, 2000; Stuss & Anderson, 2004; Stuss & Levine, 2002). It has been suggested that the prefrontal cortex can be viewed as the central executive organ for cognitive control and the orbitofrontal cortex as the central executive organ for emotional and social control. Inhibition, emotion and reward processing is mediated by the ventral medial/orbitofrontal region and thus seems implicated in behavioral self-regulation. The right frontal lobe seems particularly important in such aspects of self-awareness as the ability to reflect about one's own thoughts and events occurring in the environment, and the ability to understand the mental states of others. The left frontal lobe has been associated with memory encoding and the right frontal lobe with retrieval of episodic memory. The prefrontal cortex is involved in metamemory judgment and memory for source of information. Pathological changes in this function can be seen in patients who cannot judge whether their retrieved memory is correct, or who cannot remember the situation during which the knowledge was acquired, despite an intact memory for facts. The prefrontal cortex is further implicated in novelty processing such as new learning, creativity and adjustments to perturbations in the environment. It is devoted to complex mental integration and orchestrates extensive network interactions. Its role in inhibiting impulses and in disengaging stimuli from their customary responses seems to be related to the promotion of flexibility, foresight and planning (for a summary see Mesulam, 2000). It has further been suggested that there are distinct basic processes related to the anterior attentional system, with the bilateral superior medial frontal area (anterior cingulate region) being implicated in monitoring regulation of conflict responses and the right lateral frontal region in monitoring or checking (Stuss, Alexander, Shallicec, et al., 2005).

Despite the controversies, it seems safe to say that the frontal lobe network (with its extensive connections to other cortical and subcortical regions) plays a crucial role in pragmatic processing. However, a clearly defined contribution of the right frontal lobe to pragmatic processing remains somewhat elusive. The challenge we are facing is to define more clearly the neural circuits involved, their interaction, and the contribution of the hemispheres and subcortical regions. Some help in this endeavor may come from discussions of the neural underpinnings of social cognition and behavior. Similarly to the RHD patients described previously, patients with damage to the ventromedial frontal lobe show impairments in social reasoning and decision making, impaired social behavior and manners, a lack of concern for others and a lack of empathy, in other words, abnormalities in emotion and feelings despite intact social knowledge and intellectual functioning (Damasio, 1996). In light of these observations, Damasio has advanced the somatic marker hypothesis according to which the ventromedial frontal cortex contains convergence zones that record links between stored knowledge about situations, actors, options for actions and outcomes, and bioregulatory states such as emotions and feelings that in past experience have been associated with such situations and actions. Damage to the ventromedial frontal system prevents a normal emotional or socially relevant response from being triggered. Other structures involved in triggering emotional reactions are the amygdala and the somatosensory-related cortices in the right hemisphere. The amygdala is involved in quick and automatic responses related to potentially threatening situations or to allocating processing resources to potentially salient but ambiguous stimuli. The right somatosensory-related cortices provide access to a detailed representation of the body state associated with emotional or social behavior (Adolphs, 1999). All three structures function together and contribute to our ability to build mental models including a model about our own and other's mental states (ibid.).

Relating social cognition and brain structures is only a first tentative step in the effort to understand pragmatic processing. We should not forget that patients with damage to the frontal lobes and the right hemisphere are not a homogeneous group. Some of these patients do not show any impairments, and those who do can differ widely with respect to the nature of the impairment. Up to now, it is far from clear what the relationships between aspects of social cognition and brain functioning are. Possible routes for investigating these relationships have been opened, however, and new routes remain to be explored.

ACKNOWLEDGMENTS

This work was supported by the Canada Research Chair program. A big thanks goes to A. F. Rodden for his witty and insightful comments.

REFERENCES

Adolphs, R. (1999). Social cognition and the human brain. *Trends in Cognitive Science,* 3(12), 469–78.

Beeman, M. (1993). Semantic processing in the right hemisphere may contribute to drawing inferences from discourse. *Brain and Language,* 44, 80–120.

Bernicot, J., Lacrois, A., and Reilly, J. (2003). La narration chez les enfants atteint du syndrome de Williams: Aspects structuraux et pragmatiques. *Enfance,* 55(3), 265–81.

Bihrle, A. M., Brownell, H. H., Powelson, J. A., and Gardner, H. (1986). Comprehension of humorous and non-humorous materials by left and right brain-damaged patients. *Brain and Cognition,* 5, 399–411.

Bisset, J. D. and Novak, A. M. (1995). Drawing inferences from emotional situations: Left versus right hemisphere deficit. *Clinical Aphasiology,* 23, 217–25.

Bloom, R. L., Borod, J. C., Obler, L. K., and Gerstman, L. J. (1993). Suppression and facilitation of pragmatic performance: Effects of emotional content on discourse following right and left brain damage. *Journal of Speech and Hearing Research,* 36, 1227–35.

Body, R., Perkins, M., and McDonald, S. (1999). Pragmatics, cognition, and communication in traumatic brain injury. In S. McDonald, L. Togher, and C. Code (eds.), *Communication Disorders Following Traumatic Brain Injury* (pp. 81–112). Hove, Sussex: Psychology Press.

Borod, J. C., Rorie, K. D., Pick, L. H., Bloom, R. L., Andelman, F., Campbell, A. L., Obler, L. K., Tweedy, J. R., Welkowitz, J., and Sliwinski, M. (2000). Verbal pragmatics following unilateral stroke: Emotional content and valence. *Neuropsychology,* 14(1), 112–24.

Brownell, H. H., Carroll, J. J., Rehak, A., and Wingfield, A. (1992). The use of pronoun anaphora and speaker mood in the interpretation of conversational utterances by right hemisphere brain-damaged patients. *Brain and Language,* 43(1), 121–47.

Brownell, H. H. and Friedman, O. (2001). Discourse ability in patients with unilateral left and right hemisphere brain damage. In R. S. Berndt (ed.), *Handbook of Neuropsychology,* 2nd ed., vol. 3 (pp. 189–203). Oxford: Elsevier.

Brownell, H. H. and Gardner, H. (1988). Neuropsychological insights into humour. In J. Durant and J. Miller (eds.), *Laughing Matters* (pp. 17–34). Harlow, Essex: Longman Scientific.

Brownell, H. H. and Martino, G. (1998). Deficits in inference and social cognition: The effects of right hemisphere brain damage on discourse. In M. Beeman and C. Chiarello (eds.), *Right Hemisphere Language Comprehension: Perspectives from Cognitive Neuroscience* (pp. 309–28). Mahwah, NJ: Lawrence Erlbaum.

Brownell, H. H., Michel, D., Powelson, J., and Gardner, H. (1983). Surprise but not coherence: Sensitivity to verbal humor in right-hemisphere patients. *Brain and Language,* 18, 20–7.

Brownell, H. H., Potter, H. H., Bihrle, A. M., and Gardner, H. (1986). Inference deficits in right brain-damaged patients. *Brain and Language,* 27, 310–21.

Brownell, H. H. and Stringfellow, A. (1999). Making requests: Illustrations of how right-hemisphere brain damage can affect discourse production. *Brain and Language,* 68, 442–65.

Caplan, D. and Waters, G. (2002). Working memory and connectionist models of parsing: A reply to MacDonald and Christiansen (2002). *Psychological Review*, 109(1), 66–74.

Caspari, I., Parkinson, S. R., LaPointe, L. L., and Katz, R. C. (1998). Working memory and aphasia. *Brain and Cognition*, 37, 205–23.

Chapman, S. B., Highley, A. P., and Thompson, J. L. (1998). Discourse in fluent aphasia and Alzheimer's Disease. *Journal of Neurolinguistics*, 11, 55–78.

Coelho, C. A., Liles, B. Z., and Duffy, R. J. (1995). Impairments of discourse abilities and executive functions in traumatically brain-injured adults. *Brain Injury*, 9(5), 471–7.

Damasio, A. R. (1996). The somatic marker hypothesis and the possible functions of the prefrontal cortex. *Philosophical Transactions of the Royal Society of London – Series B: Biological Sciences*, 351, 1413–20.

Dronkers, N. F., Ludy, C. A., and Redfern, B. B. (1998). Pragmatics in the absence of verbal language: Descriptions of a severe aphasic and a language deprived adult. *Journal of Neurolinguistics*, 11, 179–90.

Foldi, N. S. (1987). Appreciation of pragmatic interpretations of indirect commands: Comparison of right and left hemisphere brain-damaged patients. *Brain and Language*, 31, 88–108.

Frederiksen, C. H. and Stemmer, B. (1993). Conceptual processing of discourse by a right hemisphere brain-damaged patient. In H. H. Brownell and Y. Joanette (eds.), *Narrative Discourse in Neurologically Impaired and Normal Aging Adults* (pp. 239–78). San Diego: Singular.

Fuster, J. M. (2002). Physiology of executive functions: The perception-action cycle. In D. Stuss and R. Knight (eds.), *Principles of Frontal Lobe Function* (pp. 96–108). Oxford: Oxford University Press.

Gibbs, R. W. (1999). Interpreting what speakers say and implicate. *Brain and Language*, 68, 466–85.

Giora, R. (2003). *On our Mind: Salience, Context, and Figurative Language*. Oxford: Oxford University Press.

Hirst, W., LeDoux, J., and Stein, S. (1984). Constraints on the processing of indirect speech acts: Evidence from aphasiology. *Brain and Language*, 23, 26–33.

Joanette, Y. and Brownell, H. H. (eds.) (1990). *Discourse Abilities and Brain Damage*. New York: Springer.

Johnson-Laird, P. N. (1983). *Mental Models: Towards a Cognitive Science of Language Inference, and Consciousness*. Cambridge: Cambridge University Press.

Johnson-Laird, P. N. (1989). Mental models. In M. I. Posner (ed.), *Foundations of Cognitive Science* (pp. 469–99). Cambridge, MA: MIT Press.

Kaplan, J. A., Brownell, H. H., Jacobs, J. R., and Gardner, H. (1990). The effects of right hemisphere damage on the pragmatic interpretation of conversational remarks. *Brain and Language*, 38, 315–33.

Kasher, A., Batori, G., Soroker, N., Graves, D., and Zaidel, E. (1999). Effects of right- and left-hemisphere damage on understanding conversational implicatures. *Brain and Language*, 68(3), 566–90.

Kee, K. S., Green, M. F., Gizer, I. R., Laack, K. A., and Zaidel, E. (2000). Hemispheric specialization and perception of emotion. *Journal of the International Neuropsychological Society (JINS)*, 6, 222.

Knight, R. T. and Stuss, D. T. (2002). Prefrontal cortex: The present and the future. In D. Stuss and R. Knight (eds.), *Principles of Frontal Lobe Function* (pp. 573–97). Oxford: Oxford University Press.

Langdon, R., Coltheart, M., Ward, P. B., and Catts, S. V. (2002). Disturbed communication in schizophrenia: The role of poor pragmatics and poor mind-reading. *Psychological Medicine*, 32(7), 1273–84.

Lehman, M. T. and Tompkins, C. A. (2000). Inferencing in adults with right hemisphere brain damage: An analysis of conflicting results. *Aphasiology*, 14(5/6), 485–99.

Martin, I. and McDonald, S. (2003). Weak coherence, no theory of mind, or executive dysfunction? Solving the puzzle of pragmatic language disorders. *Brain and Language*, 85(3), 451–66.

McDonald, S. (1999). Exploring the process of inference generation in sarcasm: A review of normal and clinical studies. *Brain and Language*, 68, 486–506.

McDonald, S. (2000). Exploring the cognitive basis of right-hemisphere pragmatic language disorders. *Brain and Language*, 75, 82–107.

McDonald, S. and Pearce, S. (1996). Clinical insights into pragmatic theory: Frontal lobe deficits and sarcasm. *Brain and Language*, 53, 81–104.

McDonald, S. and Pearce, S. (1998). Requests that overcome listener reluctance: Impairment associated with executive dysfunction in brain injury. *Brain and Language*, 61(1), 88–104.

McDonald, S. and van Sommers, P. (1993). Pragmatic language skills after closed head injury: Ability to negotiate requests. *Cognitive Neuropsychology*, 10(4), 297–315.

McDonald, S. and Wales, R. (1986). An investigation of the ability to process inferences in language following right hemisphere brain damage. *Brain and Language*, 29, 68–80.

Meilijson, S. R., Kasher, A., and Elizur, A. (2004). Language performance in chronic schizophrenia: A pragmatic approach. *Journal of Speech, Language and Hearing Research*, 47, 695–713.

Mesulam, M.-M. (2000). Behavioral neuroanatomy. In M.-M. Mesualm (ed.), *Principles of Behavioral and Cognitive Neurology* (pp. 1–120). Oxford: Oxford University Press.

Moya, K. L., Benowitz, L. I., Levine, D. N., and Finkelstein, S. (1986). Covariant deficits in visuospatial abilities and recall of verbal narrative after right hemisphere stroke. *Cortex*, 22, 381–97.

Paradis, M. (1998). The other side of language: Pragmatic competence. *Journal of Neurolinguistics*, 11(1–2), 1–10.

Prutting, C. A. and Kirchner, D. M. (1987). A clinical appraisal of the pragmatic aspects of language. *Journal of Speech and Hearing Disorders*, 52, 105–19.

Read, D. E. (1981). Solving deductive reasoning problems after unilateral temporal lobectomy. *Brain and Language*, 12, 92–100.

Rehak, A., Kaplan, J. A., Weylman, S. T., Kelly, B., Brownell, H. H., and Gardner, H. (1992). Story processing in right-hemisphere brain-damaged patients. *Brain and Language*, 42, 320–36.

Shammi, P. and Stuss, D. (1999). Humour appreciation: A role of the right frontal lobe. *Brain*, 122, 657–66.

Siegal, M., Carrington, J., and Radel, M. (1996). Theory of mind and pragmatic understanding following right hemisphere damage. *Brain and Language*, 53, 40–50.

Soroker, N., Kasher, A., Giora, R., Batori, G., Corn, C., Gil, M., and Zaidel, E. (2005). Processing of basic speech acts following localized brain damage: A new light on the neuroanatomy of language. *Brain and Cognition*, 57(2), 214–17.

Sperber, D. (2000). Metarepresentations in an evolutionary perspective. In D. Sperber (ed.), *Metarepresentations: A Multidisciplinary Perspective* (pp. 117–37). New York: Oxford University Press.

Stemmer, B. (1994). A pragmatic approach to neurolinguistics: Requests (re)considered. *Brain and Language*, 46, 565–91.

Stemmer, B. (1999a). Discourse studies in neurologically impaired populations: A quest for action. *Brain and Language*, 68(3), 402–18.

Stemmer, B. (1999b). Pragmatics: Theoretical and clinical issues. Introduction to special issue of *Brain and Language*, 68, 389–91.

Stemmer, B. and Cohen, H. (2002). Neuropragmatique et lésions de l'hémisphère droit. *Psychologie de l'Interaction*, 13–14, 15–46.

Stemmer, B., Giroux, F., and Joanette, Y. (1994). Production and evaluation of requests by right hemisphere brain-damaged individuals. *Brain and Language*, 47, 1–31.

Stemmer, B. and Joanette, Y. (1998). The interpretation of narrative discourse of brain-damaged individuals within the framework of a multilevel discourse model. In M. Beeman and C. Chiarello (eds.), *Right Hemisphere Language Comprehension: Perspectives from Cognitive Neuroscience* (pp. 329–48). Mahwah, NJ: Lawrence Erlbaum.

Stone, V. E., Baron-Cohen, S., and Knight, R. T. (1998). Frontal lobe contributions to theory of mind. *Journal of Cognitive Neuroscience*, 10(5), 640–56.

Stuss, D. T. and Alexander, M. P. (2000). Executive functions and the frontal lobes: A conceptual view. *Psychological Research*, 63, 289–98.

Stuss, D. T., Alexander, M. P., Floden, D., Binns, M. A., Levine, B., McIntosh, A. R., Rjah, N., and Hevenor, S. J. (2002). Fractionation and localization of distinct frontal lobe processes: Evidence from focal lesions in humans. In D. Stuss and R. Knight (eds.), *Principles of Frontal Lobe Function* (pp. 392–407). Oxford: Oxford University Press.

Stuss, D. T., Alexander, M. P., Shallicec, T., Picton, T. W., Binns, M. A., Macdonald, R., Borowiec, A., and Katz, D. I. (2005). Multiple frontal systems controlling response speed. *Neuropsychologia*, 43, 396–417.

Stuss, D. T. and Anderson, V. (2004). The frontal lobes and theory of mind: Developmental concepts from adult focal lesion research. *Brain and Cognition*, 55, 69–83.

Stuss, D. T., Gallup, G. G., and Alexander, M. P. (2001). The frontal lobes are necessary for 'theory of mind'. *Brain*, 124, 279–86.

Stuss, D. T. and Levine, B. (2002). Adult clinical neuropsychology: Lessons from studies of the frontal lobes. *Annual Reviews of Psychology*, 53, 401–33.

Togher, L. and Hand, L. (1998). Use of politeness markers with different communication partners: An investigation of five subjects with traumatic brain injury. *Aphasiology*, 12(7/8), 755–70.

Tompkins, C. A. (1990). Knowledge and strategies for processing lexical metaphor after right or left hemisphere brain damage. *Journal of Speech and Hearing Research*, 33, 307–16.

Tompkins, C. A., Bloise, C. G. R., Timko, M. L., and Baumgaertner, A. (1994). Working memory and inference revision in brain-damaged and normally aging adults. *Journal of Speech and Hearing Research*, 37, 896–912.

Tompkins, C. A., Lehman, M. T., and Baumgaertner, A. (1999). Suppression and inference revision in right brain-damaged and non-brain-damaged adults. *Aphasiology*, 13(9–11), 725–42.

Tompkins, C. and Mateer, C. A. (1985). Right hemisphere appreciation of prosodic and linguistic indications of implicit attitude. *Brain and Language*, 24, 185–203.

Wapner, W., Hamby, S., and Gardner, H. (1981). The role of the right hemisphere in the apprehension of complex linguistic material. *Brain and Language*, 14, 15–33.

Weylman, S. T., Brownell, H. H., Roman, M., and Gardner, H. (1989). Appreciation of indirect requests by left- and right-brain-damaged patients: The effects of verbal context and conventionality of wording. *Brain and Language*, 36, 580–91.

Winner, E., Brownell, H., Happé, F., Blum, A., and Pincus, D. (1998). Distinguishing lies from jokes: Theory of mind deficits and discourse interpretation in right hemisphere brain-damaged patients. *Brain and Language*, 62, 89–106.

Wright, H. H. and Newhoff, M. (2005). Pragmatics. In L. L. LaPointe (ed.), *Aphasia and Related Neurogenic Language Disorders*, 3rd ed. (pp. 237–48). New York: Thieme.

5 Pragmatic Impairment as an Emergent Phenomenon

MICHAEL R. PERKINS

5.1 Introduction

Transcript 1 is an extract from a conversation between John, a child with autistic spectrum disorder (ASD), aged 4;11, and Kate, a speech and language therapist. They are looking at pictures of different kinds of fruit.

Transcript 1

1	Kate:	Could you eat that? [indicating picture of oranges]
2	John:	No.
3	Kate:	Why's that?
4	John:	Because the orange is hurting me.
5	Kate:	How does it hurt you?
6	John:	He won't eat it.
7	Kate:	You don't eat oranges?
8	John:	No.
9	Kate:	Why not, John?
10	John:	Because silly.
11	Kate:	Why are they silly?
12	John:	An orange.

Most of John's contributions to the conversation don't seem to connect well with what Kate says. One might describe them as inappropriate, irrelevant or just plain odd. Assuming that such exchanges are typical of John, would we be justified in describing his conversation as showing evidence of pragmatic impairment? If we analyze his utterances using certain categories derived from pragmatic theory the answer would appear to be 'yes'. For example, John's contributions are not particularly 'cooperative' in the sense of Grice's cooperative principle (see Ahlsén, chapter 2 in this volume). More specifically, according to Grice's theory of conversational implicature, John's responses in lines 6 and 12 – from an outside observer's viewpoint, though not necessarily from

John's – could be seen as breaking the maxim of relevance (i.e. they appear to have little to do with Kate's preceding questions) and if his responses in lines 2 and 4 are indeed untrue, they break the maxim of quality. It is not clear, though, whether these 'floutings' of the maxims are intended to trigger implicatures, and if so, what they might be. Other features of John's conversation may be described using Speech Act Theory (see Müller, Guendouzi, & Wilson, chapter 1 in this volume). For example, John's responses in lines 6 and 12 could be taken as evidence of a lack of 'illocutionary uptake'; i.e., as Blank, Gessner, and Esposito (1979) put it when describing a similar child, he seems to find it hard to "interpret the . . . intent of others" (p. 351). Kate likewise appears to find some of John's utterances hard to interpret – for example, in line 7 she tries to get John to verify whether a re-explicated version of his preceding utterance is in fact what he meant. In terms of Relevance Theory (see Leinonen & Ryder, chapter 3 in this volume), this could be construed as both Kate and John having to make a significant commitment in terms of processing effort with relatively little to show for it by way of 'contextual effects' including enhanced mutual understanding. The concepts and categories provided by pragmatic theory thus provide us with a ready means of describing atypical communicative behavior.

John would also be labeled as pragmatically impaired according to various formal assessment procedures. For example, to take just two items from Bishop's *Children's Communicative Checklist* (2003), John "uses terms like 'he' or 'it' without making it clear what he is talking about" (cf. line 6) and "it is sometimes hard to make sense of what he is saying because it seems illogical or disconnected". Likewise, according to Penn's *Profile of Communicative Appropriateness* (1985), John's conversation might be described as manifesting inappropriate 'reference', 'idea sequencing' and 'topic adherence'.

These ways of characterizing pragmatic impairment are common in clinical practice and research, and have given rise to a wide range of clinical pragmatic tests, assessments and checklists. However, while providing a useful means of *describing* anomalous communicative behavior, most tests are less successful at *explaining* such behavior in a way that provides clinicians with clear targets for intervention. For example, a lack of illocutionary uptake could be an indirect consequence of a range of factors including difficulties with inferential reasoning, a syntactic parsing problem, an attention deficit, problems with short-term verbal memory or impaired auditory processing. Thus labeling the behavioral symptoms is only a first step; the likely underlying cause also needs to be identified.

In this chapter I outline an approach to the analysis of pragmatic impairment which regards it as an 'emergent' phenomenon. That is to say, rather than seeing pragmatics as a discrete component of communicative processing like syntax, phonology or lexis, it views it as an indirect, or 'epiphenomenal', consequence of the way such components are used and interact. Furthermore, rather than viewing pragmatic competence as being solely to do with language use, the 'emergentist' approach regards it as resulting from the interaction of multiple factors including language, cognition, and more besides. The emergentist account of pragmatic ability and disability has its roots in the 'interactionist' approach pioneered by Elizabeth Bates, Carol Prutting, and Claire Penn, among others (see, for example, Gallagher, 1991; Penn, 1999). The version presented here, which has been developed over the last decade or so (e.g. Perkins, 1998, 2005, 2007), draws in addition on insights from cognitive science (e.g. A. Clark, 1997), social psychology (H. H. Clark, 1996) and conversation analysis (Wilkinson, chapter 6 in this volume).

5.2　An Emergentist Model of Pragmatic Ability and Disability

John's pragmatic problems as illustrated in the transcript above stem at least partly from being unable to work out others' states of mind including their intentions, feelings and knowledge. For meaning that is linguistically encoded, this may not pose much of a problem. However, any meaning which is left unsaid, on the assumption that the hearer will be able to infer it, is bound to be problematic in cases where there is inadequate access to others' mental states. An inability to 'read' others' minds in this way is commonly described as having an impaired 'theory of mind' (ToM) (see Stemmer, chapter 4 in this volume) – i.e. a cognitive deficit – and the link between ToM competence and pragmatic impairment is now generally accepted in research on ASD, right-hemisphere brain damage (RHD) and traumatic brain injury (TBI) (Happé, Brownell, & Winner, 1999; Martin & McDonald, 2003).

However, ToM is not the only aspect of cognition to contribute to pragmatic ability. From a speaker's perspective, pragmatics may be seen as getting the balance right between what is said and what may reasonably be left to be inferred, and the hearer's role is to work this out. This interpersonal balancing act is dependent not only on ToM but in addition on the capacity to encode and decode what is expressed linguistically. If a speaker has a language-encoding problem, the hearer may be left with a difficult or even impossible inferential task. Transcript 2 is from a conversation with W, a 74-year-old man with anomic aphasia who has problems with lexical retrieval. As a result, he is unable to encode sufficient information linguistically to express what he means. The imbalance between explicit and implicit meaning is in this instance too great to be redressed through extra inferential processing on T's part, with negative consequences for mutual understanding.

Transcript 2

　T:　so what did you make? what did the factory make?
　W:　what did we make was not a lot because we only made things for the things that were [ded] so we all made things that were out our out of our um things.

In this particular case the underlying problem happens to be one of lexical access, but difficulties with phonology, syntax or prosody have similar consequences for the explicit-implicit balance. If pragmatic competence is seen as effective language *use*, ability to make the right encoding choices clearly draws not only on cognitive factors but also on linguistic ability.

Linguistic encoding ability can in turn be indirectly affected by motor speech problems as found in conditions as different as dysarthria, cleft palate and cerebral palsy where access to phonological, syntactic and semantic form is obscured by poor articulation, but the end result in terms of additional inferential processing for the hearer is the same.

Linguistic *decoding* ability also plays a significant role in pragmatic processing. If one is unable to parse incoming utterances in order to arrive at an accurate representation of their propositional content, any additional implicit meaning will be more difficult to access. Language is thus one type of input system which the inferential reasoning system draws on, though it is not the only one relevant to pragmatics. Visual impairment, for example, can affect the detection of irony via facial expression, and young blind children have been shown to perform as poorly as children with autism on ToM tasks (Hobson & Bishop, 2003). Hearing impairment, too, has been shown to have adverse effects on conversational turn-taking and initiation (Mogford-Bevan, 1993).

Inferential reasoning also draws on a range of cognitive capacities. ToM plays a particularly important role here, as noted above, but so do other areas of cognition. The conversational extract in Transcript 3, spoken by a man with traumatic brain injury, exhibits sudden topic shifts which leave the hearer unable to work out the links and see the overall coherence of what is being said.

Transcript 3

> I have got faults and . my biggest fault is . I do enjoy sport . it's something that I've always done . I've done it all my life . I've nothing but respect for my mother and father and . my sister . and basically sir . I've only come to this conclusion this last two months . and . as far as I'm concerned . my sister doesn't exist (Perkins, Body, & Parker, 1995, p. 305)

This appears to be linked to problems with short-term memory – i.e. the speaker forgets what he has just been talking about – and 'executive function' – i.e. he has problems with planning and monitoring what he is saying.

So far, it has been tacitly assumed that the sole way of making meaning explicit is via language, and indeed such an assumption is widespread in both theoretical and clinical linguistics. Semiotic systems such as prosody, gesture, gaze, facial expression and posture are often seen as secondary to spoken language, and even 'pragmatic' insofar as they enable the hearer to infer meaning not expressed linguistically. In recent years, however, a number of research studies have suggested that all of these systems have a certain equivalence in that they provide alternative ways of making meaning explicit. Furthermore, they appear to function together as a single, mutually dependent and integrated signaling system across which meaning is orchestrated (McNeill, 2000). Such a multimodal approach to communication muddies the waters of the explicit/implicit distnction made in traditional pragmatics. In the emergentist approach, on the other hand, it simply leads to the recognition of a wider range of choices which are implicated in decisions about what meanings are to be made explicit.

The ability for a speaker to maintain, and for a hearer to work out, the precise relationship between what is explicitly conveyed and what is meant can thus be seen to be dependent on a range of underlying factors, some of which are shown in table 5.1.

The semiotic elements provide alternative ways of representing meaning which may be encoded motorically and decoded sensorily. The various cognitive elements are responsible for what is and is not encoded and decoded, and how, why, when, where and whether these processes take place. Seen in this way, pragmatics is an inherent property of the communicative spectrum as a whole, rather than being exclusively subserved by a single cognitive system, i.e. ToM, in conjunction with a single semiotic system, i.e. language, as is more commonly assumed to be the case.

From a clinical perspective, such an approach has the advantage of allowing a focus on the disparate range of factors which can lead to pragmatic impairment, and thus provides the opportunity to focus on, and treat, underlying causes in addition to behavioral symptoms. This permits a detailed typology

Table 5.1 Some semiotic, cognitive and sensorimotor elements of pragmatics

Semiotic	Cognitive	Motor	Sensory
Language:	Inference	Vocal tract	Hearing
phonology	Theory of mind	Hands	Vision
prosody	Executive function	Arms	
morphology	Memory	Face	
syntax	Emotion	Eyes	
semantics	Attitude	Body	
discourse			
Gesture			
Gaze			
Facial expression			
Posture			

Source: Perkins, 2007.

Table 5.2   A simple taxonomy of pragmatic impairments

Area of underlying deficit	Type of pragmatic impairment
inference theory of mind executive function memory emotion and attitude	Cognitive
phonology morphology syntax lexis prosody discourse	Linguistic
gesture gaze facial expression posture	Non-verbal
auditory perception visual perception motor/articulatory ability	Sensorimotor

of different pragmatic impairments, rather than forcing a reliance on a single generic, but uninformative, label such as pragmatic impairment/disability/ difficulties (Perkins, 2000). Table 5.2 represents a starting point for such a taxonomy.

Even this, though, is still something of a simplification, as it leaves out a crucial dimension of pragmatic impairment that we have so far not touched upon.

5.3   Compensatory Adaptation

Most approaches to communication impairment assume a direct link between an underlying linguistic or cognitive deficit and the set of behaviors or symptoms to which it gives rise. So, for example, aphasic agrammatism and specific language impairment (SLI) are often seen as a direct consequence of damage to a grammar 'module'. An alternative view is that behavioral symptoms are often only indirectly linked to an underlying deficit, and may in fact result from compensatory adaptation. So, for example, some now see agrammatism as "message simplification on the part of the aphasic speaker in an attempt to prevent computational overload" (Kolk, 1995, p. 294), and SLI as a compensatory adaptation to a procedural memory deficit whereby linguistic rules are learned explicitly via declarative memory, as is typically the case in adult second language learners (Ullman & Pierpont, 2005).

In similar vein, the emergentist account of pragmatic impairment sees pragmatic behavior as resulting from complex interactions and trade-offs between the kinds of elements shown in table 5.1. An individual is seen as an *intra*personal domain, comprising the sum total of all his or her interacting semiotic, cognitive and sensorimotor capacities. Any malfunctioning capacity will have consequences for the entire intrapersonal domain, and any subsequent adaptation will result in a redistribution of resources across the domain as a whole. Problems with phonological encoding, for example, may be offset by more extensive use of gesture, and syntactic comprehension difficulties may lead the hearer to rely more on contextually inferred meaning. Such adaptations and trade-offs are deemed pragmatic if they are motivated by the need to communicate with others. A group of two or more individuals is seen as an *inter*personal domain in which the individuals' capacities interact with those of the other individual(s). The interacting elements are still of the same type – i.e. semiotic, cognitive and sensorimotor – but become a shared resource. A deficit within an individual may have interpersonal consequences, and any resulting adaptations will have an impact on the explicit-implicit meaning balance at an interpersonal level. This could lead, for example, to attitudinal and emotional meaning being encoded via facial expression rather than linguistically, and being decoded visually rather than auditorily. Some examples are provided in table 5.3.

To summarize: when we describe pragmatic ability and disability as emergent, we mean that pragmatics is not a discrete entity but the complex outcome of many interacting variables. When we communicate with others, we draw on a range of capacities including (1) signaling systems such as language, gesture and facial expression, (2) cognitive systems such as theory of mind, inference and memory, (3) motor output systems such as the vocal tract and hand movement and (4) sensory input systems such as hearing and vision. All of these 'elements' exist within the individual, i.e., they constitute an intrapersonal domain, but during communication they combine with those of other individuals to form an interpersonal domain. Interpersonal communication involves many choices: for example, which meanings are explicitly encoded, and which left implicit, which signaling systems are used, and which meanings are most salient and relevant. The exercise of such choices requires multiple interactions between the various underlying semiotic, cognitive and sensorimotor capacities both within and between individuals. Intrapersonal and interpersonal domains are dynamic systems whose integrity and equilibrium are maintained via a continuous process of compensatory adaptation. The effect of this is most plainly seen when one or more individual elements malfunction and create an imbalance within the system as a whole.

Table 5.3   Examples of interpersonal compensation for expressive and receptive communication impairments

Impairment of expressive resources	Compensation by interlocutor
Semiotic, e.g. syntactic formulation problems	Greater reliance on inference based on contextual clues and shared knowledge
Cognitive, e.g. attention deficit	Greater reliance on gesture, eye contact, linguistic repetition
Sensorimotor, e.g. dysarthria, dyspraxia	Repetition of what hearer thinks has been said for verification by speaker

Impairment of receptive resources	Compensation by interlocutor
Semiotic, e.g. poor parsing, word recognition	Simplified syntax, use of gesture and visual clues
Cognitive, e.g. poor short-term memory	Frequent linguistic recapitulation and use of visual reminders
Sensorimotor, e.g. hearing impairment	Greater reliance on gesture, exaggerated articulation and other visual clues

Source: Perkins, 2007.

5.4   Clinical and Theoretical Implications of an Emergentist Model of Pragmatics

Because of its holistic perspective, the emergentist account of pragmatics is much broader in scope than other approaches which focus on a single component of pragmatic processing such as intention, inference or ToM, and is effectively co-extensive with the entire spectrum of interpersonal communication. This does not mean, though, that specificity and rigor are sacrificed for comprehensiveness. Admittedly, labels such as 'pragmatic impairment' and 'pragmatic disability' are too vague to have much diagnostic value. For example, Prutting and Kirchner's *Pragmatic Protocol* (1987) includes items as disparate as variety of speech acts, topic maintenance, repair, pause time and feedback to speakers. Likewise, pragmatic impairment has been seen as an inherent property of a similarly disparate range of unrelated communication disorders including aphasia, Asperger's syndrome, autism, dementia, developmental language disorder, hearing impairment, visual impairment and schizophrenia (Perkins, 2003). However, by focusing on the entire range of underlying factors that determine the balance between explicit and implicit meaning, the emergentist approach is able to identify the different pragmatic consequences of all these conditions in terms of both their underlying causes and their communicative effects. Furthermore, in so doing it provides an explanation of the condition rather than just describing it, and makes it possible to direct intervention at causes rather than just symptoms.

It is rarely the case, though, that anomalous behavior maps directly onto a single underlying cognitive, linguistic or sensorimotor deficit. It is quite common to find behavioral symptoms resulting from attempts to compensate for a deficit elsewhere in the intrapersonal domain. So, for example, Tarling, Perkins, and Stojanovik (2006) found that a child with Williams syndrome was able to partially mask syntactic formulation and lexical retrieval difficulties by effecting smooth and well-timed turn transitions and topic changes to give the overall impression of being an attentive and effective conversational partner. Similarly, Simmons-Mackie and Damico (1996) have shown how individuals with aphasia are able to make use of posture, gesture, repetition and neologisms to signal discourse functions such as turn initiation and termination which would normally be done linguistically. By viewing individuals and groups of individuals as dynamic organisms comprising complex interactions of cognitive, linguistic and sensorimotor processes, the emergentist approach moves away from the single deficit model of pathology and sees all communication disorders as potentially complex.

Models of typical and atypical pragmatic functioning tend to focus either on the capacities of the individual (e.g. ToM) with minimal reference to properties of the interaction in which the individual is a participant, or else on the interaction itself with little account being taken of the participants' underlying cognitive and linguistic capacities (as in conversation analysis). The emergentist model, on the other hand, sees the intrapersonal and interpersonal domains as working in synergy, as is found in dynamic models of shared cognition (e.g. Clark, 1997) and joint action (e.g. Clark, 1996).

In a case study of Peter, a child with an original diagnosis of SLI, Perkins (2007) showed that a range of anomalous communicative behaviors could only be properly understood when seen simultaneously from the perspective of the individual and that of the communicating dyad. Some of Peter's conversational problems were easily describable in traditional pragmatic terms – for example, referential inadequacy, lack of coherence, poor topic introduction and maintenance, being unclear (Grice's maxim of manner), saying too little or too much (Grice's maxim of quantity), and not always making clear the illocutionary force of his utterances. In other areas, though, Peter was clearly pragmatically skilled – for example, his use of conversational repair, gaze, prosody and gesture to manage turn-taking effectively and to coordinate his own behavior with that of the interlocutor. A single diagnostic term such as 'pragmatic impairment' is therefore clearly neither adequate nor sufficiently specific. Some of these behaviors were linked to problems with lexical retrieval and syntactic formulation, i.e. a language encoding problem, which meant that his meaning was often insufficiently explicit. However, his language performance was also very variable. For example, lexical access improved when he was able to keep his syntax simple, and syntactically complex sentences were possible provided he used pro-forms such as 'it' and 'there' instead of more semantically specified forms. (These compensatory adaptations were in fact only part of a more complex picture, being linked to underlying difficulties with auditory verbal memory (i.e. remembering what he had already said, and what others had said to him) and auditory selective attention (i.e. being able to process language against background noise).) We can describe such trade-offs in intrapersonal terms (i.e. as interactions within and between Peter's linguistic, cognitive and sensorimotor systems) but they are also clearly interpersonally motivated. In addition, some compensatory adaptations were exclusively interpersonal. For example, Peter would sometimes formulate a proposition gradually and incrementally across several conversational turns, and require evidence of understanding from his interlocutor after each increment before continuing. A simple example is shown in Transcript 4.

Transcript 4

    1 Peter: you know the tickets?
    2 Sara: yeah
    3 Peter: they tell you where to go

Instead of producing the single sentence 'the tickets tell you where to go' in one turn, the subject noun phrase is specified first, and then subsequently substituted by a pronoun which reduces the processing load. Syntactic formulation across turns in this way is only possible with appropriate input from the interlocutor, making it effectively a joint activity. A further example of interpersonal adaptation is the use of eye gaze by Peter to indicate when he requires assistance from his conversational partner to find a word. Peter's word searches can sometimes take many seconds, and he pauses frequently. Although conversational pauses are often treated by interlocutors as a place where they may take a turn, this only happens in Peter's case when in addition he re-establishes eye contact. In Transcript 5, there is a gap between 'on' and 'a ship' of about 2 seconds containing both filled and unfilled pauses (underlined in the transcript). During this time, Peter's gaze is averted, and his interlocutor does nothing to help him.

Transcript 5
(°hh = in-breath; (0.1) and (1.0) = length of pause seconds.)

    Peter: know when it was a wa °hh we went on <u>erm (0.1) [tuts] (1.0)</u> a ship

On occasions when eye contact is re-established before Peter retrieves the word, on the other hand, the interlocutor either facilitates retrieval, for example by suggesting possible targets, or else produces the word herself. Lexical retrieval in conversations with Peter is therefore also a joint activity.

It is only when the complex interplay between individual elements such as syntax, lexis, memory, attention and auditory processing are seen within intrapersonal and interpersonal domains simultaneously that we are able to grasp the systematicity in Peter's variable conversational performance. His communicative strengths and weaknesses, which are superficially captured by pragmatic labels such as 'self-repair' and 'semantic underspecification', turn out to be the emergent tip of a complex iceberg. It is only through understanding this mesh of underlying variables that effectively targeted treatment becomes possible.

In addition to its clinical relevance, the emergentist model also has implications for mainstream pragmatics and pragmatic theory. The underlying complexity of pragmatic impairment as illustrated above suggests that the study of normal pragmatic functioning might benefit from extending its scope and allocating a more central role to non-linguistic semiotic systems such as gesture, eye gaze and facial expression, to cognitive systems in addition to ToM, and to motor output and sensory input systems. Most work in pragmatics focuses exclusively on the use of *language* and it is often assumed that linguistic pragmatics is all that there is. Likewise, the contribution of cognition to pragmatics is rarely seen as extending beyond inferential reasoning, and ToM in particular. As noted above, however, a typology of pragmatic abilities based on a comprehensive range of contributory factors offers a principled means of capturing both the breadth and the detail of pragmatics without being open to the charge of being nothing more than "a range of loosely related research programmes" (Sperber & Wilson, 2005, p. 468) that is sometimes leveled at the discipline as a whole.

The way in which language and other semiotic devices appear to work together as a single composite signaling system suggests that the notion of explicitness, normally seen as an exclusive property of language, could be usefully re-examined. Interestingly, this takes us back to Morris's original conception of pragmatics as "the study of the relation of signs [i.e. not exclusively linguistic signs] to interpreters" (Morris, 1938, p. 6).

Finally, by seeing pragmatics as a fusion of intrapersonal and interpersonal domains, the emergentist program provides a framework for reconciling purely cognitively based approaches to pragmatics such as relevance theory (Leinonen & Ryder, chapter 3 in this volume) with purely ethnographic approaches such as conversation analysis (Wilkinson, chapter 6 in this volume), which excludes any reference to cognitive states except insofar as they are indirectly reflected in empirically observable behaviors.

REFERENCES

Bishop, D. V. M. (2003). *The Children's Communication Checklist, version 2 (CCC-2)*. London: Psychological Corporation.

Blank, M., Gessner, M., and Esposito, A. (1979). Language without communication: A case study. *Journal of Child Language,* 6, 329–52.

Clark, A. (1997). *Being There: Putting Brain, Body, and World Together Again.* Cambridge, MA: MIT Press.

Clark, H. H. (1996). *Using Language.* Cambridge: Cambridge University Press.

Gallagher, T. M. (ed.) (1991). *Pragmatics of Language: Clinical Practice Issues.* London: Chapman Hall.

Happé, F., Brownell, H., and Winner, E. (1999). Acquired 'theory of mind' impairments following stroke. *Cognition,* 70(3), 211–40.

Hobson, R. P. and Bishop, M. (2003). The pathogenesis of autism: Insights from congenital blindness. *Philosophical Transactions of the Royal Society, Series B358,* 335–44.

Kolk, H. (1995). A time-based approach to agrammatic production. *Brain and Language,* 50, 282–303.

Martin, I. and McDonald, S. (2003). Weak coherence, no theory of mind, or executive dysfunction? Solving the puzzle of pragmatic language disorders. *Brain and Language,* 85, 451–66.

McNeill, D. (ed.) (2000). *Language and Gesture.* Cambridge: Cambridge University Press.

Mogford-Bevan, K. (1993). Language acquisition and development with sensory impairment: Hearing-impaired children. In G. Blanken, J. Dittmann, H. Grimm, J. C. Marshall, and C.-W. Wallesch (eds.), *Linguistic Disorders and Pathologies: An International Handbook* (pp. 660–79). Berlin: Walter de Gruyter.

Morris, C. W. (1938). Foundations of the theory of signs. In O. Neurath, R. Carnap, and C. Morris (eds.), *International Encyclopedia of Unified Science* (pp. 77–138). Chicago: University of Chicago Press.

Penn, C. (1985). The profile of communicative appropriateness. *South African Journal of Communication Disorders,* 32, 18–23.

Penn, C. (1999). Pragmatic assessment and therapy for persons with brain damage: What have clinicians gleaned in two decades? *Brain and Language,* 68, 535–52.

Perkins, M. R. (1998). Is pragmatics epiphenomenal? Evidence from communication disorders. *Journal of Pragmatics,* 29, 291–311.

Perkins, M. R. (2000). The scope of pragmatic disability: A cognitive approach. In N. Müller (ed.), *Pragmatics and Clinical Applications* (pp. 7–28). Amsterdam: John Benjamins.

Perkins, M. R. (2003). Clinical pragmatics. In J. Verschueren, J.-O. Östman, J. Blommaert, and C. Bulcaen (eds.), *Handbook of Pragmatics: 2001 Installment* (pp. 1–29). Amsterdam: John Benjamins.

Perkins, M. R. (2005). Pragmatic ability and disability as emergent phenomena. *Clinical Linguistics and Phonetics,* 19(5), 367–77.

Perkins, M. R. (2007). *Pragmatic Impairment.* Cambridge: Cambridge University Press.

Perkins, M. R., Body, R., and Parker, M. (1995). Closed head injury: Assessment and remediation of topic bias and repetitiveness. In M. R. Perkins and S. J. Howard (eds.), *Case Studies in Clinical Linguistics* (pp. 293–320). London: Whurr.

Prutting, C. A. and Kirchner, D. M. (1987). A clinical appraisal of the pragmatic aspects of language. *Journal of Speech and Hearing Disorders,* 52, 105–19.

Simmons-Mackie, N. and Damico, J. (1996). The contribution of discourse markers to communicative competence in aphasia. *American Journal of Speech-Language Pathology,* 5(1), 37–43.

Sperber, D. and Wilson, D. (2005). Pragmatics. In F. Jackson and M. Smith (eds.), *Oxford Handbook of Contemporary Analytic Philosophy* (pp. 468–501). Oxford: Oxford University Press.

Tarling, K., Perkins, M. R., and Stojanovik, V. (2006). Conversational success in Williams syndrome: Communication in the face of cognitive and linguistic limitations. *Clinical Linguistics and Phonetics*, 20(7–8), 583–90.

Ullman, M. T. and Pierpont, E. I. (2005). Specific Language Impairment is not specific to language: The procedural deficit hypothesis. *Cortex*, 41, 399–433.

6 Conversation Analysis and Communication Disorders

RAY WILKINSON

6.1 Conversation Analysis

6.1.1 Orientation

There has been a growing interest in conversation analysis (CA) within the field of communication disorders since clinical studies using this method started to appear in the 1990s. A major attraction of CA for researchers and clinicians working with communication disorders is that it provides a rigorous method for the analysis of naturally occurring interactive talk and other behavior within interaction including gesture, eye gaze, body movement and the deployment of alternative methods of communication such as communication aids. While its focus on social interaction and language in context means its concerns overlap to some extent with those of linguistic pragmatics (see Levinson, 1983, chapter 6), and therefore clinical pragmatics (Smith & Leinonen, 1992), CA is in the first instance a procedure for the analysis of social activities and in particular the use of talk within social activities, and can be used to investigate various features of those activities including the participants' deployment of grammar, lexis and phonology as interactional resources (e.g. Ford, Fox, & Thompson, 2002).

A strength of a CA approach to the analysis of linguistic and clinical linguistic phenomena is that it allows aspects of language such as grammar or lexis to be investigated in terms of what might be called the *dynamic* (as opposed to static) features of their deployment. Thus this chapter will be discussing ways in which CA investigations of normal and 'disordered' language as it is deployed within interactive talk allow analysis of linguistic and phonetic phenomena in terms of how they are produced by participants:

- in naturally occurring interactions
- in real time

- as part of a larger social project, such as a social action or activity, which is likely to involve more than 'communicating information'
- in terms of the particular sequential context within which the interactional behavior is produced.

And for the analysis of the interaction of people with communication disorders the following will particularly be seen to be of interest:

- ways in which people with communication disorders and their co-participants can be seen to be affected by the constraints imposed by social interaction and to adapt to deal with those constraints
- ways in which the linguistic behavior of people with communication disorders can be seen to be treated as problematic by participants themselves within the interaction.

6.1.2 *Background*

The origins of conversation analysis lie in the work carried out in the 1960s and 1970s by the American sociologist Harvey Sacks and his colleagues Emanuel A. Schegloff and Gail Jefferson. Influenced by the studies of Erving Goffman on face-to-face interaction and, in particular, the sociological movement of ethnomethodology inspired by the work of Harold Garfinkel, conversation analysis emerged as a procedure for analyzing everyday talk-in-interaction and the institutionalized structural organizations or social conventions which underlie and inform the participants' behavior in any particular interaction (Heritage, 1984).

These conventions have a normative character, and it is by their (largely unconscious) orienting to these conventions that participants in an interaction produce verbal and non-verbal behavior which can be seen by recipients to be orderly, coherent and meaningful, and which produces the orderliness in naturally occurring interaction which CA investigations describe and explicate. The view within CA work (borne out by a large body of empirical findings) that naturally occurring talk-in-interaction is an orderly activity which can be analyzed rigorously and in its own right in order to uncover linguistic and other practices means it differs markedly from other approaches which have influenced clinical linguistics, including linguistic work in the tradition of Chomsky and cognitive (neuro)psychological approaches to normal and impaired language.

CA investigations have focused on the procedures by which speakers use their turns at talk to produce social actions (questioning, requesting, news-telling, etc.) and recipients display an understanding and response to these actions in subsequent turns. Within this analytic perspective, grammar, lexis and other aspects of language production are investigated in terms of their use as resources for turn/action construction, including how their deployment at a certain point within the turn or series of turns contributes to how that turn will be heard and responded to by its recipient(s) (Schegloff, 1996). A turn is constructed and interpreted in relation to the point in the interaction at which it is being produced. To understand an utterance recipients interpret it within the context of its immediately prior utterances, as it is assumed an utterance is constructed in relation to what has immediately preceded it unless the speaker displays otherwise. This use of sequential context as a resource for understanding an utterance can be particularly important for recipients in attempting to understand the utterances of people with communication disorders since these speakers' linguistic, phonetic or other limitations can regularly make understanding their utterances problematic. As will be noted below, when this resource is less available for recipients to draw on, such as when the person with the communication disorder attempts to initiate a new topic, or even a new sequence, recipients may have more difficulty in understanding the utterance. For similar reasons the sequential context provided by the preceding turns can also be a useful resource for people with communication disorders in constructing their turns, since they may, to a greater or lesser extent, be able to compensate for their lack of linguistic resources by designing their utterances to exploit the contextual resources available, in particular the sequential context provided by preceding talk.

CA research has also highlighted how the temporality and projectability of talk are of central importance to participants in producing and interpreting utterances. For example, there is a preference for progressivity in talk (see Lerner, 1996) such that what has been projected by the talk at this juncture to occur next is expected to be produced at that point. The delay or absence of the projected item(s) at the point due is noticeable and accountable and can open the speaker up to (often negative) inferences and can result in the production of certain actions by other participants. For example, first pair parts of sequences (Heritage, 1984), such as questions or requests, project that a corresponding second pair part should be produced in response. A delay or absence of the second pair part, for example of an answer following a question, can trigger inferences about the speaker, such as that he or she is unable or unwilling for some reason to answer the question, or has not heard the question. Similarly, when a speaker is producing a turn, each part of the emerging turn projects, and is heard by the recipient as projecting, how that turn is progressing towards possible completion and thus towards the point where another participant might non-interruptively take over the floor (Sacks, Schegloff, & Jefferson, 1974). Any delay in producing the next item due, particularly if there is a silence of over one second (Jefferson, 1989), is noticeable as such to recipients. One result can be that recipients may draw inferences as to the reason for the delay (inferring, for example, that the speaker is having difficulty in accessing or producing the required item). Another result can be that a co-participant takes the opportunity afforded by the delay to enter the turn at that point and take over the floor (Lerner, 1996). The linguistic limitations of people with communication disorders mean that it is often difficult for them to act in accordance with the constraints and expectations involved in talk-in-interaction, in particular the time constraints inherent in certain conventions of conversation such as the preference for progressivity. It can be as a consequence of the inability to produce the required item in the required way at the required time that a speaker's communication impairment may become particularly highlighted and exposed in interaction and take over as the focus of the conversational activity (e.g. the 'correct production sequences' in aphasic interaction described by Lock, Wilkinson and Bryan (2001)). Indeed, it can be in this way that a speaker may be exposed in everyday interaction *as* communication-impaired (e.g. the block of a person with a stammer which delays, or makes him or her unable to produce, an item in response to a question). On a more positive note, it has been argued, as will be seen below, that certain features of the linguistic behavior of people with communication disorders and their partners can be understood as attempts to adapt to the demands of talk-in-interaction in the light of the communication disorder.

The interactional and collaborative nature of naturally occurring talk is shown within CA investigations to be an integral aspect of how it is produced and understood. Recipients of talk, by their next turn response to a speaker's turn, are crucial, for example in how the content of that turn is registered and taken up, and an understanding of it (or not) displayed within the interaction. Similarly, the establishment of a new topic within the interaction regularly relies on how a recipient responds to a speaker's attempt to generate the new topic (Button & Casey, 1985). Unlike many other approaches to talk and/or language production which explicitly or implicitly treat spoken language as the product of a single speaker putting his or her thought or intention into verbal form, work within CA has argued that even the output of a single speaker can be shown to be an interactional and collaboratively co-constructed achievement due to the fact that how a speaker constructs his or her emerging turn can be seen to be affected by various aspects of recipients' behavior (Goodwin, 1979; Schegloff, 1982). This co-constructional feature of talk can be particularly important for interactions involving people with communication disorders since these speakers may often rely on their co-participants to assist, for example, in searching for a word, or in clarifying what the speaker with the communication disorder was trying to say.

The organization of repair in talk has been an area of CA which has been particularly drawn upon by those investigating interactions involving people with communication disorders. Repair refers to the mechanisms used by participants in dealing with troubles in talk-in-interaction and can be broken down into three parts: the repair initiation, the repair completion and the trouble source in the talk which is being treated by the participants as engendering the repair and which may or may not be an 'error' (Schegloff, Jefferson, & Sacks, 1977). Both the initiation and completion of repair can be carried out by 'self' (the participant whose trouble source is being dealt with) or 'other' (a participant other than the one whose trouble is being dealt with), thus giving various repair types such as 'self-initiated self-repair' or 'other-initiated self-repair' (see Levinson, 1983 for a description of possible repair types). Repair can raise various issues of incompetence to the surface of the interaction. This is part of the reason why, if repair is done at all, self-initiated self-repair is the most common form in normal talk since the speaker both initiates and completes the repair him- or herself, usually within the same turn, thus lessening the disruption caused by the repair to the topical talk which was in progress, and avoiding the need for others to be involved in solving the speaker's trouble. Repair is on the whole quick and successful in normal talk (Schegloff, Jefferson, & Sacks, 1977) with one or two repair tries usually proving sufficient to deal with the trouble.

Work on repair in normal talk is important for clinical linguistics in that it opens up for investigation the analysis of how interactions involving people with communication disorders may be disrupted by repair, what distinctive forms the repair can take, and how it may be different in, for example, quantity or length to that seen in normal talk. It also allows investigation of how participants work together in attempting to achieve repair, what methods they use and whether they are successful on any particular occasion. Finally, a focus on 'trouble source' rather than the notion of 'error' can be useful in relation to the analysis of communication disorders in talk. While the talk of people with communication disorders may contain a significant number of errors, many of these may be 'let pass' by the participants as being unproblematic in terms of the business at hand. An analysis of trouble sources, on the other hand, allows insights into what errors or other features of the talk the participants themselves treat as problematic and worthy of remedial action in the interaction. As such, an analysis of trouble sources and repair in general can provide the clinician with particularly useful information when attempting to target therapy at the particular problems the participants are experiencing in everyday life.

6.2   Acquired Communication Disorders

6.2.1   *Aphasia*

Aphasia was the first communication disorder to which CA was systematically applied by a number of investigators and it continues to be the focus of much analytic attention. A good deal of this attention has focused on repair sequences in aphasic talk (Laakso & Klippi, 1999; Lock, Wilkinson, & Bryan, 2001; Oelschlager & Damico, 2003).

It has been found, for example, that repair can be initiated frequently in aphasic talk. One form this can take is self-initiation by the aphasic speaker, for example in response to a linguistic error (e.g. a paraphasia) which he or she has produced and wishes to correct, or as a word search for an item which the speaker with aphasia has been unable to produce when due. Another form repair can regularly take in these interactions is that the person with aphasia other-initiates repair on the talk of a conversation partner (e.g. with 'pardon?') due to the person with aphasia's comprehension and/or hearing difficulties. A third common form is where the conversation partner other-initiates repair on the talk of the person with aphasia due, for example, to a difficulty in understanding what the person with aphasia means in his or her turn. Misunderstandings can also arise, for example when the conversation partner misunderstands what the person with aphasia meant in his or her turn (Wilkinson, 1999). Unlike repair sequences in normal talk, which are usually brief and successful, repair sequences in aphasic talk-in-interaction can regularly be long and can often be unsuccessful, despite sometimes prolonged attempts. Thus repair in aphasic talk can often be severely disruptive to the ongoing topical talk which was taking place prior to the repair as both participants become involved, regularly over long periods of time, in trying to elucidate some feature of what the aphasic speaker was trying to say. At these points in the interaction, therefore, the linguistic incompetence of the speaker with aphasia is particularly exposed, and in this environment emotions such as frustration, anger or embarrassment may be shown by the speaker with aphasia (Lock, Wilkinson, & Bryan, 2001).

Another major area of investigation has been turn and sequence organization in aphasic talk. Goodwin (1995, 2003), for example, has described some of the methods by which a nonfluent aphasic man whose lexical output was limited to 'yes', 'no' and 'and' was able to take an active part in conversations in the family home. Part of the reason why the man was able to engage interactively more successfully than would be assumed from a clinical assessment of his lexical and grammatical abilities was that he could be seen to make active use of other resources such as gesture, eye gaze and prosody. However, what Goodwin noted was of particular importance was the turns of the other participants; it was by carefully designing the types of turns they directed towards him and the ways in which they responded to his turns with attempts to elucidate what he was trying to say that his co-participants were particularly able to facilitate (or on occasion hinder) him in producing particular intelligible meanings and actions. Other investigations have examined ways in which aspects of aphasic language produced in turns within talk-in-interaction may be seen to be influenced by interactional factors. Heeschen and Schegloff (1999), for example, noted that the production of 'telegraphic' speech, a feature of agrammatism, could be seen to vary in occurrence in the talk of the aphasic speaker they analyzed. They suggested that telegraphic speech was particularly deployed by the speaker as a resource to mobilize the participation of the conversation partner and that there was evidence it might be particularly used in the interactional activity of story telling. Wilkinson, Beeke and Maxim (2003) described the use of certain distinctive lexical and grammatical features of turn construction used by two fluent aphasic speakers. They suggested that these turn-constructional methods might have interactional advantages for the speakers with aphasia including allowing them to achieve relatively good progressivity in talk. These methods also allowed them to construct turns at talk without the extensive repair and highlighting of linguistic incompetence which regularly occurred when they attempted to produce turns using the types of lexical and grammatical methods they would have employed before becoming aphasic.

6.2.2   Communication impairment in dementia and traumatic brain injury

People with dementia or traumatic brain injury (TBI) have been shown to display particular patterns of behavior in talk-in-interaction which have been hypothesized to be linked to their cognitive and communicative/linguistic deficits. For example, Perkins, Whitworth and Lesser (1998) noted that people with dementia of the Alzheimer type (DAT) displayed a pattern of attributable silences (Levinson, 1983) in their talk. One form this took was silence after the person with dementia had been selected to speak, for example through being asked a question. Another sequential location in which sometimes very long attributable silences occurred was within the turn of the speaker with dementia. Perkins, Whitworth and Lesser (1998) observed that the willingness of the conversation partners to tolerate these silences was important since, for example, if the person with dementia was given the time, he or she could, at least on some occasions, proceed with his or her talk as projected. In this pattern discussed by Perkins, Whitworth and Lesser, therefore, it is possible to see the important co-constructional role of the conversation partner in determining the eventual utterance of the person with dementia.

The manner in which people with dementia or TBI manage topic has been highlighted as a distinctive feature of their talk. For instance, the speaker may initiate a topic which can be seen to be treated by the conversation partner as in some way inappropriate or problematic, an example being speakers with dementia who may initiate topics based on hallucinations or delusions (Perkins, Whitworth, & Lesser, 1998). Another distinctive behavior is topic bias or repetitiveness which has been observed as a feature of talk in both people with dementia (Perkins et al., 1998; Spilkin & Bethlehem, 2003) and people with TBI (Perkins, Body, & Parker, 1995; Body & Parker, 2005). In their investigation of topic repetitiveness in a speaker with TBI, Perkins, Body and Parker (1995) noted two categories of topic which were repeatedly returned to by the speaker. One was certain strong personal opinions of the speaker and the other was a set of autobiographical episodes. They suggest that this behavior may be the result of a strategy employed by the speaker of reverting to these topics as 'safe' ones when other topics were proving difficult for him. As such it was suggested that the speaker's topic repetitiveness was not so much a direct reflection of underlying impairments as the result of a strategy to compensate for these impairments.

These types of behaviors involving topic by people with dementia or TBI can be seen to pose a dilemma for the speakers' conversation partners in terms of how to respond, for example whether or how much to draw attention to these behaviors and perhaps challenge them. In their description of Bernard, a man with TBI who displayed topic repetitiveness in conversation, Body and Parker (2005) noted that while the man's wife sometimes actively attempted to move the topic of talk away from his favored topics, other participants interacting with Bernard tended not to do this, a fact that Body and Parker hypothesized might be linked to politeness constraints.

6.2.3 *Acquired dysarthria and AAC use*

There has been little work published so far using CA to investigate interactions involving people with acquired dysarthria. In an examination of the talk of a man with severe dysarthria due to motor neurone disease (MND) in conversation with his mother, Bloch (2005) has described a particular pattern of the co-construction of turns which is present throughout their talk at the time of the recordings. This consists of the man with dysarthria producing an element of the turn, such as a word or even a phoneme, at a time and his mother repeating this element back to display her hearing of it. This system appears to have been developed by the interactants as a means of dealing with the dysarthric speaker's poor intelligibility and, while slow and labor-intensive, it does have the advantage that the interactants can monitor on a moment-by-moment basis whether they are in intersubjective agreement about what has just been produced or whether there is an understanding problem which has to be remedied before the turn can proceed.

Another possible means of communication in everyday life for people with dysarthria is the use of augmentative and alternative communication (AAC) systems such as voice output communication aids (VOCAs). In a study of VOCA use in conversation by people with acquired dysarthria and their everyday conversation partners, Bloch and Wilkinson (2004) noted a particular sequential location in which the VOCA was regularly used in these interactions, namely following other-initiations of repair by the conversation partner when he or she had not understood something the person with dysarthria had said. Bloch and Wilkinson also draw a distinction between intelligibility and understandability, observing that even when the 'speech' produced by the VOCA was intelligible, this was not always enough to make it understandable to the recipient in the conversation, since in conversation an important aspect of understanding an utterance is in understanding how it relates to the immediately preceding utterances. Since 'spoken' utterances generated using AAC devices are regularly slow to be produced, it is often the case that the recipient can be seen to have difficulty in following how the finally produced utterance relates to preceding talk and thus has a problem in understanding the utterance despite the fact it has been intelligible to him or her.

6.3   Developmental Communication Disorders

6.3.1   *Communication impairment in people with autism and developmental pragmatic difficulties*

A common feature of CA investigations into the interactions of people with autism is a focus on how certain autistic behaviors, which may appear quite random, incompetent and/or asocial, can, when analyzed in fine-grained detail in terms of the everyday interactional environments in which they were produced, be seen to be used with some degree of systematicity as interactional resources (see e.g. Damico & Nelson, 2005). While not denying the social and communicative limitations of the people with autism being investigated, these studies, in line with the predominant focus of CA work, concentrate particularly on what the interactants within the analysis actually *do* in interaction and *how* they do it (Dickerson, Rae, Stribling, Dautenhahn, & Werry, 2005).

An aspect of autism which has been particularly investigated in these analyses is echolalia and related phenomena (Dobbinson, Perkins, & Boucher, 2003). For example, in their study of Kevin, an 11-year-old boy with autism recorded at home and at school, Local and Wootton (1995) focus on one type of echo used in his interactions, immediate echolalia (i.e. the repetition of words from the immediate context), and in particular a subset of these echoes which they term 'unusual echoes'. This type of echo, which does not appear to occur in the talk of normally developing children, is often treated by Kevin's co-participant as puzzling since it sounds like 'empty repetition'; it occurs in sequential positions in talk where repetition is not likely to be an appropriate behavior, in particular in response to questions, and appears very closely phonetically matched to what the co-participant has just said. Local and Wootton (1995) suggest that an explanation for the production of this behavior may lie in the fact that repetition is a linguistic and interactional skill which the child is able to perform and as such a resource he can deploy within interaction to take a turn without having to engage more interactively with his co-participants, for example through attempting to provide an answer to a question.

The use of another kind of echo in autism, delayed echoes, is analysed by Tarplee and Barrow (1999). A delayed echo is an utterance which in some manner repeats talk produced on a prior occasion. The delayed echoes produced by Kenneth, the 3 year 9-months-old boy with autism analyzed by Tarplee and Barrow, have one particular source – talk by the characters in a cartoon film about dinosaurs which is a favorite of Kenneth's. Tarplee and Barrow note that these echoes are typically produced in Kenneth's interactions with his mother at points in the interaction at which Kenneth is *not* in a position of having to respond, and as such occur in a different sequential location to that of the immediate echoes described in Local and Wootton's

(1995) case study of Kevin. Kenneth regularly uses delayed echoes to initiate sequences of talk with his mother and elicit a response from her, sometimes leading to quite extended sequences of interaction. As such the delayed echoes are an interactional resource for Kenneth in that they provide "a specific, script-reliant strategy which Kenneth has for engaging his mother in bouts of reciprocal talk with him" (Tarplee & Barrow, 1999, p. 481). In this interactional use of delayed echoes Kenneth appears quite different to Kevin, who also has delayed echoes in his talk (see Wootton, 1999). Tarplee and Barrow suggest that the difference between the two children may have a number of possible causes, including Kenneth being more interactionally advanced than Kevin despite being chronologically younger.

Radford and Tarplee (2000) present a case study of David, a 10-year-old boy with pragmatic difficulties, recorded in interaction with peers in his language unit for pupils with specific language impairment and in the primary school which he also attended two days a week. A feature of David's talk is that he typically initiated new topics, often in quick succession, using certain types of boundaried topic initiations (Button & Casey, 1985) rather than the stepwise topic change (ibid.) more commonly used in peer interaction. Boundaried topic changes are commonly used in institutional talk such as the talk of teachers and doctors. Thus their repeated use in peer talk can appear quite abrupt and agenda-driven, and there is evidence in these interactions of David's peers on occasion explicitly resisting David's topic initiations by refusing to answer his questions. Radford and Tarplee (2000) hypothesize that a deficit in social cognition may be part of the explanation for David's interactional behaviors. They also note, however, that some of David's topic-initiating behaviors appear similar to those used in the language unit by, for example, David's teacher to elicit talk from the pupils in certain activities such as the 'news round', and they argue that David may be adopting these models when talking to his peers. If this is the case, they suggest, such a finding might have implications for how teachers and speech and language therapists work with children with pragmatic impairments in schools and language units.

6.3.2 Stammering

One feature of conversation analytic research into stammering has been a focus on how the conventions of conversation may impose constraints and pressures on speakers who stammer and how some of the behaviors of these speakers and their conversation partners may be understood as methods of dealing with these constraints and pressures. Acton (2004), for example, notes that the use of a first pair part by a co-participant can put pressure on a person who stammers since it may put the speaker 'on the spot' to produce a certain type of response and to produce it almost immediately. It may also make it difficult for the speaker within these constraints to avoid certain words or sounds which he or she might usually work to avoid attempting to say. Acton suggests that many of the behaviors of people who stammer, such as fillers or circumlocutions, which are often simply termed 'avoidance strategies', may turn out upon further investigation to be seen to have interactional benefits as methods of gaining or holding a turn despite not being able to produce the target word or sound at that point in the talk.

In a similar vein, Tetnowski and Damico (2001) describe the interactional behavior of a man with a moderate stammer who displayed a pattern of regularly shifting his gaze from his co-participant(s) at the point where he was dysfluent. Tetnowski and Damico suggest this behavior may be an interactional method which assists him in keeping the turn. Interactional achievements such as maintaining the turn despite dysfluency may also involve the conversation partner. Tetnowski and Damico describe a pattern in the interaction of another dyad where, when the person with a stammer was dysfluent, the conversation partner regularly responded with an acknowledgment in the form of a vocalization such as 'mmhm' and/or a head nod. Tetnowski and Damico note that this behavior by the co-participant is hearable as an encouragement to the dysfluent speaker to continue with the turn (as well as implicitly displaying to the dysfluent speaker that the co-participant is not going to challenge to take over the turn at that point).

6.3.3   *Developmental dysarthria and AAC use*

The work of Collins and her colleagues (Collins, 1996; Collins, Markovà, & Murphy, 1997) has highlighted some of the methods used and problems experienced by people with cerebral palsy in everyday interaction. Collins (1996), for example, notes that a common feature of the output of participants with cerebral palsy using AAC in interaction is the production of a series of nouns. This interactional method can be successful if the recipient is able to infer how the nouns relate to each other and how they relate to the interactional activity underway. The method was also, however, shown to create problems in interaction in that, for example, an AAC user's attempt to use a noun to shift topic was not initially understood as such since, with no overt sign from the AAC that this noun constituted a topic shift, the recipient attempted to make sense of the noun in terms of the ongoing topic in which they had been engaged.

As well as topic initiations, people with cerebral palsy using AAC have been shown to experience difficulty in successfully initiating another activity in interaction: conversational closings (Collins, Markovà, & Murphy, 1997). Closings in normal everyday interaction are usually subtly and collaboratively managed over a series of turns at talk, since if the closing is not carried out in the expected manner (for example if it is too abrupt) negative inferences may be drawn about the relationship of the participants involved (Levinson, 1983). Collins, Markova, and Murphy found that one way the speakers with cerebral palsy attempted to initiate closing was with gesture, but that this was regularly not picked up by the recipient. Speakers with cerebral palsy were also seen to use their AAC device to initiate the closing of the conversation.

However, when they did so, they regularly produced turns such as 'cheerio', which by the usual conventions of initiating closings appeared abrupt. Collins, Markovà, and Murphy suggest a number of reasons for this behavior, including the pragmatic skills of the speakers with cerebral palsy and the paucity of relevant vocabulary on the AAC device which could be used for pragmatic and interactional functions such as pre-closing moves. Collins and her colleagues discuss a number of implications of findings such as these, including the training of people with cerebral palsy and of their conversation partners, and changes to the design of AAC systems to make them more effective as resources for achieving successful interaction.

6.4   Conclusion

While CA has only relatively recently been systematically used as a method of analyzing interactions involving people with communication disorders, it has proved to be a procedure which can provide insights into a wide range of disorders including some, such as learning difficulties and hearing impairment, which for reasons of space have not been discussed here.

In terms of traditional clinical linguistic concerns, it can be argued that a limitation of a CA approach is that it does not provide an account of underlying (neuro)psychological or neurological causes of communication disorders and their 'symptoms'. In practice, therefore, a CA approach can be viewed as providing information complementary to that provided by, for example, psycholinguistic or neurolinguistic approaches. However, as was noted above, some studies using CA have explored how certain linguistic features of the talk of people with communication disorders may be accounted for, at least in part, in terms of social and interactional factors. Ultimately, it can be argued (see, for example, Heeschen & Schegloff, 2003), that it is naturally occurring interactive talk, rather than the production of, for example, single words or sentences under experimental conditions, which explanatory models or theories of communication disorders and their symptoms should be aiming to provide accounts for.

It can also be argued that, in terms of therapy for output difficulties, ultimately it is analyzable changes in naturally occurring interactional behavior that therapeutic programs should be designed to achieve and against which their effectiveness should be judged. The interactional approach provided by CA is one possible way of accomplishing this since it can be used as the basis for constructing and evaluating intervention programs which directly target the interactional behaviors of the person with the communication disorder and/or their everyday conversation partners. While promising, the use of such 'interaction training' has so far been limited to people with aphasia and their conversation partners (Booth & Perkins, 1999; Lock, Wilkinson, & Bryan, 2001). There appears no reason, however, why its general principles could not be applied to other communication disorders.

REFERENCES

Acton, C. (2004). A conversation analytic perspective on stammering: Some reflections and observations. *Stammering Research*, 1(3), 249–70.

Bloch, S. (2005). Co-constructing meaning in acquired speech disorders: Word and letter repetition in the construction of turns. In K. Richards and P. Seedhouse (eds.), *Applying Conversation Analysis* (pp. 38–55). Basingstoke: Palgrave Macmillan.

Bloch, S. and Wilkinson, R. (2004). The understandability of AAC: A conversation analytic study of acquired dysarthria. *Augmentative and Alternative Communication*, 20(4), 272–82.

Body, R. and Parker, M. (2005). Topic repetitiveness after traumatic brain injury: An emergent, jointly managed behaviour. *Clinical Linguistics and Phonetics*, 19(5), 379–92.

Booth, S. and Perkins, L. (1999). The use of conversation analysis to guide individualised advice to carers and evaluate change in aphasia: A case study. *Aphasiology*, 13(4–5), 283–304.

Button, G. and Casey, N. (1985). Topic nomination and topic pursuit. *Human Studies*, 8, 3–55.

Collins, S. (1996). Referring expressions in conversations between aided and natural speakers. In S. Von Tetzchner and M. H. Jehnsen (eds.), *Augmentative and Alternative Communication: European Perspectives* (pp. 89–100). London: Whurr.

Collins, S., Markovà, I., and Murphy, J. (1997). Bringing conversations to a close: The management of closings in interactions between AAC users and 'natural' speakers. *Clinical Linguistics and Phonetics*, 11, 467–93.

Damico, J. S. and Nelson, R. L. (2005). Interpreting problematic behaviour: Systematic compensatory adaptations as emergent phenomena in autism. *Clinical Linguistics and Phonetics*, 19(5), 405–17.

Dickerson, P., Rae, J., Stribling, P., Dautenhahn, K., and Werry, I. (2005). Autistic children's co-ordination of gaze and talk: Re-examining the 'asocial' autist. In K. Richards and P. Seedhouse (eds.), *Applying Conversation Analysis* (pp. 19–37). Basingstoke: Palgrave Macmillan.

Dobbinson, S., Perkins, M., and Boucher, J. (2003). The interactional significance of formulas in autistic language. *Clinical Linguistics and Phonetics*, 17(4–5), 299–307.

Ford, C. E., Fox, B. A., and Thompson, S. A. (eds.) (2002). *The Language of Turn and Sequence*. Oxford: Oxford University Press.

Goodwin, C. (1979). The interactive construction of a sentence in natural conversation. In G. Psathas (ed.), *Everyday Language: Studies in Ethnomethodology* (pp. 97–121). New York: Irvington.

Goodwin, C. (1995). Co-constructing meaning in conversations with an aphasic man. *Research on Language and Social Interaction*, 28, 233–60.

Goodwin, C. (2003). Conversational frameworks for the accomplishment of meaning in aphasia. In C. Goodwin (ed.), *Conversation and Brain Damage* (pp. 90–116). New York: Oxford University Press.

Heeschen, C. and Schegloff, E. A. (1999). Agrammatism, adaptation theory, conversation analysis: On the role of so-called telegraphic style in talk-in-interaction. *Aphasiology*, 13(4/5), 365–406.

Heeschen, C. and Schegloff, E. A. (2003). Aphasic agrammatism as interactional artifact and achievement. In C. Goodwin (ed.), *Conversation and Brain Damage* (pp. 231–82). New York: Oxford University Press.

Heritage, J. (1984). *Garfinkel and Ethnomethodology*. Cambridge: Polity Press.

Jefferson, G. (1989). Preliminary notes on a possible metric which provides for a 'standard maximum' silence of approximately one second in conversation. In D. Roger and P. Bull (eds.), *Conversation: An Interdisciplinary Perspective* (pp. 166–96). Clevedon: Multilingual Matters.

Laakso, M. and Klippi, A. (1999). A closer look at the 'hint and guess' sequences in aphasic conversation. *Aphasiology*, 13(4–5), 345–64.

Lerner, G. (1996). On the 'semi-permeable' character of grammatical units in conversation: Conditional entry into the turn space of another speaker. In E. Ochs, E. A. Schegloff, and S. A. Thompson (eds.), *Interaction and Grammar* (pp. 238–76). Cambridge: Cambridge University Press.

Levinson, S. (1983). *Pragmatics*. Cambridge: Cambridge University Press.

Local, J. and Wootton, A. (1995). Interactional and phonetic aspects of immediate echolalia in autism: A case study. *Clinical Linguistics and Phonetics*, 9(2), 155–84.

Lock, S., Wilkinson, R., and Bryan, K. (2001). *SPPARC (Supporting Partners of People with Aphasia in Relationships and Conversation): A Resource Pack*. Bicester, Oxon: Speechmark.

Oelschlager, M. and Damico, J. (2003). Word searches in aphasia: A study of the collaborative responses of communicative partners. In C. Goodwin (ed.), *Conversation and Brain Damage* (pp. 211–30). New York: Oxford University Press.

Perkins, L., Whitworth, A., and Lesser R. (1998). Conversing in dementia: A conversation analytic approach. *Journal of Neurolinguistics*, 11, 33–53.

Perkins, M., Body, R., and Parker, M. (1995). Closed head injury: Assessment and remediation of topic bias and repetitiveness. In M. Perkins and S. Howard (eds.), *Case Studies in Clinical Linguistics* (pp. 293–320). London: Whurr.

Radford, J. and Tarplee, C. (2000). The management of conversational topic by a ten year old with pragmatic difficulties. *Clinical Linguistics and Phonetics*, 14(5), 387–403.

Sacks, H., Schegloff, E. A., and Jefferson, G. (1974). A simplest systematics for the organization of turn-taking in conversation. *Language*, 50(4), 696–735.

Schegloff, E. A. (1982). Discourse as an interactional achievement: some uses of 'uh huh' and other things that come between sentences. In D. Tannen (ed.), *Georgetown University Roundtable on Languages and Linguistics* (pp. 71–93). Washington, DC: Georgetown University Press.

Schegloff, E. A. (1996). Turn organization: One intersection of grammar and interaction. In E. Ochs, E. A. Schegloff, and S. A. Thompson (eds.), *Interaction and Grammar* (pp. 52–133). Cambridge: Cambridge University Press.

Schegloff, E. A., Jefferson, G., and Sacks, H. (1977). The preference for self-correction in the organization of repair for conversation. *Language*, 53, 361–82.

Smith, B. R. and Leinonen, E. (1992). *Clinical Pragmatics: Unravelling the Complexities of Communicative Failure*. London: Chapman and Hall.

Spilkin, M. and Bethlehem, D. (2003). A conversation analysis approach to facilitating communication with memory books. *Advances in Speech-Language Pathology*, 5(2), 105–18.

Tarplee, C. and Barrow, E. (1999). Delayed echoing as an interactional resource: A case study of a three year old child on the autistic spectrum. *Clinical Linguistics and Phonetics*, 13(6), 449–82.

Tetnowski, J. A. and Damico, J. S. (2001). A demonstration of the advantages of qualitative methodologies in stuttering research. *Journal of Fluency Disorders*, 26, 1–26.

Wilkinson, R. (1999). Sequentiality as a problem and a resource for intersubjectivity in aphasic conversation: Analysis and implications for therapy. *Aphasiology*, 13(4–5), 327–43.

Wilkinson, R., Beeke, S., and Maxim, J. (2003). Adapting to conversation: On the use of linguistic resources by speakers with fluent aphasia in the construction of turns at talk. In C. Goodwin (ed.), *Conversation and Brain Damage* (pp. 59–89). New York: Oxford University Press.

Wootton, A. (1999). An investigation of delayed echoing in a child with autism. *First Language*, 19, 359–81.

7 Clinical Sociolinguistics

JACK S. DAMICO AND
MARTIN J. BALL

7.1 Introduction

The interaction between language and society has been one of the major concerns of linguistic science over the last 40 years, but until recently the findings of sociolinguistics have not been applied to speech and language disorders. In this chapter we outline some of the areas of research subsumed under the heading of sociolinguistics, and show how they have been applied to communication disorders in recent times. However, the area of sociolinguistic concern is a broad one; covering language variation and change at the micro- and macro-levels, language planning, bilingualism, discourse, and pragmatics. Some of these topics are dealt with in other chapters in this volume (see chapters 9 by Hua & Wei, 1 by Müller, Guendouzi, & Wilson, 5 by Perkins and 6 by Wilkinson), therefore this chapter is more narrowly focused, mainly on the variationist paradigm developed in the early work of such researchers as Labov (e.g. 1963, 1966a, 1972a, b) and Trudgill (e.g. 1972, 1974) among many others.

Variationist sociolinguistics developed partly out of the long-standing dialectology tradition (concerned with preserving the older forms of regional speech), and partly in reaction to the dominant paradigm of generative linguistics with its emphasis on the 'ideal speaker-listener' and on the exclusion of variation in linguistic output in preference for describing the invariate underlying linguistic competence. Ball (1988) describes some of the forerunner studies in the 1950s, but the first major studies in this new field of sociolinguistics appeared in the 1960s (for example, Labov, 1963, 1966a). These scholars investigated linguistic variation at various levels (although phonology has been the main area of study) and looked for correlations between the patterns of variation found and both linguistic and non-linguistic factors.

In order to do this, sociolinguists devised the unit of analysis termed the *variable* (see Wardhaugh, 1998 for further details). A linguistic variable has two or more *variants*; for example, in many dialects of English there is a variable (h) which has the variants [h] and [Ø] (i.e. the [h] may be pronounced or omitted). The use of these variants can be correlated with non-linguistic (or social) variables, for example, style, speaker's social class, sex, or age.[1] Each of these social variables will also consist of variants: style can be divided into varying degrees of formality or casualness; social class into categories such as lower, middle and upper; sex into male and female; and age into different bands according to the focus of investigation. Findings, therefore, give the degree of correlation between the usage of a linguistic variant (e.g. prestige [h] or vernacular [Ø] for the (h) variable described above) and the speaker's social class, the style of the speaker's interaction, their sex, or age. Such correlations, of course, are not causative, but may be considered predictive.

Much of Labov's work (reported for example in Labov, 1972b) suggested that variables fall into three main groupings. *Indicators* are those variables that show most non-linguistic correlation in terms of class or other group member-ship, whereas *markers* are those showing most correlation to the style variable. Finally, there is the category of *stereotype*, which is a variable that (unlike indic-ators and markers) operates above the level of conscious awareness within a speech community,[2] and as a result is often stigmatized.

Both the development of variables as a methodological device, and the clas-sification of variables into indicators, markers and stereotypes, may be applied to clinical assessment. Knowledge of the range of linguistic variables available in a dialect and the correlational patterns of these linguistic indices with social variables allows us to establish a realistic set of target forms and to determine whether a client's realizations map onto them. Further, an understanding of the classification of variables allows the clinician to ascertain whether the patterns of usage correspond to those of the speech community.

Sociolinguists have also taken the study of language variation to a more macrolinguistic level, including bi- and multilingualism, and the special case of *diglossia*. Bilingualism as a term covers both societal bilingualism (a society where two languages are spoken, but where speakers themselves are not neces-sarily bilingual), and individual bilingualism (see further in Edwards, 2005). The study of individual bilingualism encompasses measures of degree of proficiency and dominance in the relevant languages by speakers, patterns of code switching (i.e. switching in and out of different languages for stylistic or other effects), interference between languages (e.g. using the grammatical structure of one language with lexis from another, or borrowing a single lexical item perhaps to fill a word gap in one of the languages), and an invest-igation of the domains of usage of the two languages (e.g., one language may be restricted to family use rather than extended to wider or official usage). Clearly, all these features may be of importance for a speech-language path-ologist, and we return to issues of assessment with bilinguals later.

Diglossia is a form of bilingualism in which one language is used for formal, educational, and official usage in a community, and another for everyday, informal use (see Müller & Ball, 2005). The classic example is Arabic, where colloquial forms of the language are unwritten, and differ widely from region to region, while standard Arabic is the written form, and is fairly homogeneous.

However, this model can also be found in parts of the US where Spanish plays the role of the colloquial variety and English the standard variety – often termed the L (Low) and the H (High) varieties respectively – or in the UK where one of the north Indian languages may be L to English as the H. Knowledge of the domain-specific features of diglossia, and the differing status and literacy abilities associated with the L and H varieties will be of help to clinicians assessing certain bilingual clients.

As we can see from this discussion, different varieties of a language (and indeed different languages in the case of bilingualism) have differing degrees of prestige in a speech community, usually reflecting different degrees of power held by particular groups. The relationship of language and power is an important area of sociolinguistic concern (see Damico, Simmons-Mackie, & Hawley, 2005). Research in this area has shed light on how interactants exercise power through language, for example through forms of address, topic management, and speaking turn negotiation. Some issues relating to language and power in the clinical context will be discussed below.

Many other aspects of sociolinguistic research have had to be omitted from this introduction for reasons of space, but readers unfamiliar with the area are recommended to consult contributions to Ball (2005). Sociophonetic variation is covered in more detail in Docherty and Khattab (chapter 37 in this volume).

A specific clinical application for sociolinguistics was first articulated in the work of Wolfram (for example, 1977, 1983, 1993). In his 1993 paper, Wolfram asks: "How does the variation model developed originally in sociolinguistics apply to communication disorders? . . . One way relates to the interpretation of normative variable behavior and the other to an understanding of change in the remediation process" (Wolfram, 1993, p. 13).

We turn our attention next to issues of assessment and normative variation.

7.2   Sociolinguistic Sensitivity in Assessment

As noted above, some of the earliest attempts to apply the insights of sociolinguistic research to the clinical situation were in the area of sociolinguistic sensitivity in assessment. We can illustrate the dangers of ignoring the sociolinguistic characteristics of a speech community at various levels of linguistic structure (taking English as our example). At the phonetic realization level, we can note the heavy affrication of fortis stops in Liverpool English (though subject to social class differentiation), the lack of aspiration in this same plosive class by bilingual Spanish- and French-English speakers (and indeed in some regional varieties of Scottish English), and the diphthongization of front lax vowels in certain phonetic environments in Southern US English, as examples of realizations that could be deemed disordered by a clinician lacking sociolinguistic awareness.

At the phonological level, the dental fricatives are either totally absent, or stylistically variable in several varieties of English (Black English of both the

US and the UK; London English, Caribbean English, and so on); /h/ dropping is common in many areas, and again is often stylistically controlled; and onset clusters with /s/+C+/r/ (especially /str-/) are realized with initial /ʃ/ in the younger persons' speech of many English speech communities (see Ball & Rutter, 2005). Lack of sociolinguistic awareness could lead to many of these non-standard variants being judged as incorrect in the assessment of clients with potential speech disorders.

At the morphophonological level, the progressive aspect marker *-ing* has two stylistically controlled variant realizations, [ɪŋ] and [ɪn], in many regional varieties of the language. Inflectional morphology is also sociolinguistically variable to some extent: Black English varieties may variably omit the *-s* morpheme to mark third person singular present tense on lexical verbs; in derivational morphology we can note that the *-ly* de-adjectival adverb marker is virtually absent in many vernacular forms of English.

Syntactically a wide range of variation may be encountered. These include, for example, double negatives ("not seen no one"), zero relativizer ("he's a lad likes his black pudding"), and double modals ("I might could do it"), among many others. Use of these forms is often correlated with both social class and style, but as with the other levels discussed above, they are all liable to mis-interpretation as incorrect forms by assessors or assessments that are not sociolinguistically sensitive.

As a final point, we need also to consider that lexical variation is also common, and that lexical items may be specific to a regional variety ('lift' versus 'elevator'), to an ethnic variety (Irish English 'guards' or *'gardaí'* for 'policemen'), or to a regional, social class and style combination ('loo', 'john', 'WC', 'lavatory', 'toilet'; 'bathroom', 'men's/ladies' room' etc). Picture-naming assessments (for example of phonology) are often problematic in this area, as lexical items that are common in one variety may not be in another. Examples include the Santa Claus/Father Christmas difference between US and UK English, and the fact that in Australia squirrels are absent, and so pictures of squirrels may elicit 'wombat' or 'possum' from Australian children. (Both these examples are from the Goldman Fristoe Test of Articulation, Goldman, & Fristoe, 2000.)[3]

Ball (1992) was an early attempt to provide a means of noting possible sociolinguistic variation in a clinical assessment of speech or language. This paper was written within the tradition of linguistic profiling, as developed by Crystal (Crystal, Fletcher, & Garman, 1976; Crystal, 1982), and suggested adding to profiling charts an extra chart allowing a fairly detailed description of the target variety of the language, including variables that were correlated with style, and other non-linguistic variables.

Clearly, a more manageable solution is to provide assessments that cover ranges of sociolinguistically acceptable target forms for specific dialects or groups of dialects; in this regard, we can note that considerable research has been undertaken on African American English (see review in Wolfram, 2005). Other dialects divergent from standard forms that should be considered include Appalachian English, Cajun English, and Southern States English in the US,

Lowland Scots in the UK, Newfoundland English in Canada, and forms of English used by indigenous peoples in North America, Australia and New Zealand. National standards of English used in countries such as India, Pakistan, Bangladesh, Sri Lanka, Singapore and the Hong Kong Special Administrative Region of China among others might also be candidates for variety-specific assessments.

Oetting (2005) describes one step along this path: the *Diagnostic Evaluation of Language Variation (DELV)*, devised by Seymour, Roeper and de Villiers (2003). This was designed to assess children with a range of American English dialects (including those noted above), and was standardized on over a thousand children, 63 percent of whom were speakers of non-standard varieties. Test items cover phonology, syntax, semantics and pragmatics, and its goal is to allow clinicians to note which variety of American English the client is a speaker of, and to allow classification of the client as impaired or not impaired in speech and/or language.

Oetting also looked at a set of three measures often used in language analysis: mean length of utterance (MLU; Brown, 1973), Developmental Sentence Score (DSS; Lee, 1974), and the Index of Productive Syntax (IPSyn; Scarborough, 1991). She notes that these language sample measures are often avoided with non-standard dialect speakers, as there is a lack of data to show normative patterns outside the mainstream variety of English. She reports on an earlier study (Oetting, Cantrell, & Horohov, 1999) which used language samples from 31 children speaking a rural variety of Southern US English, and analyzed the data using the three measures just described. IPSyn does not require the scoring of individual utterances, rather the analyst searches the sample for examples of 56 prescribed structures. As these structures occur in most varieties, the IPSyn score was not adversely affected in Oetting, Cantrell and Horohov's study. However, both MLU and DSS did show reduced scores. Oetting's (2005) work reports a similar study with African American English-speaking children, with broadly similar results. Oetting (2005) suggests that experimental probes can be developed that avoid the differences between standard and non-standard versions of a language. One example is the non-word repetition task, where children hear and repeat nonsense words of varying length. Studies reported by Oetting show that using these tasks reduces differences in scores between standard and non-standard dialect speakers, but clearly tasks such as this are limited in their evaluative potential.

Moving beyond varieties of a single language, sociolinguistic sensitivity in assessment is also important with bi- and multilingual clients. Wei, Miller, Dodd and Hua (2005) address the issue of how speech pathologists can distinguish between linguistic variation due to bilingualism and language pathology. They stress the importance of adequate assessment procedures and, referring to the work of Taylor, Payne and Anderson (1987), they describe both pre-assessment, assessment, and post-assessment desiderata. For example, before undertaking an assessment, a clinician should become familiar with the cultural, social and cognitive norms of the individual's community, and with the linguistic and communicative norms of the individual's speech community (Wei, Miller, Dodd, & Hua, 2005, p. 203). At the assessment stage, "culturally valid procedures must be employed to obtain a sample of the client's communicative behaviour" (ibid.); and at the post-assessment stage, an important consideration must be the definition of communication pathology by the client's peers and community.

Points to be stressed about bilingual clients in the training of clinicians include the facts that bilingual clients need to be compared with similar bilinguals rather than with monolinguals, that code switching and mixing is normal, and may be used playfully by bilingual children, and that bilinguals may show evidence of 'errors' in the non-dominant language that should not be considered examples of language disorders. Wei, Miller, Dodd, and Hua (2005) also list points suggestive of disorder in bilinguals and points suggestive of imperfect acquisition (perhaps of a non-dominant language). Among the former are the inability to produce sounds which are common in the speech of children of the relevant age irrespective of their target language, inabilities in the production or comprehension of words familiar to children of the relevant age irrespective of their target language, and inability to produce grammatical sentences irrespective of the language the child is trying to speak. Among the latter are an unbalanced vocabulary between the languages, speech errors in one language while the same or similar target sounds are correct in the other, and ability to produce grammatical sentences in only one language.

Due to the wide range of possible languages spoken by bi- and multilingual clients, and the different patterns of use between the client's languages, it is of course difficult to acquire the degree of sociolinguistic awareness needed to assess potential communication disorders adequately. Nevertheless, the insights of sociolinguistic research into bilingualism can go some way to helping clinicians in this regard.

Sociolinguistic awareness in assessment should be coupled (as Wolfram, 1993 noted and as referred to above) to a similar awareness in remediation. This should include not only sociolinguistically relevant targets, but also an ability to distinguish between transitional error patterns as the client moves towards a relevant target, and the ability to know when a client has reached a realization that is acceptable in their variety of the language even if not in the standard form.

7.3   Sociolinguistics of Sign Language

The area of communication disorders where classical variationist sociolinguistics has been applied most directly is the study of sign language. This is because the movements that make up the signs themselves can vary, and thus different sign variables can be established, and the variants of these variables can be correlated to non-linguistic variables, as we have described above. Early work in this regard can be found in Woodward (1980), who found that variation in signs correlated to a range of social factors, including region, age, and ethnic background. Lucas (1989) contains a collection of contributions from different scholars on the sociolinguistics of sign language from both micro- and macrosociolinguistic viewpoints, including aspects of discourse, language contact, language planning, and language attitude. Lucas (2001) also covers some of these topics, bringing in also the topics of bi- and multilingualism.

Lucas, Bailey and Kelly (2005), and the references therein, describe some of the sociolinguistic studies undertaken on American Sign Language (ASL), as well as broader sociolinguistic aspects of deaf culture. Lucas (1995) and Lucas, Bailey and Valli (2001) report on some of the findings of a large-scale quantit- ative investigation of variation in ASL, using the Labovian model of socio- linguistic methodology referred to earlier.

Data for this study were collected from seven sites in the US, covering the northeast, the south, the midwest, California, and the northwest. At each site groups of informants were recruited. These were divided into three age groups (15–25; 26–54; 55+), two social classes (middle and working), and two ethnicities (African American and White). (At three sites, no African Americans could be recruited; and there were too few African American middle-class informants over 55 to fill that category.) In total there were 207 ASL signers in the study, with each cell containing between 2 and 7 signers (a cell being a grouping of informants by region, age, class and ethnicity).

The aims of the study were to describe phonological, morphosyntactic, and lexical variation in ASL, and its correlation with regional, age, class, and ethnicity variables. Among the linguistic variables studied were phonological ones, such as the sign DEAF, and the location of signs represented by the verb KNOW, morphosyntactic ones (in this case, overt and null subject pronouns), and lexical ones: "34 signs selected to illustrate phonological change as well as lexical innovation stemming from new technology, increased contact with Deaf people in other countries, and contemporary social attitudes" (see Lucas, Bailey, & Kelly, 2005, p. 256).

Looking at the patterns of usage of the sign DEAF, one of the phonological variables studied, it was found that of all the possible forms for this sign, only three were extracted from the videotape, even though 1,618 examples were present in the data. The citation form, which appears in sign language diction- aries and is taught in sign language classes, has the sign beginning just below the ear, and ending near the corner of the mouth. A second variant begins at the corner of the mouth and moves upward to the ear (this is known as the 'chin to ear' variant). In the third variant, known as the "contact-cheek" variant, the index finger contacts the lower cheek but does not move up.

The authors note that their results indicated that variation in the form of DEAF is "systematic and conditioned by multiple linguistic and social factors, including grammatical function, the location of the following segment, dis- course genre (narrative or conversation), age and region" (ibid., p. 257). The authors also note that these results confirm the earlier finding of Lucas (1995), where it was shown that the strongest effect on a signer's choice of one of the three variants was the grammatical function of DEAF, rather than the features of the preceding or following sign. For this item, the researchers first examined the choice between the standard variant and either of the two non-standard ones; they then looked at the choice between the two non-standard variants. The choice between the standard and either of the non-standard variants correlated with grammatical function and discourse genre, whereas the choice between the two non-standard variants correlated with both grammatical function and following segment. Non-linguistic variables were also important in the choice between the variants, in particular, region and age. For example, in California, Louisiana, Virginia, and Washington, older and younger signers preferred non-standard variants, whereas those in the middle age group preferred the standard variant. In Kansas and Missouri, the non-standard variants were preferred by all age groups, with the opposite in Massachusetts. In Maryland, the older age groups preferred non-standard variants, while the other age groups preferred the standard. Lucas, Bailey and Kelly (2005) explain the age differences through looking at the history of ASL in education. The middle age group were those mostly preferring the standard variant, and they would have been schooled at a time when ASL had just been recognized as a language, and a prescriptive approach to teaching 'correct' signs was in evidence. On the other hand, the older speakers had grown up in a period of non-recognition of ASL, so would not have had exposure to 'correct' forms. Finally, younger speakers were educated when a more relaxed attitude to sign variation was in evidence, so in some areas of the country they too developed a more open attitude to non-standard variants.

7.4   Language and Power in the Clinic

Another clear linkage between sociolinguistics and communication disorders is the role that sociolinguistic knowledge plays in understanding the remediation context (Wolfram, 1977, 1983, 1993). Since the discipline of communicative disorders is an intervention-oriented profession, understanding how we accomplish various facets of therapy is serious business; we strive to understand this process because our worth as a clinical discipline rests on how well we address identified problems through therapeutic encounters. Since the 1970s, sociolinguistic research has influenced our efforts in clinical research.

As interventionists, we are concerned with how things are accomplished during therapy and what variables act upon the therapeutic context to drive the necessary (and successful) social actions. Therapy is a complex social enterprise wherein specific goals are established and the methods for approaching these goals must be initially determined and then implemented (e.g., Kovarsky & Duchan, 1997; Wells, 1999; Lahey, 2004). For this "clinical business" to occur, it is essential that someone can take the lead in the planning and execution of therapy. That is, someone must have some form of directive influence and responsibility. Additionally, since there is always a complex and dynamic negotiation of roles, responsibilities, and obligations during the thera-peutic work, there must be an understanding of how the social and interactional negotiations are handled from the perspective of both clinician and client. This is where sociolinguistics contributes some necessary insight.

Since sociolinguistics has a long history of focusing on linguistic variation and interaction as it is juxtaposed with social action within various interactive encounters, both the methodologies and the knowledge base of sociolinguis-tics can be effectively employed to better understand the therapeutic con-text. Given the importance of the directive function in therapy (e.g., Ulichny & Watson-Gegeo, 1989; Panagos, 1996), sociolinguists' work on the influences of interactional power upon the actions and reactions of participants in inter-active contexts is especially salient. This work can be (and has been) employed to increase understanding of the interactions between clinicians and clients during therapy. Specifically, sociolinguistics helps our understanding of the ways that this complex power negotiation is implemented, and it is through the investigation of interactional power within therapy that sociolinguistics effectively informs our clinical arena in communication disorders. Simply put, by employing sociolinguistic research on interactional power within the thera-peutic context, our remedial encounters become clearer to us and we can make them more effective.

There are several ways that sociolinguistic research has assisted our under-standing of interactional power in therapeutic contexts. First, it has enabled us to see this operational construct from a robust rather than a naive perspective. As discussed by Tannen (1987), interactional power is a complicated phenom-enon. It is a social construct that is more relational than discrete; rather than existing as a separate and definable social trait, it exists only as the emergent outgrowth of interactive processes between two or more interactants. In this sense, interactional power is a dynamic reflection of intersecting attitudes, expectations and behaviors across individuals; it is not a simple or direct extension of an external reality. These points are forcefully demonstrated in the sociolinguistic literature where interactional power is revealed to be multimodal and multidimensional in manifestation (e.g., Brown & Gilman, 1960; Fairclough, 1989; Grimshaw, 1990), culturally influenced (Gumperz, 1982; Tannen, 1985; Schiffrin, 1987), and contextually relative (Hymes, 1967; Halliday, 1973; Goodwin & Duranti, 1992). These characteristics and the work done in defining this interactional concept have attempted to account for the complexity of the phenomenon and, consequently, interactional studies of clinician–client dyads have benefited from this more circumspect viewpoint (Panagos, 1996). For extended discussions on the complexity of interactional powewr and its characteristics, the reader is directed to discussions in Damico, Simmons-Mackie and Hawley (2005), Kedar (1987) and Schiffrin (1994).

A second sociolinguistic influence when addressing clinical discourse was the work done in identifying many of the ways that interactional power was manifested during social activities. These manifestations became foci for much of the initial work on interactional power in clinical contexts and although subsequent research has identified a number of other manifestations, these early linguistic and interactive variables influenced clinical research focusing on power, the awareness of the power differential in therapy, and how clinicians typically manipulate this differential to guide the therapeutic enterprise (e.g., Panagos, 1996; Kovarsky & Duchan, 1997). Given our understanding of sociolinguistics, it should not be surprising that there are a number of culturally conventionalized signals that assist in the interpretation of the power dynamic during interactions. Within certain caveats (see Damico, Simmons-Mackie, & Hawley, 2005), variables like *forms of address* (e.g., Brown & Gilman, 1960; Brown & Ford, 1961), *negotiation of speaking turns* (e.g., Brown & Levinson, 1987; Fairclough, 1989), *topic selection and maintenance* (Shuy, 1987; Walker, 1987), *questioning* (Tannen, 1987), *the structuring of interaction via discourse markers* (Kovarsky, 1990) or *response structures* (Simmons-Mackie, Damico, & Damico, 1999), and the *use of evaluative statements* (e.g., Mehan, 1979; Cazden, 1988; Ulichny & Watson-Gegeo, 1989) are just some of the manifestations noted. Attention to these and other emergent manifestations of the power differential in therapeutic contexts has created greater awareness and beneficial discussions regarding this important dimension of social/therapeutic encounters.

The third sociolinguistic influence on the study of interactional power in the clinical context involved the methodologies that were made available and the creation of a research context that focused upon complex social phenomena during social and therapeutic activities. In an excellent overview of the emergence of "speech therapy discourse", John Panagos (1996) mentions how Prutting and colleagues (Prutting, Bagshaw, Goldstein, Juskowitz, & Umen, 1978), Bobkoff (1982), Ripich (1982), and Panagos himself (e.g., Panagos & Fry, 1976; Panagos & Griffith, 1981) were influenced by the work of Hymes, Labov and others who focused on the concept of "communicative competence", on models of interaction in social life (e.g., Hymes, 1967), or on therapeutic discourse itself (Labov & Fanshel, 1977). By providing both methods and a context for investigation, the discipline of sociolinguistics influenced these "pioneers" in the study of clinical discourse from a sociolinguistic perspective. Their work, in turn, gave rise to a generation of research that can point to the confluence of the ethnography of communication with sociolinguistics as an essential catalyst for much of the work done in this clinical area.

While a number of studies over the past 30 years have focused on language and power in the clinical context, only a few will be discussed in this review as an illustration of the influence of sociolinguistics. There are, however, many other studies currently available in the communication disorders literature that demonstrate a direct lineage to similar sociolinguistic work. For further information on specific studies, the reader is directed to Panagos (1996) and Ripich and Creaghead (1994).

As mentioned above, several of the earliest investigations of therapeutic discourse in the discipline of communicative disorders were influenced by the work of Hymes (1967) and Labov and Fanshel (1977). These early studies obtained similar results to some of the studies of interaction in general conversation or in targeted teaching/learning encounters (Mehan, 1979; Cazden, 1988). Indeed, many of the same social dimensions were found to be operative, with one individual within the dyad typically being more dominant than the other. For example, in perhaps the earliest published study from a sociolinguistic perspective, Prutting and colleagues (1978) investigated therapy discourse to determine how clinician and client communicated during therapy. They found a definite asymmetrical pattern in which the clinician dominated the conversational space by approximately a 2:1 ratio. Influenced by sociolinguistic research, Prutting and colleagues also noted how this asymmetry was constructed. They found that the specific types of interactions constructed, the speech acts employed (e.g., "request type communicative acts"), the way topic selection was controlled, and the clinician's evaluative statements following client response all operated to shift a large power differential in favor of the clinician. This study had an important impact on the discipline, and other studies followed, including a later study that generally replicated the findings of Prutting and colleagues (Becker & Silverstein, 1983).

Given the results of the Prutting study and having an orientation toward the importance of the clinician during therapy, a number of subsequent studies have focused on *how* the interactional power of the clinician was established and maintained during the therapeutic encounter. Letts (1985), for example, explicitly discussed the clinician's agenda for conducting therapy and defended the need for clinician therapeutic control. She found that there were a number of rules or guidelines, around which clinicians seemed to organize therapy to create therapeutic control. For example, in her investigation, the clinician controlled the activities during therapy, how long each activity ran, and the feedback provided. Additionally, this feedback was oriented to more evaluative functions than pedagogical ones. Further, the flow of information about the client's performance and about how to modify that performance was also used as "interactional currency" to establish and maintain therapeutic control. Letts emphasized that the way the therapy session was organized is one mechanism for creating and manipulating interactional power. Much of the work of Panagos and his students also focused on the structure of the therapeutic encounter and the therapy agenda as it was formulated and advanced (e.g., Ripich & Panagos, 1985; Bobkoff & Panagos, 1986; Panagos, Bobkoff, & Scott, 1986).

In another study specifically influenced by sociolinguistic research, Kovarsky (1989, 1990) employed Schiffrin's (1987) description of discourse markers as elements of speech that act to bracket units of talk, and he investigated how the discourse markers that he identified (e.g., *okay, oh, so, well, now*) were employed to organize the actual therapeutic interactions at the local level (Goodwin & Heritage, 1990). His study was a deeper analysis of the actual conversational mechanisms and how they accomplished the work of interactional power and dominance. In his analysis, Kovarsky found three purposes for the identified discourse markers: control, evaluation, and response to informative interactions. Without question, however, the *control function* predominated both the analysis and the therapeutic context; while only one function was explicitly described as *control*, to some degree the other two functions (evaluation, the acceptance of information) also pivot on control and are functions of interactional power.

Finally, Damico and Damico (1997) borrowed from the sociolinguistic insights of Ulichny and Watson-Gegeo (1989) to demonstrate how clinicians employ another interactional device – the dominant interpretive framework (DIF) – to establish and maintain both evaluative control and the impact of learning in the therapy session. Consistent with Ulichny and Watson-Gegeo, this study detailed how clinicians used various interactional strategies to shift client responses toward preferred and expected types of answers and belief systems. In doing so, the clinicians were able to force their own interpretation of the most appropriate and acceptable answers onto responses that were actually correct. That is, the clinicians demonstrated interactional power and dominance by shaping the responses of the clients to fit the clinicians' own interpretations.

Within the clinical realm, this sociolinguistic focus on the relationship between language and power has had a pervasive impact. Much of what we understand about therapeutic interaction in terms of its complexity, its systematicity, and its impact on both learning and social management has been generated by sociolinguistic influences. This, in turn, has spawned greater attention to this facet of clinical activity. The resultant research and its applications have benefited clinicians and clients alike.

7.5   Sociolinguistics and Literacy

Another area that we believe has benefited greatly from sociolinguistic research in the past and that can continue to do so in the future is literacy research and teaching. From the emergence of the field as a separate subdiscipline in the 1960s, sociolinguistics has greatly influenced general pedagogy in literacy education. In fact, one of the earliest practical successes for the field was the refutation of the "deprivation model" which was employed by some educational psychologists to explain what they considered the reduced language spoken by some disadvantaged and minority students (e.g., Bereiter & Englemann, 1966). These psychologists argued that while disadvantaged children did have command of some language, the language they spoke was stunted and caused educational problems due to sparse vocabulary and simplistic grammar. Specifically, literacy skills could be at risk. Working from the powerful variationist paradigm discussed earlier in this chapter, sociolinguistic researchers demonstrated that the language "errors" noted in the commentaries of these educational psychologists were manifestations of language/dialectal differences and not cognitive or linguistic deficits (Labov, 1966b; 1972a; Shuy, 1977). It was found that while there may be some impact from dialectal differences in literacy acquisition, the relationship between the dialectal forms and the literacy difficulties was not simple; these difficulties were often due to a number of factors, especially pedagogical adjustments due to attitudes; importantly, little evidence was found to suggest that literacy problems were due to the existence of interference from the linguistic forms (e.g., Labov, 1983; Michaels & Cazden, 1986; Delpit, 1995).

Following on from these early influences, sociolinguistics has continued to inform literacy in many ways. Given that literacy is a manifestation of language use – on the same level as verbal discourse – this should come as no surprise. Literacy is a symbolic practice linking written linguistic code with attitudes, ideologies, and other aspects of human social action and epistemology (Scribner & Cole, 1981; Gee, 1996; 2000; Smith, 2004) – ideal areas of focus for the conceptual and methodological lens of sociolinguistic investigation. While there is much that could be discussed regarding the influence of sociolinguistics on language arts in general (e.g., Heath, 1983; Beach, Green, Kamil, & Shanahan, 1992; John-Steiner, Panofsky, & Smith, 1994; Street, 1995), the remainder of this section will discuss some specific ways that sociolinguistic research on literacy has influenced or may influence clinical applications to reading and writing problems.

Over the past two decades there has been an increased interest in how speech and language disorders impact various aspects of the academic context and special attention has been directed toward literacy (e.g., American Speech-Language-Hearing Association, 2001; Catts & Kamhi, 1986; Bishop & Adams, 1990; Catts, 1993; Stothard, Snowling, Bishop, Chipchase, & Kaplan, 1998). This is because a vast majority of students who are placed into special education and other remedial education services are initially referred to these services due to reading and writing difficulties (Lyon, 1996). Consequently, our clinical interests have been particularly oriented to the remediation of literacy disorders in children who have received various types of special education labels (e.g., language-disordered, dyslexic, learning-disabled). While a number of intervention methods have been employed with these students, there is a long tradition of employing behavioristic methodologies that result in decontextualized, fragmented, and prescriptive approaches based on dated conceptions of language and human learning (Norris & Damico, 1990; Bartolome, 1994; Freppon, 1994; Coles, 1998; White, 2002; Smith, 2004); led by research in sociolinguistic and sociocultural studies, there is growing awareness that the problems faced by these children require more than a traditional and fragmented approach to literacy intervention (e.g., Kasten, 1998; Weaver, 1998; Damico, Damico, & Nelson, 2003; Dudley-Marling & Paugh, 2004). Sociolinguistics can provide some direction regarding how best to consider literacy and how to approach its remediation in populations of exceptional children.

In a recent review, Damico, Nelson and Bryan (2005) described several ways that sociolinguistics influenced clinical literacy practices. Taking as a starting point the idea that literacy is a complex symbolic and social process, these authors demonstrated how (at least) four main data sources from sociolinguistics necessitated that literacy remediation employ strategies and techniques that can address this dynamic and complicated social process. Particularly, they stated that because of the complexity demonstrated from sociolinguistics, remediation should be oriented toward social constructivist principles (e.g., Cambourne, 1988; Au, 1993; Wells, 1999). Citing a number of researchers utilizing sociolinguistic conceptions and/or methodologies in their language arts research and practices, Damico and colleagues discussed (1) the acquisition of literacy as a socially constructed process, (2) the fact that how we define literacy is also socially constructed and often is subjected to political and socio-economic pressures, (3) that successful literacy acquisition and teaching are guided by functionality within the social context, and (4) that when literacy requirements are not met, social implications are created that require various kinds of adaptations. This further underlines the importance of literacy functionality in context. On the basis of these four data sources, Damico and colleagues made the case that a more authentic and socially mediated approach to literacy intervention was required. In the remainder of this section, the functionality argument made by these authors is expanded to further demonstrate sociolinguistic influences. For more information regarding the other three data sources, the reader is directed to Ball (2005).

Inherent in any manifestation of language in use is the fact that language phenomena are always embedded within a context of meaning and a context of functionality. That is, language manifestations exist in an authentic setting for particular purposes. The theoretical orientations of sociolinguistics and the kinds of data collected in various manifestations of language use have made this abundantly clear (e.g., Halliday, 1978; Gumperz & Hymes, 1986; Schieffelin & Ochs, 1986; Bloome, 1989; Grimshaw, 1990). Regardless of their activities and the contexts within which they operate, individuals employ language to make sense of ongoing situations and circumstances so that they can successfully negotiate the world. According to Gee (1996), language in any of its manifestations creates a way of being in the world, a way of connecting to others and to the socially constructed realities that surround us. Given its significance and role as an agent of cultural transmission, literacy is especially oriented to these social and functional considerations (Vygotsky, 1978; Bruner, 1984; Gee, 1996; Wells, 1999). To the extent that literacy intervention or remediation can operate from such a functional orientation, this pedagogy should be effective.

As demonstrated by sociolinguistics, therefore, effective intervention should embrace and exploit the crucial trait of functionality; literacy remediation must have a contextualized function for effective acquisition and usage (e.g., Bruner, 1990; Wells, 1999; Gee, 2001). When literacy operates within a situated context and when there are practical objectives or goals to pursue so that the student recognizes a purpose to the intervention efforts, then the literacy activities are more robust, more effective, and more motivating for all involved (e.g., Edelsky, 1994; John-Steiner, Panofsky, & Smith, 1994; Street, 1995; Gee, 2001).

Within both literacy education and sociolinguistic/sociocultural ideology, these ideas had no more effective proponent – in practice or in print – than the

Brazilian educator Paolo Freire (1970, 1973). In his initial promotion of literacy for the construction of social transformation, Freire emphasized reading as a political act; he stressed the fact that the learner must recognize the importance of his/her own literacy development. Indeed, this recognition must be a sociocultural and political development as well (1973). Freire labored to convince students and teachers alike that literacy had no real value as a mechanical skill to be learned; rather, it had to be understood as an experience in agency and power. As students became empowered by their literacy education and the opportunities it afforded them to transform their environment, as they and their teachers collaboratively engaged in a wide variety of literacy activities in which the students have choices, as the students felt comfortable in exploring the meanings in print and what these meanings implied about their social, cultural and political contexts, so they started to recognize that literacy was not just reading the *word*, it was also about reading the *world* (Freire & Macedo, 1987). Freire employed this philosophy of literacy education during numerous literacy campaigns in third-world situations and they tended to be quite successful. The reason often stated was the functional differences that literacy made to the individuals who actually learned to read and write.

Recognizing literacy as a socially constituted act requiring functional interaction with one's context has resulted in various other pedagogical philosophies and orientations as well. For example, based upon Freire (1970), *critical literacy* has been progressively suggested as a viable and effective component of literacy instruction (e.g., Edelsky, 1994; Egan-Robertson, 1998; Morgan, 1997; Shor, 1992). Perhaps less radical than Freire's more transformative pedagogy, critical literacy is intended to get students to engage in literacy activities by making them more knowledgeable about how texts are used to reflect and advance certain struggles for knowledge, power, representation, and material resources (Cazden, Cope, Fairclough, et al, 1996). These functionally and socially based efforts typically result in better literacy skills in both general (e.g., Graman, 1988; Edelsky, 1994; Morgan, 1997) and special education populations (e.g., Kasten, 1998; Dudley-Marling, & Paugh, 2004). In a similar vein, it has been suggested that the *whole language paradigm* was also significantly influenced by the focus on language use in context (Goodman, 1989; Norris, & Damico, 1990; Stephens, 1991). Particularly, the work of Vygotsky (1978), Halliday (1978) and others (e.g., Heath, 1983; Bloome & Green, 1984) has been cited as an early influence on the development of this meaning-based literacy philosophy.

Dudley-Marling and Paugh (2004) have recently contributed a powerful argument for employing the socio-psycholinguistic perspective of whole language for the functional benefits of enabling students to infuse their identities into the curriculum. Taking up the issue of recognizing the students' voices in order to assist in the development of their social, cultural and individual identities, these researchers stress that if the students' identities are woven into the school-based literacy materials and activities the students will be better able to draw from their own personal experiences when trying to construct meaning and purpose from the texts. Since learning typically depends on an individual's ability to make sense of new situations in light of their previous experiences, a holistic approach that infuses their experiences and identities will be more effective and successful (Dudley-Marling & Searle, 1991; Smith, 2004). Other advantages of this more socially based and functional orientation to literacy education and remediation are the continued development of student self-concept as a competent learner (Egan-Robertson, 1998), and the added benefit of making literacy more contextually relevant to the students' literacy needs outside of the classroom. Guided by sociolinguistics, these teaching and remediation methodologies create more authentic learning and the consequence is more authentic learners.

7.6   Conclusion

As a clinical discipline involved with the identification and remediation of speech and language disorders, we must be realistic about the phenomena that we address on a daily basis. Language is the most complex of human abilities, enabling us to act upon the social and physical worlds while also being a part of these worlds. Language, as our primary symbolic system, is the basis for our social actions, our cultural constructions, and our communicative interactions. If we are going to be successful as clinical and remedial agents for speech and language disorders, we must be able to effectively focus on the authentic needs of our clients and students, and we must strive to make a difference in their symbolic lives. Perhaps there is no better source of information to help us fulfill our obligations than sociolinguistics.

As this brief discussion has demonstrated, this area of linguistics, focusing on the interaction between language and society, offers the clinician a way to address the complexity of language in context. Indeed, from the beginnings of this subdiscipline the focus was on actual language users in real and embedded contexts. Whether we employ the idea of variation in our linguistic code as driven by social factors, whether we employ the complex methodologies that have so effectively described elaborate psycho-social phenomena like power, authority, and identity, whether we employ the conceptualizations of this subdiscipline to address complicated linguistic manifestations like literacy, bilingualism, or compensatory adaptation to impairment (Perkins, 2002), we can rely on sociolinguistics to highlight both the complexity and some of the ways to address that complexity.

Several clinical implications follow from a focus on sociolinguistics. First, in our efforts as professionals we must strive to address the authentic speech and language behaviors of our clients and students and the implications of these behaviors in the real world. When conducting assessments or planning and implementing interventions, we should avoid the construction of convenient and simplistic phenomena as reflected by decontextualized test performances and sanitized therapy activities. Just as sociolinguists, we should embrace language embedded in the complicated contexts that make up the daily lives of our students and clients. Second, we should recognize the complexity of language in context and respect the fact that *what* we do and *how* we do it in the clinical context will never be easy. Rather, we should strive to become clinical linguists who are not afraid to address complexity and the facets of linguistic and social phenomena. While this task may seem daunting to clinicians who are not trained in linguistics, the use of sociolinguistic research and practices can assist even the most ill-equipped individual to improve their clinical skills. The brief descriptions and references provided within this chapter will serve as an excellent starting point. The key, however, is to abandon the naive conception of speech and language as simplistic, unitary, and prepackaged. Such a conception will only lead to poor clinical results. Finally, we must be circumspect in our efforts as clinicians and "experts" in linguistic and social matters. In even the best of circumstances, armed with the most recent sociolinguistic data, we will constantly be surprised by behaviors, expectations, and occurrences. While this may result in transient confusion and even a fleeting loss of confidence in our abilities, we should simply reflect on the complexity of language and the discovery procedures available to us through sociolinguistics and press forward. It is the currency of sociolinguistics to do so.

NOTES

1 Of course, linguistic variation may also correlate with other linguistic features, such as front lax vowel raising before nasals in many American English dialects. Wolfram (1993) distinguishes between *internal* and *external* constraints on variability, representing linguistic and social factors respectively.
2 We do not have the space here to explore the notion of speech community; the treatment by Britain and Matsumoto (2005) is recommended.
3 Semantic variation is often difficult to disentangle from lexical; however, British passengers on US airlines are often taken aback to hear that the plane 'will land momentarily', wondering why it will need to take off again so soon.

REFERENCES

American Speech-Language-Hearing Association. (2001). *Roles and Responsibilities of Speech-Language Pathologists with Respect to Reading and Writing in Children and Adolescents*. ASHA, 21(Suppl.) (pp. 17–27). Rockville, MD: Author.

Au, K. H. (1993). *Literacy Instruction in Multicultural Settings*. Philadelphia: Harcourt, Brace College Publishers.

Ball, M. J. (1988). Accounting for linguistic variation: Sociolinguistics. In M. J. Ball (ed.), *The Use of Welsh* (pp. 24–38). Clevedon: Multilingual Matters.

Ball, M. J. (1992). Is a clinical sociolinguistics possible? *Clinical Linguistics and Phonetics,* 6, 155–60.

Ball, M. J. (ed.) (2005). *Clinical Sociolinguistics.* Oxford: Blackwell.

Ball, M. J. and Rutter, B. (2005). Is /str-/ a cluster in contemporary English? Presented at the American Speech-Language-Hearing Association Convention, San Diego.

Bartolome, L. (1994). Beyond the methods fetish: Toward a humanizing pedagogy. *Harvard Educational Review,* 62(2), 173–94.

Beach, R., Green, J., Kamil, M., and Shanahan, T. (ed.) (1992). *Multidisciplinary Perspectives on Literacy Research.* Urbana, IL: National Council of Teachers of English.

Becker, L. B. and Silverstein, J. E. (1984). Clinician-child discourse: A replication study. *Journal of Speech and Hearing Disorders,* 49, 104–5.

Bereiter, C. and Englemann, S. (1966). *Teaching Disadvantaged Children in the Preschool.* Englewood Cliffs, NJ: Prentice-Hall.

Bishop, D. and Adams, C. (1990). A prospective study of the relationship between specific language impairment, phonological disorders and reading retardation. *Journal of Child Psychology and Psychiatry,* 21, 1027–50.

Bloome, D. (1989). *Literacy and Classrooms.* Norwood, NJ: Ablex.

Bloome, D. and Green, J. (1984). Directions in the sociolinguistic study of reading. In P. D. Pearson (ed.), *Handbook of Reading Research* (pp. 395–421). New York: Longman.

Bobkoff, K. (1982). Analysis of verbal and non-verbal components of clinician–client interaction. Unpublished doctoral dissertation, Kent State University, OH.

Bobkoff, K. and Panagos (1986). The 'point' of language intervention lessons. *Child Language Teaching and Therapy,* 2, 50–62.

Britain, D. and Matsumoto, K. (2005). Language, communities, networks and practices. In M. J. Ball (ed.), *Clinical Sociolinguistics* (pp. 3–14). Oxford: Blackwell.

Brown, P. and Levinson, S. (1987). *Politeness: Some Universals in Language Usage.* 2nd ed. Cambridge: Cambridge University Press.

Brown, R. (1973). *A First Language.* Cambridge, MA: Harvard University Press.

Brown, R. and Ford, M. (1961). Address in American English. *Journal of Abnormal and Social Psychology,* 62, 375–85.

Brown, R. and Gilman, A. (1960). The pronouns of power and solidarity. In T. Sebeok (ed.), *Style in Language* (pp. 253–76). Cambridge, MA: MIT Press.

Bruner, J. S. (1984). Language, mind, and reading. In H. Goelman, A. Oberg and F. Smith. (eds.), *Awakening to Literacy* (pp. 193–200). Portsmouth, NH: Heinemann.

Bruner, J. S. (1990). *Acts of Meaning.* Cambridge, MA: Harvard University Press.

Cambourne, B. (1988). *The Whole Story: Natural Learning and the Acquisition of Literacy in the Classroom.* New York: Ashton Scholastic.

Catts, H. (1993). The relationship between speech-language impairments and reading disabilities. *Journal of Speech and Hearing Research,* 36, 948–58.

Catts, H. and Kamhi, A. (1986). The linguistic basis of reading disorders: Implications for the speech-language pathologist. *Language, Speech, and Hearing Services in Schools,* 17, 329–41.

Cazden, C. (1988). *Classroom Discourse: The Language of Teaching and Learning.* Portsmouth, NH: Heinemann.

Cazden, C., Cope, B., Fairclough, N., Gee, J. P., Kalantzis, M., Kress, G., Luke, A., Luke, C., Michaels, S., and Nakata, M. (1996). A pedagogy of multiliteracies: Designing social futures. *Harvard Educational Review,* 66, 60–92.

Coles, G. (1998). *Reading Lessons: The Debate over Literacy.* New York: Hill and Wang.

Crystal, D. (1982). *Profiling Linguistic Disability.* London: Edward Arnold.

Crystal, D., Fletcher, P., and Garman, M. (1976). *Language Assessment, Remediation, and Screening Procedure*. London: Edward Arnold.

Damico, J. S., Damico, H., and Nelson, R. (2003). Impact of mixed instruction on meaning making in literacy. Poster presented at the Annual meeting of the American Speech-Language-Hearing Association, Chicago, IL.

Damico, J. S. and Damico, S. K. (1997). The establishment of a dominant interpretive framework in language intervention. *Language, Speech, and Hearing Services in Schools*, 28, 288–96.

Damico, J. S., Nelson, R. L., and Bryan, L. (2005). Literacy as a sociocultural process. In M. J. Ball (ed.), *Clinical Sociolinguistics* (pp. 242–9). Oxford: Blackwell.

Damico, J. S., Simmons-Mackie, N., and Hawley, H. (2005). Language and power. In M. J. Ball (ed.), *Clinical Sociolinguistics* (pp. 63–73). Oxford: Blackwell.

Delpit, L. (1995). *Other People's Children: Cultural Conflict in the Classroom*. New York: New Press.

Dudley-Marling, C. and Paugh, P. (2004). Tapping the power of student voice through whole language practices. *Reading and Writing Quarterly*, 20, 385–99.

Dudley-Marling, C. and Searle, D. (1991). *When Students Have Time to Talk: Creating Contexts for Learning Language*. Portsmouth, NH: Heinemann.

Edelsky, C. (1994). Education for democracy. *Language Arts*, 71, 252–7.

Edwards, J. (2005). Bilingualism and multilingualism. In M. J. Ball (ed.), *Clinical Sociolinguistics* (pp. 36–48). Oxford: Blackwell.

Egan-Robertson, A. (1998). Learning about culture, language, and power: Understanding relationships among personhood, literacy practices, and intertextuality. *Journal of Literacy Research*, 30, 449–87.

Fairclough, N. (1989). *Language and Power*. London: Longman.

Freepon, P. (1994). Understanding the nature of reading and writing difficulties: An alternative view. *Reading and Writing Quarterly*, 10, 227–38.

Freire, P. (1970). *Pedagogy of the Oppressed*. New York: Seabury Press.

Freire, P. (1973). *Education for Critical Consciousness*. New York: Seabury Press.

Freire, P. and Macedo, D. (1987). *Reading the Word and the World*. Westport, CT: Bergin & Garvey.

Gee, J. P. (1996). *Social Linguistics and Literacies: Ideology in Discourse*. 2nd ed. London: Taylor and Francis.

Gee, J. P. (2000). The new literacy studies: From 'socially situated' to the work of the social. In D. Barton, M. Hamilton, and R. Ivanic (eds.), *Situated Literacies: Reading and Writing in Context* (pp. 180–96). London: Routledge.

Gee, J. P. (2001). Reading as situated language: A sociocognitive perspective. *Journal of Adolescent and Adult Literacy*, 44, 714–25.

Goldman, R. and Fristoe, M. (2000). *Goldman–Fristoe Test of Articulation 2*. Circle Pines, MN: AGS Publishing.

Goodman, K. S. (1989). Whole language research: Foundations and development. *Elementary School Journal*, 90, 207–21.

Goodwin, C. and Duranti, A. (1992). Rethinking context: An introduction. In A. Duranti and C. Goodwin (ed.), *Rethinking Context: Language as an Interactive Phenomenon* (pp. 1–43). Cambridge: Cambridge University Press.

Goodwin, C. and Heritage, J. 1990. Conversational analysis. *Annual Review of Anthropology*, 19, 283–307.

Graman, T. (1988). Education for humanization: Applying Paulo Freire's pedagogy to learning a second language. *Harvard Education Review*, 58, 433–48.

Grimshaw, A. D. (ed.) (1990). *Conflict Talk: Sociolinguistic Investigations of Arguments in Conversations*. Cambridge: Cambridge University Press.

Gumperz, J. (1982). *Discourse Strategies*. Cambridge: Cambridge University Press.

Gumperz, J. J. and Hymes, H. (ed.) (1986). *Directions in Sociolinguistics: The Ethnography of Communication*. New York: Basil Blackwell.

Halliday, M. A. K. (1973). *Explorations in the Function of Language*. London: Edward Arnold.

Halliday, M. A. K. (1978). *Language as Social Semiotic*. London: Edward Arnold.

Heath, S. B. (1983). *Ways with Words: Language, Life, and Work in Communities and Classrooms*. Cambridge: Cambridge University Press.

Hymes, D. (1967). Models of the interaction of language and social setting. *Journal of Social Issues*, 23(2), 8–28.

John-Steiner, V., Panofsky, C. P., and Smith, L. W. (ed.) (1994). *Sociocultural Approaches to Language and Literacy: An Interactionist Approach*. New York: Cambridge University Press.

Kasten, W. (1998). One learner, two paradigms: A case study of a special education student in a multiage primary classroom. *Reading and Writing Quarterly*, 14, 335–54.

Kedar, L. (ed.) (1987). *Power through Discourse*. Norwood, NJ: Ablex.

Kovarsky, D. (1989). An ethnography of communication in child language therapy. Unpublished doctoral dissertation, University of Texas at Austin.

Kovarsky, D. (1990). Discourse markers in adult-controlled therapy: Implications for child centered intervention. *Journal of Childhood Communication Disorders*, 13, 29–41.

Kovarsky, D. and Duchan, J. F. (1997). The interactional dimensions of language therapy. *Language, Speech, and Hearing Services in Schools*, 28, 297–307.

Labov, W. (1963). The social motivation of a sound change. *Word*, 19, 273–309.

Labov, W. (1966a). *The Social Stratification of English in New York City*. Washington, DC: Center for Applied Linguistics.

Labov, W. (1966b). Some sources of reading problems for speakers of non-standard Negro English. In A. Frazier (ed.), *New Directions in Elementary English* (pp. 140–67). Champaign, IL: National Council of Teachers of English.

Labov, W. (1972a). *Language in the Inner City; Studies in the Black English Vernacular*. Philadelphia: University of Pennsylvania Press.

Labov, W. (1972b). *Sociolinguistic Patterns*. Philadelphia: University of Pennsylvania Press, and Oxford: Blackwell.

Labov, W. (1983). Recognizing Black English in the classroom. In J. Chambers, Jr. (ed.), *Black English: Educational Equity and the Law* (pp. 29–55). Ann Arbor, MI: Karoma Publishers.

Labov, W. and Fanshel, D. (1977). *Therapeutic Discourse*. New York: Academic Press.

Lahey, M. (2004). Therapy talk: Analyzing therapeutic discourse. *Language, Speech, and Hearing Services in Schools*, 35, 70–81.

Lee, L. (1974). *Developmental Sentence Analysis*. Evanston, IL: Northwestern University Press.

Letts, C. (1985). Linguistic interaction in the clinic: How do therapists do therapy? *Child Language Teaching and Therapy*, 1, 321–31.

Lucas, C. (ed.) (1989). *The Sociolinguistics of the Deaf Community*. San Diego, CA: Academic Press.

Lucas, C. (1995). Sociolinguistic variation in ASL: The case of DEAF. In C. Lucas (ed.), *Sociolinguistics in Deaf Communities*, vol. 1 (pp. 3–25). Washington, DC: Gallaudet University Press.

Lucas, C. (ed.) (2001). *The Sociolinguistics of Sign Languages*. Cambridge: Cambridge University Press.

Lucas, C., Bailey, R., and Kelly, A. (2005). The sociolinguistics of sign languages. In M. J. Ball (ed.), *Clinical Sociolinguistics* (pp. 250–64). Oxford: Blackwell.

Lucas, C., Bailey, R., and Valli, C. (2001). *Sociolinguistics in Deaf Communities. Volume 7: Sociolinguistic Variation in American Sign Language*. Washington, DC: Gallaudet University Press.

Lyon, G. R. (1996). Learning disabilities. *The Future of Children*, 6(1), 54–76.

Mehan, H. (1979). *Learning Lessons*. Cambridge, MA: Harvard University Press.

Michaels, S. and Cazden, C. (1986). Teacher/child collaboration as oral preparation for literacy. In B. B. Schieffelin (ed.), *The Acquisition of Literacy: Ethnographic Perspectives* (pp. 132–53). Norwood, NJ: Ablex.

Morgan, W. (1997). *Critical Literacy in the Classroom: The Art of the Possible*. New York: Routledge.

Müller, N. and Ball, M. J. (2005). Code-switching and diglossia. In M. J. Ball (ed.), *Clinical Sociolinguistics* (pp. 49–62). Oxford: Blackwell.

Norris, J. A. and Damico, J. S. (1990). The whole language movement in theory and practice: implications for language intervention. *Language, Speech, and Hearing Services in Schools*, 21, 211–20.

Oetting, J. (2005). Assessing language in children who speak a nonmainstream dialect of English. In M. J. Ball (ed.), *Clinical Sociolinguistics* (pp. 180–92). Oxford: Blackwell.

Oetting, J., Cantrell, J., and Horohov, J. (1999). A study of specific language impairment (SLI) in the context of non-standard dialect. *Clinical Linguistics and Phonetics*, 13, 25–44.

Panagos, J. M. (1996). Speech therapy discourse: The input to learning. In M. Smith and J. S. Damico (ed.), *Childhood Language Disorders* (pp. 41–63). New York: Thieme Medical Publishers.

Panagos, J. M., Bobkoff, K., and Scott, C. M. (1986). Discourse analysis of language intervention. *Child Language Teaching and Therapy*, 2, 211–29.

Panagos, J. M. and Fry, J. (1976). Code switching during language therapy communication. Paper presented at the annual convention of the American Speech-Language-Hearing Association, Houston, TX.

Panagos, J. M. and Griffith, P. L. (1981). Okay, what do educators really know about language intervention? *Topics in Learning Disabilities*, 2, 69–82.

Perkins, M. R. (2002). An emergentist approach to pragmatic impairment. In F. Windsor, M. L. Kelly and N. Hewlett (ed.), *Investigations in Clinical Linguistics and Phonetics* (pp. 1–14). New York: Lawrence Erlbaum.

Prutting, C. A., Bagshaw, N., Goldstein, H., Juskowitz, S., and Umen, I. (1978). Clinician child discourse: Some preliminary questions. *Journal of Speech and Hearing Disorders*, 43, 123–39.

Ripich, D. (1982). Children's social perception of speech-language sessions: A sociolinguistic analysis of role-play discourse. Unpublished doctoral dissertation, Kent State University, OH.

Ripich, D. N. and Creaghead, N. A. (1994). *School Discourse Problems*. San Diego, CA: College-Hill Press.

Ripich, D. N. and Panagos, J. M. (1985). Assessing children's knowledge of sociolinguistic rules for speech therapy lessons. *Journal of Speech and Hearing Disorders*, 50, 335–46.

Scarborough, H. (1991). Index of productive syntax. *Applied Psycholinguistics*, 11, 1–22.

Schieffelin, B. B. and Ochs, E. (eds.) (1986). *Language Socialization across Cultures*. New York: Cambridge University Press.

Schiffrin, D. (1987). *Discourse Markers*. London: Cambridge University Press.

Schiffrin, D. (1994). *Approaches to Discourse*. Oxford: Oxford University Press.

Scribner, S. and Cole, M. (1981). *The Psychology of Literacy*. Cambridge, MA: Harvard University Press.

Seymour, H., Roeper, T., and de Villiers, J. (2003). *Diagnostic Evaluation of Language Variation*. San Antonio, TX: Psychological Corporation.

Shor, I. (1992). *Empowering Education: Critical Teaching for Social Change*. Chicago: University of Chicago Press.

Shuy, R. (ed.) (1977). *Linguistic Theory: What Can it Say About Reading?* Newark, DE: International Reading Association.

Shuy, R. (1987). Conversational power in FBI covert tape recordings. In L. Kedah (ed.), *Power through Discourse* (pp. 43–56). Norwood, NJ: Ablex.

Simmons-Mackie, N. N., Damico, J. S., and Damico, H. L. (1999). A qualitative study of feedback in aphasia treatment. *American Journal of Speech-Language Pathology*, 8, 218–30.

Smith, F. (2004). *Understanding Reading*. 6th ed. Mahwah, NJ: Lawrence Erlbaum Associates.

Stephens, D. (1991). *Research on Whole Language: Support for a New Curriculum*. Katonah, NY: Richard C. Owens Publishers.

Stothard, S., Snowling, M., Bishop, D., Chipchase, B., and Kaplan, C. (1998). Language impaired preschoolers: A follow-up into adolescence. *Journal of Speech, Language, and Hearing Research*, 41, 407–18.

Street, B. (1995). *Social Literacies: Critical Approaches to Literacy in Development, Ethnography, and Education*. London: Longman.

Tannen, D. (1985). 'Silence: Anything but.' In D. Tannen and M. Saville-Troike (ed.), *Perspectives on Silence* (pp. 93–111). Norwood, NJ: Ablex.

Tannen, D. (1987). Remarks on discourse and power. In L. Kedar (ed.), *Power through Discourse* (pp. 3–10). Norwood, NJ: Ablex.

Taylor, O., Payne, K., and Anderson, N. (1987). Distinguishing between communication disorders and communication differences. *Seminars in Speech and Language*, 8, 415–28.

Trudgill, P. (1972). Sex, covert prestige and linguistic change in the urban British English of Norwich. *Language in Society*, 1, 179–95.

Trudgill, P. (1974). *The Social Differentiation of English in Norwich*. Cambridge: Cambridge University Press.

Ulichny, P. and Watson-Gegeo, K. A. (1989). Interactions and authority: The dominant interpretive framework in writing conferences. *Discourse Processes*, 12, 309–28.

Vygotsky, L. S. (1978). *Mind in Society: The Development of Higher Psychological Processes*. Cambridge, MA: Harvard University Press.

Walker, A. G. (1987). Linguistic manipulation, power, and the legal setting. In L. Kedah (ed.), *Power through Discourse* (pp. 57–80). Norwood, NJ: Ablex.

Wardhaugh, R. (1998). *Introduction to Sociolinguistics*. 3rd ed. Oxford: Blackwell.

Weaver, C. (1998). Reconceptualizing reading and dyslexia. In C. Weaver (ed.), *Practicing What We Know: Informed Reading Instruction* (pp. 292–324). Urbana, IL: National Council of Teachers of English.

Wei, L., Miller, N., Dodd, B., and Hua, Z. (2005). Childhood bilingualism: Distinguishing difference from disorder. In M. J. Ball (ed.), *Clinical Sociolinguistics* (pp. 193–206). Oxford: Blackwell.

Wells, G. (1999). *Dialogic Inquiry: Toward a Sociocultural Practice and Theory of Education.* Cambridge: Cambridge University Press.

White, L. F. (2002). Learning disability, pedagogies, and public discourse. *College Composition and Communication*, 53, 705–38.

Wolfram, W. (1977). On the relationship of sociolinguistics and speech pathology. In *Papers in Honor of Ann Taylor Huey* (pp. 1–11). Evanston, IL: Northwestern University.

Wolfram, W. (1983). Test interpretation and sociolinguistic differences. *Topics in Language Disorders*, 3, 21–34.

Wolfram, W. (1993). The sociolinguistic model in speech and language pathology. In Margaret M. Leafy and Jeffrey L. Kallen (ed.), *International Perspectives in Speech and Language Pathology* (pp. 1–29). Dublin: Trinity College.

Wolfram, W. (2005). African American English. In M. J. Ball (ed.), *Clinical Sociolinguistics* (pp. 87–100). Oxford: Blackwell.

Woodward, J. (1980). Sociolinguistic: Some sociolinguistic aspects of French and American Sign Languages. In H. Lane and F. Grosjean (ed.), *Recent Perspectives on American Sign Language* (pp. 103–18). Hillsdale, NJ: Erlbaum.

8 Systemic Functional Linguistics and Communication Impairment

ALISON FERGUSON AND
JULIE THOMSON

Functional approaches to language assessment and intervention are increasingly recognized as important for both children and adult clients with communication disorders. What has been lacking is a systematic way of formulating these approaches and a theoretical perspective to inform them. Systemic Functional Linguistics is a functional model of language in use that offers clinicians this theoretical perspective. Readers new to Systemic Functional Linguistics will find comprehensive information about its theory and methods of analysis, at an introductory level in Butt, Fahey, Feez, Spinks, and Yallop, 2000 and Thompson, 1996 and at an advanced level in Eggins and Slade, 2004/1997, Halliday and Matthiessen, 2004, and Martin and Rose, 2003.

Speech-language pathologists working with both child and adult caseloads over recent years have been involved in a shift to a social paradigm of assessment and intervention, which is strongly supported by recent developments within the World Health Organization's International Classification of Functioning (WHO, 2001). At the same time, within the field of sociolinguistics there have been considerable developments in what has become known as 'critical discourse analysis' (see Müller, Guendouzi, & Wilson, chapter 1 in this volume) which have highlighted the close relationship between what is said or written and its social context, and argued for the need to critically analyze the language/power relationships between all interactants (including practitioners) and their sociocultural assumptions and discourses (Fairclough, 1995, 1997; Locke, 2004). Systemic Functional Linguistics has become one of the most widely adopted linguistic methodologies for 'doing' critical linguistics, as it provides both theoretical rigor and methodological systematicity for dealing with both macro and micro aspects of language within social context (Pennycook, 2001;

Young & Harrison, 2004). In this chapter, we focus primarily on the more 'micro' aspects of language use in social contexts, as these have been the main aspects of Systemic Functional Linguistics applied to speech-language pathology to date, but we also attempt to indicate where wider aspects of this sociolinguistic theory may have relevance for speech-language pathology (Armstrong, Ferguson, Mortensen, & Togher, 2005).

8.1   Key Concepts

Systemic Functional Linguistics (SFL) is a semantic perspective on language in use, and has been recognized as having particular relevance for speech-language pathology since the 1980s (Gotteri, 1988). There are two key aspects in the SFL model: *system* and *function* (Halliday, 1994). *System* refers to the network of choices which language users have available to them; analysis of their choices allows us to investigate the dynamic (and non-deterministic) nature of discourse. As Halliday and Matthiessen explain, "What this means is that each system – each moment of choice – contributes to the formation of the structure. . . . So when we analyse a text, we show the functional organization of its structure; and we show what meaningful choices have been made, each one seen in the context of what might have been meant but was not" (Halliday & Matthiessen, 2004, p. 24).

These choices are not consciously made (although metalinguistic awareness is possible for some choices), nor do they represent a prescriptive inventory of structures. Instead, the language user creates or '*realizes*' meaning through multiple series of choices. *Function* refers to the perspective's orientation to language in use, so that it is function rather than form that is the focus of this grammar. From an SFL perspective, language is viewed as a resource with a system of options for making meaning. The system is organised stratally in terms of its content (semantics and lexicogrammar) and expression (including phonology). Meaning choices (semantics) are expressed (realized) by lexicogrammatical choices that are, in turn, realized by choices within the phonological system (Halliday, 1994; Halliday & Matthiessen, 2004). The term lexicogrammar refers to the level of wording, lexis referring to specific word meanings and grammar to more generalized structural meanings. The relationship between lexicogrammar and phonology is formal whereas that between semantics and lexicogrammar is functional, and probabilistic rather than deterministic. It is possible therefore to realize a specific meaning in more than one way, just as the same wording can yield different meanings or interpretations. One of the advantages for speech-language pathologists using SFL is that the approach allows for consideration of all levels of language, ranging from social and interactional use of language (often referred to within speech-language pathology as 'pragmatic' features) as well as wordings and grammatical features, within the one unified theoretical framework (Thomson, 2003).

Within SFL, analysts focus on how *texts* come to make meaning in *context*. A *text* is a unit of language in use, and it is the unity of meaning that defines a text rather than length or any structural features. For the speech-language pathologist this provides for flexibility in sampling depending on the area of clinical interest. So, for example, the speech-language pathologist might sample a narrative of stroke embedded in a larger unit of conversation. If the whole conversation is analyzed, then the exchange between participants will be of interest as well as how the narrative fitted into the conversation, for example who initiated what and when. Alternatively, the focus of analysis might be on the narrative itself and how the important parts of the story were drawn together through lexical and grammatical resources for cohesion, for example.

8.2   Language in Context

8.2.1   *Context of situation*

Halliday (1994) proposes that there are three aspects of the context of situation that matter most to our understanding of how language is produced and understood: the Field of discourse (what is being talked about), the Tenor of discourse (the speaker's relationship to the listener and the message), and the Mode of discourse (the part language is playing in the discourse). Hasan (Halliday & Hasan, 1985) suggests that we can characterize the *contextual configuration* of any text by describing its Field, Tenor and Mode, and this provides a succinct description of any text we select for analysis. Further, we can use the contextual configuration as a guide when considering what language samples to select in order to ensure a range of sampling across contexts (Ferguson, 2000a). A detailed description of the contextual configuration provides for a systematic way to identify the relationships between the real-world social context and the linguistic text, and thus helps the speech-language pathologist capture points where speakers may evidence social or pragmatic difficulties, for example, where mismatches occur between use of polite forms in the social power or distance relationships between interactants (Togher & Hand, 1998).

8.2.2   *Context of culture*

The cultural context in which an interaction occurs affects the particular instance of language use or 'register' (made up of the register variables Field, Tenor and Mode, which delineate the contextual configuration as described above); for example, we may adopt a more or less formal register in a particular social context (Eggins, 1994). However, cultural context is even more systematically mapped onto discourse than such particular instances, through text types or 'genres' of discourse which are likely to occur in different cultural contexts. Genres refer to texts that share common structural elements inextricably tied to the contextual configuration (Butt, Fahey, Feez, Spinks, & Yallop, 2000). Examples of written genres are letters of complaint, recipes, and novels (with of course subgenres), and examples of spoken genres are personal narratives, recounts, instructions, and therapy sessions. Each genre can be seen as having a uniquely defining *generic structure potential* (GSP) (Eggins, 1994, pp. 25–48), which is made up of a set of obligatory and optional elements, each of which has a distinct contextual configuration in an ordered sequence. So for example, therapy sessions are a type of discourse with which an experienced speech-language pathologist is highly familiar, and the medical-therapeutic cultural features increase the probability with which particular registers will be used within that genre. The cultural presumptions embedded in this genre become more visible when we observe people new to therapy interactions; for example, Ferguson argues that one of the roles of the clinical education process is to 'acculturate' speech-language pathology students to the potential resources available within therapy sessions (Ferguson & Armstrong, 2004; Ferguson & Elliot, 2001), and Simmons-Mackie has discussed what happens when our clients make different assumptions regarding allowable contributions to the therapy session (Simmons-Mackie & Damico, 1999).

8.2.3 Text and genre

An understanding of how texts relate to genre is important in deciding which genres to sample, and helps us avoid concentrating our observations and treatment on one particular genre (e.g. narrative) at the expense of others that might also be of importance to clients (e.g. writing a letter of complaint, providing a report on a science experiment at school). Language learning from childhood through adolescence requires increasing mastery of a range of genres both in terms of control of the lexicogrammatical resources and the understanding of textual resources and generic structure required. For example, in the first few years of formal education, children/students focus on narratives, while in the middle-school and high-school years there is a demand for mastery over a wide range of genres including exposition, argument, and report. These resources are developed to fulfill the purpose of the text, for example to persuade an audience or to provide specific instructions. In order to master these genres, the student is learning how to make use of the distinct linguistic resources called upon within each genre, while at the same time the student's mastery of the genre-specific language resources enables their access to the learning in the knowledge domain to which the genre contributes (Rothery, 1996); for example, the genre of 'report' plays a major role in the domain of science.

We can go beyond just acknowledging that texts are located in a context of situation and culture, in recognizing that different ethnic cultures have different genres; for example, the narrative genre in Japanese will have a different set of obligatory elements than a 'Western' narrative genre, and different cultures may have different expectations about the possibility of social chat with the clinician in a therapy session. Further still, we can begin to recognize that texts create contexts. For example, the client might begin to interview the clinician (about the clinician's qualifications and experience, say), thus shifting the genre. In other words, the specification and description of register and generic structure potential are not a prescriptive set of requirements for language use; rather they are a set of options through which speakers chart their own course to make meanings. When using these parts of the SFL framework in speech-language intervention then, we avoid setting up a predetermined checklist of elements and sequences, but instead ask ourselves what texts our clients are able to produce or understand, and in what contexts, as well as asking how they shape and use the resources from the genre and culture in which they are situated.

8.2.4   *Metafunctions*

Halliday (1994) proposes that there are three main functions of language: to convey something about the Field of information, to create or maintain the Tenor of interpersonal relationships, and to use the resources of language (Mode) to enable this to happen. As can be seen, the three main functions of language are closely related to the three main aspects seen to be most relevant in the context of situation. But it is not that some utterances express information (Field), while others express relationships (Tenor). Instead, each and every use of language expresses each of the three main functions simultaneously – and hence these functions are called *metafunctions*. The metafunction expressing Field is called the Experiential metafunction, the metafunction expressing Tenor is called the Interpersonal metafunction, and the metafunction expressing Mode is called the Textual metafunction. In other words, every utterance tells something, establishes a relationship between interactants, and uses language to do it. The importance of this notion of metafunctions is that it provides the link between each of the main aspects of context of situation and the resources available in language to make meanings. Out of all the many resources of language that are available to speakers, SFL proposes that there are certain specific language resources that are the most visible or sensitive reflectors of each metafunction and its relationship to the context of situation.

We can look at how the resources of language are used to make meanings at three main levels: content (semantics, lexicogrammar) and the level of expression (including phonology/graphology, gestures, prosody)

8.3   Levels of Language

8.3.1   *Content: Semantics*

SFL is, generally speaking, a 'semantic' perspective; within the approach, a specific level of language is identified using the term 'semantics', often also described as 'discourse-semantics'. This level will be commonly recognized by speech-language pathologists as consistent with their understanding of the level of 'discourse', in the sense that we are thinking about how meanings are made through the entire text (Halliday & Hasan, 1976), in other words, its unity of meaning. (In order to avoid confusion, we will use the term 'discourse-semantics' to describe this level of language within this chapter.)

When we analyze the text as a whole in terms of what it is about, we can look first at how meanings relate to what is being talked about in the external world (reference), and secondly at how the meaning choices relate to other options in the meaning system (lexical relations, e.g. synonymy, antonymy, meronymy and so on). Both of these systems contribute to the cohesion of the text (Halliday & Hasan, 1976). While reference is considered to realize the Textual metafunction at the discourse-semantic level, lexical relations are considered to realize the Experiential metafunction at the discourse-semantic level. The potential of cohesion analysis as a clinical tool has been the aspect of SFL most widely applied in speech-language pathology (Coelho, Liles, Duffy, Clarkson, & Elia, 1994; Ferguson, 1993; Fine, Bartolucci, Szatmari, & Ginsberg, 1994; Jordan, Murdoch, & Buttsworth, 1991; Liles, Duffy, Merritt, & Purcell, 1995; Liles & Purcell, 1987; Mentis & Prutting, 1987; Ripich & Terrell, 1988).

SFL offers a pathway at the discourse-semantic level to an expanded understanding of the relationship between spoken and written texts, and offers speech-language pathologists a range of analytic tools for assessment and planning for intervention for clients for whom written language is a high priority, for example adolescents and young adults with language-learning difficulties or acquired language impairments. The three most salient features of discourse which illuminate key aspects of spoken-written texts are considered to be: the relative lexical density and grammatical intricacy, the use of grammatical metaphor, and rhetorical structure. For adults, spoken language is typically more *grammatically intricate* (it has a higher average number of clauses per clause complex or per sentence) and less *lexically dense* (it has a lower type–token ratio) than written language, which is conversely typically more lexically dense and less grammatically intricate. One of the main ways to increase lexical density as a resource for meaning in written texts is through the use of grammatical metaphor. *Grammatical metaphor* is a resource for meaning which involves a process of rank shifting, moving from clause to phrase or clause complex to clause level, for example. The most apparent example in written texts is the use of 'nominalization', in which clauses shift to the rank of phrase level, e.g. while a speaker might say, 'The school term ended', a writer might write, 'The ending of the school term'. This ability to use the resource of grammatical metaphor marks the development toward the mature writer (Christie, 2002), as does the use of rhetorical structure. *Rhetorical structure* generally describes the typically observed pattern or sequence of 'moves' associated with particular genres. In Mortensen's research, she has demonstrated the difficulties experienced in using rhetorical structure by writers with acquired language impairment when attempting to write an argument or narrative (Mortensen, 2003).

At the discourse-semantic level in a conversational interaction, the fundamental shifts between roles of giving and receiving information or goods and services structure the exchange, and these role shifts determine the choices made within the Interpersonal metafunction, reflecting the Tenor of the interpersonal relationship between interactants. In speech-language pathology, analyses of Tenor have been used, for example, to investigate interactions between clients with traumatic brain injury and their everyday speaking partners (Togher, 2000; Togher, Hand, & Code, 1997a, 1997b, 1999; Togher, McDonald, Code, & Grant, 1999), in the autistic population (Bartlett, Armstrong, & Roberts, 2005), and in the developmentally disordered population (Fine, 1991).

8.3.2   Content: Lexicogrammar

As previously mentioned, SFL proposes that certain lexicogrammatical resources are quite specific to the realization of different metafunctions and how they reflect the context of situation. At the level of the lexicogrammar, the Field of discourse is reflected in the network of choices within the Transitivity system. Simply, the Transitivity system is the expression of who is doing what to whom, under what conditions: Participants, Processes and Circumstances and how they relate to each other (Armstrong, 2001; Mathers, 2001). At the level of the lexicogrammar, the Tenor of discourse is reflected in the network of choices within the Mood system. This network involves the expression of the probabilities and obligations that arise and are negotiable between interactants in discourse. In English, these options include the ordering of Subject and Finite (e.g., inverted in the case of Interrogatives), the form of the Finite (e.g. use of tense), and Mood Adjuncts (expressing speaker's attitude to their message, e.g. 'unfortunately') (Ferguson, 1992; Spencer, Packman, Onslow, & Ferguson, 2005; Togher & Hand, 1998). At the level of the lexicogrammar, the Tenor of discourse is also reflected in the network of choices in the Appraisal system (Eggins & Slade, 1997/2004; Martin, 2000), which involves the expression of attitudes of the speaker, through the expression of *appreciation* (the expression of evaluation of an object or process, e.g. 'the stroke education presentation was *interesting/boring*'), *affect* (the expression of feelings/emotions, e.g. 'I'm *happy/cross* that I went along'), *judgment* (the expression of judgment about people's behavior, e.g. 'the presenter was *skillful/incompetent*'), and *amplification* (resources for grading appraisal, e.g. '*very* happy', '*just a bit* sad', and use of repetition). Appraisal analysis has been applied to the discourse of people with aphasia (Armstrong, 2005), and people with non-dominant hemisphere language impairment (Sherratt, 2004, 2007).

With regard to Mode of discourse, we have already seen that at the discourse-semantic level we have resources for building cohesion, but there are further resources available at the lexicogrammatical level which contribute to overall coherence to the listener, namely, the system of Theme. Theme involves the expression of priority or importance given to elements in a clause, and may strike a chord with those who have considered given/new relationships in texts (though there are important differences between these concepts). Thomson has applied the analysis of Theme to the narrative texts of children with specific language impairment (Thomson, 2005). In English, Theme occurs in the initial position in the clause, and the major points of interest for speech-language pathologists analyzing texts produced by individuals with language impairment are the use of multiple and marked Themes, and the analysis of Thematic progression. The use of multiple Themes reflects the language user's stage of development and/or access to lexicogrammatical resources, so for example, 'The girl cried' thematizes just 'girl', whereas 'And, unfortunately, the girl cried' highlights a number of meanings. Marked Theme allows the language user to dramatize meaning, so, for example, 'After her Mother's death, the girl cried' highlights the precipitating event rather than the girl's response and reflects not only the language user's access to lexical and grammatical resources, but also the user's grasp of the situation (pragmatic understanding) and options for how to present an utterance to the listener to achieve specific purposes. Thematic progression through a text is of interest in showing how the language user tracks or draws attention to the unfolding development of main ideas, for example through iteration ('First open the door, then step through the door, and then sit down'), or linear progression ('zigzagging'):

'The boy approached the door. The door creaked open. Through the opening there was light shining.'

As previously highlighted, each instance of language use realizes each of the three metafunctions simultaneously, and this can be exemplified at the level of the lexicogrammar fairly readily. In the example below, we have provided a snapshot of the Experiential metafunction (as realized through Transitivity), the Interpersonal metafunction (as realized through Mood), and the Textual metafunction (as realized through Theme), for just one clause.

Example: Analysis at the level of content: lexicogrammar

Context	Metafunction	Analysis	**Sadly**	**we**	**won't**	**go**	**to**	**Manly**
				Participant	Process			Circumstance
Field	Experiential	Transitivity		Mood (declarative)		Residue		
					Finite: Negative, future tense, modal			
Tenor	Interpersonal	Mood		Subject				
			Theme		Rheme			
Mode	Textual	Theme	Interpersonal	Topical				

As can be seen from the example, each metafunction is realized through lexicogrammatical choices which reflect each of the aspects of context. Also, the analysis of each metafunction allows us different lenses through which to view different lexicogrammatical resources, with some parts being more visible through one than through another lens. Combined analyses allow for a total picture to emerge as to how the speaker's meanings are being expressed. These understandings of the lexicogrammatical resources for making meanings provide a framework that the speech-language pathologist can use to explicitly assist the client to consciously make use of these resources within a metalinguistic approach to intervention.

8.3.3   *Expression*

Halliday and Matthiessen describe the area of expression in the following way:

> We can divide the phonology into two regions of articulation and prosody. . . . As a general principle, articulation is 'arbitrary' (conventional), in the sense that there is no systematic relation between sound and meaning. Prosody on the other hand, is 'natural': it is related systematically to meaning, as one of the resources for carrying contrasts in grammar. (Halliday & Matthiessen, 2004, p. 11)

As well as articulation and prosody, the level of expression also includes graphology and gestural expression. To date, there has been limited direct application of SFL approaches to expression within speech-language pathology, although Ferguson and Peterson (2002) have looked at the role of prosody in the expression of social meanings conveyed by the intonation used by communication partners of people with aphasia. They suggest that prosody provides a potential resource for speakers to draw attention to key information when talking with people with comprehension problems associated with aphasia.

SFL pays particular attention to prosody, as indicated in the above quote, as a resource for grammatical contrasts, rather than seeing it as a paralinguistic feature separate from the linguistic system. For example, prosody is a major resource for indicating clause (and clause complex) boundaries, and for making given/new distinctions. Thus prosody provides speech-language pathologists with important signposts to assist in analysis. For clinical populations, prosody is potentially both an area of difficulty (for example in traumatic brain injury) or a resource for meaning in the face of lexicogrammatical compromise (for example in Wernicke's aphasia).

8.4   Clinical Issues

SFL is one approach amongst a number that speech-language pathologists are using to assess and develop interventions for children and adults with communication difficulties. SFL is a sociolinguistic perspective and so contrasts sharply with approaches to language analysis based on psycholinguistic explanation (Hand, 2005). As a sociolinguistic perspective, SFL seeks to describe and explain how language is used by speakers, and is primarily concerned with understanding the relationship between the talk and the situations in which talking occurs. SFL does not theorize regarding the relationship between language and the brain, nor does it seek to establish universal abstract rules underlying language. It is, however, worth noting that emerging developments in cognitive linguistics, and in computational linguistics in the areas of neural networks and connectionist theories (Cohen, Johnston, & Plunkett, 2000; Daniloff, 2002), are not inconsistent with SFL notions regarding the usefulness of probabilistic modeling (Halliday & Matthiessen, 1999; Lamb, 1999). In relation to other sociolinguistic perspectives, SFL offers a semantic 'lens' through which to view all aspects of language use. SFL shares with conversation analysis (CA) (see Wilkinson, chapter 6 in this volume) its interest in naturalistic sampling, and the importance of co-text in providing resources for the dynamic interaction between speakers (Prevignano & Thibault, 2003), but differs from CA in relating observations back to a 'top-down' explanatory theory and in its focus on detailed lexicogrammatical analysis (Ferguson, 2000b). SFL is close to a number of other related discourse theories which share its concerns with contextually based analysis and explanation, most notably the work of Sinclair and Coulthard (Coulthard, 1992), the ethnographic approach of Hymes (Hymes, 1995), and the interaction approach of Gumperz (Eerdmans, Prevignano, & Thibault, 2003). Arguably, SFL offers three main aspects of interest to speech-language pathologists beyond these other approaches. First, SFL's detailed lexicogrammatical analyses allow the speech-language pathologist to comprehensively describe clients' use of language. Secondly, SFL has been applied across educational, second language learning, and clinical domains (as well as across other applied fields such as stylistics and computational linguistics), and these applications provide a rich resource for speech-language pathologists working with diverse caseloads. And thirdly, SFL's characterization of the relationship between culture, context and text has provided both theoretical and methodological rigor to critical discourse analysis, seeking to explore and question relationships of power and language. Issues of critical literacy, for example of social class, ethnicity and access to literacy (Damico, Nelson, & Bryan, 2005), and issues of access to print and on-line materials for people with communication difficulties (Ghidella, Murray, Smart, McKenna, & Worrall, 2005; Rose, Worrall, & McKenna, 2003) are just two of the areas of current concern to speech-language pathologists which can be informed by critical discourse analysis in general, and Systemic Functional Linguistics in particular.

Throughout this chapter we have attempted to provide examples of applications of SFL to speech-language pathology. What we hope is clear from these examples is that SFL is not, in itself, a specific approach to treatment, in that the theory is not a theory of learning or of behavioral change. Nor does SFL provide a 'recipe' or 'checklist' for assessment or treatment targets, as the notion that language use is dynamic and involves choices in the expression of meaning is essential to the theoretical perspective. For the speech-language pathologist, SFL involves a very fundamental shift in thinking, so that rather than thinking in terms of what clients cannot do, or what errors they make, the speech-language pathologist asks what meanings are being expressed and what resources of language are available (or potentially available) to assist their expression. The assessment protocols and treatment regimes which emerge from this perspective are highly individualized, and at the same time very detailed, descriptive, and measurable in terms of intra-individual change over time.

There are many challenges for the future in the ongoing application of SFL to speech-language pathology, not the least of which is making the theoretical perspective more readily accessible to speech-language pathologists in the field. Detailed case illustrations with description of therapy applications will be needed, along with greater specification of the clinical decision-making processes involved in the development of individualized assessment protocols and treatment regimes. Analytic methodologies currently well established for research purposes need to be refined, so that subsets of them can be developed that are both valid and reliable for routine clinical use. At the same time, it will be important for speech-language pathologists to maintain close dialogue with systemic functional linguists as pathological language presents an important crucible in which to test and develop the theory itself. Speech-language pathologists typically find that SFL's basic concepts of strata, levels of language, and aspects of context (Field, Tenor, Mode) sit comfortably within their other understandings of language. However, SFL offers speech-language pathologists an important series of conceptual challenges through the constructs of the metafunctions of each and every use of language (Experiential, Interpersonal, Textual), and systemic networks. The challenge, then, extends to finding ways in which these concepts allow us to describe and explain communication disorders in children and adults in ways that allow for contextually embedded understandings of the problems and potential for enabling the exchange of meaning.

REFERENCES

Armstrong, E. (2001). Connecting lexical patterns of verb usage with discourse meanings in aphasia. *Aphasiology*, 15, 1029–46.

Armstrong, E. (2005). Expressing opinions and feelings in aphasia: Linguistic options. *Aphasiology*, 19(3/5), 285–96.

Armstrong, E., Ferguson, A., Mortensen, L., and Togher, L. (2005). Acquired language disorders: Some functional insights. In R. Hasan, J. Webster and C. Matthiessen (eds.), *Continuing Discourse on Language*, vol. 1. London: Equinox.

Bartlett, S., Armstrong, E., and Roberts, J. (2005). Linguistic resources of individuals with Asperger Syndrome. *Clinical Linguistics and Phonetics*, 19(3), 203–13.

Butt, D., Fahey, R., Feez, S., Spinks, S., and Yallop, C. (2000). *Using Functional Grammar: An Explorer's Guide*. 2nd ed. Sydney: National Centre for English Language Teaching and Research.

Christie, F. (2002). *Classroom Discourse Analysis*. London: Continuum.

Coelho, C. A., Liles, B. Z., Duffy, R. J., Clarkson, J. V., and Elia, D. (1994). Conversational patterns of aphasic, closed head injured, and normal speakers. *Clinical Aphasiology*, 21, 183–91.

Cohen, G., Johnston, R. A., and Plunkett, K. (eds.) (2000). *Exploring Cognition: Damaged Brains and Neural Networks*. New York: Psychology Press.

Coulthard, M. (ed.) (1992). *Advances in Spoken Discourse Analysis*. London: Routledge.

Damico, J. S., Nelson, R. L., and Bryan, L. (2005). Literacy as a sociolinguistic process for clinical purposes. In M. J. Ball (ed.), *Clinical Sociolinguistics* (pp. 242–9). Malden, MA: Blackwell.

Daniloff, R. G. (ed.) (2002). *Connectionist Approaches to Clinical Problems in Speech and Language*. Mahwah, NJ: Lawrence Erlbaum.

Eerdmans, S. L., Prevignano, C. L., and Thibault, P. J. (eds.) (2003). *Language and Interaction: Discussions with John J. Gumperz*. Amsterdam: John Benjamins.

Eggins, S. (1994). *An Introduction to Systemic Functional Linguistics*. London: Pinter.

Eggins, S. and Slade, D. (2004). *Analysing Casual Conversation*. London: Equinox.

Fairclough, N. (1995). *Critical Discourse Analysis: The Critical Study of Language*. London: Longman.

Fairclough, N. (1997). Discourse across disciplines: Discourse analysis in researching social change. In A. Mauranen and K. Sajavaara (eds.), *Applied Linguistics Across Disciplines* (AILA Review 12). Milton Keynes, Bucks: Association Internationale de Linguistique Appliquée.

Ferguson, A. (1992). Interpersonal aspects of aphasic communication. *Journal of Neurolinguistics*, 7(4), 277–94.

Ferguson, A. (1993). Conversational repair of word-finding difficulty. In M. L. Lemme (ed.), *Clinical Aphasiology*, vol. 21 (pp. 299–310). Austin, TX: Pro-Ed.

Ferguson, A. (2000a). Maximising communicative effectiveness. In N. Muller (ed.), *Pragmatic Approaches to Aphasia* (pp. 53–88). Amsterdam: John Benjamins.

Ferguson, A. (2000b). Understanding paragrammatism: Contributions from Conversation Analysis and Systemic Functional Linguistics. In M. Coulthard (ed.), *Working with Dialogue: Proceedings of the 7th Biennial Congress of the International Association for Dialogue Analysis, Birmingham, April 8–10* (pp. 264–74). Amsterdam: John Benjamins.

Ferguson, A. and Armstrong, E. (2004). Reflections on speech-language therapists' talk: Implications for clinical practice and education. *International Journal of Language and Communication Disorders*, 39(4), 469–77.

Ferguson, A. and Elliot, N. (2001). Analysing aphasia treatment sessions. *Clinical Linguistics and Phonetics*, 15(3), 229–43.

Ferguson, A. and Peterson, P. (2002). Intonation in partner accommodation for aphasia: A descriptive single case study. *Journal of Communication Disorders*, 35, 11–30.

Fine, J. (1991). The static and dynamic choices of responding: Toward the process of building social reality by the developmentally disordered. In E. Ventola (ed.), *Functional and Systemic Linguistics: Approaches and Uses* (pp. 213–34). New York: Mouton de Gruyter.

Fine, J., Bartolucci, G., Szatmari, P., and Ginsberg, G. (1994). Cohesive discourse in pervasive developmental disorders. *Journal of Autism and Developmental Disorders*, 24, 315–29.

Ghidella, C. L., Murray, S. J., Smart, M. J., McKenna, K. T., and Worrall, L. (2005). Aphasia websites: An examination of their quality and communicative accessibility. *Aphasiology*, 19(12), 1134–46.

Gotteri, N. (1988). Systemic linguistics in language pathology. In R. P. Fawcett and D. Young (eds.), *New Developments in Systemic Linguistics: Theory and Application*, vol. 2. London: Pinter.

Halliday, M. A. K. (1994). *An Introduction to Functional Grammar*. 2nd ed. London: Arnold.

Halliday, M. A. K. and Hasan, R. (1976). *Cohesion in English*. London: Longman.

Halliday, M. A. K. and Hasan, R. (1985). *Language, Context, and Text: Aspects of Language in a Social-semiotic Perspective*. Victoria: Deakin University.

Halliday, M. A. K. and Matthiessen, C. M. I. M. (1999). *Construing Experience Through Meaning: A Language-based Approach to Cognition*. London: Continuum.

Halliday, M. A. K. and Matthiessen, C. M. I. M. (2004). *An Introduction to Functional Grammar*. 3rd ed. London: Arnold.

Hand, L. (2005). Some comparison and contrast between systemic-functional analyses and traditional clinical linguistic analyses of the discourse of children with specific language impairment. Paper presented at the International Systemic Functional Congress 32: Discourses of Hope: Peace, Reconciliation, Learning and Change. Sydney, July 17–22.

Hymes, D. (1995). *Ethnography, Linguistics, Narrative Inequality: Toward an Understanding of Voice*. London: Taylor & Francis.

Jordan, F. M., Murdoch, B. E., and Buttsworth, D. L. (1991). Closed-head-injured children's performance on narrative tasks. *Journal of Speech and Hearing Research*, 34, 572–82.

Lamb, S. (1999). *Pathways of the Brain: The Neurocognitive Basis of Language*. Amsterdam: John Benjamins.

Liles, B., Duffy, R., Merritt, D., and Purcell, S. (1995). Measurement of narrative discourse in children with language disorders. *Journal of Speech and Hearing Disorders*, 38, 415–25.

Liles, B. and Purcell, S. (1987). Departures in the spoken narratives of normal and language-disordered children. *Applied Psycholinguistics*, 8, 185–202.

Locke, S. (2004). *Critical Discourse Analysis*. London: Continuum.

Martin, J. R. (2000). Beyond exchange: Appraisal systems in English. In S. Hunston and G. Thompson (eds.), *Evaluation in Text* (pp. 143–75). Oxford: Oxford University Press.

Martin, J. R. and Rose, D. (2003). *Working with Discourse: Meaning Beyond the Clause*. London: Continuum.

Mathers, M. (2001). Language use in Attention Deficit Hyperactivity Disorder: A preliminary report. *Asia Pacific Journal of Speech, Language and Hearing*, 6, 47–52.

Mentis, M. and Prutting, C. A. (1987). Cohesion in the discourse of normal and head-injured adults. *Journal of Speech and Hearing Research*, 30, 88–98.

Mortensen, L. (2003). Reconstructing the writer: Acquired brain impairment and letters of community membership. Unpublished PhD thesis, Macquarie University, Sydney.

Pennycook, A. (2001). *Critical Applied Linguistics: A Critical Introduction*. Mahwah, NJ: Lawrence Erlbaum.

Prevignano, C. L. and Thibault, P. J. (eds.) (2003). *Discussing Conversation Analysis*. Amsterdam: John Benjamins.

Ripich, D. and Terrell, B. (1988). Patterns of discourse cohesion and coherence in Alzheimer's Disease. *Journal of Speech and Hearing Disorders*, 53, 8–15.

Rose, T. A., Worrall, L. E., and McKenna, K. T. (2003). The effectiveness of aphasia-friendly principles for printed health education materials for people with aphasia following stroke. *Aphasiology*, 17(10), 947–64.

Rothery, J. (1996). Making changes: Developing an educational linguistics. In R. Hasan and G. Williams (eds.), *Literacy in Society*. London: Longman.

Sherratt, S. (2004). Right brain damage and affective expression in discourse. Paper presented at the 26th World Congress of the International Association of Logopedics and Phoniatrics, Brisbane, August 29–September 2.

Sherratt, S. (2007). Right brain damage and the verbal expression of emotion: A preliminary investigation. *Aphasiology*, 21, 320–39.

Simmons-Mackie, N. and Damico, J. S. (1999). Social role negotiation in aphasia therapy: Competence, incompetence, and conflict. In D. Kovarsky, J. F. Duchan and M. Maxwell (eds.), *Constructing (In)competence: Disabling Evaluations in Clinical and Social Interaction* (pp. 313–42). Mahwah, NJ: Lawrence Erlbaum.

Spencer, E., Packman, A., Onslow, M., and Ferguson, A. (2005). A preliminary investigation of the impact of stuttering on language use. *Clinical Linguistics and Phonetics*, 19(3), 191–201.

Thompson, G. (1996). *Introducing Functional Grammar*. London: Arnold.

Thomson, J. (2003). Clinical discourse analysis: One theory or many? *Advances in Speech Language Pathology*, 5, 41–9.

Thomson, J. (2005). Theme analysis of narratives produced by children with and without Specific Language Impairment. *Clinical Linguistics and Phonetics*, 19(3), 175–90.

Togher, L. (2000). Giving information: The importance of context on communicative opportunity for people with traumatic brain injury. *Aphasiology*, 14, 365–90.

Togher, L. and Hand, L. (1998). Use of politeness markers with different communication partners: An investigation of five subjects with traumatic brain injury. *Aphasiology*, 12, 755–70.

Togher, L., Hand, L., and Code, C. (1997a). Analysing discourse in the traumatic brain injury population: Telephone interactions with different communication partners. *Brain Injury*, 11, 169–89.

Togher, L., Hand, L., and Code, C. (1997b). Measuring service encounters in the traumatic brain injury population. *Aphasiology*, 11, 491–504.

Togher, L., Hand, L., and Code, C. (1999). Exchanges of information in the talk of people with traumatic brain injury. In S. McDonald, L. Togher, and C. Code (eds.), *Communication Disorders Following Traumatic Brain Injury* (pp. 113–45). Hove, Sussex: Psychology Press.

Togher, L., McDonald, S., Code, C., and Grant, S. (1999). Can training communication partners of people with TBI make a difference? Paper presented at the 22nd Annual Brain Impairment Conference, Sydney.

WHO (2001). *ICF: International Classification of Functioning, Disability and Health*. Geneva: World Health Organization.

Young, L. and Harrison, C. (eds.) (2004). *Systemic Functional Linguistics and Critical Discourse Analysis*. London: Continuum.

Appendix: Glossary of SFL terms

channel what speech-language pathologists often refer to as the 'modality' of communication, e.g. spoken, written, signed

clause complex more than one clause that exist in some type of structural dependency relationship (parataxis – coordination, hypotaxis – subordination); the spoken equivalent of a written 'sentence'

coherence the perception of unity and sense by the listener

cohesion the linguistic resources by which a text achieves unity

context the non-verbal, non-linguistic environment of the use of language

context of culture the ideological and ethnic environment of the use of language

context of situation the main aspects of the non-linguistic environment seen to affect the use of language, namely Field, Tenor, Mode

contextual configuration the unique combination of Field, Tenor and Mode for any use of language

co-text the linguistic environment of the use of language, e.g. surrounding parts of the text

delicacy the depth of the analysis of choices being made in the linguistic system

discourse any connected use of language, whether written or spoken, involving one or more interactants, hence including conversation

discourse-semantics level of language involving systems of meaning which run through the text as a whole

Experiential the metafunction of language use to be about something

Field what is being talked or written about

Generic Structure Potential the obligatory and optional elements in a genre and their sequence

genre type of discourse, culturally determined

Interpersonal the metafunction of language use to express and create the relationship between interactants

level refers to the series of strata of meaning, in which each stratum is 'realized' by the level below: extralinguistic levels of context of culture and context of situation, and linguistic levels involving discourse-semantics, lexicogrammar, and expression.

lexical relations how the words used relate to the Field and to each other in the text and in the language system

lexicogrammar level of language involving systems of meaning expressed in wordings in the clause

metafunction one of the functions of every use of language (Experiential, Interpersonal, Textual)

Mode the part language is playing in the discourse

Mood the lexicogrammatical system of expressing the relationship between the speaker and what is being said, and the relationship between the interactants, at the clause level, involving modality (e.g. declarative, interrogative, imperative), polarity (e.g. negation), and other resources for modulating meaning

move a semantic unit, reflecting one act of meaning by the speaker, akin to turn-taking in conversation, after which a speaker change could occur without being seen as an interruption. For written texts, moves are signaled through the use of conventions such as sentence punctuation and paragraphing

rank language is seen as comprising constituents which when combined form meanings at different 'ranks': thus word constituents combine to form noun and verb phrases, which combine to form clauses, which combine to form clause complexes

realized by each level of language simultaneously reflects or expresses the meanings at the level(s) above it (and each realization constructs the meanings in a similar fashion). For example, a particular culture gives rise to (is realized by) certain genres, a particular genre gives rise to (is realized by) certain registers or contextual configurations, and a particular configuration of Field, Tenor and Mode will give rise to (is realized by) particular aspects of Experiential, Interpersonal and Textual meanings respectively, and they in turn will be realized by particular resources in the lexicogrammatical system

reference how participants are introduced and tracked through the discourse

register the way an individual speaker has used the contextual configuration of Field, Tenor and Mode in a particular instance of language use

system network the choices available to the speaker from the options in the linguistic system, diagrammatically represented

Tenor the role relationship between interactants

text some use of language that forms some sort of meaningful unit, has 'textuality'

Textual the metafunction of language use to organize meaning

Theme the lexicogrammatical system of organizing message salience, into starting points (Theme) and the remainder (Rheme).

Transitivity the lexicogrammatical system of expressing who is doing what to whom

9 Cross-Linguistic and Multilingual Perspectives on Communicative Competence and Communication Impairment: Pragmatics, Discourse, and Sociolinguistics

ZHU HUA AND LI WEI

9.1 Introduction

While English remains the best-researched language in the field of communication impairment in children and adults, cross-linguistic and multilingual studies have been expanding rapidly in the last two decades. These studies contribute to our understanding of both the underlying processes of communication impairment and the various factors that affect those processes. First of all, cross-linguistic and multilingual studies evaluate and challenge theoretical claims about typical communication development and impairment as proposed with reference to English only. Secondly, they examine whether and how differences in specific languages or language combinations result in differences in patterns of communication impairment. Thirdly, they investigate whether the same impairment manifests itself in different ways from one language to another or from monolingual speakers to multilingual speakers, and whether language differences account for more variance than individual differences among speakers of the same language/language combinations. And finally, they inform assessment and intervention suitable for monolingual populations speaking languages other than English or bilingual and multilingual speakers.

In this chapter, we review cross-linguistic and multilingual studies of communication development and impairment, focusing on pragmatics, discourse and sociolinguistics. Given that these terms have different meanings to different people, we first establish what we mean by them. We then provide a critical review of recent literature, looking at cross-linguistic research first, and then multilingual studies.

9.2   Language Use: Pragmatics, Discourse, and Sociolinguistics

In broad terms, pragmatics, discourse, and sociolinguistics are all about language use. Pragmatics is often understood as the study of meaning in context. It is about explaining how speakers produce language forms in specific ways so that their intended meanings are not only expressed in a context-appropriate manner but also understood by the hearer as intended. Concepts such as intentionality, form–function mapping, relevance, and appropriacy are central to the study of pragmatics. The acquisition of pragmatics, for example, would involve learning, at a micro-level, how to convey and interpret the meaning which cannot be expressed purely and entirely by means of the phonology, morphology, syntax and semantics of a particular language, and, at a macro-level, how to use language in social interaction. Pragmatic development includes the mastery of communicative use of linguistic and non-linguistic expressions, the development of conversational skills, and the acquisition of various contextually or culturally determined rules governing linguistic interaction to achieve communication success.

Discourse has been defined by many linguists as anything 'beyond the sentence', as discussed in Schiffrin, Tannen, and Hamilton (2001). Broadly speaking, it covers two areas: at the conversational level, interactional patterns such as turn-taking, initiation of conversation exchanges, and recognition and repair of communicative breakdown, and, at connected speech level, narrative, argument, explanation, and definition. Inevitably there is overlap between pragmatics and discourse. Some critical theorists use 'discourse' to refer to a broader range of social practice that includes non-linguistic and non-specific instances of language (e.g. discourse of power). Such a definition takes the study of discourse beyond the scope of linguistics to social sciences. In this chapter, we confine ourselves to the traditional, narrower definition of discourse and focus on language use beyond the sentence level.

Sociolinguistics is the study of stylistic, dialectal and cultural variations in language use. While it shares with pragmatics and discourse the interest in language use in context, sociolinguistics typically studies it from a speaker-oriented perspective, focusing on variables such as age, gender, and socio-economic class. Sociolinguists tend to study language use by groups of speakers rather than individually, and are concerned with collective patterns of language behavior in social contexts. In other words, sociolinguistics is not only about language in use, but also about speaker in community. It also concerns what societies do with their languages, i.e. language policy, language planning, and language attitude.

Taken together, pragmatics, discourse, and sociolinguistics are the key components of communicative competence (Hymes, 1972), the ability of the language user to "select, from the totality of grammatically correct expressions available, . . . forms which appropriately reflect the social norms governing behaviour in specific encounters" (Gumperz, 1972, p. 205). As Saville-Troike (1996, p. 363) says:

> Communicative competence extends to both knowledge and expectation of who may or may not speak in certain settings, when to speak and when to remain silent, whom one may speak to, how one may talk to persons of different statuses and roles, what non-verbal behaviors are appropriate in various contexts, what the routines for turn-taking are in conversation, how to ask for and give information, how to request, how to offer or decline assistance or cooperation, how to give commands, how to enforce disciplines, and the like – in short, everything involving the use of language and other communicative dimensions in particular social settings.

9.3   Cross-Linguistic Perspective

9.3.1   *Development of pragmatics and discourse*

For many years, the study of the development of pragmatics and discourse has been predominantly focused on English. (For developmental pragmatics in English, see Leinonen, Letts, & Smith, 2000; McTear & Conti-Ramsden, 1992; Ninio & Snow, 1996; Ochs & Schieffelin, 1979. For pragmatics and discourse of the English-speaking elderly, see Coupland, Coupland, & Giles, 1991; Davis, 2005; Maxim, 1994.) Studies on other languages have only started to emerge or become available in English in the last ten years. Most of the existing studies on languages other than English seek to apply to the description and analysis of other languages theories and models in pragmatics and discourse analysis that have been developed on the basis of English. It is not surprising, therefore, that the findings from the existing studies largely confirm the applicability of the theories and models and that the overall pragmatic and discourse patterns used by speakers of others languages are the same as those by English speakers. For instance, many studies have looked at adult–child interaction in different languages. While there are some differences in the number or proportion of directives adults produce in such a context in different cultures, the general dominance by adults in adult–child interaction is universal. Similarly, aphasic patients in different languages have shown similar patterns of impairment in language use, depending on the location of the lesion rather than on linguistic structures.

Nevertheless, there are cross-cultural differences in pragmatics that can lead to different expectations of what is normal and what is impaired. For example,

Ochs (1988) in her study of language socialization in a Samoan village in the Pacific Islands found that patterns of silence and overlapping speech were very different from those found in English-speaking cultures, and they carried specific cultural meanings that needed to be interpreted differently. Guo (1995) and Ervin-Tripp, Guo, and Lampert (1990) observed that Chinese and Japanese children followed culturally specific politeness rules in controlling the topic and flow of conversation. There have also been reports of avoidance of direct questions and apparent overuse of repetition in certain languages and cultures (see Schieffelin & Ochs, 1986).

One area of pragmatics that has received some attention from cross-linguistic researchers is the communicative use of non-verbal behaviors (e.g. gestures such as pointing) in young children. Recent examples of this work include Blake, Osborne, Cabral, and Gluck's study (2003) of Japanese children's use of gesture, Rodrigo, Gonzalez, Vega, Muneton-Ayala, and Rodriguez's longitudinal study (2004) of Spanish children's use of gestural and verbal deixis, and Guidetti's study (2005) of the combined use of gestures and speech to signal their intention to agree or refuse among young French children. While research on English-speaking children also points to the importance of gestures in language acquisition, cultural differences in the meaning of gestures are an important issue for the developing child.

At a discourse level, Meng and Schrabback (1999) look at the acquisition of German interjections, in particular 'hm' and 'na', in adult–child discourse. It was found that the children aged 2;8–3;4 had already managed to acquire basic interjectional forms and functions, as well as some discourse-type constraints, but they seemed to fail to understand the plurifunctionality of interjections. Perroni (1993) reported a longitudinal, observational study of the development of narrative discourse between two Brazilian Portuguese-speaking children and identified various types of strategies underlying narrative constructions. Aviezer (2003) investigated strategies of clarification in the face of miscommunication by Hebrew-speaking children. Corsaro and Maynard (1996) examined 'format tying' (participants' strategic use of phonological, syntactic, and semantic surface-structure features of prior turns at talk) in discussion and argument among Italian and American children. Korolija (2000) investigated the accomplishment of coherence in multiparty conversations amongst Swedish-speaking elderly people. Wong and Ingram (2003) looked at the patterns of acquisition of question among Cantonese-speaking children. Jisa (1987) described French-speaking children's use of high-frequency oral-discourse connectors in their narratives.

9.3.2   Pragmatic and discourse skills of children with language and communication impairments

There is much debate on the status of pragmatic skills in English-speaking children diagnosed with SLI. This is partly to do with the difficulty of getting an agreement amongst researchers on what pragmatics means in the first place.

Shaeffer (2005, p. 90) argued that most studies of children with SLI seem to point to deficits in pragmatic abilities such as speech acts, conversational participation and discourse regulation (initiations, replies, topic maintenance, turn-taking, utterance repair, etc.). Other studies suggest that children with SLI tend to be associated with poor participation in cooperative learning and poor negotiation skills (Brinton, Fujiki, & McKee, 1998). Craig and Evans (1993) pointed out that children with SLI presenting expressive deficits and those presenting combined expressive-receptive deficits were found to vary from each other on specific measures of turn-taking and cohesion. This seems to suggest that in addition to expressive language, the receptive language ability will need to be considered in pragmatics research. Most of these studies are concerned with English-speaking children.

An issue that needs to be considered here is the status of pragmatic impairment. There is controversy as to whether children with pure pragmatic impairment exist or the so-called pragmatic impairment is a secondary consequence of SLI or other dysfunctions. In categorizing subgroups of children with language and speech impairment, Conti-Ramsden and Botting (1999) and Conti-Ramsden, Crutchley, and Botting (1997) list pragmatic difficulties as either co-existing with semantic difficulties or existing as a separate category. In contrast, in a study on subgroups of language impairment among Dutch-speaking children, pragmatic impairment did not account for group variance and therefore was not listed as a subtype of impairment (Daal, Verhoeven, & Balkom, 2004). The debate on whether pragmatics can be impaired independently has implications not only for clinical diagnosis and management, but also for linguistic theory. Shaeffer (2005, p. 90) argued that "If pragmatics can be impaired independently, without affecting other components of language, this provides support for the modularity of language, i.e. for the hypothesis that there is an independent pragmatics module."

A different approach to pragmatic impairment is proposed by Michael Perkins (chapter 5 in this volume, 2002). In this approach, pragmatic behavior is seen as an emergent consequence of interactions within and between *linguistic systems* which include phonology, prosody, morphology, syntax, lexis and discourse, *cognitive systems* and *sensorimotor systems*. Therefore, different underlying causes may result in different types of pragmatic impairment: for example, cognitive dysfunction leads to primary pragmatic impairment; linguistic or sensorimotor dysfunction may result in secondary pragmatic impairment; dysfunction in more than one of these systems may result in complex pragmatic impairment. Again, very little is known about pragmatic impairment in children speaking languages other than English.

Pragmatic deficit also occurs in various kinds of autism. Individuals with Asperger syndrome or high-functioning autism are highly susceptible to pragmatic impairments such as inappropriate speech, non-compliance with rules of conversation, difficulty in dialogue management, and failures in communication inference. Oi (2005) looked at how non-autistic interlocutors respond to pragmatic impairments in Japanese children with Asperger syndrome. He found that the autistic participants adopted a greater number of compensation strategy types than the normally functioning adults when a breakdown occurred. Interestingly, adults' judgment on whether there is communicative breakdown in the conversation and whether the interactant's compensation strategy is effective seems to be different between initial and second-round analyses of videotapes of the conversation. This finding, though based on Japanese children with autism, may have wider implications for clinical practice across different languages.

9.3.3   *Pragmatic and discourse skills of people with acquired language and communication impairments*

Pragmatic deficits can occur as a consequence of brain damage or aphasia. Some studies document the pragmatic behaviors of English speakers with brain damage. Dennis and Barnes (1990) show that children and adolescents with closed-head injury have difficulties in certain pragmatic tasks, such as knowing the alternate meanings of an ambiguous word in context or bridging the inferential gap between events in stereotyped social institutions. Eisele, Lust, and Aram (1998) noted inferential deficits in the comprehension of implications and presuppositions in children with unilateral left- or right-hemisphere damage. Bara, Bosco, and Bucciarelli (1999) argued that for young children, the resultant pragmatic impairment is less severe than for older children with brain damage, probably because the other areas are able to take over pragmatic abilities at early ages but not later.

Aphasia often leads to pragmatic deficits. In one of the very few studies of pragmatic deficits in speakers of languages other than English, Pak-Hin, and Law (2004) developed a Cantonese linguistic communication measure to quantify narrative production of Cantonese speakers with aphasia. The measure contained eight indices reflecting the amount, efficiency, and rate of information conveyed, the grammaticality of and the extent of elaboration on sentences produced, as well as the degree of erroneous production and lexical diversity in the speech output. Cantonese speakers with aphasia displayed various deficits in these measures. Wulfeck, Bates, Juarez, et al. (1989) and Rizzi (1980) compared English, Italian and German aphasia patients' ability to differentiate the given/new contrast on several aspects of linguistic expression. Severity of aphasia rather than structural differences in languages was found to account for the differences in the speakers' pragmatic abilities.

Studies of language degeneration in adults with Dementia of Alzheimer's type (DAT) suggest that whereas phonology, morphology and syntax are relatively preserved, deterioration of conceptual, semantic and pragmatic aspects is usually evident. The patients' discourse is characterized by a predominant lack of coherence (organization of ideas at the conceptual level) in spite of good preservation of cohesion (logical organization of syntactic elements at the linguistic level). St-Pierre, Ska, and Béland (2005) investigated the discourse of French-speaking DAT patients and argued that the lack of coherence in the narrative discourse of DAT patients is due to the lower proportion of relevant information it contains.

A number of researchers have looked at language impairment of people with schizophrenia. There seems to be a general agreement that the primary language deficit is manifested in the area of pragmatic performance. Based on data from Hebrew-speaking patients, Meilijson, Kasher, and Elizur (2004) showed that participants with schizophrenia had their most inappropriate performance in topic change, followed by topic maintenance.

9.3.4   *The role of culture*

The role of culture emerges as a key issue in cross-linguistic research of language and communication impairment. It is important to point out that linguistic practices are part and parcel of a specific cultural tradition. They are manifestations of cultural values. Cultural differences are often represented through differences in linguistic practices. Speakers of different languages are socialized into different cultural values and traditions through an engagement of linguistic practices and they come to represent different cultures through their linguistic practices. Cross-linguistic studies can shed light on culture-specific appropriateness or norm which is crucial to our understanding of pragmatics and discourse in the context of language and communication impairment.

Nevertheless, how children acquire culture-specific or context-specific rules governing appropriateness of interaction seems to be underresearched. These culture-specific rules, at a micro-level, involve how to use contextualized cues to interpret other people's communicative intent and communicate one's own and, at a macro-level, consist of cultural and social norms and conventions which are intertwined with interactional practices. For example, people from certain cultures may have longer gaps between turns; different cultures may have different rules of politeness in performing various speech acts; and different languages may employ different linguistic means to achieve the same pragmatic function or the same linguistic means for different pragmatic functions.

Taylor (1986) and Taylor and Clarke (1994) proposed a cultural framework which attempts to demonstrate the impact of culture on communication disorders in terms of four central topics associated with the nature, causes, assessment and treatment of communication disorders. These topics are developmental issues (such as adult–child interaction within culture, and indigenous cognitive acquisition), precursors of communication pathology (such as cultural definitions of normal and pathological interaction), assessment (i.e. culturally valid assessment and diagnosis of communication), and diagnosis and treatment (i.e. application of culturally valid treatment procedures).

An example of the importance of cross-linguistic, cross-cultural analysis in understanding interactional and language socialization processes is King and Melzi's (2004) study which explores the use of diminutives in everyday conversation between Spanish-speaking Peruvian mothers and their children and attempts to explain why and how diminutive imitation seems to promote greater overall use of diminutives in the Peruvian context. Diminutives have received little attention from language researchers, partly because English has a relatively impoverished and unproductive diminutive system, mainly relying on the suffix *–y/ie* occurring with a restricted set of common and proper nouns. However, in languages such as Spanish diminutives have much richer semantic systems and pragmatic functions. In addition to 'smallness', diminutives in Spanish convey intimacy, playfulness, politeness or humor. They reflect the Peruvian cultural value of "carino, which translates loosely as tenderness, endearment, fondness and positive affect" (p. 257). Diminutives have been found to be prevalent in female speech and in speech directed at children. Through imitation or repetition of their mothers' use of diminutives, as King and Melzi argue, Spanish children are able to acquire the system of diminutives very early despite its semantic and pragmatic complexity.

In the areas of pragmatics and discourse, where people from different cultural and language backgrounds may behave differently in interaction and have different norms towards what constitutes culturally appropriate behaviors, culture-specific expectations and procedures need to be followed in administering clinical assessment. The cross-cultural child socialization literature also suggests that children from some cultures may not be at ease in testing situation in clinics. Cheng (2004, p. 169) argues that the discourse style of Asian-Pacific American children may differ from those of other American children at home and at school. For example, this population may delay or hesitate in response, be less likely to ask questions or use discourse markers to acknowledge the interactant, and tend to use longer pauses between turns. It is important for clinicians not to interpret these differences as "deficient, disordered, aberrant and undesirable". Barrenechea and Schmitt (1989) examined Spanish-speaking preschool children for the development of seven language functions and three discourse features. A set of preliminary guidelines for the development of normal pragmatics in Hispanic preschoolers was then developed.

9.3.5 *Development of sociolinguistic competence*

As discussed earlier, sociolinguistics concerns stylistic, dialectal and cultural variations in language use by different speaker groups. Cross-linguistic studies of sociolinguistics in the context of communication disorders, similar to those of pragmatics and discourse, are predominantly concerned with how normal speakers use linguistic means (specifically dialectal and social variations) to convey meaning. Two broad types of sociolinguistic studies can be identified in the literature: comparisons of group patterns and acquisition of dialectal and social variations.

The first type – group comparisons – often overlaps with studies of pragmatics and discourse. Rice, Sell, and Hadley (1991), for example, compared the patterns of social interactions among four groups (normally developing English, specific language impairment, speech impairment, and English as a second language). They found that children with limited communication skills were more likely than their normal language peers to initiate with adults (rather than children) and to shorten their responses or use non-verbal responses. Children learning English as a second language were the least likely to initiate interactions and were the most likely to be avoided as the recipient of an initiation. Andersen, Brizuela, DuPuy, and Gonnerman (1999) examined cross-linguistic data from American English, Lyonnais French, and Chicano Spanish on the use of discourse markers to indicate social relationships between interlocutors. Striking cross-linguistic parallels were found in the way children of different language backgrounds learn to use discourse makers both to convey social meaning and to manipulate the social situation where power relationships are not pre-established. For example, all groups were found to use more lexical discourse markers and more 'stacks' (such as *well*, *now then*) to mark higher-status roles, with non-lexical variants (such as *uh*, *euh*, or *eh*) more frequent in the low-status roles.

Amongst studies of children's acquisition of dialectal and social variations, African American English (AAE) seems to have received a considerable amount of attention. AAE is a language variety whose key features closely approximate, at the surface level, those of American-English-speaking children with SLI (such as habitual *be*, copula absence, inflectional *–s*, and other grammatical, phonological and lexical features; Wolfram, 2005). The past twenty years have seen an increasing amount of research on developing and evaluating assessment instruments and establishing expectations for the language performance of young African American children. Studies in this area include (the list is by no means exhaustive): Craig and Washington (2002), Qi, Kaiser, Milan, and Hancock (2006); Thomas-Tate, Washington, Craig, and Packard (2006); Washington and Craig (1992a, 1992b, 2004); Horton-Ikard, Weismer, and Edwards (2005) (see Roberts, 2005 for a review). Several studies also point out that children from low socio-economic strata tend to perform lower than expected on standardized tests of language abilities compared with children from middle or high socio-economic background (Qi, Kaiser, Milan, & Hancock, 2006).

These works have resulted in significant breakthroughs in our understanding of the impact of dialect and of potential educational and clinical significance of language differences associated with AAE in many aspects. These include the following:

1 Consideration needs to be given to non-standard, regional and social-cultural variations of a language in clinical assessment and diagnosis.
2 Cultural sensitivity and specificity of language-screening instruments need to be rigorously tested.
3 Both standardized assessment instruments and non-standardized, criterion-referenced assessments need to be developed and appropriately selected.

Oetting (2005) reviewed a list of newly developed and/or recently validated tools for assessing children who speak a non-mainstream dialect of English and discussed the challenges facing the clinical adaptation of these tools. Laing and Kamhi (2003) presented two procedures (processing-dependent measures and dynamic assessment measures) which they believed could provide unbiased assessment for culturally and linguistically diverse populations. Carter, Lees, Murira, et al. (2005) identified the major issues in the cross-cultural adaptation of speech and language assessment and argued that awareness of cultural variation and bias, and cooperative efforts to develop and administer culturally appropriate assessment tools, are the foundation of effective, valid treatment programs.

In a study of reliability of identification of non-standard and non-native English-speaking children with speech-language delay and disorder, Gupta, Li Wei, and Dodd (1999) found that professionals such as doctors and teachers who have not had systematic training in sociolinguistics or speech and language therapy often shared with parents their perception of dialectal variations as a potential contributor to communication disorders. On the whole, they were more likely to refer children with strong dialectal and contact features in their English to speech and language therapists. Interestingly, professionals working in geographical areas where there are easily recognizable dialectal variations or close contacts between different language groups tend to underrefer children with speech-language problems, assuming that the problems were part of the non-standard and non-native features of English.

9.4 Multilingual Perspective

9.4.1 Communicative competence of multilingual speakers

In the last two decades, there has been an increased awareness that the vast majority of the world's population are bilingual or multilingual and that studies of language and communication impairment must take into account the speaker's multilingual skills. There is a growing body of literature on the language development of multilingual children and the language use of multilingual adults and the elderly. Although some of the studies deal with specific linguistic features such as word order or gender assignment, most researchers recognize that bilingualism and multilingualism are essentially a language use issue. As Mackey (1962, p. 51) put it, *"Bilingualism* is not a phenomenon of language; but a characteristic of its use. It is not a feature of the code but of the message. It does not belong to the domain of 'langue', but of 'parole'."

To a multilingual speaker, the most important issue is appropriate choice of which language to speak to whom and when (Fishman, 1965), a central question that concerns all the studies of pragmatics, discourse and sociolinguistics. There has been much debate over the notion of language differentiation in multilingual speakers. With regard to children, the issue is how and when the child develops representations of the different languages he or she is learning, as opposed to one undifferentiated system that combines both. With regard to the elderly, the issue becomes whether or not the speaker can maintain appropriate choice of language when certain aspects of his or her language and cognitive faculty have been impaired. Language differentiation occurs at different levels: phonological, lexical, morphosyntactic and, of course, whole language systems (see De Houwer, 1995; Meisel, 2004). Typically though, multilingual speakers alternate between languages in their linguistic repertoire. This is known as 'code switching'. Code switching can occur between words, phrases, clauses, sentences and speaker turns. It assumes the speaker's ability to differentiate languages. Studies have found that bilingual children as young as two years can switch from one language to another in contextually sensitive ways (e.g., Lanza, 1992).

There is increasing evidence that code switching is the norm for many multilingual children (see Zhu & Li, 2005 for a review). In a recent study of preschool Mirpuri-English bilingual children, Pert and Letts (2006) found not only that every child in the sample produced utterances containing intrasentential code switching, but also that over 40 percent of multi-word utterances contained an intrasentential code switch. The Mean Lengths of Utterances for code-switched utterances were higher than for monolingual Mirpuri or English utterances. The code-switched utterances conformed to the grammatical constraints proposed in theoretical models such as the Matrix Language Frame model (Myers-Scotton, 1993). Pert and Letts argued, on the basis of the study, that a lack of code switching in children in this population may in fact be an indicator of language delay or intrinsic disorder. Studies of this kind have wide-ranging implications for speech and language therapy.

A number of studies of multilingual adult and elderly speakers have investigated the pragmatics of language choice and code switching from an emotional and affective perspective. It has been suggested that multilinguals often associate different experiences with different languages. Feelings, emotions and attitudes are therefore coded with specific language tags (Altarriba & Soltano, 1996; Schrauf, 2000). Multilinguals have a choice as to what language to use and thereby have the ability to select the word that most clearly captures the essence of what they are trying to communicate. Appropriate use of language switching in therapeutic settings with bilingual and multilingual populations has effects both on the clients' language and communication skills and their affective development.

9.4.2   Multilingual speakers with language and communication impairment

Studies of bilingual and multilingual children with language and communicative impairment are scarce. Paradis, Crago, Genesee, and Rice (2003, p. 14) point out that "there is a dearth of research on bilingual children with SLI, even though there are many bilingual children in North America, and even world-wide." Of the published studies, few deal specifically with issues of pragmatics or discourse. A sizable body of literature does exist on the development of narrative abilities of bilingual and multilingual children, which includes samples of bilingual children with various language disorders. Gutiérrez-Clellen (2004), for example, looked at narrative structures of Spanish-English bilingual children with language disorders. Their stories omitted specific links between events and lacked referential cohesion. For example, although when new referents were first introduced appropriate noun phrases were used, subsequent references were often ambiguous due to lack of cohesive devices. However, the researcher argued that the problems were linked to the children's limited syntactic complexity. Indeed, the children in this particular study were diagnosed as having SLI, and their difficulties with pragmatics and discourse were seen to be due more to SLI than to being bilingual.

Studies of multilingual speakers with acquired language and communication disorders often include examples of the speakers' inappropriate choice of language. Friedland (1998), for example, found that her four Afrikaans-English bilingual subjects with Alzheimer's disease all had difficulties in making addressee-appropriate language choices. This was not simply a matter of word retrieval, but an issue of pragmatics. They knew which words to use but often found it difficult to decide which language should be chosen. Similarly, some bilinguals with aphasia have problems with language choice and are unable to switch from one language to another for repairs (see Ijalba, Obler, & Chengappa, 2004 for a review).

9.5 Conclusion

As we can see from this brief review, cross-linguistic and multilingual studies of pragmatics, discourse and sociolinguistics are still in their infancy. Very few published studies deal with issues of language and communication impairment from discourse and cross-linguistic perspectives. Nevertheless, research in this area has the potential to challenge the received wisdom of normal communication development. It also presents a challenge to professionals working with speakers of languages other than English or multilingual speakers. There is an urgent need for more sophisticated assessment of communicative competence that takes into account cultural and linguistic diversity. Such assessment clearly needs to be based on sound research. It is hoped that more cross-linguistic and multilingual studies will become available in the next decade.

REFERENCES

Altarriba, J. and Soltano, E. G. (1996). Repetition blindness and bilingual memory. *Memory and Cognition*, 24, 700–11.

Andersen, E. S., Brizuela, M., DuPuy, B., and Gonnerman, L. (1999). Cross-linguistic evidence for the early acquisition of discourse markers as register variables. *Journal of Pragmatics*, 31, 1339–51.

Aviezer, O. (2003). Bedtime talk of three-year-olds: Collaborative repair of miscommunication. *First Language*, 23(1), 117–39.

Bara, B., Bosco, F. M., and Bucciarelli, M. (1999). Developmental pragmatics in normal and abnormal children. *Brain and Language*, 68, 507–28.

Barrenechea, L. I. and Schmitt, J. F. (1989). Selected pragmatic features in Spanish-speaking preschool children. *Journal of Psycholinguistic Research*, 18, 353–67.

Blake, J., Osborne, P., Cabral, M., and Gluck, P. (2003). The development of communicative gestures in Japanese infants. *First Language*, 23(1), 3–20.

Brinton, B., Fujiki, M., and McKee, L. (1998). Negotiation skills of children with specific language impairment. *Journal of Speech, Language and Hearing Research*, 41, 927–40.

Carter, J., Lees, J., Murira, G. M., Gona, J., Neville, B., and Newton, C. (2005). Issues in the development of cross-cultural assessments of speech and language for children. *International Journal of Language and Communication Disorders*, 40(4), 385–401.

Cheng, L-R. L. (2004). Speech and language issues in children from Asian-Pacific backgrounds. In R. Kent (ed.), *The MIT Encyclopedia of Communication Disorders* (pp. 167–9). Cambridge, MA: MIT Press.

Conti-Ramsden, G. and Botting, N. (1999). Classification of children with specific language impairment. In W. Yule and M. Rutter (eds.), *Language Development and Disorders* (pp. 16–41). London: Mac Keith Press.

Conti-Ramsden, G., Crutchley, A., and Botting, N. (1997). The extent to which psychometric tests differentiate subgroups of children with SLI. *Journal of Speech, Language and Hearing Research*, 40, 765–77.

Corsaro, W. and Maynard, D. (1996). Format Tying in discussion and argumentation among Italian and American children. In D. Slobin, J. Gerhardt, A. Kyratzis, and J. S. Guo (eds.), *Social Interaction, Social Context, and Language* (pp. 157–74). Mahwah, NJ: Lawrence Erlbaum.

Coupland, N., Coupland, J., and Giles, H. (1991). *Language, Society and the Elderly*. Oxford: Blackwell.

Craig, H. K. and Evans, J. (1993). Pragmatics and SLI. *Journal of Speech and Hearing Research*, 36, 779–89.

Craig, H. K. and Washington, J. A. (2002). Oral language expectations for African American preschoolers and kindergartners. *American Journal of Speech-Language Pathology*, 11, 59–70.

Daal, J. V., Verhoeven, L., and Balkom, H. V. (2004). Subtypes of severe speech and language impairments. *Journal of Speech, Language and Hearing Research*, 47, 1411–23.

Davis, B. H. (ed.) (2005). *Alzheimer Talk, Text and Context: Enhancing Communication*. London: Palgrave Macmillan.

Dennis, M. and Barnes, M. A. (1990). Knowing the meaning, getting the point, bridging the gap, and carrying the message: Aspects of discourse following closed head injury in childhood and adolescence. *Brain and Language*, 39, 428–46.

De Houwer, A. (1995). Bilingual language acquisition. In P. Fletcher and B. MacWhinney (eds.), *The Handbook of Child Language* (pp. 219–50). Oxford: Blackwell.

Eisele, J. A., Lust, B., and Aram, D. M. (1998). Presupposition and implication of truth: Linguistic deficits following early brain lesions. *Brain and Language*, 61, 335–75.

Ervin-Tripp, S., Guo, J., and Lampert, M. (1990). Politeness and persuasion in children's control acts. *Journal of Pragmatics*, 14(2), 307–32.

Fishman, J. A. (1965). Who speaks what language to whom and when? *La Linguistique*, 2, 67–88.

Friedland, D. (1998). Language loss in bilingual speakers with Alzheimer's disease. Unpublished PhD thesis, University of Newcastle upon Tyne.

Guidetti, M. (2005). Yes or no? How young French children combine gestures and speech to agree and refuse. *Journal of Child Language*, 32, 911–24.

Gumperz, J. J. (1972). Sociolinguistics and communication in small groups. In J. B. Pride and J. Holmes (eds.), *Sociolinguistics: Selected Readings*. Harmondsworth: Penguin.

Guo, J. (1995). The interactional basis of the Mandarin modal *néng* (can). In J. Bybee and S. Fleischman (eds.), *Modality in Grammar and Discourse* (pp. 205–38). Amsterdam: John Benjamins.

Gupta, A. F., Li Wei, and Dodd, B. (1999). Reliability of identification of children with speech-language delay and disorder with particular reference to non-standard or non-native English speakers. End of award (R000 22 2307) report to ESRC, UK.

Gutiérrez-Clellen, V. F. (2004). Narrative development and disorders in bilingual children. In B. A. Goldstein (ed.), *Bilingual Language Development and Disorders in Spanish-English Speakers* (pp. 235–56). Baltimore, MD: Paul Brookes.

Horton-Ikard, R., Weismer, S. E., and Edwards, C. (2005). Examining the use of standard language production measures in the language samples of African-American toddlers. *Journal of Multilingual Communication Disorders*, 3, 169–82.

Hymes, Dell H. (1972). On communicative competence. In J. B. Pride and J. Holmes (eds.), *Sociolinguistics: Selected Readings*. Harmondsworth: Penguin.

Ijalba, E., Obler, L. K., and Chengappa, S. (2004). Bilingual aphasia. In T. K. Bhatia and W. C. Ritchie (eds.), *The Handbook of Bilingualism* (pp. 71–89). Oxford: Blackwell.

Jisa, H. (1987). Sentence connectors in French children's monologue performance. *Journal of Pragmatics*, 11(5), 607–21.

King, K. and Melzi, G. (2004). Intimacy, imitation and language learning: Spanish diminutives in mother–child conversation. *First Language*, 24(2), 241–61.

Korolija, N. (2000). Coherence-inducing strategies in conversation as amongst the aged. *Journal of Pragmatics*, 32, 425–62.

Laing, S. and Kamhi, A. (2003). Alternative assessment of language and literacy in culturally and linguistically diverse population. *Language, Speech and Hearing Services in Schools*, 34, 44–55.

Lanza, E. (1992). *Language Mixing in Infant Bilingualism*. Oxford: Clarendon Press.

Leinonen, E., Letts, C., and Smith, B. R. (2000). *Children's Pragmatic Communication Difficulties*. London: Whurr.

Mackey, W. F. (1962). The description of bilingualism. *Canadian Journal of Linguistics*, 7, 51–85.

Maxim, J. (1994). *Language of the Elderly: A Clinical Perspective*. London: Whurr.

McTear, M. and Conti-Ramsden, G. (1992). *Pragmatic Disability in Children*. London: Whurr.

Meilijson, S., Kasher, A., and Elizur, A. (2004). Language performance in chronic schizophrenia: A pragmatic approach. *Journal of Speech, Language and Hearing Research*, 47, 695–713.

Meisel, J. M. (2004). The bilingual child. In T. K. Bhatia and W. C. Ritchie (eds.), *The Handbook of Bilingualism* (pp. 91–113). Oxford: Blackwell.

Meng, K. and Schrabback, S. (1999). Interjections in adult–child discourse: The cases of German HM and NA. *Journal of Pragmatics*, 31, 1263–87.

Myers-Scotton, C. (1993). *Duelling Languages: Grammatical Structure of Codeswitching.* Oxford: Clarendon Press.

Ninio, A. and Snow, C. (1996). *Pragmatic Development.* Boulder, CO: Westview Press.

Ochs, E. (1988). *Culture and Language Development: Language Acquisition and Language Socialization in a Samoan Village.* Cambridge: Cambridge University Press.

Ochs, E. and Schieffelin, B. (eds.) (1979). *Developmental Pragmatics.* New York: Academic Press.

Oetting, J. (2005). Assessing language in children who speak a nonmainstream dialect of English. In M. J. Ball (ed.), *Clinical Sociolingistics* (pp. 180–92). Malden, MA: Blackwell.

Oi, M. (2005). Interpersonal compensation for pragmatic impairments in Japanese children with Asperger syndrome or high-functioning autism. *Journal of Multilingual Communication Disorders*, 3(3), 203–10.

Pak-Hin, A. K. and Law, S.-P. (2004). A Cantonese linguistic communication measure for evaluating aphasic narrative production: normative and preliminary aphasic data. *Journal of Multilingual Communication Disorders*, 2(2), 124–46.

Paradis, J., Crago, M., Genesee, F., and Rice, M. (2003). Bilingual children with specific language impairment: How do they compare with their monolingual peers? *Journal of Speech, Language and Hearing Research*, 46, 1–15.

Perkins, M. (2002). An emergentist approach to clinical pragmatics. In F. Windsor, M. L. Kelly, and N. Hewlett (eds.), *Investigations in Clinical Phonetics and Linguistics* (pp. 1–14). Mahwah, NJ: Lawrence Erlbaum.

Perroni, M. C. (1993). On the acquisition of narrative discourse: A study in Portuguese. *Journal of Pragmatics*, 20(6), 559–77.

Pert, S. and Letts, C. (2006). Codeswitching in Mirpuri speaking Pakistani heritage preschool children: Bilingual language acquisition. *International Journal of Bilingualism*, 10(3), 349–74.

Qi, C. H-Q., Kaiser, A., Milan, S., and Hancock, T. (2006). Language performance of low-income African American and European American preschool children on the PPVT-III. *Language, Speech and Hearing Services in Schools*, 37, 5–16.

Rice, M., Sell, M., and Hadley, P. (1991). Social interactions of speech and language-impaired children. *Journal of Speech and Hearing Research*, 34, 1299–1307.

Rizzi, L. (1980). A restructuring rule in Italian syntax. In S. J. Keyser (ed.), *Recent Transformational Studies in European Languages.* Cambridge, MA: MIT Press.

Roberts, J. (2005). Acquisition of sociolinguistic variation. In M. J. Ball (ed.), *Clinical Sociolinguistics* (pp. 153–64). Malden, MA: Blackwell.

Rodrigo, M., Gonzalez, A., Vega, M., Muneton-Ayala, M., and Rodriguez, G. (2004). From gestural to verbal deixis, a longitudinal study with Spanish infants and toddlers. *First Language*, 24(1), 71–90.

Saville-Troike, M. (1996). *The Ethnography of Communication.* 2nd ed. Oxford: Blackwell.

Schieffelin, B. and Ochs, E. (eds.) (1986). *Language Socialization across Cultures.* Cambridge: Cambridge University Press.

Schiffrin, D., Tannen, D., and Hamilton, H. E. (eds.) (2001). *The Handbook of Discourse Analysis.* Malden, MA: Blackwell.

Schrauf, R. W. (2000). Bilingual autobiographical memory. *Culture and Psychology*, 6, 387–417.

Shaeffer, J. (2005). Pragmatic and grammatical properties of subjects in children with specific language impairment. In R. Okabe and K. Nielsen (eds.), *Papers in Psycholinguistics 2* (UCLA Working Papers in Linguistics, 13) (pp. 87–134). Available at www.linguistics.ucla.edu/faciliti/wpl/issues/wpl13/wpl13.htm.

St.-Pierre, M.-C., Ska, B., and Béland, R. (2005). Lack of coherence in the narrative discourse of patients with dementia of the Alzheimer's type. *Journal of Multilingual Communication Disorders*, 3(3), 211–15.

Taylor, O. L. (ed.) (1986). *Nature of Communication Disorders in Culturally and Linguistically Diverse Populations*. San Diego, CA: College-Hill Press.

Taylor, O. L. and Clarke, M. (1994). Culture and communication disorders: A theoretical framework. *Seminars in Speech and Language*, 15(2), 103–13.

Thomas-Tate, S., Washington, J., Craig, H., and Packard, M. (2006). Performance of African American preschool and kindergarten students on the expressive vocabulary test. *Language, Speech and Hearing Services in Schools*, 37, 143–9.

Washington, J. A. and Craig, H. K. (1992a). Articulation test performance of low-income, African-American preschoolers with communication impairments. *Language, Speech and Hearing Services in Schools*, 23, 203–7.

Washington, J. A. and Craig, H. K (1992b). Performance of low-income, African American preschool and kindergarten children on the Peabody Picture vocabulary test-revised. *Language, Speech and Hearing Services in Schools*, 23, 329–33.

Washington, J. A. and Craig, H. K. (2004). A language screening protocol for use with young African American children in urban settings. *American Journal of Speech-Language Pathology*, 13, 329–40.

Wolfram, W. (2005). African American English. In M. J. Ball (ed.), *Clinical Sociolinguistics* (pp. 87–100). Oxford: Blackwell.

Wong, W. and Ingram, D. (2003). Question acquisition by Cantonese speaking children. *Journal of Multilingual Communication Disorders*, 1, 148–57.

Wulfeck, B., Bates, E., Juarez, L., Opie, M., Friederici, A., MacWhinney, B., and Zurif, E. (1989). Pragmatics in aphasia: Crosslinguistic evidence. *Language and Speech*, 32, 315–36.

Zhu Hua and Li Wei (2005). Bi- and multilingual language acquisition. In M. J. Ball (ed.), *Clinical Sociolingistics* (pp. 165–79). Malden, MA: Blackwell.

Part II Syntax and Semantics

10 Chomskyan Syntactic Theory and Language Disorders

HARALD CLAHSEN

10.1 Introduction

Chomsky's theory of generative grammar regards human language as a cognitive system that is represented in a speaker's mind/brain with a grammar as its core element. The theory has seen substantial revisions over time (Chomsky, 1957, 1965, 1981, 1995, 2000), and several researchers have employed concepts and notions from different versions of Chomskyan theory in their studies of language impairments. The aim of this chapter is to present an overview of some prominent generative accounts of language impairments. Relevant concepts and notions from Chomskyan theory will be briefly mentioned, but for more detailed background information, the reader is referred to one of the many introductions to Chomskyan syntax (see e.g. Haegeman, 1991; Radford, 2004).

Why should anybody who wants to study language impairments in children or adults care about linguistic theory, more specifically, about Chomskyan generative syntax? One obvious reason is that linguistic theory provides the descriptive tools for analyzing the object of inquiry, i.e. language, and that employing these tools will lead to descriptively more precise characterizations of language disorders. A case in point comes from the study of Williams syndrome (WS), a genetically determined disorder with general cognitive deficits and a relative strength in language. Until recently linguistic studies of WS were not available, and the language of people with WS was characterized in intuitive terms, as, for example, "verbose" (Udwin & Yule 1990), exibiting "morphosyntactic difficulties" (Thal, Bates, & Bellugi, 1989), and showing an "unusual semantic organization" (Bellugi, Wang, & Jernigan, 1994). This has changed in the last few years as research on WS has adopted a linguistically more informed approach and produced detailed profiles of linguistic strengths and weaknesses of people with WS across a range of languages; see, for example, Clahsen and Almazan (2001, pp. 746ff.) for WS in English, and the contributions in Bartke and Siegmüller (2004) for WS in other languages.

Another potential advantage of a linguistic approach to language disorders is that it introduces a new way of looking at impaired language which is not readily available from traditional clinical taxonomies. This is particularly true for Chomskyan theory, which regards the human language faculty as a modular cognitive system that is said to be autonomous of non-linguistic cognitive systems such as vision, hearing, reasoning, or memory. The core of the human language faculty is a mental grammar which is broken down into various components (lexicon, phonology, morphology, syntax). This view of human language makes it possible to investigate language impairments as selective *within-language* deficits. In the past, most generative studies of language disorders have dealt with aphasia and Specific Language Impairment (SLI), i.e. with relatively pure language impairments in which other cognitive systems appear to remain intact. More recently, however, several researchers have begun to investigate a wider range of acquired and developmental disorders from this perspective, including Williams syndrome (Clahsen & Almazan, 1998) and Down's syndrome (Ring & Clahsen, 2005).

This chapter will focus on production studies of agrammatic aphasia and SLI. In addition, I will briefly outline how the study of broader cognitive impairments, in this case Down's syndrome, may benefit from a generative perspective.

10.2 Agrammatic Aphasia

Agrammatism in aphasia has traditionally been defined as a disorder of language production which mainly affects function words, i.e. bound grammatical morphemes (e.g. inflectional affixes) and free-standing functional morphemes (auxiliaries, determiners, etc.), while content words, the major lexical categories (nouns, verbs, adjectives) remain intact. Agrammatic production is often characterized as 'telegraphic speech' consisting mainly of content words and frequent omissions of grammatically required bound and free functional morphemes (*boy kiss girl*); see, for example, Goodglass (1968), Marshall (1986), Leuninger (1989), and Jarema (1998). However, much research has shown that agrammatic patients also have specific comprehension problems, for example in sentences in which functional grammatical morphemes are critical for interpretation.

Several researchers have made attempts to characterize agrammatic production in terms of Chomskyan theory. The earliest account comes from Kean (1979), who relied on Chomsky and Halle's (1968) model of generative phonology and proposed an underlying deficit at the level of phonological representation for agrammatism. Kean highlighted the fact that agrammatism affects both bound morphemes, e.g. inflectional affixes, and free-standing functional morphemes, e.g. auxiliaries and determiners, and that in semantic and syntactic terms the elements that are omitted in agrammatic production are rather heterogeneous and difficult to characterize. What they all share, however, is that they are phonological clitics in terms of Chomsky and Halle's theory. The basic distinction Kean employs is between phonological words, i.e. units relevant for word-stress assignment, and phonological clitics, that are irrelevant for stress assignment. For example, the word *kissing* is represented as [#[#kiss#] ing#] with the phonological word, but not the phonological clitic (ing#), being marked by boundary symbols on the left and on the right edge (#kiss#), thereby identifying a domain for stress assignment. According to Kean, this level of representation provides for a straightforward distinction between elements that remain intact in agrammatism (phonological words) and those that are affected (phonological clitics).

10.2.1   Feature and trace deletion

A well-known *syntactic* account of agrammatism comes from Grodzinsky (1990), who adopted Chomsky's (1981) Government and Binding (GB) Theory. Grodzinsky proposed separate accounts for production and comprehension in agrammatism.

With respect to agrammatic comprehension, Grodzinsky focused on difficulties agrammatic patients experience in the comprehension of passive sentences and other constructions which according to Chomsky (1981) involve syntactic movement. Consider, for example, passive sentences such as *The fish is eaten by the man* in which the passive participle *eaten* cannot assign objective case to its internal argument (*the fish*), resulting in movement of this argument to the subject position where it can be assigned nominative case. Object-to-subject movement is said to leave behind a phonologically silent copy of the object (trace) that is coindexed with the moved object and is assigned a thematic role by the verb ([*The fish*]$_i$ *is eaten* [t]$_i$ *by the man*). Grodzinsky (1990) found that agrammatic patients have difficulty comprehending passive sentences and other constructions involving movement traces but not corresponding simple active sentences that do not involve syntactic movement. Consequently, he argued that agrammatic patients construct syntactic representations for comprehension that do not contain any movement traces, the so-called Trace-Deletion Hypothesis. Although this accounts for the agrammatics' comprehension difficulties with passives and other syntactic phenomena involving traces, the Trace-Deletion Hypothesis has been subject to much criticism, and generative accounts of agrammatic comprehension have been much refined in recent years (see, e.g., Hickok & Avrutin, 1995; Beretta & Munn, 1998; Grodzinsky, 2000).

With respect to agrammatic production, Grodzinsky's (1990) idea was that the specific values of the features associated with functional categories are lost or deleted in agrammatism. This Feature-Deletion Hypothesis was presented in terms of Chomsky (1981), in which functional categories need to be specified for a set of abstract grammatical features. The functional category INFL, for example, is specified for features such as Tense ([PresTns] or [PastTns]), which determine the temporal value of the sentence. The functional category D(eterminer), on the other hand, which requires a nominal complement, is associated with features such as number, gender, definiteness. Grodzinsky claimed that although categories such as INFL or D are present in agrammatism, their internal features are deleted. Consider, as an illustration, the syntactic representation of the sentence *The boy kissed the girl* in normal standard English (1a) and in agrammatic English (1b).

(1a)

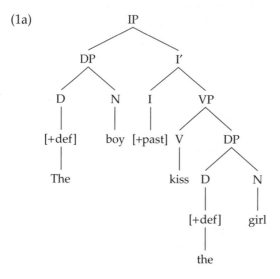

(b)

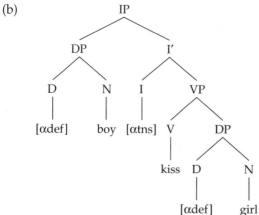

Grodzinsky (1990, p. 56) argued that the crucial property of (1b) is that the internal feature specifications of the two functional categories D and INFL are left unspecified with respect to definiteness and tense. As a consequence, English-speaking agrammatics leave the functional category slots empty, which results in telegraphic sentences such as *boy kiss girl*.

One problem for this account is that much research on agrammatic production has indicated that not all functional elements are equally affected. For example, complementizers are comparatively well retained (e.g., Goodglass, 1976; Menn & Obler, 1990), and regular noun plurals present less difficulty than possessive marking in English-speaking aphasics (Gleason, 1978), even though in phonological terms it is the same segment (-*s*). Moreover, a series of studies across a range of languages have produced evidence that tense marking is more impaired than subject–verb agreement in agrammatic production (e.g. Friedmann & Grodzinsky, 1997, 2000; Benedet, Christiansen, & Goodglass, 1998; Kolk, 2000; Wenzlaff & Clahsen, 2004). Friedmann and Grodzinsky (1997), for example, testing Hebrew- and Arabic-speaking subjects on sentence repetition and oral sentence completion tasks, found that subject–verb agreement was almost intact with error rates of less than 10 percent, whereas tense marking was severely impaired. Similar contrasts were found for English, German, Spanish, and Dutch. These findings are challenging for an account in which *all* functional categories (Grodzinsky, 1990) are said to be affected. In Chomsky (1981) both tense-marked verb forms and subject–verb agreement forms involve the specification of grammatical features of the functional element INFL, and hence according to Grodzinsky (1990) should both be affected in agrammatic production. The same is true for Ouhalla's (1993) proposal that in agrammatic speech, functional categories are completely missing. If this were correct, then the contrasts mentioned above, for example, between tense-marking and subject–verb agreement marking would be left unexplained. Likewise, in Chomsky and Halle (1968) both the past-tense *-ed* and the 3rd sg. affix *-s* are phonological clitics, and should therefore be equally affected if Kean's (1979) idea was correct that phonological clitics are impaired in agrammatic production. This prediction does not seem to hold, however, as the results mentioned above indicate. In short, the problem with these early generative accounts is that they fail to explain the subtle dissociations seen in agrammatic speech.

10.2.2 Tree-pruning

Several researchers have employed the hierarchy of functional projections posited in GB-theory to account for agrammatic production deficits (Hagiwara, 1995; Friedmann & Grodzinsky, 1997, 2000; Lee, 2003). Here our focus will be on the so-called Tree-Pruning Hypothesis (TPH; Friedmann & Grodzinsky, 1997, 2000) which explains the structural selectivity of the agrammatic production deficit in terms of Pollock's (1989) split-INFL hypothesis, according to which the category INFL is split into the functional categories TP (Tense Phrase) and AgrP (Agreement Phrase), with the former located above the latter.

Given this framework, the Tree-Pruning Hypothesis claims that in agrammatism any syntactic node from TP upwards becomes unavailable (pruned, in their terms), yielding phrase-structure representations without TP or any other functional category above TP, as illustrated in (2).

(2)

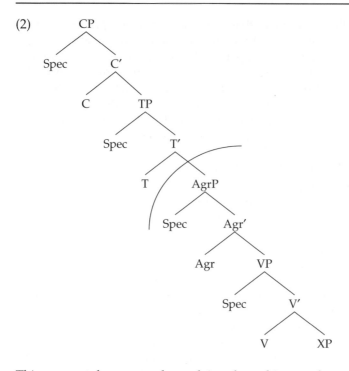

This account does not only explain why subject–verb agreement is preserved (since AgrP is lower than TP) whereas tense marking is impaired in agrammatic production; the TPH also predicts impairments in the production of *wh*-questions, embedded clauses and other CP-related phenomena in agrammatism, due to the unavailability of the CP-layer. Friedmann (2001) presents some evidence for this prediction from a series of repetition and elicited production tasks with 14 agrammatic patients, in which she found that the patients had difficulty repeating or producing sentences containing embedded complement clauses, object-relative clauses, and *wh*-questions, while at the same time they had no difficulty repeating or producing sentences with untensed complements (e.g. *John saw the woman dance*) and yes–no questions (without subject–verb inversion). Friedmann points out that these contrasts are compatible with the TPH, as the impaired phenomena all involve the CP-domain (which is unavailable for agrammatic production), and the non-impaired ones do not.

The TPH has been criticized, however, both from a theoretical perspective and on empirical grounds. Tree-pruning presupposes AgrP and TP as separate functional categories, as well as a fixed hierarchy of functional categories for CP-TP-AgrP-VP. Chomsky (2000), however, has pointed out that agreement and tense are fundamentally different syntactic concepts, with tense being an interpretable feature of the syntactic category T, and agreement not forming a functional category of its own. Instead, *Agree* is conceived of as an operation that establishes a structural relationship between, for example, the person and number features of a clausal subject and the corresponding uninterpretable features of a finite verb, which are checked by T. Thus, if T is pruned in the agrammatic phrase-structure tree (which according to the TPH accounts for impaired tense marking), *Agree* should not be able to operate because the host for a verb's person and number features (T) has been deleted. This means that an impairment of tense should co-occur with impairments in agreement, thus making it hard for the TPH to explain the observed selective impairment in tense marking.

On an empirical level, the TPH predicts that impairments in tense should coincide with impairments of CP-related phenomena. Friedmann and Grodzinsky (2000, p. 93) explicitly state that "nodes above TP do not exist in agrammatic representation". Likewise, Hagiwara (1995) predicts that there must not be any patient who can handle the elements in C(omp) but not those in T. Wenzlaff and Clahsen (2004, 2005) investigated a group of seven German-speaking agrammatic patients with respect to these predictions examining (among other phenomena) tense marking and the so-called verb-second constraint, which requires German main clauses to have a finite verb in CP. Verb-second in adverb-initial sentences such as those tested by Wenzlaff and Clahsen (2005) is clearly CP-related as it involves finite verb raising to C(omp) into a structural domain (CP) that is definitely higher than TP. And yet, in sentence-completion tasks, the patients had overall low accuracy scores for tense marking and all but one patient showed chance-level performance, while for verb-second the opposite pattern was found, i.e. overall high accuracy levels, and all but one patient performed significantly above chance level (see Wenzlaff & Clahsen, 2005, pp. 40–1). These results indicate that (contrary to what the TPH predicts) tense deficits in agrammatism are not linked to impairments with the verb-second constraint; see also Penke (1998, 2000) for converging evidence that verb-second is largely preserved in German-speaking agrammatics.

10.2.3 Underspecification of T/INFL

Wenzlaff and Clahsen (2004, 2005) proposed an interpretation of agrammatism in terms of Chomsky's (1995) Minimalist Program, claiming that in agrammatism the syntactic category T/INFL is unspecified for tense, with other features unimpaired. This account adopts the distinction between interpretable features, i.e., features relevant for semantic interpretation, and non-interpretable ones that are irrelevant for interpretation. According to Chomsky (1995), non-interpretable features must be checked and deleted in the course of the derivation, while interpretable features need not enter into checking relations. Wenzlaff and Clahsen's (2004, 2005) account rests on two crucial assumptions, (1) that T/INFL contains uninterpretable agreement features along with interpretable tense and mood features, and (2) that among the interpretable features of T/INFL, mood distinctions (between realis and irrealis forms) are primary and tense distinctions (between past and non-past forms) secondary, as illustrated in (3).

(3)

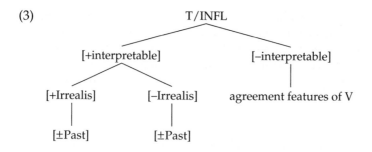

T/INFL is the host of verb finiteness features and as such contains not only agreement and tense, but also mood features, which distinguish between indicative ([–Irrealis]) and subjunctive or conditional ([+Irrealis]) finite verb forms. Mood and tense features are interpretable whereas agreement features of verbs are non-interpretable, i.e. irrelevant for the semantic interpretation of verbs. Within the interpretable features, mood distinctions are taken to be more basic than tense oppositions; mood marking is more common across languages than tense marking, and acquired earlier by children. Given these assumptions, the Tense Underspecification Hypothesis claims that agreement features and mood distinctions are maintained, while the secondary distinction between [+Past] and [–Past] is lost.

The empirical evidence for this account comes from a series of experiments investigating a group of seven German-speaking agrammatic patients with respect to subject–verb agreement and tense and mood marking. Wenzlaff and Clahsen examined these phenomena in sentence-completion tasks (to test for production deficits) as well as in grammaticality judgment tasks to determine which agrammatic symptoms extend to other modalities. It was found that all aphasic patients performed at high accuracy levels for mood and agreement in the sentence-completion and the grammaticality judgment tasks. By contrast, tense was impaired in the aphasic patients, and in both tasks. These results are consistent with the notion of an underspecification of T/INFL in agrammatism. Moreover, the finding that the grammaticality judgment and the sentence-completion tasks yielded parallel results and that no significant task effects were found indicates that T/INFL underspecification is a central representational deficit in agrammatism which can be seen not only in production, but also in other modalities; see Burchert, Swoboda-Moll, and De Bleser (2005) and Varlokosta, Valeonti, Kakavoulia, Lazaridou, and Economou (2005) for recent extensions of the T/INFL underspecification account.

10.3   Specific Language Impairment

SLI is defined as a delay or a disorder of the normal acquisition of grammar in the absence of neurological trauma, cognitive impairment, psycho-emotional disturbance, or motor-articulatory disorders (see Leonard, 1998; Levy & Kavé,

1999; Clahsen, 1999 for review). Several researchers have employed concepts and notions from Chomskyan theory in their attempts to characterize the morphosyntax of individuals with SLI and how it differs from that of typically developing children. Some accounts have posited relatively broad impairments in the underlying syntactic representations of SLI individuals to capture the kinds of difficulties they experience in morphosyntax. Other accounts have attempted to identify specific linguistic markers of SLI rather than providing a complete grammatical characterization.

One of the earliest accounts of SLI that posited a relatively broad syntactic deficit (Clahsen, 1989, 1991) claimed that the Control-Agreement Principle (Gazdar, Klein, Pullum, & Sag, 1985) is impaired in the grammars of individuals with SLI. In Gazdar and colleagues' theory, this principle is responsible for matching grammatical features of different syntactic categories within a sentence, as required for subject–verb or object–verb agreement, gender and number concord, structural case marking, and other kinds of syntactic dependencies. Another idea was that the system of *functional categories* (CP, IP, DP, etc.) is particularly vulnerable in these individuals (Eyer & Leonard, 1995; Guilfoyle, Allen, & Moss, 1991; Leonard, 1995, 1998). The third account of that ilk is van der Lely and colleagues' Representational Deficit for Dependent Relations (RDDR) hypothesis, which claims that individuals with SLI have "a deficit with building non-elementary complex syntactic dependencies between constituents" (van der Lely & Stollwerck, 1997, p. 283). What is common to these approaches is that they all posit relatively broad syntactic impairments.

Challenging for these kinds of accounts are findings indicating selective rather than broad impairments/delays in SLI grammars. Consider, for example, results from a recent study of structural case marking (Eisenbeiss, Bartke, & Clahsen, 2006), which examined large samples of production data from five German-speaking children with SLI and five control children who were matched to the children with SLI on the basis of their MLU (mean length of utterance). It was found that both the control and the children with SLI achieved high accuracy scores for all kinds of structural case marking, i.e. for nominative subjects, for accusatives on direct objects and complements of prepositions, and for datives on indirect objects, and that they overgeneralized structural case markers to exceptions, i.e. when lexical case marking was required in the adult language. For subject–verb agreement marking, on the other hand, the same children with SLI (with the exception of one child who was not available for the earlier study) performed considerably worse, with low accuracy scores relative to their MLU scores (Rothweiler & Clahsen, 1994). Structural selectivity of this kind is hard to explain by any of the three syntactic deficit accounts mentioned above, as in terms of Chomsky (1981) both case and agreement involve functional categories and a 'syntactic dependency' between grammatical features (feature checking/valuing). Thus, if any of these mechanisms were affected in SLI, we should see impairments for both structural case marking and agreement.

Another family of accounts of SLI has aimed at identifying linguistic markers of SLI, i.e. those aspects of the linguistic system that are most consistently affected across different individuals, different age groups and different languages. Several researchers working from this perspective have relied on Chomskyan theory. The following will provide a brief overview of these accounts with a focus on tense, agreement, and case marking in SLI.

10.3.1   *Optional tense*

The most widely known proposal of this kind is the Extended Optional Infinitive (EOI) hypothesis of Rice, Wexler and collaborators. The initial version of the EOI hypothesis (Rice, Wexler, & Cleave, 1995; Rice & Wexler, 1996) claimed that the functional category T(ense) is not obligatory in SLI children's grammars and that difficulties with tense marking constitute "a clinical marker" for SLI. Rice, Wexler and Cleave (1995) found, for example, that English-speaking children with SLI omitted, in obligatory contexts, 70 percent of the 3rd sg. -*s* forms and 78 percent of the past tense -*ed* forms – significantly more than non-impaired controls did. They also reported that the finite verb forms of *BE* and *DO* produced by the children with SLI were most often correctly inflected. In addition, the children with SLI did not use non-finite forms of auxiliaries when finite forms were required; for example, they did not produce sentences such as *He be sleeping*. The same pattern of errors was seen for past-tense forms, i.e., if the children used a past-tense form, it appeared in a past-tense context. Rice and colleagues noted that the common property of the 3rd sg. -*s* and the past-tense -*ed* is that they encode tense, and that they appear to be equally problematic for children with SLI. Their idea that T is optional in SLI children's grammars accounts for the fact that the children alternate between using bare verb stems and tense-marked verb forms in obligatory contexts for finite verbs, and that if a tense-marked form is used, it is correctly inflected. In more recent work, Rice (2003) presented analyses of longitudinal data showing a selective delay of the development of tense markers in children with SLI compared with unimpaired children. Rice showed that although other grammatical morphemes, e.g. the plural -*s* in English, develop within normal limits, children with SLI start using tense markers at a later age than unimpaired children, and even after several years do not achieve the same high accuracy scores as unimpaired children.

Although the idea that T is optional in the SLI grammar accounts for the pattern of results found in the children with SLI studied by Rice and colleagues, it does not seem to hold cross-linguistically. For languages such as German and Greek in which (unlike in English) tense and agreement marking can be clearly distinguished, tense marking was found to be almost error-free in children with SLI, whereas the same children showed significantly lower accuracy scores for subject–verb agreement (Clahsen, Bartke, & Göllner, 1997; Clahsen & Dalalakis, 1999). Moreover, these studies reported a fair number of true agreement errors in children with SLI, which according to the EOI hypothesis should be non-existent. There are even English SLI data which are problematic for the original version of the EOI hypothesis. Given that nominative subject case is assigned by Agr(eement) in English, the EOI hypothesis predicts that children with SLI should not produce any subject case errors, as agreement was said to be unimpaired. However, as shown in several studies, English-speaking preschool children with SLI do in fact produce many non-nominative subjects (Leonard, 1995; Loeb & Leonard, 1991; Schütze, 1997). In response to these challenges, the original version of the EOI hypothesis has been revised. The current version (Wexler, Schütze, & Rice, 1998; Wexler, 2003) claims that both tense and agreement are selectively delayed in SLI.

10.3.2   The Agreement/Tense Omission model

In order to explain that both tense and agreement are affected in SLI, this account draws on the assumption that the functional categories Agr and T both contain a D-feature that needs to be checked against the D-feature of the subject-DP to satisfy the Extended Projection Principle (Chomsky, 1995). Wexler (1998, 2003) claimed that the grammars of typically developing children (when they are in the 'optional-infinitive stage') are subject to a developmental constraint, the so-called Unique Checking Constraint (UCC), according to which formal features can only be checked once. UCC prevents a D-feature on the subject-DP from checking more than one D-feature on functional categories, thus forcing either Agr or T to be omitted.

Wexler, Schütze, and Rice (1998) and Wexler (2003) proposed a two-factor account according to which children with SLI sometimes leave T/Agr unspecified. This account allows for four options:

1   full specification of tense and agreement,
2   underspecified tense and agreement,
3   underspecified tense only,
4   underspecified agreement only.

Wexler and colleagues argue that these possibilities can all be found in data from English-speaking children with SLI. Option 1 underlies instances in which children get subject case, tense and agreement marking right and produce adult-like utterances. Sentences in which neither T nor Agr is specified (i.e., option 2) may have a null subject or a subject in the default (objective) case and a bare verb stem, e.g. *(him) fall down*. Option 3, when Agr is specified and T is unspecified, covers cases of correct nominative subject case and uninflected bare verb forms, such as *he bite me*. Finally, option 4, unspecified Agr and specified T, is for incorrect non-nominative subjects in sentences with tense-marked verbs, e.g. *me falled in grave*. In this way, Wexler, Schütze, & Rice (1998) capture the optional occurrence of finite and non-finite verb forms and of nominative and non-nominative subjects in the speech of English-speaking preschool children with SLI.

One problem with the Agreement/Tense Omission model is that it does not explain the distribution of case and finiteness markings in older English-speaking subjects with SLI. Clahsen, Bartke, and Göllner (1997) found that the group of 10- to 13-year-old children with SLI they studied had 100 percent correct nominative case marking, and past tense marking correctness scores of around 80%, but chance-level scores for the 3rd sg. -*s*. To derive the correct case marking from Wexler and colleagues' typology, one would have to say that, for these children with SLI, Agr is always specified. If this is the case, however, then the low correctness scores of the 3rd sg. -*s* remain unexplained. Moreover, if Agr was tied up with nominative case, as argued by Wexler et al., one would expect to find more instances of non-nominative subjects in sentences in which T is present but Agr is not than in sentences with the reverse distribution. Schütze and Wexler (1996) reported data from unimpaired children in which this contrast did in fact hold. In the SLI data, however, there is no such contrast. Clahsen, Bartke, and Göllner (1997) found that the children with SLI did not produce any non-nominative subject, even in the 311 sentences that contained a verb form that was specified for tense but not for agreement. The lack of non-nominative subjects in sentences with past-tense verb forms (**me falled in grave*) in these data is not what one would expect from the typology of Wexler and colleagues.

10.3.3   The agreement-deficit account

The idea of a grammatical agreement deficit in SLI has been couched in terms of Chomsky's (1995) theory of formal features (Clahsen, Bartke, & Göllner, 1997). Recall that Chomsky distinguishes interpretable features, i.e., features relevant for semantic interpretation, from non-interpretable ones that are irrelevant for interpretation. Agreement features of verbs (and adjectives) form a natural class in Chomsky's system of formal features in that they are non-interpretable and need to be checked off in the course of the derivation. The agreement-deficit hypothesis claims that these features are specifically affected in SLI. This account is not meant to provide a complete characterization of the language problems of people with SLI. Clearly, several linguistic phenomena which have been observed to cause difficulty for subjects with SLI fall outside of what is covered by an impairment of agreement, for example impaired comprehension of reversible passive sentences and reflexive anaphors (van der Lely, 1996; van der Lely & Stollwerck, 1997), difficulties with tense marking (Rice, Wexler, & Cleave, 1995), and other functional elements (Leonard, 1998).

The agreement-deficit account has received empirical support from a range of SLI data indicating that subject–verb agreement causes difficulty for people with SLI across different languages and different age groups, and even for children for whom tense marking functions normally (see Clahsen & Dalalakis, 1999 for review). On the other hand, the reverse pattern, i.e. impaired tense marking and intact subject–verb agreement marking, does not seem to exist in SLI. Moreover, structural case marking for direct and indirect objects, a phenomenon outside the domain of agreement features of verbs (and adjectives), was found to be unimpaired in SLI (Eisenbeiss, Bartke, & Clahsen, 2006).

Chomsky (1995) distinguishes between two separate components of the language faculty, a lexicon of stored entries and a computational system of combinatorial operations and principles to form larger linguistic expressions. Given this distinction one may think of two possible sources for the problems that people with SLI have with grammatical agreement. The first possibility would be an impairment of the computational system such that agreement features would be supplied from the lexicon, but not be properly checked, because the particular computational mechanism that normally checks agreement features is missing from the SLI grammar. The effect of this would be that agreement features of verbs cannot be deleted in the course of the derivation and have to be ignored for the purposes of interpretation. Consequently, a child with SLI would be free to use any person and number form of a given verb, yielding many agreement errors. This, however, is not what we typically find in SLI data. Even though children with SLI do indeed produce agreement errors (see, e.g., Clahsen, Bartke, & Göllner, 1997), it is true that most of the occurring finite verb forms are correctly marked for agreement and that verbs which do carry an agreement inflection have a subject with correctly matching person and number features; this suggests that abstract (computational) knowledge of agreement is unlikely to be missing completely.

Another possibility is that an impairment of agreement affects the lexicon. Effects of this can be seen most clearly in languages with rich agreement paradigms. For SLI in Greek, for example, Clahsen and Dalalakis (1999) found that 2nd sg. and 2nd pl. contexts accounted for most of the agreement errors, whereas for other combinations of person and number features (e.g. in 1st sg., 1st pl., and 3rd pl. contexts) correctness scores were much higher (80 to 90 percent). For SLI in German, several studies have shown particularly low accuracy scores and many errors in cases in which the 2nd person singular suffix -*st* is required in the adult language (Rothweiler & Clahsen, 1994; Bartke, 1998). For Italian, Leonard, Bertolini, Caselli, McGregor, & Sabbadini (1992) found that with respect to 3rd pl. subject–verb agreement suffixes, the mean percentage of correct usage in obligatory contexts was significantly lower for children with SLI than for MLU controls (49.9% vs. 82.3%), whereas for 3rd sg. forms children with SLI achieved the same high correctness score (92.7%) as the MLU controls. For Hebrew-speaking children with SLI, Dromi, Leonard, Adam, and Zadunaisky-Ehrlich (1999) reported significantly more agreement errors for children with SLI than for MLU-matched unimpaired children in one verb class (binyan), whereas in the three other binyanim they studied, children with SLI achieved similar correctness scores to MLU-matched controls. These findings suggest that agreement is not completely absent in SLI, but that the adult agreement paradigm seems to be incomplete, with problems focusing on particular forms or verb classes. These cases are likely to be the result of incomplete acquisition of the morphological paradigm of subject–verb agreement. The consequences of that are that agreement features are not always fully specified on verbs taken from the lexicon, and that a child with SLI may produce non-finite (default) forms or incorrect agreement markings when a verb is taken from the lexicon without any agreement features or with an incomplete feature set.

10.4 Down's Syndrome

Concepts from Chomskyan theory have recently also been applied to developmental disorders such as Down's syndrome and Williams syndrome, in which language impairments coincide with more general cognitive delays and deficits (see, e.g., Clahsen & Almazan, 1998; Perovic, 2004; Ring & Clahsen, 2005). Here our focus is on Down's syndrome.

Down's syndrome (DS) is a congenital neurodevelopmental disorder resulting from the triplication of (part of) chromosome 21, with an approximate incidence of 1 in 800 live births (Lubec, 2002). Several previous studies have indicated that language abilities are relatively more impaired than other areas of cognition in this population (Fowler, Gelman, & Gleitman, 1994; Miller, 1996; Mervis & Bertrand, 1997; Tager-Flusberg, 1999; Clibbens, 2001), and that within the language system, morphosyntax is more impaired than other linguistic domains (see Miller, 1988; Fabretti, Pizzuto, Vicari, & Volterra, 1997; Schaner-Wolles, 2004). Several studies have also reported asynchronous patterns of linguistic development in DS, for example enhanced levels of lexical skill relative to reduced levels of morphosyntax (Miller, 1988; Chapman, Schwarz, & Kay-Raining Bird, 1991; Kernan & Sabsay, 1996; Vicari, Caselli, & Tonucci, 2000, among others). Moreover, there are studies of DS that discovered patterns of morphosyntactic skill that are qualitatively different from those observed in normally developing children (Fabretti, Pizzuto, Vicari, & Volterra, 1997). Taken together, these results suggest the possibility of within-language impairments in people with DS.

Two recent studies have employed Chomskyan theory to characterize language impairments in DS. Perovic (2004) was the first to report an unusual pattern of performance in the comprehension of anaphoric pronouns in four English-speaking adolescents with DS. She found (near) perfect accuracy scores in sentences with non-reflexive pronouns and reduced accuracy scores of around 60 percent in sentences with reflexives for her participants with DS, which led her to suggest "a specific syntactic deficit" in DS.

Ring and Clahsen (2005) presented results from a somewhat larger study investigating anaphoric binding and passivization in eight adolescents diagnosed with DS and, for control purposes, groups of 5-, 6-, and 7-year-old children whose chronological ages were matched to the mental ages of the impaired participants but who had no known learning impairments. For anaphoric binding, Ring and Clahsen replicated Perovic's results showing that for reflexive pronouns the participants with DS performed significantly worse than the controls, whereas on non-reflexive pronouns they achieved the same high accuracy scores as the controls. With respect to active and passive sentences, Ring and Clahsen found that the DS participants' accuracy scores for actives were significantly higher than for passives, and that the participants with DS gave significantly more reversal responses than the controls, i.e., they incorrectly took the first NP they heard as the agent argument.

Ring and Clahsen (2005) offered a syntactic interpretation of these findings, adopting accounts of binding and passivization from Chomskyan syntax. Specifically, they followed Reuland (2001), who showed that the binding properties of reflexive pronouns follow from independently needed conditions on A-chains, as both the reflexive and the antecedent are in argument positions and share the same syntactic features, and the antecedent c-commands the reflexive, whereas the interpretation of non-reflexive pronouns is determined by semantic principles. Moreover, A-chain formation is also involved in the derivation of passive sentences, in order to syntactically link the nominal expression in subject position to its underlying object position. Ring and Clahsen claim that A-chain formation is impaired in DS, which not only accounts for difficulties in interpreting sentences with reflexives but also for the relatively low accuracy scores in comprehending passive sentences.

Clearly, research on developmental disorders has only fairly recently begun to employ notions and concepts from linguistic theory, and more empirical studies are required before any strong conclusions can be drawn. The two studies mentioned on DS, for example, raise several questions, which have to be left to future research. Does the impairment affect other syntactic constructions that involve A-chains, e.g. raising constructions (*John seems to be a nice guy*), to infinitives (*John is believed to be a nice guy*), or unaccusatives (*The book arrived yesterday*)? Does the impairment extend to other syntactic dependencies, e.g. A'-chains, as required for *wh*-questions or relative clauses? Are the difficulties with passives and reflexives that people with DS experience more readily explicable in terms of broader (non-linguistic) deficits? Although these questions have to be left open, the studies mentioned above illustrate that a Chomskyan perspective can be helpful in characterizing language impairments, even in people who have other known impairments outside the domain of language.

ACKNOWLEDGMENTS

I am grateful to Sonja Eisenbeiss, Claudia Felser, Andrew Radford, and Stavroula Stavrakaki for helpful comments on an earlier draft.

REFERENCES

Bartke, S. (1998). *Experimentelle Studien zur Flexion und Wortbildung. Pluralbildung und lexikalische Komposition im unauffälligen Spracherwerb und im Dysgrammatismus.* Tübingen: Niemeyer.

Bartke, S. and Siegmüller, J. (eds.) (2004). *Williams Syndrome across Languages*. Amsterdam: Benjamins.

Bellugi, U., Wang, P., and Jernigan, T. (1994). Williams syndrome: an unusual neuro-psychological profile. In S. Broman and J. Grafman (eds.), *Atypical Cognitive Deficits in Developmental Disorders: Implications for Brain Function* (pp. 23–56). Hillsdale, NJ: Lawrence Erlbaum.

Benedet, M. J., Christiansen, J. A., and Goodglass, H. (1998). A cross-linguistic study of grammatical morphology in Spanish- and English-speaking agrammatic patients. *Cortex*, 34, 309–36.

Beretta, A. and Munn, A. (1998). Double-agents and trace-deletion in agrammatism. *Brain and Language*, 65, 404–21.

Burchert, F., Swoboda-Moll, M., and De Bleser, R. (2005). Tense and agreement dissociations in German agrammatic speakers: Underspecification vs. hierarchy. *Brain and Language*, 94, 188–99.

Chapman, R., Schwarz, S., and Kay-Raining Bird, E. (1991). Language skills of children and adolescents with Down syndrome. I: Comprehension. *Journal of Speech and Hearing Research*, 34, 1106–20.

Chomsky, N. (1957). *Syntactic Structures*. The Hague: Mouton.

Chomsky, N. (1965). *Aspects of the Theory of Syntax*. Cambridge, MA: MIT Press.

Chomsky, N. (1981). *Lectures on Government and Binding*. Dordrecht: Foris.

Chomsky, N. (1995). *The Minimalist Program*. Cambridge, MA: MIT Press.

Chomsky, N. (2000). Minimalist inquiries: The framework. In R. Martin, D. Michaels, and J. Uriagereka (eds.), *Step by Step* (pp. 89–155). Cambridge, MA: MIT Press.

Chomsky, N. and Halle, M. (1968). *The Sound Pattern of English*. New York: Harper & Row.

Clahsen, H. (1989). The grammatical characterization of developmental dysphasia. *Linguistics*, 27, 897–920.

Clahsen, H. (1991). *Child Language and Developmental Dysphasia: Linguistic Studies of the Acquisition of German*. Amsterdam: Benjamins.

Clahsen, H. (1999). Linguistic perspectives on specific language impairment. In W. C. Ritchie and E. K. Bhatia (eds.), *Handbook of Child Language Acquisition* (pp. 675–704). London: Academic Press.

Clahsen, H. and Almazan, M. (1998). Syntax and morphology in children with Williams syndrome. *Cognition*, 68, 167–98.

Clahsen, H. and Almazan, M. (2001). Compounding and inflection in language impairment: Evidence from Williams Syndrome (and SLI). *Lingua*, 111, 729–57.

Clahsen, H., Bartke, S., and S. Göllner (1997). Formal features in impaired grammars: A comparison of English and German SLI children. *Journal of Neurolinguistics*, 10, 151–71.

Clahsen, H. and Dalalakis, J. (1999). Tense and agreement in Greek SLI: A case study. *Essex Research Reports in Linguistics*, 24, 1–25.

Clibbens, J. (2001). Signing and lexical development in children with Down Syndrome. *Down Syndrome Research and Practice*, 7, 101–5.

Dromi, E., Leonard, L., Adam, G., and Zadunaisky-Ehrlich, S. (1999). Verb agreement morphology in Hebrew-speaking children with specific language impairment. *Journal of Speech, Language, and Hearing Research*, 42, 1414–31.

Eisenbeiss, S., Bartke, S., and Clahsen, H. (2006). Structural and lexical case in child German: Evidence from language-impaired and typically-developing children. *Language Acquisition*, 13(1), 3–32.

Eyer, J. and Leonard, L. (1995). Functional categories and specific language impairment: A case study. *Child Language Teaching and Therapy*, 10, 127–38.

Fabretti, D., Pizzuto, E., Vicari, S., and Volterra, V. (1997). A story description task in children with Down's syndrome: Lexical and morphological abilities. *Journal of Intellectual Disability Research*, 41, 165–79.

Fowler, A., Gelman, R., and Gleitman, L. (1994). The course of language learning in children with Down syndrome. In H. Tager-Flusberg (ed.), *Constraints on Language Acquisition: Studies of Atypical Children* (pp. 91–140). Hillsdale, NJ: Erlbaum.

Friedmann, N. (2001). Agrammatism and the psychological reality of the syntactic tree. *Journal of Psycholinguistic Research*, 30, 71–90.

Friedmann, N. and Grodzinsky, Y. (1997). Tense and agreement in agrammatic production: Pruning the syntactic tree. *Brain and Language*, 56, 397–425.

Friedmann, N. and Grodzinsky, Y. (2000). Split inflection in neurolinguistics. In M.-A. Friedemann and L. Rizzi (eds.), *The Acquisition of Syntax* (pp. 84–104). Harlow: Longman.

Gazdar, G., Klein, E., Pullum, G., and Sag, I. (1985). *Generalized Phrase Structure Grammar*. Cambridge, MA: Harvard University Press.

Gleason, J. B. (1978). The acquisition and dissolution of the English inflectional system. In A. Caramazza and E. B. Zurif (eds.), *Language Acquisition and Language Breakdown: Parallels and Divergences* (pp. 109–20). Baltimore, MD: Johns Hopkins University Press.

Goodglass, H. (1968). Studies in the grammar of aphasics. In S. Rosenberg and J. Koplin (eds.), *Developments in Applied Psycholinguistic Research* (pp. 177–208). New York: Macmillan.

Goodglass, H. (1976). Agrammatism. In H. Whitaker and H. A. Whitaker (eds.), *Studies in Neurolinguistics*, vol. 1. New York: Academic Press.

Grodzinsky, Y. (1990). *Theoretical Perspectives on Language Deficits*. Cambridge, MA: MIT Press.

Grodzinsky, Y. (2000). The neurology of syntax: Language use without Broca's area. *Behavioral and Brain Sciences*, 23, 1–71.

Guilfoyle, E., Allen, S., and Moss, S. (1991). Specific language impairment and the maturation of functional categories. Paper presented at the Boston University Conference on Language Development, Boston, MA.

Haegeman, L. (1991). *Introduction to Government and Binding Theory*. Oxford: Blackwell.

Hagiwara, H. (1995). The breakdown of functional categories and the economy of derivation. *Brain and Language*, 50, 92–116.

Hickok, G. and Avrutin, S. (1995). Representation, referentiality, and processing in agrammatic comprehension: Two case studies. *Brain and Language*, 50, 10–26.

Jarema, G. (1998). The breakdown of morphology in aphasia: A cross-language perspective. In B. Stemmer and H. A. Whitaker (eds.), *Handbook of Neurolinguistics* (pp. 221–34). San Diego: Academic Press.

Kean, M.-L. (1979). Agrammatism: A phonological deficit. *Cognition*, 7, 69–83.

Kernan, K. and Sabsay, S. (1996). Linguistic and cognitive ability of adults with Down Syndrome and mental retardation of unknown etiology. *Journal of Communication Disorders*, 29, 401–22.

Kolk, H. (2000). Canonicity and inflection in agrammatic sentence production. *Brain and Language*, 74, 558–60.

Lee, M. (2003). Dissociations among functional categories in Korean agrammatism. *Brain and Language*, 84, 170–88.

Leonard, L. (1995). Functional categories in the grammars of children with specific language impairment. *Journal of Speech and Hearing Research*, 38, 1270–83.

Leonard, L. B. (1998). *Children with Specific Language Impairment*. Cambridge, MA: MIT Press.

Leonard, L., Bertolini, U., Caselli, M., McGregor, K. and Sabbadini, L. (1992). Morphological deficits in children with specific language impairment: The status of features in the underlying grammar. *Language Acquisition*, 2, 151–79.

Leuninger, H. (1989). Modulare Sprachverarbeitung: Evidenz aus der Aphasie. *Frankfurter Linguistische Forschungen, Sondernummer 2*.

Levy, Y. and Kavé, G. (1999). Language breakdown and linguistic theory: A tutorial overview. *Lingua*, 107, 95–143.

Loeb, D. and Leonard, L. (1991). Subject case marking and verb morphology in normally-developing and specifically-language-impaired children. *Journal of Speech and Hearing Research*, 34, 340–6.

Lubec, G. (2002). The brain in Down Syndrome (Trisomy 21). *Journal of Neurology*, 249, 1347–56.

Marshall, J. C. (1986). The description and interpretation of aphasic language disorder. *Neuropsychologia*, 24, 5–24.

Menn, L. and Obler, L. K. (1990). Cross-language data and theories of agrammatism. In L. Menn and L. K. Obler (eds.), *Agrammatic Aphasia: A Cross-language Narrative Sourcebook*, vol. 2 (pp. 1369–89). Amsterdam: John Benjamins.

Mervis, C. and Bertrand, J. (1997). Developmental relations between cognition and language: Evidence from Williams syndrome. In L. Adamson and M. Romski (eds.), *Communication and Language Acquisition: Discoveries from Atypical Development* (pp. 75–106). Baltimore, MD: Brookes.

Miller, J. F. (1988). The developmental asynchrony of language development in children with Down's syndrome. In L. Nadel (ed.), *The Psychobiology of Down Syndrome* (pp. 167–98). Cambridge, MA: MIT Press.

Miller, J. F. (1996). The search for a phenotype of disordered language performance. In M. Rice (ed.), *Toward a Genetics of Language* (pp. 297–314). Hillsdale, NJ: Erlbaum.

Ouhalla, J. (1993). Functional categories, agrammatism, and language acquisition. *Linguistische Berichte*, 143, 3–36.

Penke, M. (1998). *Die Grammatik des Agrammatismus*. Tübingen: Niemeyer.

Penke, M. (2000). Controversies about CP. *Brain and Language*, 77, 351–63.

Perovic, A. (2004). Knowledge of binding in Down syndrome: Evidence from English and Serbo-Croatian. Unpublished doctoral dissertation, University College London.

Pollock, J.-Y. (1989). Verb movement, Universal Grammar, and the structure of IP. *Linguistic Inquiry*, 20, 365–424.

Radford, A. (2004). *Minimalist Syntax: Exploring the Structure of English*. Cambridge: Cambridge University Press.

Reuland, E. (2001). Primitives of binding. *Linguistic Inquiry*, 32, 439–92.

Rice, M. (2003). A unified model of specific and general language delay: Grammatical tense as a clinical marker of unexpected variation. In Y. Levy and J. Schaeffer (eds.), *Language Competence across Populations* (pp. 63–95). Mahwah, NJ: Erlbaum.

Rice, M. and Wexler, K. (1996). Toward tense as a clinical marker of specific language impairment in English-speaking children. *Journal of Speech and Hearing Research*, 39, 1239–57.

Rice, M., Wexler, K., and Cleave, P. (1995). Specific language impairment as a period of extended optional infinitive. *Journal of Speech and Hearing Research*, 38, 850–63.

Ring, M. and Clahsen, H. (2005). Distinct patterns of language impairment in Down's Syndrome and Williams Syndrome: The case of syntactic chains. *Journal of Neurolinguistics*, 18, 479–501.

Rothweiler, M. and Clahsen, H. (1994). Dissociations in SLI children's inflectional systems: A study of participle inflection and subject–verb-agreement. *Journal of Logopedics and Phoniatrics*, 18, 169–79.

Schaner-Wolles, C. (2004). Domain-general or domain-specific cognitive capacities? Language acquisition in Williams syndrome and Down syndrome. In S. Bartke and J. Siegmüller (eds.), *Williams Syndrome across Languages* (pp. 93–124). Amsterdam: Benjamins.

Schütze, C. (1997). Infl in Child and Adult Language: Agreement, Case and Licensing. PhD dissertation, MIT, Cambridge, MA.

Schütze, C. and Wexler, K. (1996). Subject case licensing and English root infinitives. In A. Stringfellow, D. Cahan-Amitay, E. Hughes, and A. Zukowski (eds.), *Proceedings of the 20th Boston University Conference on Language Development*. Boston: Cascadilla Press.

Tager-Flusberg, H. (1999). Language development in atypical children. In M. Barrett (ed.), *The Development of Language* (pp. 311–48). Hove, Sussex: Psychology Press.

Thal, D., Bates, E., and Bellugi, U. (1989). Language and cognition in two children with Williams syndrome. *Journal of Speech and Hearing Research*, 32, 489–500.

Udwin, O. and Yule, W. (1990). Expressive language of children with Williams Syndrome. *American Journal of Medical Genetics Supplement*, 6, 108–14.

van der Lely, H. (1996). Specifically language impaired and normally developing children: Verbal passive vs. adjectival passive sentence interpretation. *Lingua*, 98, 243–72.

van der Lely, H. and Stollwerck, L. (1997). Binding theory and grammatical specific language impairment in children. *Cognition*, 62, 245–90.

Varlokosta, S., Valeonti, N., Kakavoulia, M., Lazaridou, M., and Economou, A. (2005). The breakdown of functional categories in Greek aphasia: Evidence from agreement, tense and aspect. Unpublished MS.

Vicari, S., Caselli, M., and Tonucci, F. (2000). Asynchrony of lexical and morphosyntactic development in children with Down syndrome. *Neuropsychologia*, 24, 138–49.

Wenzlaff, M. and Clahsen, H. (2004): Tense and agreement in German agrammatism. *Brain and Language*, 89, 57–68.

Wenzlaff, M. and Clahsen, H. (2005). Finiteness and verb-second in German agrammatism. *Brain and Language*, 92, 33–44.

Wexler, K. (1998). Very early parameter setting and the unique checking constraint: A new explanation of the optional infinitive stage. *Lingua*, 106, 23–79.

Wexler, K. (2003). Lenneberg's dream: Learning, normal language development, and specific language impairment. In Y. Levy and J. Schaeffer (eds.), *Language Competence across Populations* (pp. 11–62). Mahwah, NJ: Erlbaum.

Wexler, K., Schütze, C., and Rice, M. (1998). Subject case in children with SLI and unaffected controls: Evidence for the Agr/Tns omission model. *Language Acquisition*, 7, 317–44.

11   Formulaic Sequences and Language Disorder

ALISON WRAY

11.1   Introduction

The term 'formulaic sequence' was coined to refer to a wide range of subtypes of multi-word strings that "[are] or appear . . . to be, prefabricated: that is, stored and retrieved whole from memory at the time of use, rather than being subject to generation or analysis by the language grammar" (Wray, 2002b, p. 9). Formulaic sequences have long been recognized as a feature of language disorders. Early clinicians remarked on their resilience in aphasia, where they often remain when other linguistic capabilities have been lost. However, they occur in a number of other conditions too. Only by putting all the different manifestations together, and locating them within the nature of normal communication practice, can we see the whole picture. It is for theoretical models to explain how and why certain word strings should have the status of 'formulaic' when others do not, and why different subtypes are found in different language disorders.

In clinical linguistics, as in second language acquisition research, identifying formulaic sequences is assisted by the contrast between normal (or native-like) language and abnormal (or non-native-like) language. Nevertheless, identification is by no means uncontroversial, even with a chosen definition (Wray, 2002b, chs. 2–3), and one major reason is that the vast majority of formulaic sequences are not fully fixed. Any sequence that contains a finite verb will be able to take paradigmatic morphological variation, but lexical variation is also common, whether highly constrained (e.g. *I haven't (got) the faintest/foggiest/slightest idea*) or potentially infinite, as with *the X-er the Y-er*. Such variation must be accommodated naturally within a plausible theoretical model.

The amount and nature of variation in formulaic sequences appears to be a variable in the clinical domain, indicative of progress in autism, and of deterioration in Alzheimer's disease. Overall the occurrence of formulaicity in disordered language is probably best viewed as an extreme manifestation of what happens in normal usage. However, it is necessary also to consider the range of ways in which extraordinary needs might trigger extraordinary strategies in linguistic processing, resulting in new forms or functions for formulaic material.

11.2   Formulaic Sequences in Aphasia

Accounts of islands of complex language in dysfluent aphasia date back several centuries. An individual only otherwise capable of *yes* and *no* might retain: deliberately memorized material such as prayers, chants, Bible verses, nursery rhymes, or song lyrics; lists such as the numbers to ten, the start of the alphabet, the days of the week; some sentence-initial phrases; swearwords; and speech formulas such as greetings (Benton & Joynt, 1960; Van Lancker Sidtis, 2004). Idiosyncratic expressions are also common (Critchley, 1970), including repeated nonsense strings (Code, 1994). The material within the items cannot be used creatively, only reproduced verbatim.

Broca's and transcortical sensory aphasias are particularly characterized by formulae, which can sometimes be so effectively deployed as to disguise the extent of the linguistic deficit (Van Lancker Sidtis, 2004). However, formulaic sequences appear in most forms of aphasia to some degree (Code, 1982) and it has been hypothesized that part-fixed formulaic frames could underlie some fluent aphasic output (Wray, 2002b, pp. 221–4).

Most commentators assume that the multi-word strings retained in aphasia are retrieved whole from memory, so that their intact form is achieved without the temporary restoration of impaired linguistic abilities. However, access to the lexical store is not sufficient explanation on its own: something is determining why this handful of internally complex lexical items is available when most single words and the vast majority of formulaic sequences are not. Function is the preferred explanation – that is, the surviving formulaic sequences play a role in supporting interaction and the needs of the speaker. A function-based account does not in itself predict multi-word strings, just the retention of the ability to express key interactional messages. However, since complete messages tend to have a form more than one word long, it follows that there will be a disproportionate retention of multi-word strings.

The functional role of an expression in aphasia may not always be the same as in normal usage, with pro-forms or idiosyncratic 'fillers' often carrying a range of meanings (see Wray, 2002b, pp. 230–1 for a review). Sometimes there may appear to be no intention behind formulaic sequences at all – one reason why Hughlings Jackson (1958b) termed them 'non-propositional' (but see Wray, 2002b, pp. 238ff. for problems with this term). Formal tests, particularly, often underestimate linguistic ability in aphasia (see discussion below), and do not pick up improvements in communication over time (Edwards & Knott, 1994). However, research directly examining conversational exchanges (e.g., McElduff & Drummond, 1991; Oelschlaeger & Damico, 1998) confirms what carers frequently report, namely, that formulaic sequences can be effectively employed to achieve significant communicatory functions.

11.3   Formulaic Sequences in Alzheimer's Disease

Classic symptoms of speech in Alzheimer's disease include difficulties with reference, resulting in pronouns without antecedents, paraphrasis, repetition and empty phrases (Davis & Bernstein, 2005, pp. 64–5; see also Orange, 2001). Some of the nuns in Snowdon's (2001) study "could barely articulate a sentence, yet many managed to answer the priest with appropriate responses" (p. 22). According to Orange (2001), as Alzheimer's progresses there is increasing reliance on "stereotyped social greetings and phrases . . . [used] to engage in and maintain conversations" until, in the later stages, there are "continuous spoken streams of nonsense words and utterances" (see also Hamilton, 1994, p. 44). These formulaic features occur within a general trajectory of increasing word-finding difficulties and a reduction in focus during story telling, in idea density, and in grammatical complexity (Kemper, Greiner, Marquis, Prenovost, & Mitzner, 2001; Orange, 2001; Venneri, Forbes-Mckay, & Shanks, 2005). If anything, measures of grammatical complexity in production may overestimate ability, since a formulaic sequence might be quite complicated internally, yet produced without any grammatical processing.

Formulaic responses can obscure the level of the speaker's comprehension and engagement. For example, Brewer's (2005, p. 91) transcripts of conversations in which RB is told by her son that her husband has died, include the following, where RB might be using formulaic sequences that are automatically triggered – and thus effectively deployed in the discourse structure – to disguise a lack of understanding about what is being said.

CB: . . . He was my Daddy too, right?
RB: **That might be possible.** (p. 91)

CB: I told you yesterday.
RB: **I didn't hear you.** (p. 92)

CB: . . . I just wanted to be sure you knew about it. That's why I'm telling you again. Okay?
RB: **Well, who's to blame for it?** (p. 92)

CB: We're going to have a funeral for him Monday.
RB: **Well, I can't help that either** (p. 93).

In the extract below (from Davis & Bernstein, 2005, p. 75), formulaic sequences appear to be maintaining the exchange, even at the expense of the truth (cf. Tannen, 1984, pp. 76, 95; Wray, 2002c, p. 123). LW responds appropriately, but with an apparent level of distraction that we might compare to that of someone being asked questions while trying to concentrate on another task. His replies are plausible but, as subsequently revealed, untrue, since he had in fact got a bad cold.

BD: How have you been – feeling okay?
LW: Yeah. I'm improving right along.
BD: That's great.
LW: Sure is.
BD: Of the people I come here to see, a lot of them have colds and you don't –
you look well.
LW: It's my iron will.

As with aphasia, assessments of linguistic abilities in Alzheimer's are argued to be much more revealing in genuine communicative settings than in tests (Davis, 2005, p. xi). Indeed Davis and Bernstein (2005) report that LW "refused ... to participate in any interaction where the conversation partner carried notebooks or picture cards or asked content-seeking questions" (p. 60).

As Alzheimer's progresses, there is increasing use of fillers, or 'empty words', which, although often short, seem to be a type of formulaic sequence (Wray, 2002b, pp. 230–1). Davis and Bernstein (2005) observed increasing use of "clichéd phrases" in initial position by one patient: "It is as if she were buying a fraction of time to think, retaining the floor as a means of maintaining social connection" (p. 67).

In Alzheimer's disease, formulaic sequences contribute to a situation in which production is possible when comprehension (even of the same material) is significantly impaired (Van Lancker Sidtis, 2004, p. 27). This presumably comes about because the retrieval of formulaic sequences is sufficiently automatic and holistic to bypass any encounter with the disrupted linguistic faculties, enabling a response in which performance outstrips competence (cf. Wray, 2002a, pp. 129ff.).

11.4 Formulaic Sequences in Autism

According to Prizant (1983, p. 299), "due to specific linguistic deficits, autistic persons must often rely on utterances 'borrowed' from others in order to express their needs and intentions, even though the internal structure (i.e., semantic-syntactic relationships) of such utterances may not be analyzed or fully comprehended". In autism, formulaic language occurs in the context of a general stereotypy in behavior based around "routines and rituals always to be carried out in precisely the same way" (R. Paul, 2004, p. 117). Typically, an autistic person will have a specific way of opening a conversation, and may have a routinized script for continuing it, covering the same topics in the same order and using the same words (Prizant, 1983, p. 299). Because of the likelihood that linguistic behavior in autism is a manifestation of a broader tendency to behave formulaically, formulaic language in autism needs to be viewed in inclusive terms in order to catch everything. Thus, Dobbinson, Perkins and Boucher (2003, p. 305) identify voice quality and tone as formulaic markers of discourse functions.

The most notable type of formulaic language in autism is echolalia. According to R. Paul (2004, p. 116), echolalia is observed in 40 percent of people with autism, though earlier estimates have been as high as 75 percent (Rutter, 1968). Despite the implication that echolalia is meaningless repetition, in fact structural change is a variable (Prizant & Duchan, 1981, p. 241). Dobbinson, Perkins and Boucher (2003) speak of a "continuum of productivity-formulaicity rather than a repertoire in which items are either distinctly formulaic or available for productive usage" (p. 305). At the extreme end of fixedness, echoes will feature 'pronominal reversal', that is, usually, use of the second person to refer to self. This comes about because of the failure to replace the pronouns from the original, something also observed in beginner learners of a second language (Myles, Mitchell, & Hooper, 1999), where it tends to indicate insufficient knowledge of the forms in the word string. The same may apply in autistic speech, though it is difficult to be sure. As Roberts (1989) demonstrates, less fixed, or 'mitigated', echolalia can accommodate the pronoun change, so that the question *Do you want a drink?* elicits *Do I want a drink?* Other kinds of mitigated echolalia include repetition with affirmation or negation (*Do you want a drink, yes please*), and less apparently principled changes (*Do you want the drink?*), including telegraphic echo (*What do you play at home? – What I play home?*) (p. 277). Other than unmodified telegraphic echo, which, again, is reminiscent of early second language learners (Wray, 2002b, chapter 9), such changes indicate that the linguistic form is at least somewhat understood.

Echolalia, however, cannot be judged on its form alone. Prizant and Duchan (1981) identify seven functions: non-focused, turn-taking, declarative, rehearsal, self-regulatory, yes-answer and request (pp. 246–7). These uses come with considerable variation in apparent intentionality and comprehension of the preceding input. Rydell and Mirenda (1991), taking the perspective of 'information-processing', view echolalia as "a language that can be used in situations where the cognitive demands exceed the child's linguistic capacity" (p. 135). Borrowed words are, of course, a bulky, unsubtle tool for communication, and knowing what to say in certain types of situation is insufficient to avoid problems with fine tuning in usage (Prizant, 1983, p. 302).

A further function of echolalia is learning. Prizant and Duchan (1981) note that "Typical comments of those who interact with echolalic autistic children include 'he tells himself what to do', 'he learns language through repeating', and 'echoing helps him to understand'" (p. 242). McEvoy, Loveland and Landry (1988) found that as language comprehension improved, so echolalia decreased. Again, it behoves us not to view this learning strategy as particularly alien, for it has a long and successful pedigree in language learning (e.g. Ding, 2007). Prizant (1983), indeed, cites gestalt (holistic) learning in first and second language acquisition as the reference point for understanding the gradual evolution away from echolalia.

Learning does not occur in all echolalic individuals, however, and Prizant and Duchan (1981) recommend different approaches where echolalia is a permanent state and where it appears to be transitory. In the former case, "the . . . child may need to be taught rote verbal routines that would be useful for daily functioning", while in the latter, "a well-trained clinician can help an autistic child develop more effective communication with people and the environment, . . . motivat[ing] the autistic child to want to learn language, initiate interaction with others, and become an active member of the world around him" (p. 248).

Dobbinson, Perkins and Boucher (2003, p. 305) speculate that "the social deficit in autism may be the root cause of . . . inflexibility [in formula usage]", but Prizant (1983) sees things the other way round, suggesting that difficulties of coping with generative language might account for the autistic person's avoidance of social situations (see also Prizant & Duchan, 1981).

11.5   Holistic Processing, the Right Hemisphere and Interhemispheric Communication

It has long been understood that "Portions of the right hemisphere may . . . be activated for tasks presumed to require holistic or global processing" (Tompkins, Fassbinder, Lehman-Blake, & Baumgaertner, 2002, p. 439), and Hughlings Jackson (1958a, 1958b) was one of the first to suggest that formulaic sequences might be managed from the right hemisphere. Ideas about hemispheric specialization have moved on since then, as has our understanding of linguistic processing. Nevertheless, there is a sizable literature drawing on evidence from both left- and right-hemisphere damage, which continues to implicate the right hemisphere in certain aspects of language comprehension and production. Typically disrupted in right-hemisphere damage are relevance, inference, prosody and pragmatics, including humor and the comprehension of idioms and metaphors (Chantraine, Joanette, & Ska, 1998; Heath & Blonder, 2005; Jung-Beeman, 2005; Tompkins, Fassbinder, Lehman-Blake, & Baumgaertner, 2002). Furthermore, Brownell, Pincus, Blum, Rehak, and Winner (1997), examining how people with right-hemisphere damage used terms of personal reference, conclude that "their language performance . . . [was] aberrant at the level of social interaction and in terms of narrative and conversational discourse" (p. 75).

It is tempting to speculate, as Hughlings Jackson did, that certain complete word strings are holistically stored in the right hemisphere, complete with their intonation contour and pragmatic color. However, as noted earlier, formulaic sequences are subject to considerable internal variation, making a simple holistic store-and-retrieve arrangement insufficient, unless every conceivable realization is separately stored. What has been considered more plausible is the operation of two systems: holistic processing for fixed material, and full grammatical and lexical processing (often termed 'analytic') for novel material. Several such 'dual systems' models have been proposed, including those of Sinclair (1991), Van Lancker Sidtis (2002), Wray (1992) and, for reading, Coltheart, Rastle, Perry, Langdon, and Ziegler (2001).

To be effective, dual-systems processing must normally favor the holistic route over the analytic one, with concomitant benefits of speed and simplicity. In a model in which processing is serial, the analytic route is called in whenever the holistic one fails. If parallel, the two systems operate simultaneously, the holistic route being faster. Information can be fed between them, to achieve the optimal balance of efficiency and accuracy. Parallel dual-systems processing, especially if there is a feedback mechanism ('cascading' in Coltheart and colleagues' (2001) model of reading), would enable a holistically retrieved frame to be edited analytically, using morphology and lexis to tailor-make it to its context.

However, dual-systems processing is not the only model that can explain how large and small units combine to express messages in idiomatic ways. Wray (2002b) concludes that formulaic sequences are simply lexical units like any other, retrieved from the lexicon holistically because, like a morpheme or a simple word, they have a semantic entry attached to them. Holistic processing, as a separate activity, is not necessary in this view. Rather, it is a consequence of handling lexical units that have, in some instances, an internal composition. Formulaic sequences that contain gaps are completed using insertion rules. In place of the idea that the right hemisphere is dedicated to holistic processing, Wray proposes that the lexicon can be notionally divided into five parts, on the basis of function: grammatical, referential, interactional, memorized (mnemonic) and reflexive (pp. 261ff.; compare Altmann, Kempler, & Andersen, 2001). She hypothesizes that one or more of these five sublexicons might be supported and/or accessed from outside of the left-hemisphere 'language areas' (thus, conceivably, from the right hemisphere), with the result that left-hemisphere damage affects the different sublexicons to different degrees. Although all five sublexicons can contain morphemes, polymorphemic words and multi-word strings, the balance will be different: there are relatively few multi-word grammatical operators, and relatively few monomorphemic interactional routines or mnemonics.

As the technology available for neurolinguistic measuring has improved, it has become increasingly evident that the original notion of the left and right hemispheres having clearly demarcated tasks and styles is not well supported (Damasio, Tranel, Grabowski, Adolphs, & Damasio, 2004; Efron, 1990; Poeppel & Hickok, 2004), and much more attention is now being paid to the communication between the two hemispheres. The new emphasis is justified by evidence that the impaired interhemispheric communication arising from agenesis of the corpus callosum results in linguistic deficits reminiscent of those seen in right-hemisphere damage: "difficulty with the pragmatic and paralinguistic aspects of communication" including the tendency to interpret non-literal expressions literally (L. K. Paul, Van Lancker Sidtis, Schieffer, Dietrich, & Brown, 2003, p. 314).

Substantial support for a model of integrated activity comes from experiments exploring the interpretation of idioms, proverbs and metaphors, a popular paradigm for clinical investigations, though not unproblematic (see below). As the traditional view of the holistic right hemisphere would predict, people with right-hemisphere damage tend to choose a literal interpretation over the conventional non-literal one (Hillert, 2004; Van Lancker & Kempler, 1987). However, contrary to that model, the same is also true in other conditions:

Alzheimer's (Papagno, Lucchelli, Muggia, & Rizzo, 2003), agenesis of the corpus callosum (Huber-Okrainec, Blaser, & Dennis, 2005; L. K. Paul, Van Lancker Sidtis, Schieffer, Dietrich, & Brown, 2003), autism (Qualls, Lantz, Pietrzyk, Blood, & Hammer, 2004), and, most notably, left-hemisphere damage (Papagno & Genoni, 2004; Papagno, Tabossi, Colombo, & Zampetti, 2004), where the left–right dichotomous model might have predicted the favoring of holistic over literal readings.

One hypothesis is that the right hemisphere "weakly activates large diffuse semantic fields, including information distantly related to the words" while the left hemisphere "strongly activates small and focused semantic fields" (Jung-Beeman, 2005, p. 514). Bilateral activity ensures 'semantic integration', which is necessary for natural language comprehension because both precise and broader associative information is encoded in linguistic forms when used in a communicative context. In other words, the right hemisphere facilitates the conceptual abstraction that enables a collection of words to be interpreted non-literally, but both hemispheres must communicate effectively in order to achieve the correct balance of information for an appropriate interpretation (L. K. Paul, Van Lancker Sidtis, Schieffer, Dietrich, & Brown, 2003, p. 318).

In this view, literal interpretations of idioms will arise when there is a 'suppression deficit' of the non-literal meaning, leading to "a tendency to hold on too long to interpretations that become contextually irrelevant" (Tompkins, Fassbinder, Lehman-Blake, & Baumgaertner, 2002, p. 224; see also Dressler, Stark, Vassilakou, et al., 2004; Orange, 2001; L. K. Paul, Van Lancker Sidtis, Schieffer, Dietrich, & Brown, 2003; Tompkins & Fassbinder, 2004). Since suppression entails a chain of processes (generating the alternatives, juxtaposing them, selecting one over the others), it is possible to account for how different conditions result in the same effect, by hypothesizing that the chain has been broken in different places. In Alzheimer's, working memory deficits could prevent competing interpretations from being compared (see also Grossman & Rhee, 2001; Papagno, Lucchelli, Muggia, & Rizzo, 2003). In agenesis of the corpus callosum, poor interhemispheric communication would be responsible. The same applies for autism and Developmental Language Disorder (or SLI), where there is reduced interhemispheric white matter in the corpus callosum relative to white matter within each hemisphere (Herbert, Ziegler, Deutsch, et al., 2005, p. 214). Because of their suppression function, the basal ganglia are also implicated, with the prediction that in Parkinson's disease non-literal meanings will be increasingly dispreferred as the literal meanings encounter less resistance (Van Lancker Sidtis, 2004, p. 33).

The suppression model does not offer any explanation, however, for echolalic behavior in autism or for the use of formulaic interactional routines in Alzheimer's and aphasia. This suggests that the two rather contradictory features of these conditions – the easy or compulsive use of holistic language on the one hand, and the difficulty with appreciating holistic meanings on the other – may be independently motivated, the latter by neurological structures and the former, as indicated earlier, by social need.

11.6   Issues with Testing Methodology

The issue of how to test linguistic knowledge, always a challenge in the clinical domain, requires particular caution where formulaic sequences are concerned, because they are so contextually sensitive. In research on Alzheimer's it has been noted that data from tests and data from real conversation are markedly different in kind (e.g. Bucks, Singh, Cuerden, & Wilcock, 2000; Davis, 2005; Davis & Bernstein, 2005; Perkins, Whitworth, & Lesser, 1998; Snowdon, 2001), and similar observations have been made about aphasia (Edwards & Knott, 1994; McElduff & Drummond, 1991; Oelschlaeger & Damico, 1998). In fact a nest of related hazards pervade formulaic language in clinical and non-clinical testing.

Firstly, language demarcated for a testing purpose carries its own pragmatic agenda: a proverb cited in a test does not carry the pragmatics of a proverb, but of a citation. Gathering information about naturalistic language in an unnatural situation relies on the testee's ability to understand the pretence inherent in testing and to instate a particular pragmatic agenda. For instance, providing the 'correct' picture match for the idiom *he paid an arm and a leg for it* entails understanding that humorous worlds in which limb-bartering occurs are not relevant. Furthermore, subjects must share the tester's assumption that a non-literal interpretation is 'better', even though folk linguistic beliefs could classify the non-literal meaning, like slang, as less correct, and therefore less acceptable in a test. In short, the pragmatics of testing are complex and cannot safely be ignored, particularly when the tests are used on individuals who have a pragmatic impairment. Irrespective of any 'suppression deficit', deciding what should be suppressed is dependent on what you think is expected of you.

Secondly, it should not be assumed that people with pragmatic difficulties will have acquired the holistic meaning of idioms, metaphors and proverbs in the first place, and if they have not, then they will not be able to access them in tests (Huber-Okrainec, Blaser, & Dennis, 2005).

Thirdly, testing demands a focus on language that is rarely necessary or useful in normal communication (Wray, 1992). Actions and reactions that are normally effortless can become confusing and difficult when attended to, even perhaps because that attention prevents them from being achieved using the normal processing routes.

Fourthly, people who are self-conscious about their communication problems may find it especially difficult to perform well in tests, and may have developed strategies that are not optimal for the intentions of the test. A person with impaired grammatical ability, for instance, may find it preferable only to attend to recognizable lexical items, filtering out the rest of the detail because there is little point in trying to deal with it. In real interaction, it could mean that the grammar-impaired person filters out most of *Let's get your shoes on, 'cos we're going to the shops*, to end up with *** shoes *** shops, and relies on the literal meaning of those items, plus pragmatics, to extract a likely interpretation. The same strategy, when faced with the test stimulus *he paid an arm and a leg for it*, will render *** *arm* *** *leg* ***. With such a minimal representation, which could underlie many different sentences, it would be safer to point at a picture featuring images of an arm and a leg than one that does not. In fact, it can be argued that all of us, given only *** *arm* *** *leg* *** to work with, would not easily think of the idiom, because those lexical items are not salient within the meaning of the whole. It would be little different from giving someone ***sing and expecting them to come up with *browsing*, or ***pet*** and expecting them to think of *competition*. Thus, when a clinical test subject with a grammatical impairment selects the picture representing the literal meaning of an idiom, it will be worth considering whether this necessarily means that the idiom has been interpreted literally, or perhaps only means that the form has been selectively attended to.

The very linguistic nature of the idiom creates a fifth challenge for clinical research. Much discussion revolves around whether the literal meaning of an idiom is accessed before, after or at the same time as the non-literal meaning, but this takes for granted that the literal meaning is normally accessed *at all*, other than in test conditions where attention to form may ensure that it is. Wray's (2002b) 'needs-only analysis' model proposes that meaning is assigned to the largest possible configuration, and that once the meaning has been assigned, no more analysis need take place unless a situation arises in which it becomes desirable to do so (see also Van Lancker Sidtis, 2002, p. 10). In this way, the 'literal' composition of an idiom might never be noticed, or only by chance many years after first encountering it.

Needs-only analysis predicts that items such as *dog collar* (as worn by a priest) and *toad-in-the-hole* (a savory dish of sausages and pudding) have long since lost their original 'literal' roots and now have these meanings as primary, so that identifying the 'literal' meaning is post hoc linguistic game-playing, not the tapping of existing knowledge or customary processing. If this view is correct, then some investigations may not have been testing what they claimed. For instance, Hillert (2004) expected subjects to access the 'literal' meanings of *Bienenstich*, a cake but literally 'bee sting', and *Eselohren*, literally 'donkey-ears', the folds in a page that in English make a book 'dog-eared'. It is not that individuals may not have noticed at some point that there is a 'literal' meaning to these words, but rather that the 'literal' meaning is actually etymological, and unnecessary for understanding the customary meaning. As such, it is not possible to be sure that any given individual *has* previously noticed the 'literal' meaning, any more than it can be guaranteed that everyone has noticed that *Mediterranean* refers to the middle of the earth, that a *bullet point* in a document 'literally' means the tip of a lethal missile, or that *forget* is a historical compound of *get*. In short, the difference between 'literal meaning' and etymology is a continuum, and will vary from person to person (Wray, 2002b). It is not an absolute upon which experiments can safely be designed.

11.7   Conclusion

Making sense of why formulaic sequences are so prominent in language disorders requires a model of the dynamic way in which the demands of processing and communicative function are met in normal language use. Wray (2002b) proposes that all formulaic sequences – including phatic routines, memorized rhymes, proverbs and idioms, turns of phrase and preferred collocations – share a single underlying function: that of promoting the speaker's interests (pp. 95ff.). Formulaic sequences variously ensure easy access to information, fluent delivery (which helps retain the turn), the effective conveying of messages, the meeting of physical and emotional needs, and self-presentation as a group member and as an individual. A sophisticated recognition of what formulaic sequences are and do will help to ensure that appropriate questions are asked when researching language disorders. The resilience of formulaic sequences in aphasia and Alzheimer's, and their role in anchoring interaction and learning in autism, make more sense when formulaicity is placed at the center of normal language, rather than at its periphery. This central role then signals that those with right-hemisphere damage or poor interhemispheric connections may be experiencing greater difficulties with language than their surface coping behavior easily reveals. To be deprived of formulaicity in language may be like knowing all the moves but no longer knowing the dance, and if formulaic language is as pervasive and central to human communication as it now seems to be, research into the effects of its absence, and its preservation, may have barely scratched the surface.

REFERENCES

Altmann, L. J. P., Kempler, D., and Andersen, E. S. (2001). Speech errors in Alzheimer's disease: Reevaluating morphosyntactic preservation. *Journal of Speech, Language and Hearing Research*, 44, 1069–82.

Benton, A. L. and Joynt, R. J. (1960). Early descriptions of aphasia. *Archives of Neurology*, 3, 109–26, 205–22.

Brewer, J. P. (2005). Carousel conversation: Aspects of family roles and topic shift in Alzheimer's talk. In B. H. Davis (ed.), *Alzheimer Talk, Text and Context: Enhancing Communication* (pp. 87–101). Basingstoke: Palgrave Macmillan.

Brownell, H., Pincus, D., Blum, A., Rehak, A., and Winner, E. (1997). The effects of right-hemisphere brain damage on patients' use of terms of personal reference. *Brain and Language*, 57(1), 60–79.

Bucks, R. S., Singh, S., Cuerden, J. M., and Wilcock, G. K. (2000). Analysis of spontaneous, conversational speech in dementia of Alzheimer type: evaluation of an objective technique for analysing lexical performance. *Aphasiology*, 14(1), 71–91.

Chantraine, Y., Joanette, Y., and Ska, B. (1998). Conversational abilities in patients with right-hemisphere damage. *Journal of Neurolinguistics*, 11, 21–32.

Code, C. (1982). Neurolinguistic analysis of recurrent utterances in aphasia. *Cortex*, 18, 141–52.

Code, C. (1994). Speech automatism production in aphasia. *Journal of Neurolinguistics*, 8(2), 135–48.

Coltheart, M., Rastle, K., Perry, C., Langdon, R., and Ziegler, J. (2001). DRC: A dual route cascaded model of visual word recognition and reading aloud. *Psychological Review*, 108, 204–56.

Critchley, M. (1970). *Aphasiology and Other Aspects of Language*. London: Arnold.

Damasio, H., Tranel, D., Grabowski, T., Adolphs, R., and Damasio, A. (2004). Neural systems behind word and concept retrieval. *Cognition*, 92(1–2), 179–229.

Davis, B. (2005). Introduction: Some commonalities. In B. H. Davis (ed.), *Alzheimer Talk, Text and Context: Enhancing Communication* (pp. xi–xxi). Basingstoke: Palgrave Macmillan.

Davis, B. and Bernstein, C. (2005). Talking in the here and now: reference and politeness in Alzheimer conversation. In B. H. Davis (ed.), *Alzheimer Talk, Text and Context: Enhancing Communication* (pp. 60–86). Basingstoke: Palgrave Macmillan.

Ding, Y. (2007). Text memorization and imitation: The practices of successful learners of English. *System*, 35, 271–80.

Dobbinson, S., Perkins, M. R., and Boucher, J. (2003). The interactional significance of formulas in autistic language. *Clinical Linguistics and Phonetics*, 17(4), 299–307.

Dressler, W. U., Stark, H. K., Vassilakou, M., Rauchensteiner, D., Tosic, J., Weitzenauer, S. M., Wasner, P., Pons, C., Stark, J., and Brunner, G. (2004). Textpragmatic impairments of figure-ground distinction in right-brain damaged stroke patients compared with aphasics and healthy controls. *Journal of Pragmatics*, 36, 207–35.

Edwards, S. and Knott, R. (1994). Assessing spontaneous language abilities of aphasic speakers. In D. Graddol and J. Swann (eds.), *Evaluating Language* (pp. 91–101). Clevedon: Multilingual Matters.

Efron, R. (1990). *The Decline and Fall of Hemispheric Specialization*. Hillsdale, NJ: Lawrence Erlbaum.

Grossman, M. and Rhee, J. (2001). Cognitive resources during sentence processing in Alzheimer's disease. *Neuropsychologia*, 39, 1419–31.

Hamilton, H. E. (1994). *Conversations with an Alzheimer's Patient*. Cambridge: Cambridge University Press.

Heath, R. L. and Blonder, L. X. (2005). Spontaneous humor among right hemisphere stroke survivors. *Brain and Language*, 93, 267–76.

Herbert, M. R., Ziegler, D. A., Deutsch, C. K., O'Brien, L. M., Kennedy, D. N., Filipek, P. A., Bakardjiev, A. I., Hodgson, J., Takeoka, M., Makris, N., and Caviness, V. S. J. (2005). Brain asymmetries in autism and developmental language disorder: A nested whole-brain analysis. *Brain*, 128(1), 213–26.

Hillert, D. G. (2004). Spared access to idiomatic and literal meanings: A single-case approach. *Brain and Language*, 89, 207–15.

Huber-Okrainec, J., Blaser, S. E., and Dennis, M. (2005). Idiom comprehension deficits in relation to corpus callosum agenesis and hypoplasia in children with spina bifida meningomyelocele. *Brain and Language*, 93, 349–68.

Hughlings Jackson, J. (1958a). Notes on the physiology and pathology of language. In J. Taylor (ed.), *Selected Writings of John Hughlings Jackson*, vol. 2 (pp. 121–8). London: Staples Press. (Originally published 1866.)

Hughlings Jackson, J. (1958b). On the nature of the duality of the brain. In J. Taylor (ed.), *Selected Writings of John Hughlings Jackson*, vol. 2 (pp. 129–45). London: Staples Press. (Originally published 1874.)

Jung-Beeman, M. (2005). Bilateral brain processes for comprehending natural language. *Trends in Cognitive Sciences*, 9(11), 512–18.

Kemper, S., Greiner, L. H., Marquis, J. G., Prenovost, K., and Mitzner, T. L. (2001). Language decline across the life span: Findings from the nun study. *Psychology and Aging*, 16(2), 227–39.

McElduff, K. and Drummond, S. S. (1991). Communicative functions of automatic speech in non-fluent dysphasia. *Aphasiology*, 5, 265–78.

McEvoy, R. E., Loveland, K. A., and Landry, S. H. (1988). The functions of immediate echolalia in autistic children: A developmental perspective. *Journal of Autism and Developmental Disorders*, 18(4), 657–68.

Myles, F., Mitchell, R., and Hooper, J. (1999). Interrogative chunks in French L2: A basis for creative construction? *Studies in Second Language Acquisition*, 21(1), 49–80.

Oelschlaeger, M. L. and Damico, J. S. (1998). Spontaneous verbal repetition: A social strategy in aphasic conversation. *Aphasiology*, 12(11), 971–88.

Orange, J. B. (2001). Family caregivers, communication and Alzheimer's Disease. In M. L. Hummert and J. F. Nussbaum (eds.), *Aging, Communication and Health* (pp. 225–48). Mahwah, NJ: Lawrence Erlbaum.

Papagno, C. and Genoni, A. (2004). The role of syntactic competence in idiom comprehension: A study on aphasic patients. *Journal of Neurolinguistics*, 17, 371–82.

Papagno, C., Lucchelli, F., Muggia, S., and Rizzo, S. (2003). Idiom comprehension in Alzheimer's disease: The role of the central executive. *Brain*, 126, 2419–30.

Papagno, C., Tabossi, P., Colombo, M. R., and Zampetti, P. (2004). Idiom comprehension in aphasic patients. *Brain and Language*, 89, 226–34.

Paul, L. K., Van Lancker Sidtis, D., Schieffer, B., Dietrich, R., and Brown, W. S. (2003). Communicative deficits in agenesis of the corpus collosum: Non-literal language and affective prosody. *Brain and Language*, 85, 313–24.

Paul, R. (2004). Autism. In R. D. Kent (ed.), *The MIT Handbook of Communication Disorders* (pp. 115–19). Cambridge, MA: MIT Press.

Perkins, L., Whitworth, A., and Lesser, R. (1998). Conversing in dementia: A conversation analytic approach. *Journal of Neurolinguistics*, 11(1–2), 33–53.

Poeppel, D. and Hickok, G. (2004). Towards a new functional anatomy of language. *Cognition*, 92(1–2), 1–12.

Prizant, B. M. (1983). Language acquisition and communicative behavior in autism: Toward an understanding of the 'whole' of it. *Journal of Speech and Hearing Disorders*, 48, 296–307.

Prizant, B. M. and Duchan, J. F. (1981). The functions of immediate echolalia in autistic children. *Journal of Speech and Hearing Disorders*, 46(3), 241–9.

Qualls, C. D., Lantz, J. M., Pietrzyk, R. M., Blood, G. W., and Hammer, C. S. (2004). Comprehension of idioms in adolescents with language-based learning disabilities compared to their typically developing peers. *Journal of Communication Disorders*, 37, 295–311.

Roberts, J. M. A. (1989). Echolalia and comprehension in autistic children. *Journal of Autism and Developmental Disorders*, 19(2), 271–81.

Rutter, M. (1968). Concepts of autism. *Journal of Child Psychology and Psychiatry*, 9, 1–25.

Rydell, P. J. and Mirenda, P. (1991). The effects of two levels of linguistic constraint on echolalia and generative language production in children with autism. *Journal of Autism and Developmental Disorders*, 21(2), 131–57.

Sinclair, J. M. (1991). *Corpus, Concordance, Collocation*. Oxford: Oxford University Press.

Snowdon, D. (2001). *Aging with Grace*. London: Fourth Estate.

Tannen, D. (1984). *Conversational Style: Analysing Talk among Friends*. Norwood, NJ: Ablex.

Tompkins, C. A. and Fassbinder, W. (2004). Right hemisphere language disorders. In R. D. Kent (ed.), *The MIT Encyclopedia of Communication Disorders* (pp. 388–92). Cambridge, MA: MIT Press.

Tompkins, C. A., Fassbinder, W., Lehman-Blake, M. T., and Baumgaertner, A. (2002). The nature and implications of right hemisphere language disorders: Issues in search of answers. In A. E. Hillis (ed.), *The Handbook of Adult Language Disorders* (pp. 429–48). New York: Psychology Press.

Van Lancker, D. and Kempler, D. (1987). Comprehension of familiar phrases by left- but not by right-hemisphere damaged patients. *Brain and Language*, 32, 265–77.

Van Lancker Sidtis, D. (2002). Toward a dual processing model of language: normal and neurologic studies. Paper presented at the Language and Cognition Seminar Series, Columbia University.

Van Lancker Sidtis, D. (2004). When novel sentences spoken or heard for the first time in the history of the universe are not enough: Toward a dual-process model of language. *International Journal of Language and Communication Disorders*, 39(1), 1–44.

Venneri, A., Forbes-Mckay, K. E., and Shanks, M. F. (2005). Impoverishment of spontaneous language and the prediction of Alzheimer's disease. *Brain*, 128(4), E27.

Wray, A. (1992). *The Focusing Hypothesis: The Theory of Left-lateralised Language Reexamined*. Amsterdam: John Benjamins.

Wray, A. (2002a). Dual processing in protolanguage: Performance without competence. In A. Wray (ed.), *The Transition to Language* (pp. 113–37). Oxford: Oxford University Press.

Wray, A. (2002b). *Formulaic Language and the Lexicon*. Cambridge: Cambridge University Press.

Wray, A. (2002c). Formulaic language in computer-supported communication: theory meets reality. *Language Awareness*, 11(2), 114–31.

12 Syntactic Processing in Developmental and Acquired Language Disorders

THEODOROS MARINIS

12.1 Introduction

One of the major debates within developmental language disorders concerns whether children's impaired language is caused by incomplete linguistic knowledge or by processing limitations. A similar debate exists within the area of acquired language impairment. Given that in acquired language disorders the language impairment has a physiological cause, e.g. a lesion, and the language system was fully developed prior to that, the debate here is about whether the physiological cause has affected the language system itself or the processing mechanisms that enable language performance.

The present chapter addresses this issue by reviewing literature on syntactic processing in developmental and acquired language disorders with a focus on Specific Language Impairment (SLI) and aphasia. I will demonstrate that, although the vast majority of research uses off-line methods that, by definition, are not able to distinguish between impairment in linguistic knowledge and processing mechanisms, within the last decade there has been a breakthrough in this research area. Several studies have started to look at how children with SLI and adults with aphasia process language in real time using on-line methodologies. These have revealed thought-provoking findings about the nature of the disorders, and promise that if more systematic research on syntactic processing is conducted, this issue may be resolved fairly soon.

12.2 What is Syntactic Processing?

Adult non-impaired native speakers of a language can effortlessly understand what other people say when they listen to them, and, similarly, trained readers can easily understand the sentences they read. This ease of comprehension conceals the different processes and cognitive demands involved in sentence comprehension. For example, when we listen to a sentence, such as *The zebra was kissing the camel*, we have to decode the sounds, segment and recognize words from the speech stream (the/zebra/was/kissing/ . . .), assign syntactic categories to words (the = determiner, zebra = noun), combine words into constituents (the zebra = Noun Phrase), assign thematic roles (e.g., the zebra = agent, the camel = patient/theme), and interpret the sentence. In sentences such as *The monkey was combing him*, we also have to link the pronoun *him* to the entity it refers to from the discourse, and in sentences such as *Who did Balloo give the long carrot to at the farm?*, we have to keep the *wh*-word *who* in working memory, and then link it to the verb *give* and the preposition *to*. Thus, sentence processing involves rapid integration of different types of information (lexical/semantic, structural, discourse/pragmatic, etc.), storage and retrieval from working memory, and building up the grammatical structure of the sentence. Research in *syntactic processing* or *parsing* investigates the mental processes involved when we comprehend sentences in real time, and the way different types of information are utilized to build up the grammatical structure of the sentence, and thus sentence interpretation.

12.3 Syntactic Processing in Typically Developing Children

A large body of research on syntactic processing by healthy adults shows that mature readers/listeners are able to utilize and rapidly integrate different types of information when they read or listen to sentences in real time (Gibson & Pearlmutter, 1998; Pickering, 1999).

Recently, an increasing number of studies have started to look at how children process sentences in real time, in order to establish how syntactic processing develops in children, and whether children use the same processing routines and strategies as adults do. These have shown that, at least by the age of four, typically developing (TD) children are capable of utilizing structural/syntactic information in the same way as adults. A study by Tyler and Marslen-Wilson (1981) was one of the first to show that 5-, 7-, and 10-year-old children show the same processing pattern as adults when they monitored sentences to detect a word in three conditions: normal prose, semantically anomalous, and syntactically anomalous sentences. A further study by McKee, Nicol, and McDaniel (1993) looked at the processing of syntactic dependencies involving pronouns and reflexives in 4 to 6-year-old children using a cross-modal picture-priming task. In this task, children listened to sentences such as (1) below.

(1) The alligator knows that the leopard with the green eyes is patting himself/him/the nurse on the head with a soft pillow

At the offset of *himself/him/the nurse* children saw a picture on a computer screen that corresponded to the second noun phrase of the sentence (*the leopard*). Upon encountering the picture of the leopard and before the end of the sentence, children had to make an aliveness decision for the picture by pressing a button. This provided a measure of how fast in milliseconds they decided for the animacy of the picture. In the sentences with the reflexive pronoun, the picture was the antecedent of the reflexive pronoun (*himself*), whereas in the other sentences, there was no link between the pronoun (*him*) or the noun phrase (*the nurse*) and the picture. Similar tasks with adults have revealed that a pronoun reactivates its syntactically possible antecedents. This speeds up the judgment for the animacy of the picture. Thus, reaction times to the picture of the leopard in the sentences with reflexives are shorter compared to the ones with the noun phrase (*the nurse*) because the leopard is the antecedent of the reflexive. In contrast, no such differences are attested between the sentences with the pronoun and the noun phrase because the leopard is not the antecedent of either of the two. These predictions were borne out in the McKee and McDaniel study, indicating that children as young as four years process reflexives in a similar way to adults: when they encounter a reflexive, they rapidly reactivate its antecedent. This provides additional evidence that at this age they have acquired the grammar that enables binding of reflexives.

The same task was employed by Roberts, Marinis, Felser, and Clahsen (2007) to investigate how children process object relative clauses such as (2).

(2) John saw [the peacock]$_i$ to which the small penguin gave the nice birthday present t$_i$ in the garden last weekend.

In this sentence, according to linguistic theory within the generative framework, the noun phrase *the peacock*, which is the indirect object of the verb *gave*, has moved out of the relative clause to the main clause leaving a gap or trace (*t$_i$*) behind. Thus, there is a syntactic dependency between the noun phrase *the peacock* and the gap. In this study, children heard a sentence, and at the gap or at a control position (after *nice*), they saw a picture corresponding to the noun phrase that has moved to the main clause (*peacock*) or an unrelated picture (*carrot*), and had to perform an aliveness decision for the picture by pressing a button. If children are capable of establishing a syntactic dependency between the dislocated noun phrase (*the peacock*) and the gap, then, at the gap position, reaction times for the picture of the peacock should be shorter than for the picture of the carrot. This difference should not occur at the control position because there is no syntactic dependency between the peacock and the control position. The underlying assumption here is similar to the one in the study by McKee, Nicol, and McDaniel. At the gap position, a syntactic dependency is established between the dislocated phrase (*the peacock*) and the gap, which should reactivate the dislocated phrase. This reactivation should speed the judgment for the animacy of the picture. This prediction was borne out in the study by Roberts, Marinis, Felser, and Clahsen (2007) for both adults and 6- to 7-year-old children and shows that children as young as six years of age are capable of utilizing structural/syntactic information and constructing syntactic dependencies involving movement.

Syntactic dependencies involving movement, such as the one above, involve storing some part of the sentence (*the peacock*) in working memory, retrieving it from working memory at a syntactically relevant position later in the sentence (the gap), and integrating it in the structure of the sentence. This increases processing demands, and predicts that working-memory capacity may impact on the children's performance in this task, and in general on sentence comprehension of syntactic dependencies involving movement. This has indeed been demonstrated in some recent studies. In the study by Roberts, Marinis, Felser, and Clahsen (2007) discussed above, reactivation was attested in adults and children with high working memory. Adults and children with low working memory did not show this effect, although they were able to comprehend the sentences as accurately as the adults and children with high working memory. Participants with low working memory may have required more time to retrieve the words from working memory and to establish the syntactic dependency, and maybe this is why no effect was attested at the gap. In addition, a study by Booth, MacWhinney, and Harasaki (2000) showed a different pattern of performance in 8- to 11-year-old children with high vs. low working memory when they processed sentences involving an object relative clause, a subject relative clause, or a conjoined verb phrase. Thus, although there is evidence that children as young as four are able to utilize structural/syntactic information when they process sentences in real time, it seems that working-memory limitations can affect their performance in on-line tasks that put increased demands on their processing system. This issue is very important when looking at results from on-line experiments in language-impaired children and adults, because these populations seem to have limitations in their working-memory capacity.

12.4 Sentence Processing in Developmental Language Disorders

Developmental language disorders are disorders that occur in children before the language system has been fully developed. For example, children with Williams syndrome, or Down's syndrome have atypical development in cognitive and non-cognitive domains, among others in language. Another group with a developmental language disorder constitutes children with Specific Language Impairment (SLI). This is a heterogeneous group of language-impaired children who do not seem to have an impairment in any cognitive or non-cognitive domain apart from language (Leonard, 1998). The group is heterogeneous because it is defined by exclusion. Children classified as having SLI are the ones that have a language impairment but perform within the norms in non-verbal cognitive tasks. Their inclusion in this group is not based on the aetiology of the impairment because this is still unknown. Therefore, as it stands, this group consists of children with a very mixed profile.

Research on the language abilities of children with SLI has revealed deficits in morphosyntax, phonology, and the lexicon (Leonard, 1998). This has led to the development of theories arguing that SLI is caused by a deficit in grammar. However, several studies have also shown that children with SLI seem to have deficits in some non-linguistic abilities, such as symbolic play (Johnston, 1994) and motor skills (Hill, 2001). Finally, a rich body of research has revealed that children with SLI show deficits in phonological memory (Gathercole & Baddeley, 1990) and process linguistic but also non-linguistic information at a slower rate than TD children (Miller, Kail, Leonard, & Tomblin, 2001). Thus, there is a lack of agreement on the nature and cause of SLI, with some theories arguing that SLI is caused by a deficit in grammar, and others that it is caused by general processing-capacity limitations (Joanisse & Seidenberg, 1998).

The majority of studies investigating the linguistic abilities of children with SLI have used off-line comprehension, production and grammaticality judgment tasks. For example, the most widely used tasks tapping sentence comprehension are picture-selection and picture-verification tasks. In a picture-selection task, children typically see a set of two to four pictures and listen to a sentence; after the end of the sentence, they have to select the picture that matches the sentence. In the picture-verification task, children see only one picture. Then they listen to one sentence and have to say whether the sentence matches the picture. In both tasks, children have to listen and build up the grammatical structure of the sentence, store it in memory, observe pictures, and then make a decision. To select a picture out of two, four or even more pictures, the child also requires good observation skills, and the ability to spot differences between pictures. In addition, as the number of pictures increases, so does the processing capacity required from the child to decide which picture matches the sentence. Thus, these tasks involve not only sentence comprehension but also memory and observation skills, and they place attentional demands and variable processing-capacity demands, depending on the number of pictures. Given that it is impossible to separate these factors, these tasks cannot genuinely disentangle whether SLI results from a grammatical impairment or processing-capacity limitations. In contrast, on-line sentence-processing tasks are able to address this debate because they are implicit; they tap how children process sentences as they unfold, and they rely less on memory.

A series of studies from the 1990s until now have looked at how children with SLI process sentences using word-monitoring tasks (Montgomery, 2000, 2002; Montgomery & Leonard, 1998; Montgomery, Scudder, & Moore, 1990). In a word-monitoring task, participants are presented with the picture of a target word, and then have to detect it in a sentence. Upon encountering the target word in the sentence, they have to press a button as fast as possible. This provides information about how fast they detect words, and can inform us about lexical retrieval. In addition, given that children have to detect a word within a sentence, this task can inform us about how children process sentences in real time.

Studies using word-monitoring tasks have revealed that children with SLI are slower to detect words than TD children matched on age or language abilities. However, they also demonstrated that children with SLI, although slower, do not differ in their processing pattern from TD children. For example, Montgomery, Scudder, and Moore (1990) investigated how 7- to 12-year-old language-impaired children and language controls monitor words in three types of sentences: normal sentences, as in (3) below, sentences that maintain semantic-syntactic relational integrity (syntactic sentences) but do not conform to real-world expectation, as in (4) below, and sentences devoid of syntactic, semantic, and real-world information (acoustic sentences), as in (5) below.

(3)   Jessie likes to dress in bright colors. His blue *socks* and purple shoes are some of his favorite clothes.

(4)   Some yards are all glass. A pretty *fish* under the table was sleeping in some heavy paper.

(5)   Long were cool nail star. She very *boots* her the got swim green slow ugly dirt bad.

Overall, language-impaired children were slower than language controls in word detection. However, both groups were faster in normal than in syntactic and acoustic sentences, and also in syntactic than in acoustic sentences. This shows that, similarly to TD children, children with SLI are making use of both syntactic, semantic and real-world information when they process sentences in real time.

Two further studies by Montgomery (2000, 2002) revealed that English children with SLI follow the same processing pattern as TD children. Both studies used a word-monitoring task, and children had to detect words at the beginning, middle, or end of sentences. If children with SLI are not able to process and integrate syntactic or other types of information, their response times (RTs) should be similar in the three positions or should decrease as words occurred later in the sentence. The study by Montgomery (2000) revealed that, in 7- to 10-year-old children with SLI, RTs decreased as words occurred later in the sentence, which was similar to age and language controls. This indicates that although children with SLI are slower overall, their sentence processing is facilitated by the accumulation of sentential information. The study by Montgomery (2002) compared word monitoring in sentences with a high proportion of stop consonants to sentences with a high proportion of non-stop consonants in 6- to 10-year-old children with SLI, age- controls and language-matched controls. Children with SLI showed overall slower responses, but their pattern of processing did not differ from that of TD children. All three groups showed similar responses to sentences with a high proportion of stop consonants and a high proportion of non-stop consonants.

In contrast to the above studies, a study by Montgomery and Leonard (1998) and a study by Marinis and van der Lely (2007) showed qualitative differences between TD children and children with SLI. Montgomery and Leonard (1998) using a word-monitoring task investigated how 6- to 10-year-old children with SLI-, age- and language-matched controls process verbs with low perceptual saliency morphemes (third person singular -*s* and past tense -*ed*) as opposed to verbs with a high perceptual saliency morpheme (present-progressive -*ing*). In this task, children had to detect words following an inflected verb, as in (6), or an uninflected verb, as in (7) below.

(6)   Jerry can't wait to get home from school. Every day he races home and eats *cookies* before dinner.

(7)   Becky loves Saturday mornings. She always gets up early and eats *breakfast* before she watches cartoons.

If children are able to process the morphosyntactic information encoded at the verb inflection, they are predicted to show longer RTs in sentences with uninflected verbs than in inflected verbs, because the ungrammaticality will slow them down. Children with SLI showed overall longer RTs than age-matched controls, and there were also qualitative differences between TD children and children with SLI. TD children showed longer reaction times when both types of inflectional morphemes were missing; in contrast, children with SLI did not show this effect in the sentences involving morphemes with low perceptual salience; i.e., children with SLI showed longer RTs when -*ing* was missing compared to -*ing* present, but there was no difference in RTs between verbs with -*ed/-s* missing and verbs with -*ed/-s* present. This has been taken as evidence in favour of the Surface Account, according to which children with SLI have greater difficulty processing low perceptual saliency morphemes than high perceptual saliency morphemes.

Finally, Marinis and van der Lely (2007) investigated how 10- to 17-year-old children with SLI-, age- and language-matched controls process *wh*-questions, as in (8) below, using a cross-modal picture-priming experiment.

(8)   Balloo gives a long carrot to the rabbit$_i$. Who$_i$ did Balloo give the long carrot to t$_i$ at the farm?

This task was similar to the one by Roberts, Marinis, Felser, and Clahsen (2007). Children heard sentences, such as in (8), that involve a dislocated *wh*-word (*who*) that has moved leaving a gap or trace (t$_i$) behind. Children saw a picture while listening to the question, and had to press a button for animacy decision. The picture was either the antecedent of *who*, i.e. a picture of a rabbit, or an unrelated picture. This picture was presented at the position of the gap (offset of the preposition *to*), at the offset of the verb, or at a control position. Similarly to the study by Roberts, Marinis, Felser, and Clahsen, if children are capable of establishing a syntactic dependency between the dislocated *wh*-word (*who*) and the gap, then RTs at the gap for the picture of the rabbit should be shorter than for the unrelated picture (reactivation). This difference could also be present at the verb because studies in adults have revealed that processing of verbs reactivates their possible arguments (Nicol, 1996). However, this should not occur at the control position. Children with SLI showed overall longer RTs than age-matched controls. In addition, age and language controls showed reactivation at the gap, in contrast to children with SLI who showed reactivation at the verb, but not at the gap. This was taken as evidence that children with SLI are not able to establish a syntactic dependency between the *wh*-word and the gap. These data were interpreted within van der Lely's model (2005), according to which children with SLI have an impairment at the computational system. However, this is not the only possible interpretation of the data. As far as the effect at the verb is concerned, this is not surprising given that studies with adults have found the same effect. Children with SLI may try to integrate the *wh*-word at the verb *give* as an indirect object. When they subsequently encounter the preposition *to*, they should revise this hypothesis and postulate a gap. Lack of reactivation at the offset of the preposition does not necessarily mean that the children were not able to establish a syntactic dependency between the *wh*-word and the gap. Given that children with SLI show slower RTs overall, they could have shown reactivation slightly later, for example at the next word after the gap, a position that was not tested in this experiment. Two possible alternatives can account for the fact that children with SLI did not show reactivation at the gap. The first one relates to processing-capacity limitations: children with SLI may lack the processing capacity to revise their initial hypothesis. A second explanation could relate to slower processing and lexical retrieval. A large number of word-monitoring studies have shown that children with SLI show longer RTs, which could be linked to problems with lexical retrieval. Given that the cross-modal priming involves lexical retrieval, slower lexical retrieval could have caused lack of priming at the gap rather than an inability to construct syntactic dependencies, which is in line with previous findings from on-line studies on children with SLI.

In summary, children with SLI show longer RTs than TD children, but the overwhelming majority of studies show that their pattern of processing does not differ from the one in TD children. This implies that children with SLI are capable of processing and integrating different types of information (syntactic, semantic, world-knowledge). Slower RTs are more likely to result from a general processing-capacity limitation affecting lexical retrieval than from a deficit in the grammatical system.

12.5   Sentence Processing in Acquired Disorders

In contrast to developmental language disorders, acquired language disorders result from damage to the brain after the language system has been established. This section focuses on sentence processing in aphasia. Similarly to research in SLI, the great majority of research in aphasia is based on off-line methods. These have shown that Broca's patients perform above chance in the comprehension of canonical sentences, such as actives and subject clefts; in contrast they perform at chance level in sentences with non-canonical word-order, such as passives and object clefts. This has led to the formulation of several theories for the nature of the impairment, some of which argue that the impairment is at the structural level (Grodzinsky, 2000), while others argue that it is caused by a pathologically fast decay rate of representations (Haarman & Kolk, 1994), or by processing limitations (Pinango, 2000). However, off-line methods are affected by memory and attentional demands and contaminate the participants' performance on the language tasks. Therefore, on the basis of only off-line data it is not possible to disentangle the two types of hypotheses. Recently, several studies have used on-line methodologies to examine how aphasic patients process sentences in real time. In the rest of this section, I first review these studies, and then address the implications of these results for theories of aphasia and the nature of the impairment.

In a case study, Tyler (1985) used an on-line word-monitoring task with an agrammatic patient, DE, who in an off-line task showed lower accuracy in the judgment of anomalous sentences than controls. In the word-monitoring task, DE showed longer RTs for syntactically correct but semantically anomalous prose than for normal prose, and even longer RTs for word salad (acoustic sentences). This indicates that DE had some sensitivity to sentential meaning and syntactic structure. In addition, RTs were shorter at later points in normal prose, and there were normal effects of semantic and syntactic anomalies on the RTs for the words following an anomalous word. This also indicates sensitivity to syntactic and semantic information. However, in contrast to the control group, RTs were not shorter at later points in anomalous prose, which suggests reduced sensitivity to syntactic structure. Further evidence that agrammatic patients have some sensitivity to syntactic structure was provided in a study by Shankweiler, Crain, Gorrell and Tuller (1989). They conducted a study with six agrammatic patients, four of whom performed poorly on an off-line comprehension task with reversible passives. However, in an on-line grammaticality judgment participants showed faster reaction times as each sentence progressed, which is similar to the finding by Tyler (1985). In addition, RTs were faster when there was a short distance between the anomalous and the licensing segments. The agrammatic patients' overall accuracy was lower than in the control group but above chance, and their accuracy in detecting ungrammaticalities was better in sentences involving between-grammatical-class substitutions than in sentences involving within-grammatical-class substitutions. This provides further evidence for their sensitivity to syntactic information. Thus, these two studies show that although agrammatic patients are not able to use syntactic information to determine the meaning of sentences off-line, they are capable of using syntactic information on-line. This is in contrast to a series of studies by Swinney, Zurif and colleagues using the cross-modal priming paradigm (Balogh, Zurif, Prather, Swinney, and Finkel,

1998; Swinney, Zurif, Prather, & Love, 1996; Zurif, Swinney, Prather, Solomon, & Bushell, 1993).

These studies focused on subject and object relative clauses, as shown in (9) and (10) respectively.

(9)   The gymnast loved the professor$_i$ from the northwestern city who$_i$ t$_i$ complained about the bad coffee.

(10)   The priest enjoyed the drink$_i$ that the caterer was serving t$_i$ to the guests.

Studies using off-line tasks have revealed that Broca's patients showed relatively normal comprehension for subject relative clauses, but Wernicke's patients showed comprehension at chance level. In contrast, both groups showed comprehension at chance level for object relative clauses. The on-line cross-modal priming experiments revealed different results for the two groups of patients. Although Wernicke's participants performed at chance in the off-line task for both subject and object relative clauses, they showed reactivation of the antecedent at the trace in both subject and object relative clauses. Broca's participants who in the off-line task performed relatively well for subject relative clauses, in the on-line task did not show reactivation at the trace in any of the two sentence types. According to Swinney, Zurif and colleagues, the on-line results by Wernicke's participants reflect their ability to establish syntactic dependencies; their chance-level comprehension in off-line tasks reflects difficulties with accessing the argument structure of verbs and thematic role assignment. The lack of reactivation at the trace by Broca's participants was interpreted as a processing problem due to either abnormally slow linking of antecedents and traces or failure to link the two. Non-grammatical strategies, such as the agent-first strategy (Caplan & Futter, 1986), were argued to compensate for their inability to establish dependency relations. By linking these results to results showing slower than normal lexical activation (Prather, Shapiro, Zurif, & Swinney, 1991), Swinney, Zurif and colleagues proposed that the brain region implicated in Broca's aphasia is not the locus of syntactic representations *per se*. Instead, they suggested that this brain region provides the resources necessary to sustain lexical activation and its syntactic ramifications. However, they acknowledged alternative ways to interpret these data. Given that long-distance dependencies in object relative clauses rely on working memory, they recognized that this region could accommodate memory storage demands arising during comprehension.

A subsequent study by Blumstein, Byma, Kurowski, et al. (1998) using the same technique showed very different results. Blumstein and colleagues investigated the processing of filler-gap dependencies in Broca's and Wernicke's patients using several types of sentences involving movement (subject and object relative clauses, simple and embedded *wh*-questions). Using two tasks similar to the ones presented above, Blumstein and colleagues found reactivation of the antecedent at the trace in Broca's but not in Wernicke's participants.

However, there were two crucial differences between the tasks used by Blumstein et al. and the ones used by Swinney, Zurif and colleagues. The first difference regards the modality used in the tasks. Whereas Swinney, Zurif and colleagues used the cross-modal lexical priming, in which participants heard a sentence (auditory modality), and saw a word on a computer screen (visual modality), Blumstein and colleagues used a single-modality lexical priming task, in which both the sentence and the word were presented through the auditory modality. According to Blumstein and colleagues, the single-modality presentation reduces attentional demands, and they argue that this could be the reason why in their task Broca's participants showed reactivation of the antecedent at the trace. The second difference regards the timing of the presentation of the word. In the studies by Swinney, Zurif and colleagues, the word was presented in the middle of the sentence, which is the general practice in this paradigm. In contrast, in the study by Blumstein and colleagues, the word was presented at the end of the sentence, which is the locus for another effect, a wrap-up effect. Balogh, Zurif, Prather, Swinney, and Finkel (1998) argue that this is the decisive reason for the differences between the results of the two studies. According to Balogh and colleagues, the effect attested in the study by Blumstein and colleagues for Broca's and Wernicke's participants does not reflect syntactically driven gap-filling, but is a wrap-up effect at the end of the sentence. Wrap-up effects implicate semantics and discourse information and result from the integration of different types of information at the end of the sentence when participants build up the meaning of the sentence. Broca's patients may have been successful in showing this effect because it is likely to be less temporally restrained than a filler-gap effect in the middle of the sentence. Wernicke's patients, on the other hand, may have shown no end-of-the-sentence effect because they have more difficulties in activating the argument structure of verbs, and problems at the level of semantics.

A further study looking at syntactic processing in aphasic patients was conducted by Caplan and Waters (2003). They used a self-paced listening task with sentences of different syntactic complexity – cleft subject sentences (11), cleft object sentences (12), right-branching object–subject relative clauses (13), and center-embedded subject–object relative clauses (14).

(11)   It was the food that nourished the child.

(12)   It was the woman that the toy amazed.

(13)   The father read the book that terrified the child.

(14)   The man that the fire injured called the doctor.

Cleft object sentences (12) and center-embedded subject–object relative clauses (14) are more complex than cleft subject sentences (11) and right-branching object–subject relative clauses (13). In this study, 28 aphasic patients and 28 controls listened to sentences of the types above in a phrase-by-phrase fashion by pushing a button. At the end of the sentence they had to judge the plausibility of the sentence they had just heard. RTs were recorded for pressing the button after each phrase. The underlying assumption in this task is that RTs reflect the time it takes for the participants to integrate the words/phrases into the syntactic structure, and longer RTs reflect integration difficulties.

Results from the plausibility judgment showed that both aphasic patients and controls took longer for the judgment of more complex sentences (12, 14) than for less complex ones. Controls were equally good at judging the plausibility of all sentence types, but aphasic patients were less accurate in the judgment of more complex than of less complex sentences. RTs showed that aphasics were overall slower than controls, and the pattern of processing differed as a function of their level of comprehension. Good comprehenders performed similarly to controls; in center-embedded subject–object relative clauses they showed longer RTs at the end of clauses and at points of syntactic complexity than at right-branching object–subject relative clauses. These effects were not attested in poor comprehenders, suggesting that they did not assign the syntactic structure of center-embedded subject–object relative clauses on-line. Poor comprehenders also showed a different pattern of processing from good comprehenders in cleft sentences; poor comprehenders' RTs on the verb were longer in sentences that were incorrectly judged to be implausible than in those that were correctly judged to be so. This effect was not attested in good comprehenders. This indicates that when poor comprehenders made errors, they spent more time trying to build up the structure of the sentence, and allocated additional time to process the most demanding phrase of the sentence. Finally, Caplan and Waters found that the pattern of processing differed as a function of the patients' clinical diagnosis. RTs in Broca's aphasics indicated that they were not processing complex syntactic structures on-line. In contrast, fluent aphasics' RTs indicated that their comprehension impairment occurred after on-line processing was accomplished.

Summarizing, studies on syntactic processing in aphasia using on-line methods have provided invaluable insight into the nature of the patients' impairment. Patients with chance-level performance in off-line tasks have been shown to have some sensitivity to syntactic information. This shows that performance at chance in off-line sentence comprehension tasks does not always coincide with an inability to assign syntactic structure in real time. Poor performance in off-line tasks could have different causes. Aphasic patients may have some sensitivity to syntactic information, but they may not have a critical level of sensitivity that would allow them to perform above chance. Alternatively, performance at chance in off-line tasks may reflect difficulties in a review stage at the end of the sentence. Further research combining off-line and on-line tasks with the same sentences in the same populations is essential for the characterization of the nature of the deficits in different groups of patients with aphasia.

REFERENCES

Balogh, J., Zurif, E., Prather, P., Swinney, D., and Finkel, L. (1998). Gap-filling and end-of-sentence effects in real-time language processing: Implications for modeling sentence comprehension in aphasia. *Brain and Language*, 61, 169–82.

Blumstein, S., Byma, G., Kurowski, K., Hourihan, J., Brown, T., and Hutchinson, A. (1998). On-line processing of filler-gap constructions in aphasia. *Brain and Language*, 61, 149–68.

Booth, J. R., MacWhinney, B., and Harasaki, Y. (2000). Developmental differences in visual and auditory processing of complex sentences. *Child Development*, 71, 981–1003.

Caplan, D. and Futter, C. (1986). Assignment of thematic roles by an agrammatic aphasic patient. *Brain and Language*, 27, 117–35.

Caplan, D. and Waters, G. (2003). On-line syntactic processing in aphasia: Studies with auditory moving window presentation. *Brain and Language*, 84, 222–49.

Gathercole, S. and Baddeley, A. (1990). Phonological memory deficits in language disordered children: Is there a causal connection? *Journal of Memory and Language*, 29, 336–60.

Gibson, E. and Pearlmutter, N. (1998). Constraints on sentence comprehension. *Trends in Cognitive Science*, 2, 262–8.

Grodzinsky, Y. (2000). The neurology of syntax: Language use without Broca's area. *Behavioural and Brain Sciences*, 23, 1–71.

Haarman, J. and Kolk, H. (1994). On-line sensitivity to subject–verb agreement violations in Borca's aphasics: The role of syntactic complexity and time. *Brain and Language*, 46, 493–516.

Hill, E. L. (2001). Non-specific nature of specific language impairment: A review of the literature with regard to concomitant motor impairments. *International Journal of Language and Communication Disorders*, 36, 149–71.

Joanisse, M. and Seidenberg, M. (1998). Specific language impairment: A deficit in grammar or processing? *Trends in Cognitive Sciences*, 2, 240–7.

Johnston, J. R. (1994). Cognitive abilities of children with language impairment. In R. Watkins and M. Rice (eds.), *Specific Language Impairments in Children: Current Directions in Research and Intervention*. Baltimore, MD: Paul H. Brookes.

Leonard, L. (1998). *Children with Specific Language Impairment*. Cambridge, MA: MIT Press.

Marinis, T. and van der Lely, H. (2007). On-line processing of wh-questions in children with G-SLI and typically developing children. *International Journal of Language and Communication Disorders*, 42, 557–82.

McKee, C., Nicol, J., and McDaniel, D. (1993). Children's application of binding during sentence processing. *Language and. Cognitive Processes*, 8(3), 265–90.

Miller, C., Kail, R., Leonard, L., and Tomblin, B. (2001). Speed of processing in children with specific language impairment. *Journal of Speech, Language and Hearing Disorders*, 44, 416–33.

Montgomery, J. (2000). Relation of working memory to off-line and real-time sentence processing in children with specific language impairment. *Applied Psycholinguistics*, 21, 117–48.

Montgomery, J. (2002). Examining the nature of lexical processing in children with Specific Language Impairment: Temporal processing or processing capacity deficit. *Applied Psycholinguistics*, 23, 447–70.

Montgomery, J. and Leonard, L. (1998). Real-time inflectional processing by children with specific language impairment: Effects of phonetic substance. *Journal of Speech, Language and Hearing Research*, 41, 1432–43.

Montgomery, J., Scudder, R., and Moore, C. (1990). Language-impaired children's real-time comprehension of spoken language. *Applied Psycholinguistics*, 11, 273–90.

Nicol, J. L. (1996). Syntactic priming. *Language and Cognitive Processes*, 11, 675–9.

Pickering, M. (1999). Sentence comprehension. In S. Garrod and M. Pickering (eds.), *Language Processing*. Hove, Sussex: Psychology Press.

Pinango, M. (2000). Canonicity in Broca's sentence comprehension: The case of psychological verbs. In J. Grodzinsky, L. Shapiro, and D. Swinney (eds.), *Language and the Brain*. San Diego, CA: Academic Press.

Prather, P., Shapiro, L., Zurif, E., and Swinney, D. (1991). Real-time examination of lexical processing in aphasia. *Journal of Psycholinguistic Research*, 23, 271–81.

Roberts, L., Marinis, T., Felser, C., and Clahsen, H. (2007). Antecedent priming at gap positions in children's sentence processing. *Journal of Psycholinguistic Research*, 36, 175–88.

Shankweiler, D., Crain, S., Gorrell, P., and Tuller, B. (1989). Reception of language in Broca's aphasia. *Language and Cognitive Processes*, 4, 1–33.

Swinney, D., Zurif, E., Prather, P., and Love, T. (1996). Neurological distribution of processing operations underlying language comprehension. *Journal of Cognitive Neuroscience*, 8, 174–84.

Tyler, L. (1985). Real-time comprehension processes in agrammatism: A case study. *Brain and Language*, 26, 259–75.

Tyler, L. K. and Marslen-Wilson, W. D. (1981). Children's processing of spoken language. *Journal of Verbal Learning and Verbal Behavior*, 20, 400–16.

van der Lely, H. K. J. (2005). Domain-specific cognitive systems: Insight from grammatical specific language impairment. *Trends in Cognitive Sciences*, 9, 53–9.

Zurif, E., Swinney, D. A., Prather, P. A., Solomon, J. A., and Bushell, C. (1993). An on-line analysis of syntactic processing in Broca's and Wernicke's aphasia. *Brain and Language*, 45, 448–64.

13 Morphology and Language Disorder

MARTINA PENKE

Morphology is concerned with the structure of words. Traditionally, morphological operations are divided into word formation, i.e. the processes by which we can create new words with new meanings, and inflection, i.e. the processes by which grammatical information such as PERSON, NUMBER, or TENSE is realized on a word. All morphological operations can be affected in language disorders. However, research on morphological deficits has mostly been concerned with inflectional morphology (for research on word-formation deficits see Miceli & Caramazza, 1988; Luzzatti & de Bleser, 1996; Libben & Jarema, 2006). Deficits with inflectional morphology are a symptom frequently observed in acquired and developmental language disorders. Such deficits have been reported for developmental language deficits such as Specific Language Impairment (SLI), Williams syndrome, Down's syndrome and autism, and for acquired language deficits such as aphasic language disorders (Broca's aphasia, anomic aphasia) and degenerative (Parkinson's disease, Alzheimer's disease, Huntington's disease, semantic dementia) or inflammatory (herpes simplex encephalitis) brain diseases. Whereas inflectional deficits have been the subject of intense research in Broca's aphasia and SLI during the last 20 years, other language disorders such as Down's syndrome, Parkinson's syndrome, and autism have only recently come into focus, and our knowledge of inflectional disorders in these diseases is still very limited. Also, whereas impairments of inflectional morphology are characteristic of diseases such as Broca's aphasia, the observed deficits do not seem to be specific to a given language disorder in such a way that a given deficit is always and only observed in this type of disorder, but similar observations are made and similar accounts for these deficits are discussed across different language disorders. The goal of this chapter, therefore, is not to list language disorders and the inflectional deficits that have been reported for these disorders, but to provide an overview of how inflectional systems are affected in language impairments.

13.1 Factors Influencing Errors with Inflectional Morphology

The last 20 years have seen a growing interest in investigating language disorders across languages. This research has led to some important findings about factors that influence which inflectional systems or inflected forms are especially vulnerable in language disorders.

13.1.1 Typology and complexity of inflectional systems

Much research on inflectional deficits has been concerned with Broca's aphasia in English-speaking individuals. Since the omission of inflectional affixes is a core symptom of English speakers with Broca's aphasia, omissions of inflectional markers were for a long time seen as a characteristic sign of this disorder across languages. However, the cross-language investigation of aphasic disorders that started in the 1980s revealed that typological differences in inflectional systems affect the type of inflectional errors that will be observed in language disorders. In a seminal work, Yosef Grodzinsky (1984) pointed out that omissions of inflectional markers only occur in aphasic speech if the remaining word stem is a possible word in the language in question. Thus, the omission of the plural marker -s in the English word *books* results in the form *book* which is a possible word in English. Corresponding omissions of the inflectional markers in languages such as Russian or Italian would, in contrast, result in stems which cannot surface as possible words in these languages (Italian *libr-* instead of *libri*, Russian *knig-* instead of *knigi*). Grodzinsky provides evidence that – although omission errors are characteristic of English-speaking Broca's aphasics – omission errors do not occur in languages like Russian or Italian where the omission would result in an illegal word. The finding that omissions of inflectional elements will only occur where licensed by the grammar of a language constitutes an important generalization on inflectional deficits in language disorders.

  Grodzinsky's claim that inflectional affixes will be omitted if the remaining stem constitutes a possible word in the language, however, turned out to be too strong. Research across languages has provided evidence that the number of inflectional elements omitted by aphasic speakers is related to the amount of syntactically relevant information expressed by these elements. Whereas in English – an analytic language with a largely reduced inflectional component – inflectional markers tend to be omitted, in languages where inflectional systems are more elaborate and express more syntactic information (such as Finnish, German, Italian, Polish or Spanish) omission rates are markedly lower than in English (e.g. Bates, Friederici, & Wulfeck, 1987; Dromi, Leonard, Adam, & Zadunaisky-Ehrlich, 1999). Thus, whereas, for instance, the English 3rd person singular marker -s is omitted in about half of the obligatory contexts for this marker by children with SLI (Clahsen, Bartke, & Göllner, 1997) and adult Broca's aphasics (Goodglass & Berko, 1960), omission rates for subject–verb agreement inflection in German-speaking subjects are considerably lower (20 percent for the German SLI children in Clahsen, Bartke, and Göllner, 1997, 2 percent for the Broca's aphasics in Penke, 1998).

Cross-language comparisons have moreover suggested that the number of forms contained in an inflectional paradigm influences the number of inflectional errors where one inflectional form is substituted by another. The more forms an inflectional system contains, i.e. the larger the inventory of forms from which to choose the correct form, the more substitution errors are likely to occur (Bates, Friederici, & Wulfeck, 1987; Dromi, Leonard, Adam, & Zadunaisky-Ehrlich, 1999). Whereas substitution errors made up 7.5 percent in an elicitation task on Italian article inflection, which differentiates between nine article forms inflected for gender and number, the substitution rate increased to 16 percent for German Broca's aphasics who have twelve different forms to choose from in the paradigm of article inflection (Bates, Friederici, & Wulfeck, 1987).

The investigation of inflectional deficits across languages has thus shown that language-specific factors related to the complexity and importance of inflectional systems, and to whether or not uninflected forms are permitted, critically affect type and amount of inflectional errors in language-impaired speakers.

13.1.2   Inflection type

Inflectional processes are restricted to words of a certain grammatical category. Tense inflection, for example, can only appear on verbs, comparative inflection is restricted to adjectives, and case inflection occurs on nominal elements. Moreover, inflection encodes information on a number of different morphosyntactic categories such as TENSE, ASPECT, NUMBER, GENDER, and CASE. That inflectional morphology is classified according to the word category it applies to and to the morphosyntactic information it provides suggests that deficits with inflectional morphology might not affect all inflectional systems of a language in parallel, but might selectively affect only some inflectional systems of a language. Indeed, such deficits are observed in aphasic speakers and children with SLI.

Inflectional deficits selective for a specific grammatical class of words have been observed across languages in a small number of aphasic subjects (e.g. Laiacona & Caramazza, 2004). In elicitation tasks where subjects have to produce inflected forms for verbs and nouns that are homophones (e.g., 'This is a guide; these are ___', 'This person guides, these people ___'), the subjects show a dissociation in their capability to produce correctly inflected noun or verb forms: whereas some of the tested aphasic subjects display significantly more problems in producing inflected verb forms than in producing homophone noun forms, others show the opposite pattern.

Developments in syntactic theory that led to the split-up of the functional projection INFL into an AGR node relevant for subject–verb agreement and a T node relevant for tense inflection have drawn research interests to differential deficits of agreement and tense inflection in Broca's aphasia and SLI. Depending on which type of syntactic deficit is invoked to capture the language deficits in these disorders (cf. section 13.2), selective deficits of tense inflection sparing agreement inflection (Friedmann & Grodzinsky, 1997; Rice, Wexler, & Cleave, 1995) or, conversely, selective deficits of agreement inflection sparing tense inflection (Clahsen, Bartke, & Göllner, 1997) have been reported.

That inflectional affixes can be selectively affected in language disorders, even when homophonous such as plural -s, possessive -s, and 3rd person singular -s in English, was shown by Goodglass and Berko (1960). They found that their aphasic subjects experienced more problems in providing forms inflected with the possessive -s (error rate 56%) than with 3rd person singular (error rate 43%) and plural forms (error rate 21%).

All these findings suggest that inflectional forms or inflectional affixes that belong to different inflectional systems are independent of each other. Selective deficits might then occur because different classes of grammatical words (noun or verb) or different morphological processes (such as agreement inflection or plural inflection) are subserved by different brain areas selectively affected by brain damage (Laiacona & Caramazza, 2004). Whether this suggestion will prove valid or whether other factors such as the frequency of affixes (subsection 13.1.4) might account for these observations, is a matter of future research.

13.1.3 Regularity

In many languages and inflectional systems, regular and irregular inflected forms exist side by side. Consider for instance English past-tense formation, where we find regular forms inflected with -ed (*laughed*) and irregular ones like *went* that are idiosyncratic and largely unpredictable. According to an influential view in linguistics and psycholinguistics – defended most prominently by Pinker (e.g. 1999) – regular inflected forms are built by application of a mental symbolic rule (add -ed), whereas irregular forms are stored in the mental lexicon. A central tenet of such a dualistic approach to inflection is that the representations and mechanisms involved in the production and comprehension of regular and irregular inflectional forms are fundamentally different and thus should be selectively affected by different types of language disorders. Research during the last 10 years has indeed provided ample evidence that deficits with inflectional morphology might selectively affect only regular or only irregular inflection.

Selective deficits of regular inflection have been reported for English-speaking subjects with Broca's aphasia, Parkinson's disease, SLI, Down's syndrome and autism (e.g. Laws & Bishop, 2003; Tager-Flusberg, 2003; Ullman, Corkin, Coppola, et al., 1997; van der Lely & Ullman, 2001). In elicitation tasks that test the production of regular and irregular inflected past tense forms (e.g.

Every day, I wash my car. Just like every day, yesterday I ____.), speakers with such language disorders typically display more problems in providing correctly inflected regular forms than irregular forms. Moreover, these subjects rarely overapply the regular past-tense affix *-ed* to irregular verbs (e.g. *goed* instead of *went*), and do not use the regular affix to produce past-tense forms for pseudo-verbs as unimpaired subjects will typically do (e.g. *ploamphed*). Selective deficits of irregular inflection have conversely been reported for children with Williams syndrome, fluent anomic aphasic speakers and speakers suffering from herpes simplex encephalitis or degenerative brain disease (e.g. Alzheimer's disease, semantic dementia) (see, e.g., Clahsen & Almazan, 1998; Tyler, deMornay-Davies, Anokhina, et al., 2002; Ullman, Corkin, Coppola, et al., 1997). In these cases, speakers display significantly more problems in providing irregular inflected forms than regular inflected forms and overapply regular inflectional markers to irregular inflected stems (e.g. *goed* instead of *went*).

The validity of the reported selective deficits of regular as opposed to irregular inflectional morphology has, however, been questioned. For some language impairments the existing evidence for a selective deficit – especially with regular inflection – is rather scarce. This is because reports of such deficits are some-times based on just a few individuals, display only small differences between regular and irregular inflected forms, and are not replicated in other studies. Thus, whereas children with Down's syndrome display deficits with inflec-tional morphology, there is conflicting evidence on the question whether this deficit is especially pronounced for regular inflected forms (Eadie, Fey, Douglas, & Parsons, 2002). Similarly, several studies failed to replicate the finding of a selective deficit of regular inflection in speakers with Parkinson's disease (Longworth, Keenan, Barker, Marslen-Wilson, & Tyler, 2005; Penke, Janssen, Indefrey, & Seitz, 2005).

Another line of criticism addresses the issue of whether selective deficits are simply artifacts of the experimental design chosen. Thus, it has been proposed that English regular inflected past-tense forms are of greater phonological complexity than irregular ones, since they display complex consonant clusters (e.g. *walked*) whereas irregular forms often do not (e.g. *ran*). Bird, Lambon Ralph, Seidenberg, McClelland, and Patterson (2003), for instance, have provided evidence that a selective deficit with regular inflection observed in English-speaking subjects with Broca's aphasia disappeared when the test material was controlled for phonological complexity.

And finally, it has been questioned whether selective deficits observed in language-impaired speakers of English do hold across languages. Thus, whereas a selective vulnerability of irregular inflection has been confirmed for subjects with Williams syndrome and degenerative brain disease across languages (e.g. Cholewa & de Bleser, 1995; Penke & Krause, 2004), a selective deficit of regular inflection, which is characteristic of English-speaking sub-jects with Broca's aphasia and SLI, is not found in other languages such as German, Dutch, Italian, or Spanish (e.g. Clahsen & Rothweiler, 1993; de Diego Balaguer, Costa, Sebastián-Galles, Juncadella, & Caramazza, 2004; Luzzatti & de Bleser, 1996; Penke & Westermann, 2006).

13.1.4 Frequency

A major factor in determining how error-prone inflected word forms are in language disorders is frequency. As a rule of thumb, infrequent inflected forms are more error-prone than frequent ones – in normal and impaired speakers. Frequency effects are seen as indicative of processes of lexical storage and access. Memory traces get stronger with each exposure, making frequently occurring forms easier and quicker to access than infrequent ones. A frequency effect, however, will only affect inflected forms or components of inflected forms that are stored in the mental lexicon. Irregular inflected forms, for instance, are stored as fully inflected whole word forms in the mental lexicon. In production experiments error rates for stored irregular inflected forms are typically correlated with the frequency of the inflected form: the less frequent the inflected irregular form, the higher the error rate observed for language-impaired speakers (Penke, Janssen, & Krause, 1999).

A notable exception to this observation might occur in Williams syndrome. In an elicitation task with German Williams-syndrome children the error rates for irregular inflected participles appeared not to be dependent on the frequency of the inflected forms (Penke & Krause, 2004). This is not only in contrast to normally developing children, but is reminiscent of other findings in Williams syndrome where performance seems unaffected by the frequency of occurrence of a word. Thus, for instance, in word-fluency tasks where subjects have to give as many animals as come to mind during a minute, subjects with Williams syndrome typically produce more infrequent animal names than control children (Bellugi, Lichtenberger, Mills, Galaburda, & Korenberg, 1999). These findings indicate that organization of and/or access to entries stored in the mental lexicon might be different in subjects with Williams syndrome.

First results also point to an influence of affix frequency on error rates of language impaired speakers. Some morphological theories propose that regular inflectional affixes have independent entries in the mental lexicon (Wunderlich, 1996). If this assumption is correct, access to these affix entries should also be dependent on frequency: the more often a specific affix is encountered, the greater its accessibility. In a series of experiments on inflectional morphology in German Broca's aphasia, we have tested the production of inflected forms for a range of different regular inflectional affixes and observed a close correspondence between the number of words an affix is used with and the aphasic speakers' error rates. The more words an inflectional affix occurs with, the lower the error rate obtained. The frequency of the inflected regular forms, in contrast, did not influence error rates. Thus, the regular participle affix *-t* can be found on about 1000 German simplex verbs and only about 9 percent of these forms are produced incorrectly by our 13 aphasic subjects. In contrast, the regular plural suffix *-s* occurs with only 208 simplex nouns and the error rate for *-s*-plurals is about 62 percent (cf. Penke, 2006). This correlation suggests that the problems of language-impaired speakers with the production of some regular inflected forms result from difficulties in accessing the entries of these affixes. Problems in lexical access could thus cause impairments of infrequent irregular inflected forms as well as deficits with the application of infrequent regular affixes.

13.1.5   *Morphosyntactic specifications and markedness*

Inflectional affixes are organized in inflectional paradigms. Such paradigms are structured along morphosyntactic dimensions such as PERSON, NUMBER, GENDER or CASE. In morphological theory, these dimensions are generally represented in terms of binary features with marked (positive) and unmarked (negative) values. Whether forms are marked or unmarked with respect to a specific feature is determined on the basis of typological, morphological, syntactic, or conceptual arguments, and might vary between languages. Plural forms (e.g. *books*), for instance, are generally considered to be marked in comparison to singular forms (e.g. *book*), since plural forms are often marked by a morphological element (e.g. *-s*), whereas singular markers are very rare in the languages of the world.

Several studies on inflectional errors (in Broca's aphasia and SLI) have indicated that errors within one inflectional system do not result in random exchanges of one inflected form of the paradigm by another. Instead, errors rarely deviate in more than one morphosyntactic feature from the correct target (Bates, Friederici, & Wulfeck, 1987; Clahsen, Sonnenstuhl, Hadler, & Eisenbeiss, 2001; Menn & Obler, 1990), and they display a strong tendency to replace forms with a marked feature specification by forms with an unmarked feature specification within the same dimension of the paradigm (Janssen & Penke, 2002). As an example, consider the paradigm of German subject–verb agreement inflection which is organized along the dimensions PERSON (with the specification [±2nd]) and NUMBER (with the specification [±PLURAL]).

(1)

| | | NUMBER | |
		[–PLURAL]	[+PLURAL]
	[–2nd]	möchte	möchte-n
PERSON	[+2nd]	möchte-st	möchte-t

A substitution error might replace the German plural verb form *möchten* 'want' marked for the feature [+PLURAL] by the singular form *möchte* which encodes the unmarked feature value [–PLURAL]. The reverse error – a substitution of the unmarked singular form *möchte* by the more marked plural form *möchten* – is in contrast very rare, as is the substitution of the [+2nd, +PLURAL] form *möchtet* by the form *möchte* which is specified for [–2nd, –PLURAL] and thus differs in both morphosyntactic features from the target.

These findings indicate that the morphosyntactic features that structure an inflectional paradigm affect the type of errors that occur within a given inflectional system. Moreover, the tendency to replace marked forms by unmarked ones might turn out to be a core property of inflectional deficits (cf. Lapointe, 1985). It not only captures which substitution errors are likely to occur within an inflectional paradigm, but it also accounts for the frequently made observation that language-impaired speakers display a preference for substituting inflected finite verbs forms, marked for PERSON, NUMBER and TENSE, with nonfinite forms, such as infinitives or participles unmarked for these morphosyntactic properties, and to replace marked case-inflected forms by citation forms, typically unmarked nominative forms.

Moreover, inflectional errors are affected by morphophonological markedness. Inflectional affixes often are consonants. What if a consonantal inflectional ending is affixed to a stem that ends in the very same consonant? Adding the English past-tense ending /d/ to a stem such as *land-* which already ends in [d] would result in a sequence of two adjacent identical phones *landd*. Such sequences are, however, avoided in languages. One option – chosen in English (*landed*) or German (*heft-* + -$t_{3.SG}$ = *heftet* 'staples') – is to insert an epenthetic vowel between the two identical segments. Another option is chosen in Dutch, for instance, where only one of the two identical segments is realized (*ge+land-* + -*d* = *geland* 'landed'). Data from language acquisition indicate that the English/German solution is more marked than the Dutch solution, taking more time in acquisition (Grijzenhout & Penke, 2005). In an analysis of inflection errors produced by German Broca's aphasics in regular participle formation, we found that the marked German solution is prone to error. Only 50% of the regular verbs ending in a stem-final segment [t] were correctly inflected with the regular participle ending -*t* (e.g. *ge+heft-* + -*t* = *geheftet* 'stapled'), as opposed to 92.3% for regular verbs with stem-final segments other than [t]. Moreover, for verbs with stem final [t], 79% of the errors were omissions of the participle affix -*t* (**geheft* instead of *geheftet*). In contrast, omission errors made up only 2% of the errors for verbs ending in segments other than [t] (**geleb* instead of *gelebt* 'lived'). These data show that morphophonologically marked forms are prone to error, and they suggest that language-impaired speakers opt for the unmarked, Dutch, solution where only one of the identical segments is realized (cf. Grijzenhout & Penke 2005).

13.1.6 Language-external factors

Factors external to the grammatical system of a language have also been shown to exert some influence on inflectional deficits. Kolk and Heeschen (1992) have demonstrated that the number of omission errors is dependent on the task the subject has to perform. Whereas their German Broca's aphasic subjects displayed relatively high omission rates for inflected forms in spontaneous speech, omission rates dropped markedly when the very same subjects had to produce inflected forms in an elicitation task. The number of substitution errors, in contrast, increased. Kolk and Heeschen argue that omission errors result from a strategy of avoiding areas of potential problem – such as choosing the correct inflected form from the paradigm (subsections 13.1.1 and 13.1.5). How effective such an avoidance strategy can be is illustrated by some of my data on German participle inflection in Broca's aphasia. In spontaneous speech, where subjects can choose what to produce, only one percent of the irregular participles produced by five German Broca's aphasics were incorrectly inflected (Penke, 1998). Direct testing in an elicitation task reveals, however, that irregular participle inflection is affected (mean error rate of 13 subjects = 33%; Penke & Westermann, 2006). Specifically, the data indicate that the aphasic subjects suffer from a deficit accessing infrequent irregular participles in the mental lexicon, a deficit which would never become apparent in spontaneous speech where the production of difficult forms can be avoided.

Other external factors that influence the performance of language-impaired subjects relate to the testing situation (familiarity with the investigator, formality of the testing) and to how demanding a task is for the language-impaired subject. Tasks which minimize processing load, such as cloze tasks where the subject has to inflect a word presented in a sentential context, often lead to better performance than more unrestrained tasks. To control for such influences, inflectional deficits should be explored by using different methodologies and tasks.

13.2   Accounting for the Deficits

How inflection should be captured in linguistic theory, and to which component of the language capacity it belongs, are still matters of debate, since inflection has close connections to syntax, phonology and the mental lexicon. Accordingly, inflectional deficits have been attributed to deficits in syntactic, phonological, and morphological components of the language faculty as well as to deficits in lexicon organization and lexical access.

According to an influential view, our language capacity contains a mental lexicon, where words are stored together with learned idiosyncratic information, and a mental grammar component that contains the rules to generate composite structures such as sentences and complex words out of the stored elements in the mental lexicon (Pinker, 1999). Under this view, regular inflection belongs to the rule component of the grammar, while irregular inflected forms are stored in the mental lexicon. Selective deficits of regular inflection consequently result from damage to the rule component and co-occur with other 'rule'-deficits such as syntactic deficits (e.g. Gopnik, 1994; Ullman, Corkin, Coppola, et al., 1997). Selective deficits with irregular inflected forms, in contrast, are due to the lexical component and will, for instance, result from problems with lexical access. While such models account for selective deficits of regular or irregular inflection and for the observation that error rates for irregular inflected forms are strongly dependent on the frequency of these forms, they neglect issues such as the category dependency of inflectional deficits (affecting only verbal morphology or only tense morphology) or the influence of markedness and paradigm complexity on error rates.

Inflectional morphology realizes morphosyntactic information concerning NUMBER, PERSON, TENSE, CASE, etc., and thus encodes information about the participants, the temporal situation of events and the argument roles of the involved participants. This information is vital for syntactic representations since it expresses the grammatical functions (e.g. subject, object) of arguments and establishes agreement relationships between sentence constituents. In generative syntactic theories, the relevant morphosyntactic information is provided by or checked in functional categories in the syntactic tree. Stems like a verb have to move to functional categories such as AGR and TENSE to collect or check inflectional features encoding information on tense and subject–verb agreement. Concordant with this syntactic view of inflection are deficit accounts that attribute impairments with inflection to syntactic deficits. In such accounts, either the functional categories relevant for the realization of inflectional markers can no longer be projected, resulting in pruned syntactic trees (Friedmann & Grodzinsky, 1997), or the morphosyntactic information that is hosted in specific functional nodes is left unspecified (Clahsen, Bartke, & Göllner, 1997; Grodzinsky, 1990). Differing assumptions about which functional node is affected by the assumed deficit account for the different inflectional deficits proposed. Thus, assuming a syntactic tree such as (2), a deficit at the functional node TENSE will account for a deficit that selectively affects tense inflection, but spares agreement inflection (cf. Friedmann & Grodzinsky, 1997; Rice, Wexler, & Cleave, 1995). Accounts assuming that agreement features are underspecified will, on the other hand, capture selective deficits with verbal agreement morphology that spare tense inflection (e.g. Clahsen, Bartke, & Göllner, 1997). Whereas these approaches can account for category specific deficits – such as deficits affecting only verbal morphology or only tense morphology – they do not address other issues, such as deficits selectively affecting only regular or only irregular inflection, or the influence of frequency or markedness on inflectional errors.

(2)

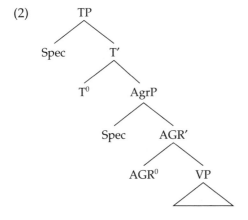

In more recent syntactic theories such as the Minimalist Program, the lexicon projects fully inflected forms into syntax and the morphosyntactic properties of these lexical elements determine the building up of syntactic structure. In such an account, problems with inflection might not be due to problems with functional categories, but they might already arise in the lexicon where the inflected form is built. Under a lexicalist account, inflectional deficits might stem from difficulties in accessing inflected forms or affixes in the mental lexicon. Processing limitations might lead to problems in accessing lexical entries that are less frequently activated or are more marked (e.g. Lapointe, 1985; Stemberger, 1984). Processing limitations might also lead to problems in identifying affixes or inflected forms with the correct morphosyntactic specifications in an inflectional paradigm, thus accounting for the observation that the number of inflected forms organized in an inflectional paradigm and the architecture of an inflectional paradigm affect number and type of the occurring inflectional errors (Bates, Friederici, & Wulfeck, 1987; Dromi, Leonard, Adam, & Zadunaisky-Ehrlich, 1999; Janssen & Penke, 2002).

Inflectional affixes typically display phonological characteristics that make them difficult to perceive and produce. Affixes, for instance, are shorter than other lexemes, are typically restricted to a small set of phonemes such as coronal consonants and the vowel schwa, and are often unstressed. Accordingly, accounts that see problems in perception and production of inflectional affixes as the basis of disorders such as SLI or Broca's aphasia have a long tradition in the field (e.g. Kean, 1977; Tallal, 2000). Recently an attempt has been made to put the deficit with regular inflection that is characteristic for English-speaking subjects with Broca's aphasia down to the greater phonological complexity of regular than of irregular past-tense forms (Bird, Lambon Ralph, Seidenberg, McClelland, & Patterson 2003). Since regular past-tense forms, unlike many irregulars, involve the addition of phonetic material (the past-tense affix) leading to complex consonant clusters at words' ends (compare *walked* vs. *ran*), they place greater demands on the phonological system and are consequently more difficult to produce and perceive for speakers suffering from a phonological deficit. However, a look at Broca's aphasia across languages casts some doubt on this proposal. Consider regular past-tense formation in English and regular participle formation in German and Dutch. Regular past-tense as opposed to participle forms are of similar phonological complexity in all three languages, since in all three languages a coronal stop ([t] or [d]) is added to the verb stem resulting in similarly complex final consonant clusters in regular inflected forms (compare English *danced* [da:nst] with German *getanzt* [. . . tanst] and Dutch *gedanst* [. . . danst]). Despite similar phonological complexity, error rates for the production of regular English past-tense forms are high in English-speaking subjects with SLI or Broca's aphasia (70 to 80 percent; cf. Bird, Lambon Ralph, Seidenberg, McClelland, & Patterson, 2003; Ullman, Corkin, Coppola, et al., 1997), whereas regular participle formation in German and Dutch speakers is unimpaired (error rates less than 10 percent, Penke & Westermann, 2006). Also, in contrast to English aphasic subjects, who hardly ever overapply the regular past-tense marker to irregular verbs (e.g. *goed* instead of *went*), German and Dutch subjects readily over-apply the regular participle ending to irregular verbs, despite the complex consonant clusters that result (e.g. *gesingt* instead of *gesungen*). These findings cannot be explained by the proposed phonological-deficit account. Moreover, theories that see phonological deficits as the basis of inflectional deficits cannot capture differential deficits of homophone affixes and leave the influence of paradigm structure, markedness and frequency on inflectional errors unexplained.

13.3   The Relevance of Inflectional Disorders for Linguistic Theory

The investigation of language breakdown can be looked at from two different perspectives. Whereas the central goal certainly is to describe and explain the observed deficits, the study of language disorders can also provide insights into the structure and organization of the normal language system. The value of erroneous forms was probably first noticed in speech-error research. A linguistic investigation of speech errors quickly revealed that such errors were not random, but were constrained by the architecture of the language system (Fromkin, 1971). A similar logic can be applied to erroneous forms produced in language impairments. Consider, for instance, the issue whether or not regular and irregular inflection are qualitatively distinct. According to dualistic approaches to inflection (Pinker, 1999), the representations and mechanisms involved in the processing of regular and irregular inflectional forms are fundamentally different. If the dualistic view holds, then we should find language disorders that either selectively affect the regular inflectional component with the irregular inflectional module spared or, conversely, selectively affect the irregular inflectional component leaving the regular component unimpaired. A failure to find such a selective deficit, on the other hand, would weaken the dualistic view on inflection. Whether or not selective deficits of regular or irregular inflection can be found thus constitutes a test for the dualistic approach to inflection. That such deficits have meanwhile been observed across languages in a number of acquired and developmental language disorders (subsection 13.1.3) confirms a central prediction of the dualistic view of inflection.

Moreover, the finding that regular and irregular inflection often dissociate in language disorders can be used as diagnostic for which inflectional markers are regular or irregular. Consider as an example the rather intricate system of German noun plurals where we find five different plural markers (*-e*, *-er*, *-n*, *-s* or unmarked). There has been a long-standing debate on which of these forms are regularly inflected and which are stored irregular forms. A case in point is *-n* plurals. We were able to show that two types of *-n* plurals dissociate in subjects with Broca's aphasia, with the *-n* plural on feminine nouns significantly better retained than the -*n* plural on masculine/neuter nouns (Penke & Krause, 2002). That the two types of -*n* plurals can be differentially affected in Broca's aphasia suggests a qualitative distinction between these two types of -*n* plurals and confirms theoretical approaches which claim that the -*n* plural on feminine nouns is regular, whereas -*n* plurals on masculine/ neuter nouns are stored irregular forms.

The investigation of inflectional deficits has also provided some evidence on the status of inflectional morphemes (subsection 13.1.4). Whether or not inflectional affixes have independent entries in the mental lexicon is a matter of controversy in theoretical morphology. Whereas in strong lexicalist approaches stems and regular inflectional affixes have independent entries in the mental lexicon that can be productively combined via affixation (e.g. Wunderlich, 1996), other morphological theories argue against independent affix entries in the mental lexicon (e.g. Bybee, 1995). The observation that error rates of aphasic speakers are closely related to the number of words an affix is used with suggests that regular inflectional affixes have lexical entries in the mental lexicon and that the problems aphasic speakers exhibit in the production of certain regular inflected forms result from difficulties in accessing these affix entries.

13.4   Conclusion

The aim of this chapter was to highlight in which ways inflectional morphology can be impaired in language disorders. Theoretically founded cross-language comparisons of inflectional deficits have been and will be of central importance in furthering our understanding of inflectional deficits. The investigation of inflectional deficits across languages has provided important insights into how different grammatical systems might affect manifestations of a particular language disorder. Whether a language disorder will result in omission or substitution errors, and how many and which type of errors are likely to occur seem to be crucially dependent on language-specific characteristics of inflectional systems. Cross-language comparisons of language disorders also enable us to determine which deficits are characteristic for a given language disorder across languages and which are not. This enhances our understanding of what is going wrong in a particular language disorder and, thus, also has consequences for language therapy. Whereas, for example, a deficit with irregular inflection seems to be a characteristic sign of Williams syndrome across languages, the deficit with regular inflection observed in English-speaking subjects with Broca's aphasia is not. Moreover, a phonological-deficit account stating that such a deficit with regular inflection is due to problems with complex consonant clusters can be ruled out by data on German and Dutch Broca's aphasics who display no deficit with regular inflection despite similar phonological complexity of the inflected forms.

Secondly, morphological theory has played and will play an important role in the investigation of inflectional deficits. Morphological theory points out areas of potential problems in language-impaired speakers, such as complex inflectional paradigms or marked forms. It helps in designing experiments and in accounting for the observed behavior. However, to sound a word of caution, an experiment or analysis of inflectional deficits is often only as good as the morphological analysis underlying it. Determining what is a marked or an unmarked, a regular or an irregular form requires expertise that exceeds traditional school or grammar-book knowledge. Nevertheless, theoretically guided investigations of inflectional deficits will not only further our understanding of language disorders, they might also be profitable for theoretical linguistics.

REFERENCES

Bates, E., Friederici, A., and Wulfeck, B. (1987). Grammatical morphology in aphasia. *Cortex*, 23, 545–74.

Bellugi, U., Lichtenberger, L., Mills, D., Galaburda, A., and Korenberg, J. R. (1999). Bridging cognition, the brain and molecular genetics: Evidence from Williams syndrome. *Trends in Neurosciences*, 22, 197–207.

Bird, H., Lambon Ralph, M. A., Seidenberg, M., McClelland, J. L., and Patterson, K. (2003). Deficits in phonology and past-tense morphology. *Journal of Memory and Language*, 48, 502–26.

Bybee, J. L. (1995). Regular morphology and the lexicon. *Language and Cognitive Processes*, 10, 425–55.

Cholewa, J. and de Bleser, R. (1995). Neurolinguistische Evidenz für die Unterscheidung morphologischer Wortbildungsprozesse [Neurolinguistic evidence on word formation]. *Linguistische Berichte*, 158, 259–97.

Clahsen, H. and Almazan, M. (1998). Syntax and morphology in Williams syndrome. *Cognition*, 68, 167–98.

Clahsen, H., Bartke, S., and Göllner, S. (1997). Formal features in impaired grammars. *Journal of Neurolinguistics*, 10, 151–71.

Clahsen, H. and Rothweiler, M. (1993). Inflectional rules in children's grammars. *Yearbook of Morphology*, 1992, 1–34.

Clahsen, H., Sonnenstuhl, I., Hadler, M., and Eisenbeiss, S. (2001). Morphological paradigms in language processing and language disorders. *Transactions of the Philological Society*, 99, 247–83.

de Diego Balaguer, R., Costa, A., Sebastián-Galles, N., Juncadella, M., and Caramazza, A. (2004). Regular and irregular morphology and its relationship with agrammatism. *Brain and Language*, 91, 212–22.

Dromi, E., Leonard, L. B., Adam, G., and Zadunaisky-Ehrlich, S. (1999). Verb agreement morphology in Hebrew speaking children with specific language impairment. *Journal of Speech and Hearing Research*, 42, 1414–31.

Eadie, P. A., Fey, M. E., Douglas, J. M., and Parsons, C. L. (2002). Profiles of grammatical morphology and sentence imitation in children with Specific Language Impairment and Down's syndrome. *Journal of Speech, Language, and Hearing Research*, 45, 720–32.

Friedmann, N. and Grodzinsky, Y. (1997). Tense and agreement in agrammatic production. *Brain and Language*, 56, 397–425.

Fromkin, V. (1971). The non-anomalous nature of anomalous utterances. *Language*, 47, 27–52.

Goodglass, H. and Berko, J. (1960). Agrammatism and inflectional morphology in English. *Journal of Speech and Hearing Research*, 3, 257–67.

Gopnik, M. (1994). Impairments of tense in a familial language disorder. *Journal of Neurolinguistics*, 8, 109–33.

Grijzenhout, J. and Penke, M. (2005). On the interaction of phonology and morphology in German and Dutch first language acquisition and Broca's aphasia. *Yearbook of Morphology*, 2005, 49–81.

Grodzinsky, Y. (1984). The syntactic characterization of agrammatism. *Cognition*, 16, 99–120.

Grodzinsky, Y. (1990). *Theoretical Perspectives on Language Deficits*. London: MIT Press.

Janssen, U. and Penke, M. (2002). How are inflectional affixes organized in the mental lexicon? *Brain and Language*, 81, 180–91.

Kean, M.-L. (1977). The linguistic interpretation of aphasic syndromes. *Cognition*, 5, 9–46.

Kolk, H. H. J. and Heeschen, C. (1992). Agrammatism, paragrammatism and the management of language. *Language and Cognitive Processes*, 7, 89–129.

Laiacona, M. and Caramazza, A. (2004). The noun/verb dissociation in language production. *Cognitive Neuropsychology*, 21, 103–23.

Lapointe, S. G. (1985). A theory of verb form use in the speech of agrammatic aphasics. *Brain and Language*, 24, 100–55.

Laws, G. and Bishop, D. (2003). A comparison of language abilities in adolescents with Down's syndrome and children with Specific Language Impairment. *Journal of Speech, Language, and Hearing Research*, 46, 1324–39.

Libben, G. and Jarema, G. (2006). *The Representation and Processing of Compound Words*. Oxford: Oxford University Press.

Longworth, C. E., Keenan, S. E., Barker, R. A., Marslen-Wilson, W., and Tyler, L. (2005). The basal ganglia and rule-governed language use. *Brain*, 128, 584–96.

Luzzatti, C. and de Bleser, R. (1996). Morphological processing in Italian agrammatic speakers. *Brain and Language*, 54, 26–74.

Menn, L. and Obler, L. K. (1990). Cross-language data and theories of agrammatism. In L. Menn and L. Obler (eds.), *Agrammatic Aphasia: A Cross-language Narrative Sourcebook* (pp. 1369–88). Amsterdam: Benjamins.

Miceli, G. and Caramazza, A. (1988). Dissociation of inflectional and derivational morphology. *Brain and Language*, 35, 24–65.

Penke, M. (1998). *Die Grammatik des Agrammatismus* [The grammar of agrammatism]. Tübingen: Niemeyer.

Penke, M. (2006). The representation of inflectional morphology in the mental lexicon: An overview on psycho- and neurolinguistic methods and results. In D. Wunderlich (ed.), *Advances in the Theory of the Lexicon* (pp. 389–428). Berlin: Mouton De Gruyter.

Penke, M., Janssen, U., Indefrey, P., and Seitz, R. (2005). No evidence for a rule/procedural deficit in German patients with Parkinson's disease. *Brain and Language*, 95, 139–40.

Penke, M., Janssen, U., and Krause, M. (1999). The representation of inflectional morphology: Evidence from Broca's aphasia. *Brain and Language*, 68, 225–32.

Penke, M. and Krause, M. (2002). German noun plurals: A challenge to the Dual-Mechanism Model. *Brain and Language*, 81, 303–11.

Penke, M. and Krause, M. (2004). Regular and irregular inflectional morphology in German Williams syndrome. In S. Bartke and J. Siegmüller (eds.), *Williams Syndrome across Languages* (pp. 245–70). Amsterdam: Benjamins.

Penke, M. and G. Westermann (2006). Broca's area and inflectional morphology: Evidence from Broca's aphasia and computer modeling. *Cortex*, 42, 563–76.

Pinker, S. (1999). *Words and Rules*. New York: Basic Books.

Rice, M., Wexler, K., and Cleave, P. (1995). Specific Language Impairment as a period of extended optional infinitives. *Journal of Speech and Hearing Research*, 38, 850–63.

Stemberger, J. P. (1984). Structural errors in normal and agrammatic speech. *Cognitive Neuropsychology*, 1, 281–313.

Tager-Flusberg, H. (2003). Language impairment in children with complex neuro-developmental disorders. In Y. Levy and J. Schaeffer (eds.), *Language Competence across Populations* (pp. 297–322). London: Lawrence Erlbaum.

Tallal, R. (2000). Experimental studies of language learning impairments. In D. Bishop and L. Leonard (eds.), *Speech and Language Impairments in Children* (pp. 131–56). Hove, Sussex: Psychological Press.

Tyler, L., deMornay-Davies, P., Anokhina, R., Longworth, C., Randall, B., and Marslen-Wilson, W. (2002). Dissociations in processing past tense morphology. *Journal of Cognitive Neuroscience*, 14, 79–94.

Ullman, M. T., Corkin, S., Coppola, M., Hickok, G., Growdon, J., Koroshetz, W., and Pinker, S. (1997). A neural dissociation within language. *Journal of Cognitive Neuroscience*, 9, 266–76.

van der Lely, H. and Ullman, M. T. (2001). Past tense morphology in specifically language impaired and normally developing children. *Language and Cognitive Processes*, 16, 177–217.

Wunderlich, D. (1996). A minimalist model of inflectional morphology. In C. Wilder (ed.), *The Role of Economy Principles in Linguistic Theory* (pp. 267–98). Berlin: Akademie-Verlag.

14 Normal and Pathological Semantic Processing of Words

KARIMA KAHLAOUI AND YVES JOANETTE

14.1 Introduction

How the brain processes the meanings of words has been puzzling the human mind ever since it was acknowledged that the brain is responsible for this amazing ability. In trying to understand how the brain processes word meanings, it soon became obvious that one basic characteristic of the brain was very important: the human brain is made up of two hemispheres, the left (LH) and the right (RH), which differ not only functionally but also anatomically. These differences are particularly important when it comes to the semantic processing of words. Although the LH's superiority for language processing is indisputable, it is now clear that the processing of word meanings occurs bilaterally. Empirical evidence from neurologically intact and brain-injured participants indicates that both hemispheres process word meanings, although not necessarily in the same way (Chiarello, 1998; Joanette, Goulet, & Hannequin, 1990). The fact that both hemispheres seem to be involved in language comprehension raises important questions about the role each hemisphere plays in processing word semantics, and how it carries out that role. The main objective of this chapter is to offer an overview of the neural bases of word semantics, with a focus on the specific contributions of the left and right cerebral hemispheres. First, the brain organization sustaining normal word semantics will be summarized, mainly through behavioral studies (e.g., divided visual-field experiments). Then, the impact of acquired brain lesions on word semantic abilities will be addressed.

14.2   Hemispheric Asymmetries in Semantic Processing: An Overview

A fundamental question in cognitive neuropsychology and neurolinguistics is how semantic networks are functionally organized across the cerebral hemispheres. One informative approach for tackling this complex issue is the use of a semantic priming paradigm. This technique allows one to measure time-limited information-processing events that occur during access to word semantics. One major model of semantic processing conceptualizes the lexicon as a spatially distributed network of semantic elements, with increased distance representing decreased degree of association (Collins & Loftus, 1975). A robust and convergent effect that has been recurrently demonstrated in neurologically intact participants is that lexical decisions are made faster and more accurately on targets (e.g., *doctor*) that are primed by a preceding word that is related in meaning (e.g., *nurse*) than on words that are preceded by an unrelated word (e.g., *cat*; for a review, see Neely, 1991). These priming effects reflect, directly or indirectly, the fact that lexical concepts in semantic memory are clustered according to a matrix of semantic similarity (Collins & Loftus, 1975). At the semantic level of representation, the network is thought to be organized according to the degree of semantic similarity between the nodes. Nodes representing semantically related words are assumed to be more strongly connected, via direct links, than nodes for unrelated words. The presence of a priming effect usually indicates that the semantic network is structurally largely unaffected.

Two general mechanisms have been proposed to account for the semantic priming effect: automatic spreading activation and controlled semantic processing (Neely, 1991; Posner & Snyder, 1975). According to the first approach, semantic priming reflects an automatic spread of activation in semantic memory. It is thought to be automatic in that it onsets and offsets rapidly, occurs without effort, and places few demands on central processing resources. The presentation of a prime stimulus is thought to activate the corresponding conceptual representation in a semantic network; activation spreads to related nodes, through the links, increasing their activation level. Hence, if a word denoting a related concept is presented, its recognition (i.e., target decision making) will be facilitated (Collins & Loftus, 1975). According to the second approach – controlled semantic processing – the semantic priming is a result of effortful or attentional processes. Attentional processing occurs when participants are encouraged to attend to the relationship between the prime and target stimuli and to consciously use this information to aid in target decision making. In contrast to automatic spreading activation, attentional priming is relatively slow to onset, lasts over longer intervals, and places a drain on central processing resources (Posner & Snyder 1975). Consequently, processing of a related word is facilitated while processing of an unrelated word is inhibited. A number of factors determine whether automatic or controlled priming mechanisms are the main contributors to the overall priming effect (Neely, 1991). Three main factors are the relatedness pair proportion, the stimulus-onset asynchrony (SOA) between prime and target, and the instructions given to participants. It has been suggested that automatic spread of activation is the relevant mechanism with a low proportion of related targets, a short SOA, and instructions to participants that are devoid of any allusion to related pairs in the stimulus set. Controlled processes are generally engaged with a high proportion of related targets, SOAs of greater than 400 milliseconds (ms), and task instructions that specifically draw attention to the presence and use of category exemplar pairs in the stimulus set (Neely, 1991). Such semantic priming results have been taken to reflect aspects of the organization of word meaning in semantic memory. Generally, in order to study these processes, decision making involves either a lexical decision task, in which participants decide whether the presented stimulus is a real word or not, or a semantic judgment task, in which participants decide whether the prime and the target are semantically related.

Insight into the role of the cerebral hemispheres in semantic processing has also come from semantic priming studies using divided visual field techniques (Burgess & Simpson, 1988; Collins, 2002). This technique allows us to infer how each cerebral hemisphere understands and processes language because of the brief, lateralized presentation of the stimuli. In a typical experiment, participants view words presented to either the left visual field (LVF) or the right visual field (RVF). Because of the anatomy of the visual system, stimuli presented in the LVF are directly transmitted to the RH, while stimuli presented in the RVF are directly transmitted to the LH. Both response speed and accuracy are considered as indices of hemispheric capabilities.

In the last few decades, a number of studies have contributed to our understanding of how word meanings are activated in both hemispheres. For example, Chiarello, Burgess, Richards, and Pollock (1990) discovered that the hemispheres differ in their sensitivity to different types of semantic relationships at an SOA of 575 ms. Hemispheres show equivalent levels of priming for lexically associated members of a semantic category (e.g., *dog – cat*), and no priming when primes and targets are closely related but do not share category members (i.e., associated category members; *bee – honey*). However, only the RH shows significant priming for lexically unassociated category members (e.g., *dog – goat*). These findings were confirmed in a subsequent study by Chiarello and Richards (1992), which investigated the possibility that the category dominance of primes was instrumental in influencing the direction and magnitude of lateral differences in priming. These authors systematically varied the category dominance of pairs projected to the LVF and RVF. They were also careful to ensure that their prime-target pairs were as free from associative links as possible. Their results showed no significant effects of category dominance but a priming effect was once again reliably obtained only in the LVF. Chiarello, Burgess, Richards, and Pollock (1990) suggest that these results support the view that the RH's semantic system operates diffusely, with activation spreading to a broad range of semantic candidates over an extended time course. Similarly, Beeman and colleagues (Beeman & Chiarello, 1998; Beeman, Friedman, Grafman, et al., 1994) refined this hypothesis in the context of a more comprehensive account of the differences between the hemispheres in language processing, and proposed the *depth of activation hypothesis*. According to this hypothesis, the neural networks sustained by the RH do not process words semantically in the same way as those in the LH. Indeed, only a small set of closely related information is activated when the LH initiates processing. In contrast, a large set of related information may be activated, including distantly related information, when the RH initiates the processing. In other words, not only associated but also remotely related information is activated in the RH, whereas activation in the LH is restricted to a smaller set of highly related information. Thus, these authors suggest that the RH processes the semantics of words through a *coarse semantic coding* process while the LH uses *fine-grained coding*. This hypothesis is consistent with the findings in brain-damaged populations, which suggest that right-hemisphere-damaged patients have problems drawing inferences, understanding humor, and interpreting ambiguous phrases (Brownell, Potter, Bihrle, & Gardner, 1986; Grindrod & Baum, 2005; Tompkins, Fassbinder, Lehman-Blake, Baumgaertner, & Jayaram, 2004; Tompkins, Lehman-Blake, Baumgaertner, & Fassbinder, 2001), all of which require the activation of multiple word meanings.

Hemispheric differences also have been reported in the time course of the meaning activation. For example, the study by Abernethy and Coney (1996) challenges the RH advantage in semantic category priming, using two different SOAs: 250 ms and 450 ms. With a shorter SOA (250 ms), the results showed only LH priming. At a longer SOA (450 ms), the results showed priming for targets presented to both hemispheres, but only when the prime was presented to the LH. The authors concluded that semantic categories are represented in the LH but that this categorical information may be relayed from left to right, with a long enough SOA. These contradictory results concerning the hemispheric contributions to semantic processing, and more specifically to the processing of semantic categories, led Koivisto (1997) to study this question in relation to the SOA used and to propose the *time course hypothesis*. In his study, Koivisto presented non-associated primes and targets from the same categories (e.g., *sister – aunt*) unilaterally to the RVF and the LVF with SOAs of 165 vs. 250 vs. 500 vs. 750 ms. At 165 ms, only the LH was primed. In contrast, at 750 ms, only the RH presentations resulted in priming. The intermediate SOAs produced an increase in priming in the RH, while there was a decrease in the LH with longer SOAs. Koivisto concluded that both closely and distantly related kinds of information are initially activated in the LH. In the RH, the activation of distantly related information is assumed to start later than in the LH. Consequently, both LH and RH may have similar spreads of activation, but over different lengths of time. The LH may prime quickly and its arousal may decrease fast, while the RH may prime more slowly. Recently, other studies have confirmed the differential organization of the two cerebral hemispheres using both short and long SOAs (Chiarello, Liu, Shears,

Ouan, & Kacinik, 2003; Collins, 1999; Yochim, Kender, Abeare, Gustafson, & Whitman, 2005).

In summary, the majority of studies outlined in this section support the position that both hemispheres can play a role in semantic processing. Studies concerning the time course of activation using short SOAs show that both close and distant information is automatically activated in the LH. With time, the attention is focused on close, expected relations in the LH, suppressing the activation of more distantly related information. However, in the RH, both close and distant relations stay active for a longer time, although the onset of semantic processing may be slower than in the LH. Taken together, these data suggest that the hemispheres have access to similar lexicons, but operate somewhat differently. However, there is a distinction to be made between studies on each hemisphere's specific capacity for semantic processing, and studies describing their actual contribution to language abilities. Thus, additional evidence concerning each hemisphere's contribution to semantic processing comes from the study of patients with focal brain damage.

14.3   Hemispheric Asymmetries in Semantic Processing: Brain Lesion Studies

14.3.1   *Semantic impairments following a left-hemisphere lesion*

Impairments in the processing of word meanings have long been known to be one of the possible consequences of brain damage. In particular, semantic deficits were believed to be one of the dimensions that clearly separated the symptom space of Broca's and Wernicke's aphasia. These two types of aphasia are usually the consequence of a left-hemisphere lesion in right-handers (Lecours & Lhermitte, 1979). Individuals with Broca's aphasia have damage to the frontal lobe of the brain. They frequently speak in short, meaningful phrases that are produced with great effort. Broca's aphasia is thus characterized as a nonfluent aphasia. In contrast to Broca's aphasia, damage to the temporal lobe may result in a fluent aphasia that is called Wernicke's aphasia. Individuals with Wernicke's aphasia show a considerable impairment in comprehension; they may speak fluently but their output is difficult to understand since they produce numerous paraphasias, add unnecessary words, and even produce neologisms.

Studies in which participants were required to explicitly judge semantic relations obtained evidence of severe disruptions of semantic processing in Wernicke's aphasics (Grober, Perecman, Kellar, & Brown, 1980; Whitehouse, Caramazza, & Zurif, 1978). In contrast to the Wernicke's aphasics, the performance of patients with Broca's aphasia in these studies was close to that of neurologically intact participants. This led to the claim that, in Wernicke's aphasia, the semantic lexicon was structurally affected, whereas in Broca's aphasics it was largely unaffected (Grober, Perecman, Kellar, & Brown, 1980).

Thus, comprehension deficits in Wernicke's patients were initially attributed to a partial degradation of stored linguistic representations (Caramazza & Zurif, 1976). However, in recent decades, this claim has been challenged by a number of word-priming studies of aphasic patients (e.g., Hagoort, 1993, 1997; Milberg, Blumstein, Giovanello, & Misiurski, 2003; Prather, Zurif, Love, & Brownell 1997; Prather, Zurif, Stern, & Rosen, 1992; Swaab, Brown, & Hagoort, 1998), which reported results that are suggestive of processing impairments rather than of a loss of knowledge. These studies showed that, despite significantly longer response latencies, Wernicke's aphasics consistently showed the same pattern of results as the neurologically intact participants; that is, both neurologically intact participants and Wernicke's aphasics needed less time to recognize the target as a word when it was preceded by an associatively related word (Blumstein, Milberg, & Shrier, 1982; Hagoort, 1993; Milberg, Blumstein, & Dworetzky, 1987). However, for Broca's aphasics, the results are contradictory. In the majority of priming studies, semantic priming effects have been found in patients, especially when prime–target pairs were highly associated (Blumstein, Milberg, & Shrier, 1982; Hagoort, 1993). In contrast, when the semantic relationship between the prime and the target was more subtle, or when the stimuli were presented as triplets (i.e., participants made a lexical decision on the third word of a series), no priming effects were obtained in these patients (Milberg & Blumstein, 1981; Milberg, Blumstein, & Dworetzky, 1987). Milberg and colleagues concluded that the Broca's aphasics are impaired in their automatic access to semantic representations of words. However, the fact that the Broca's aphasics can make semantic judgments indicates that, although the activation level of lexical entries may be reduced, the lexical entries are accessed and the organization of the semantic network appears to be intact. Consequently, these patients are able to use strategies in an off-line task to judge the semantic relationship between prime–target pairs.

Two claims can be made on the basis of these studies. On one hand, because of the evidence of semantic facilitation in Wernicke's aphasics, it has been suggested that the semantic impairments in these patients are not due to a loss of stored linguistic representations but rather to the patient's inability to use or manipulate semantic information. On the other hand, the second claim is that Broca's aphasics might have an impairment affecting their automatic routines for accessing semantic information. However, the theoretical weakness of this claim resides in the implicit assumption that word-priming studies mainly tap into the automatic processing of semantic information, including word meanings. As was argued for in the first part of this chapter, priming effects may be attributed to both automatic and controlled priming mechanisms (Neely, 1991). In the studies in which no priming effects were observed in Broca's aphasics, the authors used relatively long intervals between primes and targets. For example, Milberg, Blumstein and Dworetzky (1987) used a single interval of 500 ms, making it difficult to dissociate the automatic and controlled aspects of semantic processing. In order to investigate the contribution of automatic and controlled aspects of semantic processing, Hagoort (1993) extended the study by Milberg, Blumstein, & Dworetzky (1987) to include short (300 ms) and long (1,400 ms) SOAs. Both Broca's and Wernicke's aphasics were able to automatically access the semantic lexicon, but had difficulties with controlled processing. The results of these studies support the notion that LH damage may disrupt semantic processing, but are limited in several respects. Overall, the results of the reaction-time priming studies with aphasic patients suggest that a more likely functional focus of reduced or absent priming effects is at the postlexical level of semantic matching of primes and targets. This ability to track the time course of semantic processing in terms of rapid automatic and slower controlled processes is very important, given that both LH and RH contribute to semantic processing over time and in automatic and controlled processes (e.g., Collins, 1999; Koivisto, 1997; Yochim, Kender, Abeare, Gustafson, & Whitman, 2005). Prather and colleagues (1997) studied the slowed-activation hypothesis of automatic processing in both Broca's and Wernicke's aphasia by examining the time course of semantic activation with a list-priming paradigm (LPP). Temporal delays between successive words were manipulated, ranging from 300 to 2,100 ms. In contrast to neurologically intact participants, who prime at relatively short inter-stimulus intervals (ISI) beginning at 500 ms, the Broca's aphasic participants showed reliable automatic priming only at a long ISI of 1,500 ms. That is, Broca's aphasics can access semantic information automatically if allowed sufficient time to do so. This result may help explain their disrupted comprehension of normally rapid conversational speech. In contrast, the Wernicke's aphasics showed normally rapid initial activation but continued slow priming over an abnormally long range of periods, from 300 to 1,100 ms. This protracted priming suggests a failure to dampen activation and might explain the semantic confusion exhibited by fluent Wernicke's patients.

Another field of research has provided additional insights into how semantic knowledge may be organized across the cerebral hemispheres, namely the study of category-specific deficits. Although the usual pattern is that the processing of living items (e.g., animals, fruits) is found to be impaired compared to that of nonliving items (e.g., furniture, tools), aphasic individuals showed the opposite pattern, that is, a deficit for nonliving compared to living items (for reviews, see Capitani, Laiacona, Mahon, & Caramazza, 2003; Humphreys & Forde, 2001). Clinical and neuroimaging studies show that the processing of nonliving items appears to be confined to the LH, suggesting that a LH lesion will lead to an impairment of nonliving items (Devlin, Moore, Mummery, et al., 2002; Tranel, Damasio, & Damasio, 1997; Warrington & McCarthy, 1983, 1987). More recently, convergent data from functional neuroimagery, in addition to the systematic description of brain-lesioned individuals, suggest that the left anteromedial temporal cortex plays a crucial role in the differentiation of semantic concepts (Moss, Rodd, Stamatakis, Bright, & Tyler, 2005). The latter suggest that, since living items are more similar between themselves than nonliving items, this area of the temporal lobe would play a greater role in sustaining semantic representations of living items. Conversely, the manipulation knowledge (i.e., knowledge of how items are used) associated with nonliving items might also result in their semantic representations' involving more fronto-parietal based neural networks (Bub, 2003; Buxbaum & Saffran, 2002). In other words, the nature of the semantic representation (e.g., living/nonliving) appears to influence the specific neurobiological 'inscriptions' of such concepts in the LH, and hence results in distinctive impacts on object-naming abilities and the semantic processing of words in general when these regions are individually lesioned.

In summary, a large number of studies have provided further insights into the dichotomy between automatic and controlled processing as they may contribute to the semantic deficits of Wernicke's and Broca's aphasics. On one hand, because of the evidence of semantic facilitation in Wernicke's aphasics, it has been suggested that at least some aspects of the representations of word meanings are preserved in this kind of aphasia. These patients' language-comprehension deficits seem to reflect their inability to overtly access, use or manipulate semantic information rather than a loss of the underlying semantic representations of words. On the other hand, Broca's aphasics sometimes show a deficit affecting postlexical integration processes. However, the claim that there is a deficit affecting automatic access to semantic information remains without empirical support. Thus, the comprehension deficits found in Wernicke's and Broca's aphasics appear to be related to the method of assessment used. Indeed, the way in which semantic information is used in tasks requiring explicit semantic judgments might differ from access to semantic information under implicit task conditions, which do not focus the participants' attention on the semantics of the words presented visually. In addition, the sites of lesions in the left hemisphere may have a specific impact on the nature of the semantic concepts that will be most affected. In particular, it appears that semantic representations of living things are particularly dependent upon the integrity of the anteromedial temporal cortex, whereas semantic representations of nonliving items might depend on the integrity of the fronto-parietal cortex.

14.3.2   Semantic impairments following a right-hemisphere lesion

Since the seminal contributions of pioneers such as Jon Eisenson (1962), numerous studies have allowed us to better understand the RH's contribution to language processing. Most of the evidence for RH involvement in language processing comes from studies of right-hemisphere-damaged (RHD) individuals; there is also evidence from neuroimaging studies. RHD individuals are reported to be impaired in retrieving or using semantic information. Such impairments affect the semantic processing of words more than their formal dimensions (e.g., phonological, morphological), and they appear to particularly affect words that are infrequent, abstract or non-imageable (for a review, see Beeman & Chiarello, 1998; Joanette, Goulet, & Hannequin, 1990; Tompkins, 1990).

In addition to semantic priming paradigms, verbal fluency tasks have been reported to assess semantic abilities and thus to be sensitive to acquired RH lesions. Numerous studies have suggested that RHD individuals perform worse than matched controls on word-naming tasks in which the production criterion is semantic (e.g., naming animals) but not when it is orthographic (e.g., words starting with the letter 'L' or 'B') (Goulet, Joanette, Sabourin, & Giroux, 1997; Joanette & Goulet, 1986). This observation is consistent with a number of neuroimaging studies reporting RH activation for the semantic processing of words, but not for their phonological processing (Gernsbacher & Kashack, 2003; Walter, Jbabdi, Marrelec, Benali, & Joanette, 2005). Moreover, such impairments appear to stem from problems affecting the use of recall strategies. Joanette, Goulet and Le Dorze (1988) compared both RHD and neurologically intact participants on a word-fluency task using a semantic criterion. An analysis of responses over a two-minute production period showed no significant difference between groups in the first 30 seconds of recall, but significant differences did emerge subsequently. This has been interpreted as suggesting that, in the first period, subjects recall highly automatic, closely associated items. Once these are exhausted, subjects need to guide their recall by making use of retrieval strategies. Collectively, these findings implicate the RH in the exhaustive retrieval of semantic category members, particularly those that are not highly accessible. Le Blanc and Joanette (1996) reported that RHD individuals had a specific tendency to produce less prototypical words in an unconstrained oral naming task. In addition, studies on RHD patients have revealed their difficulties in maintaining or in imparting coherence, as well as a deficit in their ability to access and/or report more distantly related category members.

Another approach to the right hemisphere's semantic capacities has been proposed with reference to the nature of semantic relationships, with similar outcomes. These studies used lateralized presentation of word pairs in semantic judgment tasks supposed to induce controlled processing to assess the differences between hemispheres. Their results, elicited in neurologically intact participants, showed that the RH is particularly efficient at activating interconceptual links, while the LH is more efficient at activating intraconceptual links (Drews, 1987). More recently, Nocentini, Goulet, Roberts, and Joanette (2001) examined the differential sensitivity of the two hemispheres to various types of semantic relationships, comparing both RHD and LHD participants. In their study, three kinds of intraconceptual and two kinds of interconceptual relationships were devised. The intraconceptual relationships were the following: Superordinate (e.g., *eagle – bird*), Categorical (e.g., *eagle – penguin*), and Whole–Part (e.g., *eagle – beak*) relationships. The interconceptual relationships were Locative (e.g., *eagle – sky*), and Same location (e.g., *eagle – sun*). Pairs of common words were given to participants, who indicated whether or not there was any relationship between the words. The results showed that a clear dissociation only exists in the sensitivity of the LHD and RHD groups to Whole–Part and Same location relations. These results do not support the existence of a general, rule-governed difference in sensitivity between the two hemispheres, according to Drews's (1987) inter- and intraconceptual framework. Another dimension of word semantics to which the RH is suspected of making a specific contribution has to do with the metaphorical alternative meanings of polysemic words (Brownell, Simpson, Bihrle, Potter, & Gardner, 1990; Gagnon, Goulet, Giroux, & Joanette, 2003). Though somewhat contradictory, the results of the studies addressing this question do suggest that an RH lesion may affect the processing of some polysemic words in a qualitatively unique way. However, it remains to be demonstrated that this presumed specificity does not simply represent a specific case of a more general characteristic of word semantics sustained by the RH, such as its propensity to sustain more remote and distant semantic associates (Beeman & Chiarello, 1998).

In addition to the question of the semantic specificity of word-level impairments following an RH lesion, another research direction has attempted to determine whether they constitute impairments to a somewhat conscious access to semantic knowledge or disruptions of the automatic activation of this knowledge. In studies by Gagnon, Goulet, and Joanette (1990, 1994), the objective was to determine whether the RH's contribution relates to the automatic activation of the semantic organization of lexical items or to the strategic use of the semantic knowledge. Both RHD and neurologically intact participants were given three tasks with varying activation requirements: two lexical-decision tasks with semantic priming, one with a short SOA and the other with a long one, and a semantic judgment task. The results showed that RHD subjects were impaired on the semantic judgment task, whereas they showed normal priming effects. These findings are congruent with other studies, which reported normal semantic priming effects (automatic and controlled) in RHD participants (Tompkins, 1990), but also problems with semantic judgment tasks involving cohyponymic relationships (Chiarello & Church, 1986).

In summary, a number of word semantic impairments following an RH lesion have been described in the literature. According to Beeman and Chiarello (1998), studies of RHD individuals have shown that they tend to have problems accessing and/or processing more distantly related category members. In addition, an RH lesion appears not to be associated with deficits in automatic and controlled processing, but it is associated with impaired access to explicit semantic information. Indeed, the RH's possible contribution mainly seems to become prominent when an attentional or conscious access to semantic processing is needed. Overall, these studies suggest that the RH's integrity is crucial for the full semantic processing of words.

14.3.3 *Semantic impairments in Alzheimer's disease*

Dementia of the Alzheimer's type (DAT) is usually, if not invariably, associated with progressive language impairment. For that reason, DAT represents an interesting model of central nervous system dysfunction upon which to base a study of semantic representation. Despite individual differences, the pathological alterations DAT gives rise to within the cerebral hemispheres follow a fairly predictable time sequence and affect neuronal subsets within fairly predictable regions of the brain (Kemper, 1994). In DAT, medial temporal structures are implicated early. The neocortex is involved next, with the posterior association cortex altered to a greater extent than frontal association regions. Both left and right cerebral hemispheres are usually affected in parallel and to comparable extents. The importance of the study of semantic processing in patients with DAT thus becomes straightforward: the pathological changes of DAT consistently affect brain regions in which semantic information is believed to be represented. However, despite the evidence of semantic deficits in Alzheimer's disease (AD), the nature of these deficits remains to be clarified. A major controversy remains as to whether the semantic deficit stems from a loss of information in the semantic store (Binetti, Magni, Cappa, et al., 1995; Chertkow, Bub, Bergman, et al., 1994; Chertkow, Bub, & Seidenberg, 1989; Hodges, Salmon, & Butters., 1992), or whether the store of semantic memory remains intact in DAT, and the deficit is related to an inability to access and manipulate semantic information (Ober & Shenaut, 1999). In addition to neuropsychological tests, the semantic priming paradigm is often used to investigate semantic memory. A number of studies have investigated semantic priming effects in patients with DAT, often with conflicting results. At first, some studies showed a lower than normal priming effect (Ober & Shenaut, 1988; Silveri, Monteleone, Burani, & Tabossi, 1996), suggesting a deficit affecting semantic information storage. Then other studies reported an equivalent semantic priming effect for both patients with DAT and neurologically intact participants (Nebes, Martin, & Horn, 1984; Ober, Shenaut, Jagust, & Stillman, 1991), which suggested that some patients with DAT have attention deficits related to semantic impairments. Finally, some studies showed a hyperpriming phenomenon (i.e., an increased semantic priming effect), which evolves in a dynamic manner depending on the level of semantic memory deterioration (Chertkow, Bub, Bergman, et al., 1994; Chertkow, Bub, & Seidenberg, 1989; Giffard, Desgranges, Nore-Mary, et al., 2002). The hyperpriming effect reflects the hierarchical organization of semantic knowledge. Given the conceptual structure of hierarchical models of semantic memory, both general and specific semantic information is supposed to be stored at different levels. Thus, the presence of semantic priming does not necessarily mean that the semantic representations of concepts are entirely preserved (Moss, Tyler, Hodges, & Patterson, 1995). In the case of a semantic loss, specific information represented at lower hierarchical levels could therefore be disrupted even if general information represented at a higher superordinate level remained intact. Moreover, normal priming effects may reflect partial semantic degradation; damage to stored representations may result in the loss of some of the specific attribute information. Thus, semantic priming effects supported by the remaining intact features only can be observed. This hyperpriming effect seems to reflect a deterioration in semantic memory and, more specifically, a deficit affecting storage of specific attribute information: from the onset of the disease, semantic representations deteriorate progressively, affecting the specific attributes first, with retention of general semantic knowledge. This makes it more and more difficult to distinguish between coordinate concepts since they share the same preserved superordinate category while their specific attributes, which allow them to be distinguished, are lost (Giffard, Desgranges, & Eustache, 2005; Giffard, Desgranges, Nore-Mary, et al., 2002; Martin & Fedio, 1983).

Another research avenue has undertaken to determine whether the deterioration of semantic knowledge in DAT has an equivalent effect across semantic categories. Although there is a debate as to the putative nature of this dissociation, one of the main hypotheses, the domain-specific hypothesis (Caramazza & Shelton, 1998), explains that category-specific deficits arise because information about living and nonliving items is processed by different parts of the brain. A specific impairment of the processing of either living or nonliving items may arise as the consequence of a focal lesion selectively involving the corresponding substrate. As was argued in the preceding section, category-specific effects should be attributed to variations in the location of cortical atrophy in DAT individuals. In addition, Gonnerman, Andersen, Devlin, Kempler, & Seidenberg (1997) showed a progression of category-specific effects as a function of different degrees of impairment in DAT. In the first phase, when the damage is light, DAT individuals showed a selective difficulty with nonliving items but no impairment with living items. In the second phase, the opposite pattern is observed, with a significant and selective problem with living items, while the deficit affecting processing of nonliving items remains stable. In the last phase, damage is extensive enough that the processing of both living and nonliving items is significantly impaired, so that no category-specific effects arise. However, most researchers argue that the distinction between living and nonliving items is not a primary principle of neural organization, but reflects a more fundamental distinction between different types of information. For example, Warrington and McCarthy (1987) proposed that the dissociation between the processing of living and nonliving items could be related to their differing reliance on perceptual versus functional information. Similarly, Whatmough, Chertkow, Murta, et al. (2003) found an advantage for nonliving items when they investigated category-specific effects in DAT individuals. The ability of DAT participants to name living and nonliving items declined progressively, but the performance on nonliving items tends to decline less rapidly. According to Dixon, Bub, Chertkow, and Arguin (1999), category deficits are due to a greater structural and conceptual similarity between items within the living category. The classical advantage for the nonliving category (e.g., *car*) over the living category (e.g., *dog*) is not due to a semantic category dichotomy. Rather, it results from the fact that a *dog* closely resembles other animals both physically and semantically, whereas a *car* is an object that is quite distinct in its structure and its use. Thus, the greater semantic and structural distinctiveness of nonliving items makes them more resistant to the gradual degradation of semantic knowledge in DAT and gives nonliving items a small but significant advantage in object identification tasks.

In summary, several studies have shown that semantic impairments represent a major feature of DAT. These deficits are mainly observed in semantic priming paradigms, which represent privileged tools for investigating the integrity of semantic networks in brain-lesioned individuals. Overall, studies investigating processing of word semantics in DAT provide evidence that the loss of semantic knowledge in DAT does not occur randomly. Indeed, a progressive deterioration of semantic memory is demonstrated, affecting specific attributes first, with a perseveration of general semantic knowledge. Similarly, representations of semantic categories in the brain are differently affected, with the category of living items deteriorating first.

14.4   Conclusion

The purpose of this chapter was to review the specific contributions the cerebral hemispheres make to semantic processing. A large body of studies based on behavioral and clinical approaches has led to the conclusion that both hemispheres may be differentially involved in the representation and/or processing of different kinds of semantic knowledge. These findings have also indicated substantial hemispheric differences in the nature and time course of information retrieval during word processing. In conclusion, the studies reviewed here suggest that the processing of word semantics by the RH is unique and complements and enriches processing in the LH (Chiarello, 1998). In fact, language abilities represent a key example of the need for the two hemispheres of the brain to cooperate fully (Sergent, 1994).

REFERENCES

Abernethy, M. and Coney, J. (1996). Semantic category priming in the left cerebral hemisphere. *Neuropsychologia*, 34, 339–50.

Beeman, M. J. and Chiarello, C. (1998). *Right Hemisphere Language Comprehension: Perspectives from Cognitive Neuroscience*. Mahwah, NJ: Erlbaum.

Beeman, M. J., Friedman, R., Grafman, J., Perez, E., Diamond, S., and Lindsay, M. (1994). Summation priming and coarse semantic coding in the right hemisphere. *Journal of Cognitive Neuroscience*, 6, 26–43.

Binetti, G., Magni, E., Cappa, S. F., Padovani, A., Bianchetti, A., and Trabucchi, M. (1995). Semantic memory in Alzheimer's disease: An analysis of category fluency. *Journal of Clinical and Experimental Neuropsychology*, 17, 82–9.

Blumstein, S. E., Milberg, W., and Shrier, R. (1982). Semantic processing in aphasia: Evidence from an auditory lexical decision task. *Brain and Language*, 17, 301–15.

Brownell, H. H., Potter, H. H., Bihrle, A. M., and Gardner, H. (1986). Inference deficits in right brain-damaged patients. *Brain and Language*, 27, 310–21.

Brownell, H. H., Simpson, T. L., Bihrle, A. M., Potter, H. H., and Gardner, H. (1990). Appreciation of metaphoric alternative word meanings by left and right brain-damaged patients. *Neuropsychologia*, 28, 375–83.

Bub, D. N. (2003). Measuring the activation and causal role of motor affordances in object identification. *Brain and Language*, 87, 92–3.

Burgess, C. and Simpson, G. (1988). Cerebral hemispheric mechanisms in the retrieval of ambiguous word meanings. *Brain and Language*, 33, 86–103.

Buxbaum, L. J. and Saffran, E. M. (2002). Knowledge of object manipulation and object function: Dissociations in apraxic and nonapraxic subjects. *Brain and Language*, 82, 179–99.

Capitani, E., Laiacona, M., Mahon, B., and Caramazza, A. (2003). What are the facts of semantic category-specific deficits? A critical review of the clinical evidence. *Cognitive Neuropsychology*, 20, 213–61.

Caramazza, A. and Shelton, J. R. (1998). Domain-specific knowledge systems in the brain: The animate–inanimate distinction. *Journal of Cognitive Neuroscience*, 10, 1–34.

Caramazza, A. and Zurif, E. B. (1976). Dissociation of algorithmic and heuristic processes in language comprehension: Evidence from aphasia. *Brain and Language*, 3, 572–82.

Chertkow, H., Bub, D., Bergman, H., Bruemmer, A., Merling, A., and Rothfleich, J. (1994). Increased semantic priming in patients with dementia of the Alzheimer's type. *Journal of Clinical and Experimental Neuropsychology*, 16, 608–22.

Chertkow, H., Bub, D., and Seidenberg, M. (1989). Priming and semantic memory loss in Alzheimer's disease. *Brain and Language*, 36, 420–46.

Chiarello, C. (1998). On codes of meaning and the meaning of codes: Semantic access and retrieval within and between hemispheres. In M. J. Beeman and C. Chiarello (eds.), *Right Hemisphere Language Comprehension: Perspectives from Cognitive Neuroscience* (pp. 141–60). Mahwah, NJ: Erlbaum.

Chiarello, C., Burgess, C., Richards, L., and Pollock, A. (1990). Semantic and associative priming in the cerebral hemispheres: Some words do, some words don't . . . sometimes, some places. *Brain and Language*, 38, 75–104.

Chiarello, C. and Church, K. L. (1986). Lexical judgments after right- or left-hemisphere injury. *Neuropsychologia*, 24, 623–30.

Chiarello, C., Liu, S., Shears, C., Ouan, N., and Kacinik, N. (2003). Priming of strong semantic relations in the left and right visual fields: A time course investigation. *Neuropsychologia*, 41, 721–32.

Chiarello, C. and Richards, L. (1992). Another look at categorical priming in the cerebral hemispheres. *Neuropsychologia*, 30, 381–92.

Collins, A. M. and Loftus, E. F. (1975). A spreading-activation theory of semantic processing. *Psychological Review*, 82, 407–28.

Collins, M. (1999). Differences in semantic category priming in the left and right cerebral hemispheres under automatic and controlled processing conditions. *Neuropsychologia*, 37, 1071–85.

Collins, M. (2002). Interhemispheric communication via direct connections for alternative meanings of ambiguous words. *Brain and Language*, 80, 77–96.

Devlin, J. T., Moore, C. J., Mummery, C. J., Gorno-Tempini, M. L., Phillips, J. A., Noppeney, U., Frackowiak, R. S. J., Friston, K. J., and Price, C. J. (2002). Anatomic constraints on cognitive theories of category specificity. *Neuroimage*, 15, 675–85.

Dixon, M. J., Bub, D. N., Chertkow, H., and Arguin, M. (1999). Object identification deficits in dementia of the Alzheimer type: Combined effects of semantic and visual proximity. *Journal of the International Neuropsychology Society*, 5, 330–45.

Drews, E. (1987). Qualitatively different organizational structures of lexical knowledge in the left and right hemisphere. *Neuropsychologia*, 25, 419–27.

Eisenson, J. (1962). Language dysfunction associated with right-brain damage. *Language and Speech*, 5, 49–53.

Gagnon, J., Goulet, P., and Joanette, Y. (1990). Utilisation active et passive du savoir lexico-sémantique chez les cérébrolésés. *Langages*, 96, 95–111.

Gagnon, J., Goulet, P., and Joanette, Y. (1994). Automatic and controlled activation of lexical-semantic knowledge in right-brain-damaged right-handers. *Linguistische Berichte* (special issue: Neurolinguistics), 6, 33–48.

Gagnon, L., Goulet, P., Giroux, F., and Joanette, Y. (2003). Processing of metaphoric and non-metaphoric alternative meanings of words after right- and left-hemispheric lesion. *Brain and Language*, 87, 217–26.

Gernsbacher, M. A. and Kashack, M. P. (2003). Neuroimaging studies of language production and comprehension. *Annual Review of Psychology*, 54, 91–114.

Giffard, B., Desgranges, B., and Eustache, F. (2005). Semantic memory disorders in Alzheimer's disease: Clues from semantic priming effects. *Current Alzheimer Research*, 2, 425–34.

Giffard, B., Desgranges, B., Nore-Mary, F., Lalevee, C., Beaunieux, H., de la Sayette, V., Pasquier, F., and Eustache, F. (2002). The dynamic time course of semantic memory impairment in Alzheimer's disease: Clues from hyperpriming and hypopriming effects. *Brain*, 125, 2044–57.

Gonnerman, L. M., Andersen, E. S., Devlin, J. T., Kempler, D., and Seidenberg, M. S. (1997). Double dissociation of semantic categories in Alzheimer's disease. *Brain and Language*, 57, 254–79.

Goulet, P., Joanette, Y., Sabourin, L., and Giroux, F. (1997). Word fluency after a right-hemisphere lesion. *Neuropsychologia*, 35, 1565–70.

Grindrod, C. M. and Baum, S. R. (2005). Hemispheric contributions to lexical ambiguity resolution in a discourse context: Evidence from individuals with unilateral left and right hemisphere lesions. *Brain and Cognition*, 57, 70–83.

Grober, E., Perecman, E., Kellar, L., and Brown, J. (1980). Lexical knowledge in anterior and posterior aphasics. *Brain and Language*, 10, 318–30.

Hagoort, P. (1993). Impairments of lexical-semantic processing in aphasia: Evidence from the processing of lexical ambiguities. *Brain and Language*, 45, 189–232.

Hagoort, P. (1997). Semantic priming in Broca's aphasics at a short SOA: No support for an automatic access deficit. *Brain and Language*, 56, 287–300.

Hodges, J. R., Salmon, D. P., and Butters, N. (1992). Semantic memory impairment in Alzheimer's disease: Failure of access or degraded knowledge? *Neuropsychologia*, 30, 301–14.

Humphreys, G. W. and Forde, E. M. (2001). Hierarchies, similarity, and interactivity in object recognition: 'Category-specific' neuropsychological deficits. *Behavioral and Brain Sciences*, 24, 453–76.

Joanette, Y. and Goulet, P. (1986). Criterion-specific reduction of verbal fluency in right brain-damaged right-handers. *Neuropsychologia*, 24, 875–9.

Joanette, Y., Goulet, P., and Hannequin, D. (1990). *Right Hemisphere and Verbal Communication*. New York: Springer-Verlag.

Joanette, Y., Goulet, P., and Le Dorze, G. (1988). Impaired word naming in right-brain-damaged right-handers: Error types and time-course analyses. *Brain and Language*, 34, 54–64.

Kemper, T. L. (1994). Neuroanatomical and neuropathological changes during aging and in dementia. In M. L. Albert and E. J. E. Knoepfel (eds.), *Clinical Neurology of Aging* (pp. 3–67). New York: Oxford University Press.

Koivisto, M. (1997). Time course of semantic activation in the cerebral hemispheres. *Neuropsychologia*, 35, 497–504.

Le Blanc, B. and Joanette, Y. (1996). Unconstrained oral naming in left- and right-hemisphere-damaged patients: An analysis of naturalistic semantic strategies. *Brain and Language*, 55, 42–5.

Lecours, A. R. and Lhermitte, F. (1979). *L'Aphasie*. Paris: Flammarion.

Martin, A. and Fedio, P. (1983). Word production and comprehension in Alzheimer's disease: The breakdown of semantic knowledge. *Brain and Language*, 19, 124–41.

Milberg, W. and Blumstein, S. E. (1981). Lexical decision and aphasia: Evidence for semantic processing. *Brain and Language*, 14, 371–85.

Milberg, W., Blumstein, S. E., and Dworetzky, B. (1987). Processing of lexical ambiguities in aphasia. *Brain and Language*, 31, 138–50.

Milberg, W., Blumstein, S. E., Giovanello, K. S., and Misiurski, C. (2003). Summation priming in aphasia: Evidence for alterations in semantic integration and activation. *Brain and Cognition*, 51, 31–47.

Moss, H. E., Rodd, J. M., Stamatakis, E. A., Bright, P., and Tyler, L. K. (2005). Anteromedial temporal cortex supports fine-grained differentiation among objects. *Cerebral Cortex*, 15, 616–27.

Moss, H. E., Tyler, L. K., Hodges, J. R., and Patterson, K. (1995). Exploring the loss of semantic memory in semantic dementia: Evidence from a primed monitoring study. *Neuropsychology*, 9, 16–26.

Nebes, R. D., Martin, D. C., and Horn, L. C. (1984). Sparing of semantic memory in Alzheimer's disease. *Journal of Abnormal Psychology*, 93, 321–30.

Neely, J. H. (1991). Semantic priming effects in visual word recognition: A selective review of current findings and theory. In D. Besner and G. W. Humphreys (eds.), *Basic Processes in Reading: Visual Word Recognition* (pp. 264–336). Hillsdale, NJ: Erlbaum.

Nocentini, U., Goulet, P., Roberts, P. M., and Joanette, Y. (2001). The effects of left- versus right-hemisphere lesions on the sensitivity to intra- and interconceptual semantic relationships. *Neuropsychologia*, 39, 443–51.

Ober, B. A. and Shenaut, G. K. (1988). Lexical decision and priming in Alzheimer's disease. *Neuropsychologia*, 26, 273–86.

Ober, B. A. and Shenaut, G. K. (1999). Well-organized conceptual domains in Alzheimer's disease. *Journal of the International Neuropsychological Society*, 5, 676–84.

Ober, B. A., Shenaut, G. K., Jagust, W. J., and Stillman, R. C. (1991). Automatic semantic priming with various category relations in Alzheimer's disease and normal aging. *Psychology and Aging*, 6, 647–60.

Posner, M. I. and Snyder, C. R. R. (1975). Attention and cognitive control. In R. L. Solso (ed.), *Information Processing and Cognition: The Loyola Symposium*. Hillsdale, NJ: Erlbaum.

Prather, P. A., Zurif, E., Love, T., and Brownell, H. (1997). Speed of lexical activation in nonfluent Broca's aphasia and fluent Wernicke's aphasia. *Brain and Language*, 59, 391–411.

Prather, P. A., Zurif, E., Stern, C., and Rosen, T. J. (1992). Slowed lexical access in nonfluent aphasia: A case study. *Brain and Language*, 43, 336–48.

Sergent, J. (1994). Spécialisation fonctionnelle et coopération des hémisphères cérébraux. In X. Seron and M. Jeannerod (eds.), *Neuropsychologie humaine* (pp. 105–25). Liège: Mardaga.

Silveri, M. C., Monteleone, D., Burani, C., and Tabossi, P. (1996). Automatic semantic facilitation in Alzheimer's disease. *Journal of Clinical and Experimental Neuropsychology*, 18, 371–82.

Swaab, T. Y., Brown, C., and Hagoort, P. (1998). Understanding ambiguous words in sentence contexts: Electrophysiological evidence for delayed contextual selection in Broca's aphasia. *Neuropsychologia*, 36, 737–61.

Tompkins, C. A. (1990). Knowledge and strategies for processing lexical metaphor after right or left hemisphere brain damage. *Journal of Speech, Language and Hearing Research*, 33, 307–16.

Tompkins, C. A., Fassbinder, W., Lehman-Blake, M., Baumgaertner, A., and Jayaram, N. (2004). Inference generation during text comprehension by adults with right hemisphere brain damage: Activation failure versus multiple activation. *Journal of Speech, Language and Hearing Research*, 47, 1380–95.

Tompkins, C. A., Lehman-Blake, M. T., Baumgaertner, A., and Fassbinder, W. (2001). Mechanisms of discourse comprehension impairment after right hemisphere brain damage: Suppression in inferential ambiguity resolution. *Journal of Speech, Language and Hearing Research*, 44, 400–15.

Tranel, D., Damasio, H., and Damasio, A. R. (1997). A neural basis for the retrieval of conceptual knowledge. *Neuropsychologia*, 35, 1319–27.

Walter, N., Jbabdi, S., Marrelec, G., Benali, H., and Joanette, Y. (2005). FMRI functional connectivity of the phonological and semantic processing of words. Paper presented at the Organization for Human Brain Mapping (OHBM) 11th Annual Meeting, June 12–16, Toronto.

Warrington, E. K. and McCarthy, R. (1983). Category specific access dysphasia. *Brain*, 106, 859–78.

Warrington, E. K. and McCarthy, R. (1987). Categories of knowledge: Further fractionations and an attempted integration. *Brain*, 110, 1273–96.

Whatmough, C., Chertkow, H., Murta, S., Templeman, D., Babins, L., and Klener, N. (2003). The semantic category effect increases with worsening anomia in Alzheimer's type dementia. *Brain and Language*, 84, 134–47.

Whitehouse, P., Caramazza, A., and Zurif, E. (1978). Naming in aphasia: Interacting effects of form and function. *Brain and Language*, 6, 63–74.

Yochim, B. P., Kender, R., Abeare, C., Gustafson, A., and Whitman, R. D. (2005). Semantic activation within and across the cerebral hemispheres: What's left isn't right. *Laterality*, 10, 131–48.

15 Neural Correlates of Normal and Pathological Language Processing

STEFAN FRISCH, SONJA A. KOTZ, AND ANGELA D. FRIEDERICI

15.1 The Classical Models and Beyond

In 1874, the German neuroanatomist Eduard Hitzig presented his ideas on language and the brain to the Berlin Anthropological Society (cf. Hagner, 2000). He interpreted aphasia as a loss of 'motor images of words' very similar to neuronal representations of other types of motor activity in humans and non-human animals. Hitzig was sharply criticized by Heymann Steinthal, a linguist, who had analyzed most of the aphasiological data available at that time. Steinthal was convinced that the leading view of language in the second half of the nineteenth century completely underestimated the complexity of language as a psychological function. He concluded that language had to be conceived as a complex psychological mechanism beyond the current view of the leading neurologists and neuroanatomists.

Although Steinthal discussed his ideas with many important scientists at the time, the leading theoretical views on aphasia and language prevailed. These views had begun to gain influence after the scientific descriptions of motor aphasia by Paul Broca and of sensory aphasia by Carl Wernicke. Wernicke (1977) incorporated both findings into a model of a motor speech center in the inferior frontal and a sensory speech center in the superior temporal cortex, the two being connected by a massive fiber bundle (arcuate fasciculus). Lichtheim (1885) added a 'concept center' to this model and arrived at his famous 'house model' of language that supposedly made it possible for all types of aphasic syndromes to be explained. Although the so-called *Wernicke–Lichtheim model* of language has been very influential as a heuristic for both research and therapy, it is faced with a number of problems (see also Hickok & Poeppel, 2004): the idea of a few aphasic syndromes is not sufficient to explain the variety of aphasic phenomena; nor is their association to different anatomical areas as clear as the classical model suggests. Furthermore, the model is (psycho)linguistically strongly underspecified. Today, Steinthal's claim that the complex structure of language is inherently tied to a differentiated neural basis has gained much influence. Neuronal models of language are inextricably bound to (psycho)linguistic theories. Furthermore, new techniques to measure brain activity *in vivo* give us an idea of how complex the neuronal basis of language is and how the different language functions are supported by a distributed network of cortical as well as subcortical areas. Through these new methods, we gain understanding about language being processed *in time*. When the lexical entry of a word is retrieved, many different types of linguistic information (phonological, syntactic and semantic) need to be integrated into a sentence representation. This happens very fast, even though the process engages multiple interactions between information types. Thus, a model of language not only has to describe anatomically and functionally distinct language-related areas in the brain, it must also explain when these different areas come into play and interact with each other so that language is produced and understood under the time-critical conditions of real life communication.

15.2   Language Processing and the Timing Issue

Numerous studies have described time as a critical parameter of aphasic language. For example, Friederici and Kilborn (1989) reported that Broca's aphasics showed longer lexical decision times for target words in sentence contexts rather than in isolation than did age-matched controls. Also unlike those of controls, decision times were longer when there was no pause between a context and a target word. As grammatical knowledge of a sentence was preserved, results suggest that sentence processing under strong time restrictions was impaired. In a recent study in English conducted by Burkhardt, Piñango, and Wong (2003), Broca's aphasics showed a priming effect in a cross-modal lexical decision task at the original position of a moved argument such as 'the cheese' in (1), as do controls (the concept of movement will be explained in more detail below). However, patients showed a priming effect for a word related to *cheese* in (1) (such as *cheddar*) compared to an unrelated word (such as *album*) only when this target word was presented with a considerable delay (650 ms) relative to its original position (i.e. at trace position 't').

(1)   The kid loved the cheese$_i$ which$_i$ the new microwave melted t$_i$ yesterday afternoon . . .

By contrast, normal controls already showed a comparable effect 100 ms after the critical position. These results as well as those from Friederici and Kilborn (1989) highlight the importance of a dynamic view of pathological language processing. They clearly emphasize the limits of representational accounts that assume loss of grammatical knowledge for sentences such as (1) (as, e.g., Grodzinsky, 2000).

In addition to reaction-time experiments, time-sensitive neurophysiological measures receive increasing attention in research on both normal and pathological language processing. In particular, *event-related brain potentials* (ERPs), which allow the electrophysiological correlates of cognitive processes to be monitored continuously with a very high time resolution (millisecond-by-millisecond), have attracted a lot of interest over recent decades. ERPs are obtained by averaging epochs of spontaneous EEG activity which are time-locked to the onset of critical stimulus events (e.g. syntactically or semantically mismatching words). The averaging procedure results in a wavelike pattern consisting of typical peaks which are positive or negative relative to a control condition (e.g. syntactically and/or semantically legal words). These peaks are termed *components*. They are defined not only by their *polarity* (positive or negative), but also by the time delay after onset of the critical stimulus (*latency*) and the area over the skull where they are maximal (*topography*). An *N400 component*, for example, is a negative (hence 'N') deflection which occurs approximately 400 milliseconds after a critical stimulus. Although ERP components are defined by their topographic distribution over the skull, this does not enable cognitive processes to be related to specific brain areas. This is because EEG activity is oriented orthogonally to the sulcated cortex surface and not to the skull surface. Therefore, for each ERP pattern which is recorded on the surface of the skull, there is an infinite number of possible sources (*generators*).

There are several ways to determine the neuronal basis of a specific component and therefore of the specific step in language processing it represents. One possibility is to test patients with circumscribed brain lesions and to find out whether they show the component in question or not. Another possibility is to test similar experimental manipulations with neuroimaging methods which allow a high spatial resolution. These methods trace changes in the cerebral blood flow either via a radioactive substance in *positron emission tomography* (PET) or via changes in the magnetic field in *functional magnetic resonance imaging* (fMRI). The problem with these methods, however, is that the physiological mechanism they depend upon (i.e. cerebral blood flow) changes relatively slowly in comparison to electrophysiological activity. Thus, there seems to be a trade-off between spatial and temporal resolution in the different methods. ERPs on the one hand and fMRI/PET on the other can thus be seen as complementary methods that play important roles in the development of a neurocognitive model of language processing.

In the following, we present some of the ERP and fMRI evidence on syntactic and semantic processing at the sentence level and integrate them into a model. Please keep in mind that this is an area of active and ongoing research. Accordingly, sentence processing-models are very much 'in flux'. Due to space limitations, we will not discuss results on early processes of speech segmentation (see Hickok & Poeppel, 2000) or on phonological processing (see Friederici & Alter, 2004).

15.3   Semantic Integration

Kutas and Hillyard (1980) were the first to find that semantically anomalous sentences such as (2) lead to a specific ERP response.

(2)   He spread the warm bread with <u>socks</u>.

In comparison to correct sentences, Kutas and Hillyard found a negative ERP deflection occurring approximately 400 ms after the word *socks* was presented, rendering (2) semantically inappropriate. Since then, the N400 has been the focus of numerous studies. There is some debate about what the N400 exactly reflects, but there is good evidence that it can best be characterized as a marker of semantic integration (Chwilla, Brown, & Hagoort, 1995). The N400 has also been shown to reflect thematic mismatch of argument-structure violations (Osterhout, Holcomb, & Swinney, 1994; Frisch, Hahne, & Friederici, 2004) as well as hierarchic thematic interpretation problems (Frisch & Schlesewsky, 2001, 2005).

In order to determine the brain areas which support the semantic processes reflected in the N400, several studies with brain-damaged patients have been carried out. In these studies, patients were selected on the basis of either their functional deficits (i.e. behavioral impairment) or their structural deficits (i.e. lesion location). One example of the former type of study was conducted by Swaab, Brown, and Hagoort (1997) in a passive listening paradigm. They found the N400 effect in aphasic patients with low comprehension scores (measured on an independent test) to be delayed in comparison to aphasic patients with high comprehension scores, patients with right-hemisphere damage and normal controls. Neither the exact site of lesion within the left hemisphere nor the specific aphasic syndrome (Broca's versus Wernicke's aphasia) was crucial. The authors took their results as evidence that aphasics with low comprehension abilities are delayed in lexical integration.

While comprehension performance was the critical criterion in the experiments just described, there are also studies which have subgrouped their patients according to lesion location.

Friederici, Hahne, and von Cramon (1998) found that an aphasic patient with a left-temporoparietal lesion did not show an N400 effect in semantically anomalous sentences such as (3).

(3)   Der Honig wurde <u>ermordet</u>.
       the honey was murdered

A further study by Friederici, von Cramon, and Kotz (1999) showed that the N400 for sentences such as (3) was preserved in patients with left inferior-frontal lesions as well as in patients with subcortical lesion of the left basal ganglia. This was taken to show that the respective structures do not play a crucial role in processes of semantic integration.

Since most fMRI studies on semantic processing in healthy subjects focus on the single-word level, there are only a few studies that use sentences as a testing ground. These studies have found activation of a network of inferior-frontal as well as temporal loci when subjects are confronted with semantically anomalous sentences.

Ni, Constable, Menci, et al. (2000) presented semantically anomalous sentences such as (4) to their subjects.

(4)   Trees can eat.

Sentences such as (4) lead to more activation in the posterior superior temporal gyrus (STG), the middle temporal gyrus (MTG), the angular gyrus, and the inferior frontal gyrus (IFG) than do sentences with morphosyntactic violations. Higher activations in the MTG (BA[1]21), the angular gyrus and the inferior frontal region (BA46/BA9), but also the medial temporal cortex, for semantically incongruent sentences were also reported by Newman, Pancheva, Ozawa, Neville and Ullman (2001).

Kuperberg, McGuire, Bullmore, et al. (2000) tested sentences with semantic violations in the strict sense, i.e. selectional restriction violations, such as (5).

(5)   The young man drank the guitar.

The authors found enhanced activation differences in the (right) STG as well as the (right) MTG compared to syntactic violations. In comparison to both syntactic and selectional restriction violations, pragmatically anomalous sentences such as (6) lead to higher activation differences in the left STG.

(6)   The young man buried the guitar.

Friederici, Rüschemeyer, Hahne and Fiebach (2003) found enhanced activity for semantic anomalies in comparison to a baseline condition in the middle to posterior STG and the insular cortex bilaterally, but no IFG activation.

Rüschemeyer, Fiebach, Kempe, and Friederici (2005) contrasted semantically anomalous with correct sentences and found the lateral prefrontal cortex (BA44/45) and an area including the posterior MTG and the superior temporal sulcus (STS) to be specifically active.

Both (posterior) superior and middle temporal areas seem to be involved in semantic integration processes, but also an inferior frontal area (namely BA47) anterior to Broca's area which has traditionally been associated with syntactic processing. As has been suggested by Dapretto and Bookheimer (1999), these two regions may serve different aspects of language processing. In a study testing identical sentences in a syntactic and a semantic task the authors found the anterior portion of left IFG (mainly BA47) more active in the semantic task than in the syntactic task. On the other hand, activation differences were stronger in the posterior portion of left IFG (mainly BA44) in the syntactic task than the semantic task. These results suggest that the IFG may respond as a function of the strategic aspects of the task employed.

In sum, studies on the processing of semantic information converge in the finding that processes of semantic integration take place around 400 ms after a critical stimulus and that these processes are subserved by a (bilateral) cortical network including the MTG, the middle and posterior portions of STG and the anterior IFG, whereby the involvement of the latter is presumably tied to strategic aspects of processing.

15.4   Syntactic Processes: Word Category Integration, Processing of Morphosyntactic Information and Syntactic Repair/Reanalysis

Apart from semantic information, syntactic information (word category, morphosyntax, argument structure, case, etc.) is entailed in a word's lexical entry. During on-line sentence processing this information has to be linked with syntactic restrictions provided by the sentence context. As ERP studies have shown, syntactic processes take place in three different time windows.

One ERP effect in response to morphosyntactic violations which can be observed in the same time window (300–500 ms) as the N400 is the so-called *left-anterior negativity* (LAN). LAN effects have been observed for number-agreement violations in different languages such as English (Osterhout & Mobley, 1995) and Dutch (Gunter, Stowe, & Mulder, 1997). They have also been observed for violations of gender (Gunter, Schriefers, & Friederici, 2000) and case (Coulson, King, & Kutas, 1998; Friederici & Frisch, 2000). The LAN can therefore be characterized as reflecting unsuccessful integration of morpho-syntactic information. There is little systematic evidence on the neuronal basis of morphosyntactic integration processes, but the STG and possibly the IFG seem to play an important role (Ni, Constable, Menci, et al., 2000; Raettig, Kotz, Frisch, & Friederici, 2005).

Furthermore, there are two other time phases in which syntactic violations lead to characteristic ERP effects, one preceding and one following the LAN/N400 time window. In the earlier phase (around 150 ms) words are integrated into the ongoing sentence structure on the basis of their syntactic category. In (7), for example, such an integration is impossible as only nouns and adjectives, but not verbs (such as *gegessen*) can follow a preposition (such as *im*) in German.

(7)   Der Honig wurde im gegessen.
      the honey was in-the eaten

(8)   Der Honig wurde gegessen.
      the honey was eaten

Verbs such as *gegessen* in (7) create a word-category violation. In comparison to a correct sentence such as (8) (without the preposition), they elicit a very early negative ERP deflection peaking at around 150 ms. The component has its topographical maximum over (left-)anterior electrode sites and is therefore termed *early left anterior negativity* (ELAN). In the model of Friederici (2002), word-category integration temporally and functionally precedes the integration of all other types of information (syntactic and semantic) associated with a word. This seems to be warranted since the ELAN occurs irrespective of simultaneous violations based on other types of syntactic or semantic information, for example verb-argument structure (Frisch, Hahne, & Friederici, 2004) or selectional restrictions (Friederici, Steinhauer, & Frisch, 1999; Hahne & Friederici, 2002). In addition, the ELAN is independent of non-linguistic factors such as the predictability of a word-category violation (Hahne & Friederici, 2002). By contrast, the electrophysiological correlates of other types of violation (such as a verb-argument structure or a semantic violation) are not found if the sentence contains an additional word-category violation (Friederici, Steinhauer, & Frisch, 1999; Hahne & Friederici, 2002; Frisch, Hahne, & Friederici, 2004). This finding is independent of whether the word category of the violating word is available before or after its semantic properties (Friederici, Gunter, Hahne, & Mauth, 2004). An early negativity in response to a word-category violation was found not only in German, but also in English (Neville, Nicol, Barss, Forster, & Garrett, 1991), Dutch (Hagoort, Wassenaar, & Brown, 2003), Japanese (Kubota, Ferrari, & Roberts, 2003) and Chinese (Ye, Lou, Friederici, & Zhou, 2006).

Sentences that contain a word-category violation, such as (7), not only elicit an ELAN component on the mismatching verb but also a positive deflection component peaking around 600 ms, the so-called *P600* (Friederici, Steinhauer, & Frisch, 1999; Hahne & Friederici, 2001). It was first reported by Osterhout and Holcomb (1992) for words that create a syntactic violation in a sentence. In contrast to the ELAN, the P600 is not specific for word-category violations, but occurs with most other syntactic violations. Among others, these include violations of agreement (Gunter, Stowe, & Mulder, 1997; Gunter, Schriefers, & Friederici, 2000; Osterhout & Mobley, 1995), case (Coulson, King, & Kutas, 1998; Friederici & Frisch, 2000; Frisch & Schlesewsky, 2001, 2005) and verb-argument structure (Osterhout, Holcomb, & Swinney, 1994; Friederici & Frisch, 2000; Frisch, Hahne, & Friederici, 2004).

Apart from outright violations, the P600 is also sensitive to processing differences between sentences which are all syntactically legal. Osterhout and Holcomb (1992) reported P600 effects in locally ambiguous sentences such as (9).

(9)   The broker persuaded to sell the stock was . . .

Up to the preposition 'to', sentence (9) can be parsed as a main clause structure consisting of a subject and a verb. The preposition requires that this preferred (as structurally simplest) reading is given up in favor of a more complex reduced relative clause (*the broker who had been persuaded to* . . .). The finding that the revision of a preferred reading of a locally ambiguous sentence induces a P600 has been replicated many times (Mecklinger, Schriefers, Steinhauer, & Friederici, 1995; Frisch, Schlesewsky, Saddy, & Alpermann, 2002; Frisch, beim Graben, & Schlesewsky, 2004). A P600 has also been found for differences in syntactic integration difficulty between different non-ambiguous sentences (Kaan, Harris, Gibson, & Holcomb, 2000) as well as for local ambiguities compared to unambiguous structures (Frisch, Schlesewsky, Saddy, & Alpermann, 2002).

With respect to the different experimental contexts in which late positivities have been found, the P600 can be seen as a marker of enhanced syntactic processing cost, due to either repair, revision/reanalysis, integration cost or ambiguity. In contrast to the ELAN, the P600 amplitude decreases with increasing probability of the syntactic violation (Hahne & Friederici, 2001; Coulson, King, & Kutas, 1998; Gunter, Stowe, & Mulder, 1997) and can be modulated by additional (non-syntactic) violations (Gunter, Stowe, & Mulder, 1997). These findings emphasize the role of the P600 as reflecting stages of controlled evaluative processing.

Can these different types of syntactic processes (reflected by ELAN and P600) be located in the brain? An answer to this question provides a good example of how evidence from different resources has to be integrated in order to get a more complete picture of the dynamic character of language processing in the brain. In an fMRI study, Friederici, Rüschemeyer, Hahne, and Fiebach (2003) tested word-category violations such as (7) which elicit an ELAN–P600 pattern in the ERP. Compared to a correct condition, these violations activated superior temporal (the anterior and posterior part of left STG), inferior frontal (the left deep frontal operculum) as well as subcortical areas (the putamen of the left basal ganglia). As previously stated, the problem with fMRI is its relatively low time resolution that does not allow subsequent subprocesses to be distinguished. However, there is evidence from ERP studies on patients with circumscribed brain lesions. In the aforementioned study by Friederici, Hahne, and von Cramon (1998), a patient with a temporoparietal lesion did not show an N400 effect for semantic violations, but did show both an ELAN and a P600 for word-category violations. Furthermore, the authors found no ELAN, but a P600 for the same type of violation (as well as an N400 for a semantic violation) in a second patient with a left inferior frontal lesion (see also Friederici, von Cramon, and Kotz, 1999, for a similar result with a larger sample of patients with left-frontal lesions). The same pattern (a P600, but no ELAN) was found in a study with patients who had suffered a lesion of the anterior temporal lobe (Kotz, von Cramon, & Friederici, 2003). Further evidence that a word-category mismatch activates a network of inferior frontal (deep frontal operculum) and anterior temporal areas comes from a study using magnetoencephalography (MEG), a technique which traces changes in the magnetic fields of neurone assemblies as they depolarize. MEG has the same temporal resolution as ERPs but a higher spatial resolution. In a MEG study with healthy participants, Friederici, Wang, Herrmann, Maess, and Oertel (2000) conducted a dipole source localization and found that the ELAN was best explained by two generators, one in the anterior part of the STG (planum polare) and a second one in the inferior frontal cortex.

These regions do not seem to be crucial for late, controlled syntactic processes, as P600 effects were found in patients with lesions in the anterior temporal or inferior frontal area. However, a P600 for a word-category violation (or other syntactic violation) was reduced or absent in patients with lesions in the left basal ganglia (Friederici, von Cramon, & Kotz, 1999; Frisch, Kotz, von Cramon, & Friederici, 2003; Kotz, Frisch, von Cramon, & Friederici, 2003). Obviously, syntactic processes are not exclusively hosted by cortical areas, but subcortical structures also play an important role (see also Ullman, 2004).

Taken together, all these results suggest that word-category integration (as reflected by the ELAN) takes place early and is supported by a network of inferior frontal and anterior temporal areas. By contrast, late controlled processes of syntactic repair (as reflected by the P600) may possibly be regulated in the basal ganglia and the posterior STG.

15.5   Violations and Beyond

In the preceding section we have demonstrated that language processing in the brain takes place in different subsequent phases. These phases are supported by different parts of a large cortico-subcortical network which is summarized in figure 15.1. In the first phase (at around 150 ms), the syntactic category of a word is integrated into a sentence context. If this fails, an ELAN is elicited. The neuronal basis for this process seems to be a perisylvian network of (anterior) STG and IFG (deep frontal operculum). Although most of the fMRI activity is found in left-hemisphere regions, right-hemisphere homologues are often coactivated. In a second phase (approximately between 300 and 500 ms), the integration of lexical-semantic/thematic information (reflected in an N400) as well as morphosyntactic information (reflected in a LAN) takes place. Semantic integration is provided by the (posterior) STG and MTG as well as the IFG, whereas the STG and the IFG also play a role in the integration of morphosyntactic information. A third phase follows in which a general (largely syntactic) evaluation of the sentence takes place. It seems to be supported by a cortico-subcortical network including (posterior) STG and the basal ganglia.

The studies we have presented here are largely based on the processing of violations. Especially with respect to syntax, however, there is another type of experimental manipulation which has attracted increasing interest, namely, the processing of sentences with non-canonical word orders. Syntactic theories make the assumption that each language has a basic ('canonical') order of core constituents (i.e. verb and arguments). Sentences that do not follow this order are not necessarily illegal, but associated with enhanced processing cost. In English, for example, the canonical order is subject–verb–object, as in (10a).

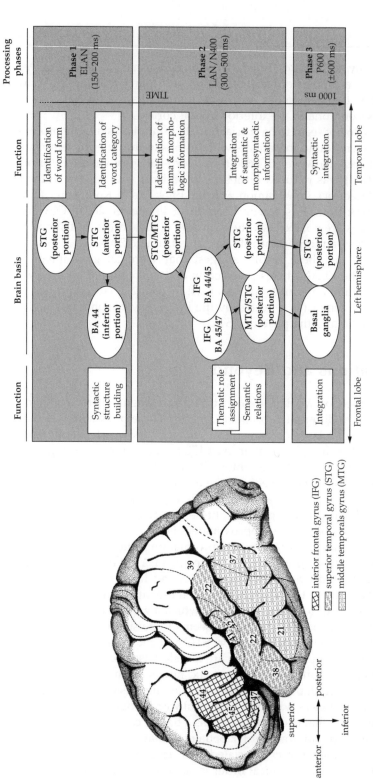

Figure 15.1 Left-hand side: View of the left hemisphere with the cortical gyri (IFG, STG and MTG) that are most relevant for language processing. The respective Brodmann areas (BA) are numbered.
Right-hand side: Adapted version of the neurocognitive model of Friederici (2002) showing the different, subsequent phases of syntactic and semantic processing (associated with the different language-related ERP components) and the brain areas that support them. Note that early processes of speech segmentation and phonological processing are not considered here, since they are not discussed in the present chapter. For further explanation see text.

(10a)   The girl called [the boy]$_i$ who t$_i$ sold the ice cream.

(10b)   [The boy]$_i$ who the girl called t$_i$ sold the ice cream.

In (10a), the NP 'the boy' is the object of the main clause, where it follows the subject ('the girl') and the verb ('called'). At the same time, it is the subject of the relative clause where it precedes the verb and the object. In (10b), by contrast, 'the boy' is the object of the relative clause but precedes the subject and the verb. Therefore, (10b) is an object relative clause, whereas (10a) is a subject relative clause. Some syntactic theories assume that 'the boy' has been *moved* from its original object position in (10b) (and from the subject position in 10a) in order to derive the 'surface' structure object–subject–verb. This is indicated by the 't' (for 'trace') in both (10a) and (10b) and by the 'i' that coindexes trace and moved constituent.

Sentences in which the constituent order deviates from the canonical one have played an important role in research involving aphasic patients. It was shown that Broca's aphasics not only have characteristic impairments in language production (nonfluent, 'telegram-style' output) but also experience severe comprehension problems with non-canonical sentences, at least if it is not clear on grounds of plausibility alone which constituent is the subject and which the object (Caramazza & Zurif, 1976). Thus in examples (10a) and (10b), it is plausible that a boy sells ice cream, but not that ice cream sells a boy, whereas a girl can call a boy and vice versa. It has been proposed that Broca's aphasics lack the knowledge about the original position of the moved NP ('the boy') and therefore they cannot reconstruct a movement (cf. Grodzinsky, 2000). As Broca's aphasia is a syndrome often associated with the left IFG (BA44 and 45, Broca's area), it was proposed that this cortical area plays a key role in the processing of the dependencies between the moved sentence constituents on the 'surface' of the sentence and their original positions in the underlying canonical order. Accordingly, imaging research has been undertaken in order to find out which areas are activated when confronted with a non-canonical sentence structure. In two PET studies, Stromswold, Caplan, Alpert, and Rauch (1996) and Caplan, Alpert, and Waters (1998) found more activation in the left IFG (BA44) for sentences such as (10b) than for sentences such as (10a). However, as the authors admit, these results are not necessarily due to the different word orders. They could also be caused by the fact that a relative clause interrupts a main clause in (10b), whereas it follows a main clause in (10a). Just, Carpenter, Keller, Eddy, and Thulborn (1996), however, found that BA44 was also more active for an object relative clause (11b) than for a subject relative clause (11a) when both relative clauses were embedded.

(11a)   [The reporter]$_i$ who t$_i$ attacked the senator admitted the error.

(11b)   [The reporter]$_i$ who the senator attacked t$_i$ admitted the error.

Obviously, these activation differences must depend on differences in constituent order. However, it is not clear whether object-before-subject *per se* is crucial or whether there is yet another explanation for the difference between (11a) and (11b) or for the one between (10a) and (10b): In the object relative clauses (10b) and (11b), the distance between the moved constituent ('the reporter') and its original position is necessarily longer than in their subject relative counterparts (10a and 11a) as subject and verb intervene in the former, but not in the latter. Thus, the increased difficulty for the (b)-sentences may be due to higher working-memory demands, as the moved constituent has to be rehearsed until it can be assigned to its original position. Since all the studies mentioned above were conducted in English, which relies on strong word order constraints, the two possible explanations cannot be resolved. Grewe, Bornkessel, Zysset, Wiese, von Cramon, and Schlesewsky (2005) have addressed this question in German, a language with more flexibility in word order than English. They presented sentences such as (12) with three arguments, namey a subject ('SUB'), an indirect object ('IOB') and a direct object ('DOB'). In one condition, these arguments occurred in their canonical order (SUB>IOB>DOB, see 12a). In another condition, the indirect object was moved in front of the subject (IOB>SUB>DOB, see 12b). Note that, in German, word-order variations such as in (12b) are marked, but nevertheless grammatical, in contrast to English. Translating (12a) and (12b) into English would give identical results.

(12a)   Dann hat [der Lehrer] [dem Gärtner] [den Spaten] gegeben.
        then has [the teacher]SUB [the gardener]IOB [the spade]DOB given

(12b)   Dann hat [dem Gärtner] [der Lehrer] [den Spaten] gegeben.
        then has [the gardener]IOB [the teacher]SUB [the spade]DOB given

The authors found bilateral IFG (pars opercularis/BA44) activation for scrambled sentences such as (12b) compared to sentences with a canonical order (12a). Could this result not be explained in terms of higher working-memory cost?

Grewe, Bornkessel, Zysset, et al. looked at two further conditions. One had the same word order as in (12b), but the indirect object was replaced by a pronoun ('ihm'/'him') such as in (12c).

(12c)   Dann hat [ihm] [der Lehrer] [den Spaten] gegeben.
        then has [him]IOB [the teacher]SUB [the spade]DOB given

Crucially, there is a strong tendency for pronouns in German to precede all non-pronomial arguments, probably for phonological reasons, irrespective of whether they are the subject or the object of the sentence. In other words, they enforce argument permutations (here, indirect object before subject). Interestingly, the authors found no activation differences in IFG (or anywhere else) between (12c) and a sentence such as (12a) but with a pronominal subject.

Results question the working memory account. They are also hard to reconcile with approaches that assume that IFG activation increases with the number of transformations that have to be computed in order to receive a non-canonical surface order (Ben-Shahar, Hendler, Kahn, Ben-Bashat, & Grodzinsky, 2003). Grewe, Bornkessel, Zysset, et al. (2005) instead argue that the IFG, and more specifically Broca's area, is sensitive to hierarchical linguistic dependencies (i.e. subject>object, pronoun>non-pronoun, etc.) which are spelled out differently in the world's languages. On the basis of these data and especially with respect to another study by Fiebach, Schlesewsky, Bornkessel and Friederici (2004) who directly contrasted grammatical scrambled sentences with ungrammatical ones, there is evidence that ungrammaticality activates not the IFG, but the deep frontal operculum. This seems also to be true for most of the above-cited studies on the processing of syntactic violations, at least as long as the violation is created via two adjacent elements. By contrast, word-order variations lead to IFG activation but do not alter activity in fronto-opercular areas. Since the latter are probably older phylogenetic territory than the former, this suggest a more profound functional differentiation between these two brain regions (see Friederici, Bahlmann, Heim, Schubotz, & Anwander, 2006).

To conclude, the variety of empirical results in the field of neuronal language processing is enormous. This is due not only to the inherent differences in the methods employed (electrophysiological vs. brain imaging), but also to the variety of linguistic manipulations, experimental designs, tasks, languages, etc. Nevertheless, we have shown that the picture becomes much more coherent if we analyze similar questions under different perspectives, i.e. with different methods, which cover both the temporal and the spatial parameters of language processing in the brain.

NOTE

1   The best-known and most widely used parcellation of the human cortex based on its cytoarchitecture goes back to the German neuroanatomist Korbinian Brodmann (1868–1918). Resulting cortical areas are therefore termed 'Brodmann areas' ('BA').

REFERENCES

Ben-Shahar, M., Hendler, T., Kahn, I., Ben-Bashat, D., and Grodzinsky, Y. (2003). The neural reality of syntactic transformations: Evidence from fMRI. *Psychological Science*, 14, 433–40.

Burkhardt, P., Pinango, M. M., and Wong, K. (2003). The role of the anterior left hemisphere in real-time sentence comprehension: Evidence from split intransitivity. *Brain and Language*, 86, 9–22.

Caplan, D., Alpert, N., and Waters, G. S. (1998). Effects of syntactic structure and propositional number on patterns of regional cerebral blood flow. *Journal of Cognitive Neuroscience*, 10, 541–52.

Caramazza, A. and Zurif, E. (1976). Dissociation of algorithmic and heuristic processes in language comprehension: evidence from aphasia. *Brain and Language*, 3, 572–82.

Chwilla, D. J., Brown, C. M., and Hagoort, P. (1995). The N400 as a function of the level of processing. *Psychophysiology*, 32, 274–85.

Coulson, S., King, J. W., and Kutas, M. (1998). Expect the unexpected: Event-related brain responses to morphosyntactic violations. *Language and Cognitive Processes*, 13, 21–58.

Dapretto, M. and Bookheimer, S. Y. (1999). Form and content: Dissociating syntax and semantics in sentence comprehension. *Neuron*, 24, 427–32.

Fiebach, C. J., Schlesewsky, M., Bornkessel, I., and Friederici, A. D. (2004). Distinct neural correlates of legal and illegal word order variations in German: How can fMRI inform cognitive models of sentence processing? In M. Carreiras and C. Clifton, Jr. (eds.), *The On-Line Study of Sentence Comprehension* (pp. 357–70). New York: Psychology Press.

Friederici, A. D. (2002). Towards a neural basis of auditory sentence processing. *Trends in Cognitive Sciences*, 6, 78–84.

Friederici, A. D. and Alter, K. (2004). Lateralization of auditory language functions: A dynamic dual pathway model. *Brain and Language*, 89, 267–76.

Friederici, A. D., Bahlmann, J., Heim, S., Schubotz, R. I., and Anwander, A. (2006). The brain differentiates human and non-human grammars: Functional localization and structural connectivity. In *Proceedings of the National Academy of Sciences of the USA*, 103, 2458–63.

Friederici, A. D. and Frisch, S. (2000). Verb argument structure processing: The role of verb-specific and argument-specific information. *Journal of Memory and Language*, 43, 476–507.

Friederici, A. D., Gunter, T. C., Hahne, A., and Mauth, K. (2004). The relative timing of syntactic and semantic processes in sentence comprehension. *NeuroReport*, 15, 165–9.

Friederici, A. D., Hahne, A. and von Cramon, D. Y. (1998). First-pass versus second-pass parsing processes in a Wernicke's and a Broca's aphasic: Electro-physiological evidence for a double dissociation. *Brain and Language*, 62, 311–41.

Friederici, A. D. and Kilborn, K. (1989). Temporal constraints on language processing: Syntactic priming in Broca's aphasia. *Journal of Cognitive Neuroscience*, 1, 262–72.

Friederici, A. D., Rüschemeyer, S.-A., Hahne, A. and Fiebach, C. J. (2003). The role of left inferior frontal and superior temporal cortex in sentence comprehension: Localizing syntactic and semantic processes. *Cerebral Cortex*, 13, 170–7.

Friederici, A. D., Steinhauer, K., and Frisch, S. (1999). Lexical integration: Sequential effects of syntactic and semantic information. *Memory and Cognition*, 27, 438–53.

Friederici, A. D., von Cramon, D. Y., and Kotz, S. A. (1999). Language related brain potentials in patients with cortical and subcortical left hemisphere lesions. *Brain*, 122, 1033–47.

Friederici, A. D., Wang, Y., Herrmann, C. S., Maess, B., and Oertel, U. (2000). Localization of early syntactic processes in frontal and temporal cortical areas: A magnetoencephalographic study. *Human Brain Mapping*, 11, 1–11.

Frisch, S., beim Graben, P., and Schlesewsky, M. (2004). Parallelizing grammatical functions: P600 and P345 reflect different costs of reanalysis. *International Journal of Bifurcation and Chaos*, 14, 431–550.

Frisch, S., Hahne, A., and Friederici, A. D. (2004). Word category and verb-argument structure information in the dynamics of parsing. *Cognition*, 91, 191–219.

Frisch, S., Kotz, S. A., von Cramon, D. Y., and Friederici, A. D. (2003). Why the P600 is not just a P300: The role of the basal ganglia. *Clinical Neurophysiology*, 114, 336–40.

Frisch, S. and Schlesewsky, M. (2001). The N400 reflects problems of thematic hierarchizing. *NeuroReport*, 12, 3391–4.

Frisch, S. and Schlesewsky, M. (2005). The resolution of case conflicts: A neurophysiological perspective. *Cognitive Brain Research*, 25, 484–98.

Frisch, S., Schlesewsky, M., Saddy, D., and Alpermann, A. (2002). The P600 as an indicator of syntactic ambiguity. *Cognition*, 85, B83–B92.

Grodzinsky, Y. (2000). The neurology of syntax: Language use without Broca's area. *Behavioral and Brain Sciences*, 23, 1–71.

Grewe, T., Bornkessel, I., Zysset, S., Wiese, R., von Cramon, D. Y., and Schlesewsky, M. (2005). The emergence of the unmarked: A new perspective on the language-specific function of Broca's area. *Human Brain Mapping*, 26, 178–90.

Gunter, T. C., Schriefers, H., and Friederici, A. D. (2000). Syntactic gender and semantic expectancy: ERPs reveal early autonomy and late interaction. *Journal of Cognitive Neuroscience*, 12, 556–68.

Gunter, T. C., Stowe, L. A., and Mulder, G. (1997). When syntax meets semantics. *Psychophysiology*, 34, 660–76.

Hagner, M. (2000). *Homo cerebralis*. Frankfurt/Leipzig: Insel.

Hagoort, P., Wassenaar, M., and Brown, C. M. (2003). Syntax-related ERP effects in Dutch. *Cognitive Brain Research*, 16, 38–50.

Hahne, A. and Friederici, A. D. (2001). Processing a second language: Late learners' comprehension strategies as revealed by event-related brain potentials. *Bilingualism: Language and Cognition*, 4, 123–41.

Hahne, A. and Friederici, A. D. (2002). Differential task effects on semantic and syntactic processes as revealed by ERPs. *Cognitive Brain Research*, 13, 339–56.

Hickok, G. and Poeppel, D. (2000). Towards a functional neuroanatomy of speech perception. *Trends in Cognitive Sciences*, 4(4), 131–8.

Hickok, G. and Poeppel, D. (2004). Dorsal and ventral streams: A framework for understanding aspects of the functional anatomy of language. *Cognition*, 92, 67–99.

Just, M., Carpenter, P., Keller, T., Eddy, W., and Thulborn, K. (1996). Brain activation modulated by sentence comprehension. *Science*, 274 (5284), 114–16.

Kaan, E., Harris, A., Gibson, E., and Holcomb, P. J. (2000). The P600 as an index of syntactic integration difficulty. *Language and Cognitive Processes*, 15, 159–201.

Kotz, S. A., Frisch, S., von Cramon, D. Y., and Friederici, A. D. (2003). Syntactic language processing: ERP lesion data on the role of the basal ganglia. *Journal of the International Neuropsychological Society*, 9, 1053–60.

Kotz, S. A., von Cramon, D. Y., and Friederici, A. D. (2003). Differentiation of syntactic processes in the left and right anterior temporal lobe: ERP evidence from lesion patients. *Brain and Language*, 87, 135–6.

Kubota, M., Ferrari, P., and Roberts, T. P. L. (2003). Magnetoencephalography detection of early syntactic processes in humans: Comparison between L1 speakers and L2 learners of English. *Neuroscience Letters*, 353, 107–10.

Kuperberg, G. R., McGuire, P. K., Bullmore, E. T., Brammer, M. J., Rabe-Hesketh, S., Wright, I. C., Lythgoe, D. J., Williams, S. C. R., and David, A. S. (2000). Common and distinct neural substrates for pragmatic, semantic, and syntactic processing of spoken sentences: An fMRI study. *Journal of Cognitive Neuroscience*, 12, 321–41.

Kutas, M. and Hillyard, S. A. (1980). Reading senseless sentences: Brain potentials reflect semantic incongruity. *Science*, 207, 203–5.

Lichtheim, L. (1885). On aphasia. *Brain*, 7, 433–84.

Mecklinger, A., Schriefers, H., Steinhauer, K., and Friederici, A. D. (1995). Processing relative clauses varying on syntactic and semantic dimensions: An analysis with event-related potentials. *Memory and Cognition*, 23, 477–94.

Neville, H., Nicol, J., Barss, A., Forster, K., and Garrett, M. (1991). Syntactically based sentence processing classes: Evidence from event-related potentials. *Journal of CNS Neuroscience*, 3, 151–65.

Newman, A. J., Pancheva, R., Ozawa, K., Neville, H. J., and Ullman, M. T. (2001). An event-related fMRI study of syntactic and semantic violations. *Journal of Psycholinguistic Research*, 30(3), 337–61.

Ni, W., Constable, T., Menci, W. E., Pugh, K. R., Fulbright, R. K., Shaywitz, S. E., Shaywitz, B. A., Gore, J. C., and Schankweiler, D. (2000). An event-related neuroimaging study: Distinguishing form and content in sentence processing. *Journal of Cognitive Neuroscience*, 12, 120–33.

Osterhout, L. and Holcomb, P. J. (1992). Event-related brain potentials elicited by syntactic anomaly. *Journal of Memory and Language*, 31, 785–806.

Osterhout, L., Holcomb, P., and Swinney, D. (1994). Brain potentials elicited by garden-path sentences: Evidence of the application of verb information during parsing. *Journal of Experimental Psychology: Learning, Memory and Cognition*, 20, 786–803.

Osterhout, L. and Mobley, L. A. (1995). Event-related brain potentials elicited by failure to agree. *Journal of Memory and Language*, 34, 739–73.

Raettig, T., Kotz, S. A., Frisch, S., and Friederici, A. D. (2005). Neural correlates of verb-argument structure and semantic processing: An efMRI study. *Journal of Cognitive Neuroscience*, Supplement, 77.

Rüschemeyer, S.-A., Fiebach, C. J., Kempe, V., and Friederici, A. D. (2005). Processing lexical semantic and syntactic information in first and second language: fMRI evidence from German and Russian. *Human Brain Mapping*, 25, 266–86.

Stromswold, K., Caplan, D., Alpert, N., and Rauch, S. (1996). Localization of syntactic comprehension by positron emission tomography. *Brain and Language*, 52, 452–73.

Swaab, T. Y., Brown, C. M., and Hagoort, P. (1997). Spoken sentence comprehension in aphasia: Event-related potential evidence for a lexical integration deficit. *Journal of Cognitive Neuroscience*, 9(1), 39–66.

Ullman, M. T. (2004). Contributions of memory circuits to language: The declarative/procedural model. *Cognition*, 92, 231–70.

Wernicke, C. (1977). *The Aphasia Symptom Complex: A Psychological Study on an Anatomical Basis*. Wernicke's works on aphasia. The Hague: Mouton. (Original work published 1874.)

Ye, Z., Lou, Y., Friederici, A. F., and Zhou, X. (2006). Semantic and syntactic processing in Chinese sentence comprehension: Evidence from event-related potentials. *Brain Research*, 1071, 186–96.

16 Bilingualism and Language Impairment

JAN DE JONG

16.1 Introduction

This chapter deals with two types of language impairment, specific language impairment (SLI) in children and aphasia in adults. Bilingual language impairment in children has only recently been studied in some depth. The study of bilingual cases of aphasia has a longer history. In this chapter, the focus is on bilingual SLI; a brief discussion of bilingual aphasia serves comparative and contrastive purposes. For obvious reasons, bilingualism has to be placed in different contexts in developmental and acquired disorders. Important differences concern the processes of language acquisition (or learning) relative to the onset of disorder, and the nature of bilingualism. Bilingual language development may be either simultaneous or successive. In simultaneous bilingualism, the two languages are learned from the start. In characteristic cases of successive (or sequential) bilingualism, the child begins to grow up monolingual, but encounters a second language in kindergarten or primary school. SLI in bilingual children affects developing language systems, whether a child is exposed to two (or more) languages simultaneously, or a second language is introduced at some time during early childhood.

Adult-acquired aphasia, on the other hand, affects established language systems. While an aphasic bilingual may have acquired two (or more) languages either simultaneously or successively, by the time of onset, we can assume that all languages have been mastered (though not necessarily to the same degree of fluency), and language-use patterns for all languages have been established. Here there is loss of language, whereas in language-impaired children we witness the growth of two languages, albeit in the context of an underlying problem with language.

16.2   Bilingual SLI

As we will see, there is major overlap between diagnostic concerns and scientific research in the field of bilingual SLI. In their book, *Dual Language Development and Disorders*, Genesee, Paradis, and Crago (2004; Paradis, 2005) describe two types of potential misclassification of bilingual children. On the one hand, poor insight into second language learning in typically developing children can sometimes lead to the placement of children in special education when there is no true need for that (in Genesee, Paradis and Crago's words these are cases of 'mistaken identity'). On the other hand the problems of a language-impaired child can be overlooked ('missed identity') because his or her slow development is simply seen as the natural consequence of learning a second language and of the time it takes to master it. The latter mistake often causes late referral of children for language intervention (Salameh, Nettelbladt, Håkansson, & Gullberg, 2002). These two sorts of misdiagnosis exemplify the problems involved when employing the label 'specific language impairment' (SLI) with children who speak two languages. They correspond to the dilemma that faces researchers who investigate bilingual SLI: researchers are also concerned with the boundaries between typical second language learners and language pathology. (It should be noted that by definition SLI should express itself in both languages. However, the child's first language often cannot be assessed for lack of a diagnostician who is a native speaker. This adds to the diagnostic quagmire sketched above.)

A caveat is needed when we address bilingualism. It is well known that every term to be used for children learning two languages is debatable. Each label has its advantages, disadvantages and connotations. Here it is accepted that bilingualism can refer to simultaneous and successive learning of two languages. We also recognize that the distinction between the two is not watertight. This is one of the reasons why Genesee, Paradis, and Crago (2004) prefer to apply the cover term 'dual language impairment' to both. In this chapter, the word 'bilingual' will be used as an 'agnostic' term for either type. When research on either type of bilingualism is referred to, it will be made clear which type is involved.

16.2.1   Group comparisons in SLI

A key issue in the study of SLI (and one that is intrinsically relevant to the topic of this chapter) concerns the nature of the difference between children with SLI and normally developing children. Leonard (1998) describes several ways in which the difference between the two groups can be characterized. The most obvious relationship between the two groups is one of delay: children with SLI are like children without language problems, but their language development starts later and it takes them longer to master the grammar of their native language. Another possibility is that the difference reaches beyond simple delay. There is a general consensus that the latter is the case with SLI. Several patterns are found in language-impaired children. Leonard (1998, pp. 31–6) lists the following: a developmental plateau, a different profile across language skills, an abnormal frequency of error and a qualitative difference (deviant forms). A crucial determinant of such group differences is the choice of a control group. It has been shown early on that, when one merely takes chronological age peers as a reference point, the outcome is a descriptive variant of 'delay' that cannot bring to light specific weaknesses in the children's language performance (Morehead & Ingram, 1973). By definition, children with SLI will simply fall behind on most language measures. In order to refine the comparison, different matching criteria have been introduced. The most frequently used measure is language level as indicated by mean length of utterance (MLU, counted in either words or morphemes). The rationale is that, MLU being an index of morphosyntactic growth, differences between groups matched on MLU (in which the typically developing children are by definition younger) will disclose the vulnerable areas in language-impaired children's grammar. This procedure can be criticized, though, and with every matching tool the question must be answered what the results actually signify (Plante, Swisher, Kiernan, & Restrepo, 1993; DeThorne, Johnson, & Loeb, 2005). Other indices of language level have been used, as well as mental age measures. The choice of a matching measure is crucially determined by the dependent variable targeted, and every comparison generates different information.

What is relevant about the research practice of matching language-impaired and non-impaired children is that it raises issues of comparability. Within every group comparison, the first question must be: what are the implications, and what do these commonalities or differences tell us? And if there is a difference, what is the nature of the difference?

If we wished to present a description of monolingual SLI in a particular language, the most obvious way to do it would be to outline the symptoms by linguistic level, using comparisons of impaired and non-impaired children matched for language level. In studies on bilingual SLI, however, matching paradigms are manifold. The question what bilingual SLI is and how it compares to monolingual SLI is answered by a composite of group comparisons in which bilingualism and/or SLI feature. We will therefore present empirical findings for each type of comparison. For every comparison, we will try to formulate what it contributes to our understanding of bilingual SLI. Together, these efforts mark out the domain of our question. They also highlight the dilemmas that both the researcher and the diagnostician are faced with.

16.2.1.1 *Monolingual SLI across languages*
There is a rich tradition of research into cross-linguistic differences in the symptoms of monolingual SLI. Leonard, who has pioneered comparisons between a range of languages, gives a survey in his seminal book (Leonard, 1998). His conclusion from the cross-linguistic research so far is that grammatical morphology is impaired in every language studied, but the nature of

the impairment varies with the typological characteristics of the language. For instance, in languages with a rich morphology substitutions are found in the output of children with SLI; in languages with a sparse morphology omissions predominate. The relevance for bilingual language impairment is clear. When considering the bilingual child with SLI, one possible view is that we are dealing with two-monolinguals-in-one. If that is the case, the logical assumption is that cross-linguistic differences will show up in a single child and that "the same child with SLI will show two different grammatical profiles depending on the language being spoken" (Leonard, in his introduction to Genesee, Paradis, & Crago, 2004, p. xvi). Even if one does not accept this position, the typological difference between the languages spoken by the child must be considered.

16.2.1.2   Monolingual children with SLI and typically developing L2 learners

In several studies, SLI and second language (L2) acquisition have been compared. The rationale for this comparison is that the areas that are vulnerable in both groups of language learners are similar.

For instance, Håkansson (2001) investigated inflectional morphology and verb placement. Swedish is a verb-second language and word order has proven to be a problem for Swedish children with SLI. In Håkansson's study, both second language learners and monolingual children with SLI had difficulty producing the inverted word order (verb–subject instead of subject–verb) that is obligatory with topicalization (for instance, after a preposed adverb) in Swedish. Håkansson and Nettelbladt (1996) refer to similar patterns in adult L2 learners that have been explained by transfer from the first language (L1) (where word order is subject–verb). The finding that monolingual children with SLI also prefer this order leads the authors to speculate that markedness might be involved, i.e., subject–verb might be the unmarked order.

Paradis and Crago (2000) also found similarities between monolingual French-speaking children with SLI and English-speaking L2 learners of French. Their difficulties concerned the marking of finiteness, tense and subject–verb agreement, as well as the production of object clitics. Paradis (2005) extended this comparison to include L2 learners whose first language is a minority language, "meaning that their L1s were not high-status and widely spoken languages in the community in which they were living at the time of study" (p. 173). She found that this linguistically diverse group exhibited difficulties with the grammatical morphology of English (their L2). Their error patterns and accuracy rates resembled those of monolingual English children with SLI.

These comparisons suggest that there are vulnerable areas in the target language that are a challenge for monolingual children with SLI and typically developing L2 learners alike. The results present a significant diagnostic dilemma. After all, if the same 'symptom' is identified in children with SLI as well as in second language learners, how does one correctly diagnose bilingual children with SLI, based, that is, on their second language skills? Consequently, Paradis (2005) suggests that typically developing L2 learners can be mistaken for children with SLI precisely because both groups of children show similar problems with grammatical morphology.

Because in this type of study only typically developing bilingual children are included, the outcomes can only be tangentially related to bilingual SLI. Nevertheless, it highlights the potential confusion that makes it harder to apply the diagnostic label. The clear implication is that the monolingual symptoms of SLI in the target language cannot be taken as valid markers for *bilingual* SLI (in the children's L2 output). In L2 learners, these are part of typical development. This is not a trivial conclusion in a situation where the identification of SLI in bilingual children is (owing to lack of diagnostic tools for L1) often based on their L2 performance.

16.2.1.3   *Successive bilingual children with SLI (L2) and monolingual children with SLI*

When speech therapists deal with bilingual children with language impairment, what may draw their clinical attention is the way in which the L2 of these children (which usually is also the language the therapists speak themselves) resembles or differs from that of monolingual children with SLI for whom the same language is their L1.

If there is a difference (in terms of the severity of the disorder) between monolingual and bilingual children with SLI, this may indicate that bilingualism is an additional burden for language-impaired children (a claim that not everybody subscribes to, witness the two-monolinguals-in-one assumption). Another hypothesis is that differences may point at specific markers of *bilingual* SLI in the L2. Of course, for both these hypotheses an additional control group of typically developing bilingual children must be entered into the comparison.

Crutchley, Botting, and Conti-Ramsden (1997) undertook a large cohort study among English children with language delay. Their aim was primarily an educational one: to identify the factors that led to placement in special education. Monolingual English-speaking children and bilingual children were compared. Both groups were attending language units. Linguistically, it appeared that the bilingual children were more likely to have problems with syntax and also morphology and less likely to have difficulties only with phonology and articulation. Moreover, their problems tended to be receptive as well as expressive. Crutchley (1999) hypothesized that the differences might also be a matter of diagnostic bias. The morphosyntactic symptoms might be more obvious to the observer – and thus lead to referral to special care – whereas phonological problems might at first glance reflect typical patterns in second language learners rather than pathology.

16.2.1.4   *Successive bilingual children with SLI (L1) and monolingual children with SLI*

Comparisons with monolingual speakers of L1 should be considered with some caution, since there are factors at work that may contaminate the data. It is common in Western Europe that successive bilinguals are children from immigrant families, whereas their monolingual peers live in their country of origin. The language environment with regard to L1 for both populations is often quite different. The L1 input may be affected by attrition in the immigrant adults. In addition, the child may in time show a relative preference for L2 and in so doing neglect the L1 to some extent. Schiff-Myers (1992) even mentions the possibility of 'arrested development' in L1.

A practical problem in comparing the L1 of monolingual and bilingual speakers is that for many languages information on monolingual SLI is extremely sparse. This is certainly true for minority languages in Western Europe like Turkish, Arabic and Berber. The results of a comparison of two bilingual groups (with and without SLI) in the immigrant country may be in fact the first indication of the form of monolingual SLI in the L1.

16.2.1.5   *Simultaneous bilingual children with SLI and monolingual children with SLI*

Paradis, Crago, Genesee, and Rice (2003) also compared monolinguals and bilinguals. However, their subjects were French-English simultaneous bilingual children with SLI, who were compared to French children without SLI and to monolingual children with SLI in either language. Of course, in simultaneous bilingualism, there is no real distinction between L1 and L2. Paradis and colleagues found similarities between the two groups. Tense problems appeared in all language-impaired children, both the bilingual group and the monolingual groups. Non-tense morphemes fared better in both groups. The authors conclude that this suggests that (given the absence of disproportionate problems among the bilinguals) children with SLI can learn two languages. Bilingualism is not a 'risk factor' (cf. Genesee, 1987), even for children with SLI.

Paradis, Crago, and Genesee (2005/2006) investigated acquisition of object pronouns in French-English bilingual children with SLI. They used monolingual controls for both languages. Interestingly, they were also able to include a group of younger typically developing bilingual children matched on MLU in words. This type of matching is not yet common practice in research on bilingual SLI, for reasons outlined below. For the French data, they also included monolingual controls (with and without SLI). The bilingual children with SLI resembled the younger typically developing bilinguals and the monolingual children with SLI. The resemblance showed in the vulnerability of French object clitics across groups. As in their earlier research, the claim that bilingualism is an extra burden for children with SLI was not supported. If that were the case, bilingual children with SLI should differ from their typically developing counterparts and from the monolingual children with SLI.

The conclusion that SLI is not an impediment for learning two languages may be premature, though. After all, this claim has not yet been tested within a similar design for successive L2 learners whose first language is a minority language. The outcome in such groups might be different, since the situation for those language learners seems to be more adverse (see Genesee, Paradis, & Crago, 2004).

16.2.1.6   Bilingual children with SLI and typically developing bilinguals

In research on monolingual SLI, comparison with normal controls is used to identify characteristics that form a profile of SLI. As mentioned before, this is usually done by matching the groups on a language measure. The resulting hallmarks of impairment are seen as 'clinical markers' or even 'phenotypic markers' of SLI. Similar comparisons in bilingual children have a related aim. In such studies, group comparisons are undertaken to find symptoms of bilingual SLI in the L2 (e.g. Jacobson & Schwartz, 2005). However, the research here is, as it were, one step behind. Whereas in monolingual SLI a difference with chronological age peers is often taken for granted and matching by language age (LA) is favored, studies on bilingual children with language delay usually include only a control group matched on chronological age (CA). Only when differences with CA peers have been established can a language-matching paradigm be considered. The Paradis, Crago, and Genesee (2005/2006) study is a notable exception. Since they could make a comparison between two languages for which symptoms of monolingual SLI are well known, MLU matching was feasible.

Jacobson and Schwartz (2005) focused on English past-tense morphology in two groups of sequential bilingual Spanish-English speakers (age 7;0–9;0). They found differences in the profiles of language-impaired (LI) and typically developing children (the study did not refer to SLI "because standardized test scores necessary to meet the criterion for classification of SLI were not available" (Jacobson & Schwartz, 1995, p. 314[1]). Not only did the LI children produce more errors, there was also a qualitative difference between the two groups. Children with LI performed better on irregular verbs, the typically developing group on regular verbs. The normally developing children also produced more productive error types (overregularizations) while the LI children produced more omissions. The authors propose that an error analysis based on these findings may be helpful in the diagnosis of LI in bilingual children.

Salameh, Håkansson, and Nettelbladt (2004; see also Håkansson, Salameh, & Nettelbladt, 2003) investigated Swedish-Arabic preschool children with SLI and CA-matched controls longitudinally. They investigated both L1 and L2. Their comparison was done within the framework of processability theory (PT; Pienemann, 1998). In PT, a hierarchy of processing requisites is assumed. The levels differ in the extent to which grammatical information is exchanged. Grammatical development starts with no exchange (unanalyzed forms), via marking of plurals on nouns and agreement within the phrase to exchange of information between phrases (as in subject–verb agreement). The top level is subordination of clauses. For each of the two languages, structures were elicited that represented each of the PT levels. For Arabic, this was only possible for the first three levels, due to characteristics of the language (Arabic is a pro-drop language where overt subject is optional; subordination is not obligatory). The ordering of the levels is implicational by hypothesis: children should master one level before the next. The children with SLI did indeed develop each language in the same implicational way that the controls showed. However, they showed delay in both of their languages, although there were individual differences. Direct comparison across languages is notoriously difficult. The PT model, Salameh et al. (2004) suggest, allows for an assessment of progress in L1 and L2.

The study of Salameh, Håkansson, and Nettelbladt (2004) is a rare example of a comparison between two languages in successive bilinguals with SLI. As mentioned before, research on monolingual SLI has a strong cross-linguistic tradition (Leonard, 1998). It is worth noting that gathering data from two languages from a single child has a significant benefit: "the bilingual child comes close to being the 'perfect matched pair'" (De Houwer, 1990, p. 1). Paradis, Crago, Genesee, and Rice (2003) quote this line because it is highly relevant for research on SLI. SLI is known for its heterogeneity. This heterogeneity is multiplied in cross-linguistic comparison and augmented by other subject variables. Comparing two languages in the same (impaired) child offers a partial resolution of the problem. Therefore, in current projects in Hamburg and Amsterdam, L1 (i.e. Turkish) data are collected as well as data from L2 (German and Dutch, respectively). A comparison between the two data sets will add information about cross-linguistic discrepancies and similarities in SLI.

16.2.2   What do these approaches contribute to our understanding of bilingual SLI?

Bilingual SLI has only recently become a research topic in its own right. As the discussion of the research above shows, much of the literature is of a very recent date. The research field is gradually expanding, for various reasons. The languages studied are different across countries and this is often due to demographic developments that create distinct diagnostic needs. The research focus illustrates this. In Europe much attention is devoted to immigrant children whose L1 is a minority language (an increasing part of the population). In the United States, the many children who speak Spanish and English are widely investigated. In Canada, the same is true for bilingual French-English speakers (whether simultaneous or successive), who naturally constitute a large part of the population.

The comparisons reviewed above illuminate part of the puzzling question of what bilingual SLI is. So far, more similarities than differences have been identified between monolingual SLI and bilingual SLI (or even typical bilinguals),[2] although it is too early to consider the evidence conclusive. Some researchers (e.g. Jacobson & Schwartz, 2005) have found differential patterns for bilingual children with SLI. Pert and Letts (2006) propose that code-switching patterns may also be indicative of SLI: since children with SLI have difficulties with grammatical morphology, they may face problems in code switching. The body of evidence on unique patterns in bilingual SLI is still extremely limited and more direct comparisons between successive bilinguals with and without SLI await us. It seems that there is a movement away from comparisons between monolingual SLI and second language learning towards research that directly addresses bilingual SLI (impaired vs. normal).

The similarities found between bilingual SLI on the one hand and monolingual SLI and typical L2 on the other seem to disprove the claim that bilingualism has a taxing effect on children with SLI. Therefore researchers have volunteered the opinion that children with SLI can indeed learn a second language (Genesee, Paradis, & Crago, 2004). This position is at odds with the advice sometimes given to parents to withhold a second language from the language-impaired child because it has enough trouble dealing with one language. Of course, parents from immigrant families do not have that choice in the first place since they and their children have to acquire the L2 in order to be able to lead their lives in the host country.

An intriguing question is what sort of theory will guide future research. So far, part of the research has started from theories about second language learning or normal development as in the case of Pienemann (1998). Other studies test hypotheses that have been formulated for the linguistic explanations of monolingual SLI. An example is the Paradis, Crago, Genesee, and Rice (2003) study, which departs from the Extended Optional Infinitive account (Rice, Wexler, & Cleave, 1995). So far, theories for L2 acquisition or for SLI have been applied to bilingual SLI, but not in tandem. It is not yet clear what type of theory will explain bilingual SLI. Of course, explanations of bilingual SLI should also outline the role of familiar factors in L2 success, like language dominance, language attitude, language status, and time of exposure.

16.3   Bilingual Aphasia

There are parallels between issues in the study of bilingual SLI and in that of bilingual aphasia. Grosjean's (1989) exhortation "Neurolinguists, beware! The bilingual is not two monolinguals in one person" defines an issue that is also addressed in SLI research: is the language impairment simply equivalent in both languages? In aphasia as well as SLI, cross-linguistic comparisons have been made of the symptoms of the disorder (see the review by Bates, Wulfeck and MacWhinney, 1991).

The most pertinent issue in bilingual aphasia is the different recovery patterns that are encountered in aphasic bilinguals (see the survey in Paradis, 2004). The most common pattern is one where both languages are equally affected and recovery is similar: 'parallel recovery'. If there *is* a difference in recovery, this may reflect a difference in premorbid fluency between the two languages. Recovery can also be 'differential'. If so, the recovery *contradicts* the premorbid situation: the language least mastered recovers best. In the case of 'antagonistic recovery' only one language is available first, then to be replaced by the other, and so on. In the case of 'blending recovery' the two languages are mixed in a way that does not occur in healthy speakers. Finally, in 'selective aphasia' only one language is affected at all; this is, of course, an aphasia type, not a recovery pattern. It should be noted that very few cases have been described of the less common (non-parallel) recovery patterns, so the evidence for their status is not yet conclusive.

A major factor in the recovery process is the premorbid language status: the level of fluency in two languages is seldom identical. One language was usually stronger than the other. But what does 'stronger' mean? The native language? The language most familiar? The language most useful? Paradis (2004) considers several explanations for the recovery of language function in bilingual aphasics that all depend on the answer given to these questions. There is a parallel to similar discussions in the development of L2 in children, where the notion of a stronger language also surfaces. Is L1 the first language? The stronger language, the one best mastered? The language of the mother? The language belonging to the domestic culture?

Some authors have argued for the existence of 'differential aphasia', in which a different type of aphasia would be present in the two languages of the aphasic person. Paradis (2004) critically reviews several cases of differential bilingual aphasia (aphasia research, more than research in SLI, has a rich tradition of case studies).[3] He does not find the evidence convincing. An example is the case of a patient who spoke English and Hebrew. Agrammatism in English results in the omission of morphemes. Substitution of morphemes, on the other hand, is characteristic of paragrammatism in English. In Hebrew, however, substitution of morphemes is seen as part of agrammatism. Traditionally, agrammatism is associated with Broca's aphasia; paragrammatism is identified with Wernicke's aphasia. It is thus clear how differential diagnoses, and the use of certain diagnostic labels, can be debatable. The cross-linguistic difference compares to those found in SLI studies, where omission errors are found in languages with a sparse morphology and commission errors in languages with a rich morphology.

Research on bilingual aphasia – connected as it is to information about brain pathology – has drawn much attention because it adds to our knowledge of how language (in this case: *two* languages) is organized in the brain. Paradis's (2004) monograph provides an in-depth discussion of these contributions. This, however, is beyond the scope of this chapter.

16.4   Assessment

16.4.1   Assessment in children

In establishing the nature of language impairment in bilingual children, one has to carefully document the child's language history and present language situation. The subsequent formal measurement assessment of language, however, is a matter for discussion. The problems of misclassification mentioned earlier are naturally associated with shortcomings in the available diagnostic tools. Again, these concern the instruments for L2. If diagnosis on the basis of L1 were universally possible, the diagnostic confusion would probably not be so serious.

Gutiérrez-Clellen (1996) gives a review of assessment in the context of language diversity. It is worth listing some of her reservations. First of all, language tests often show a major lack of sensitivity and specificity when dealing with bilingual children. This results, for instance, in the common finding that on language tests an ample majority of bilingual children score one or more standard deviations below the mean for typically developing children of their age group. Of course, the test should specifically isolate only children with language delay and no others. Failure to do so leads to many cases of 'mistaken identity'. This effect was demonstrated by Paradis (2005) for the *Test of Early Grammatical Impairment* (Rice & Wexler, 2001). The majority of her typically developing bilingual subjects fell within the clinical range on this test (an effect, by the way, predicted by the test's manual). Gutiérrez-Clellen (1996) shows that even when tests are translated and the reference database is made to include children who share the language background of the child, the bias remains.

There are also problems with the use of spontaneous language. The domain in which this becomes apparent in the most obvious way is grammatical morphology. Any morphological measure covers different ingredients in different languages. The calculation of MLU across languages is a good example. The MLU of children who learn a language with a rich morphology is not equivalent to the MLU of children who learn a more analytic language like English (for an extensive review of this and other problems that affect language samples in bilinguals, exemplified by Spanish and English, see Gutiérrez-Clellen, Restrepo, Bedore, Peña, & Anderson, 2000).

Because direct measures of language may be biased or because their content is language-specific, language-independent ways of testing performance have been suggested. In the literature it has been hypothesized that deficits in processing speed, working memory or temporal processing underlie the language problems of (monolingual) children with SLI (for a review of the evidence for and against such hypotheses, see Bishop, 1997; Leonard, 1998). As Kohnert, Windsor and Yim (2006) argue, provided the hypothesis makes sense, measures that address such processing skills could be useful in identifying bilingual children with SLI since they are not language-specific. However, their attempt to apply two processing tasks to distinguish bilingual children with LI from typically developing children showed that "performance on these tasks does not provide compelling diagnostic power for separating typically developing bilinguals from monolingual children with LI" (Kohnert, Windsor, & Yim, 2006, p. 19). Still, the results in this study were not unambiguous and it is to be expected that this route for assessment will be explored further.

Another useful approach is dynamic assessment ('test–teach–test'), where the child's capacity to learn is probed instead of language level *per se* (Crutchley, 1999; Peña, Quinn, & Iglesias, 1992).

16.4.2   Assessment of bilingual aphasia

For aphasia, an instrument has been developed that is only intended for use with bilinguals: The Bilingual Aphasia Test (BAT; Paradis & Libben, 1987). The aim is to broaden the diagnostics of aphasia: in aphasia, as in SLI, assessment is often done for one language only.

The BAT consists of three parts. Part A contains a questionnaire about the patient's language history. The aim is to make an inventory of the premorbid language situation. Part B assesses the proficiency in each of the two languages separately. It contains numerous tasks addressing all modalities: hearing, speaking, reading, writing. Part C focuses on bilingualism directly and explicitly. For instance, grammaticality judgments are elicited for features where the languages contrast, and the patients are asked to translate words or sentences between the two languages. Test materials are available for numerous languages and language pairs.

One of the considerations underlying the structure of the BAT is also valid for (S)LI in children. It picks up an issue discussed earlier in this chapter. Paradis (2004, p. 74) argues that if one wants to measure two languages with comparable instruments, equivalency criteria should be adopted: "a sentence with structural complexity equivalent to an English passive . . . may require an altogether different construction in another language (e.g., a cleft object construction). In other words, if the equivalence criterion is syntactic complexity, a structure of similar complexity (quite possibly not the passive) must be selected." This recalls the study by Salameh, Håkansson, and Nettelbladt (2004), who attempted to pinpoint structures of similar complexity in order to assess the level of the two languages spoken by their bilingual subjects.

NOTES

1   This hiatus affects many other studies of bilingual (S)LI as well, although not all researchers shy away from the term SLI.
2   Kay-Raining Bird, Cleave, Trudeau, et al. (2005) compared bilingual and monolingual children with Down syndrome. There was no difference between the groups on the English language tests used in this study.
3   Fabbro (1999) also gives an overview of the history of research in bilingual aphasia, and summarizes the 'classic' cases in the literature.

REFERENCES

Bates, E., Wulfeck, B., and B. MacWhinney (1991). Cross-linguistic research in aphasia: An overview. *Brain and Language*, 41, 123–48.
Bishop, D. V. M. (1997). *Uncommon Understanding: Development and Disorders of Language Comprehension in Children*. Hove: Psychology Press.

Crutchley, A. (1999). Bilingual children with SLI attending language units: Getting the bigger picture. *Child Language Teaching and Therapy*, 15, 201–17.

Crutchley, A., Botting, N., and Conti-Ramsden, G. (1997). Bilingualism and specific language impairment in children attending language units. *European Journal of Disorders of Communication*, 32, 226–36.

De Houwer, A. (1990). *The Acquisition of Two Languages from Birth: A Case Study*. Cambridge: Cambridge University Press.

DeThorne, L. S., Johnson, B. W., and Loeb, J. (2005). A closer look at MLU: What does it really measure? *Clinical Linguistics and Phonetics*, 19, 635–48.

Fabbro, F. (1999). *The Neurolinguistics of Bilingualism: An Introduction*. Hove, Sussex: Psychology Press.

Genesee, F. (1987). Bilingual language development in preschool children. In D. Bishop and K. Mogford (eds.), *Language Development in Exceptional Circumstances*. Hove, Sussex: Erlbaum.

Genesee, F., Paradis, J., and Crago, M. B. (2004). *Dual Language Development and Disorders: A Handbook on Bilingualism and Second Language Learning*. Baltimore, MD: Brookes.

Grosjean, F. (1989). Neurolinguists, beware! The bilingual is not two monolinguals in one person. *Brain and Language*, 36, 3–15.

Gutiérrez-Clellen, V. F. (1996). Language diversity: implications for assessment. In K. N. Cole, P. S. Dale, and D. J. Thal (eds.), *Assessment of Communication and Language*. Baltimore, MD: Brookes.

Gutiérrez-Clellen, V. F., Restrepo, M. A., Bedore, L., Peña, E., and Anderson, R. (2000). Language sample analysis in Spanish-speaking children: Methodological considerations. *Language, Speech and Hearing Services in Schools*, 31, 88–98.

Håkansson, G. (2001). Tense morphology and verb-second in Swedish L1 children, L2 children and children with SLI. *Bilingualism: Language and Cognition*, 4, 85–99.

Håkansson, G. and Nettelbladt, U. (1996). Similarities between SLI and L2 children: evidence from the acquisition of Swedish word order. In C. E. Johnson and J. H. V. Gilbert (eds.), *Children's Language*, vol. 9. Mahwah, NJ: Erlbaum.

Håkansson, G., Salameh, E.-K., and Nettelbladt, U. (2003). Measuring language development in bilingual children: Swedish-Arabic children with and without language impairment. *Linguistics*, 41, 255–88.

Jacobson, P. F. and Schwartz, R. G. (2002). Morphology in incipient bilingual Spanish-speaking preschool children with specific language impairment. *Applied Psycholinguistics*, 23, 23–41.

Jacobson, P. F. and Schwartz, R. G. (2005). English past tense use in bilingual children with language impairment. *American Journal of Speech-Language Pathology*, 14, 313–23.

Kay-Raining Bird, E., Cleave, P., Trudeau, N., Thordardottir, E., Sutton, A., and Thorpe, A. (2005). The language abilities of bilingual children with Down Syndrome. *American Journal of Speech-Language Pathology*, 14, 187–99.

Kohnert, K., Windsor, J., and Yim, D. (2006). Do language-based processing tasks separate children with language impairment from typical bilinguals? *Learning Disabilities Research and Practice*, 21, 19–29.

Leonard, L. B. (1998). *Children with Specific Language Impairment*. Cambridge, MA: MIT Press.

Morehead, D. and Ingram, D. (1973). The development of base syntax in normal and linguistically deviant children. *Journal of Speech and Hearing Research*, 16, 330–52.

Paradis, J. (2005). Grammatical morphology in children learning English as a second language: Implications of similarities with specific language impairment. *Language, Speech and Hearing Services in Schools*, 36, 172–87.

Paradis, J. (2006). Differentiating between child SLA and SLI: Focus on functional categories. Plenary address given at GASLA (Generative Approaches to Second Language Acquisition), Banff, Alberta.

Paradis, J. and Crago, M. (2000). Tense and temporality: Similarities and differences between language-impaired and second-language children. *Journal of Speech, Language and Hearing Research*, 43, 834–48.

Paradis, J., Crago, M., and Genesee, F. (2005/2006). Domain-general versus domain-specific accounts of specific language impairment: Evidence from bilingual children's acquisition of object pronouns. *Language Acquisition*, 13, 33–62.

Paradis, J., Crago, M., Genesee, F., and Rice, M. (2003). French-English bilingual children with SLI: How do they compare with their monolingual peers? *Journal of Speech, Language and Hearing Research*, 46, 1–15.

Paradis, M. (2004). *A Neurolinguistic Theory of Bilingualism*. Amsterdam/Philadelphia, PA: John Benjamins.

Paradis, M. and Libben, G. (1987). *The Assessment of Bilingual Aphasia*. Hillsdale, NJ: Erlbaum.

Peña, E., Quinn, R., and Iglesias, A. (1992). The application of dynamic methods to language assessment: A nonbiased procedure. *Journal of Special Education*, 26, 269–80.

Pert, S. and Letts, C. (2006). Codeswitching in Mirpuri speaking Pakistani heritage preschool children: Bilingual language acquisition. *International Journal of Bilingualism*, 10, 349–74.

Pienemann, M. (1998). *Language Processing and Second Language Development: Processability Theory*. Amsterdam: John Benjamins.

Plante, E., Swisher, L., Kiernan, B., and Restrepo, M. A. (1993). Language matches: Illuminating or confounding? *Journal of Speech and Hearing Research*, 36, 772–6.

Rice, M. and Wexler, K. (2001). *Test of Early Grammatical Impairment*. New York: Psychological Corporation.

Rice, M., Wexler, K., and Cleave, P. (1995). Specific language impairment as a period of extended optional infinitive. *Journal of Speech, Language and Hearing Research*, 38, 850–63.

Salameh, E.-K., Håkansson, G., and Nettelbladt, U. (2004). Developmental perspectives on bilingual Swedish-Arabic children with and without language impairment: A longitudinal study. *International Journal of Language and Communication Disorders*, 39, 65–90.

Salameh, E.-K., Nettelbladt, U., and Gullberg, B. (2002). Risk factors for language impairment in Swedish bilingual and monolingual children relative to severity. *Acta Paediatrica*, 91, 1379–84.

Salameh, E.-K., Nettelbladt, U., Håkansson, G., and Gullberg, B. (2002). Language impairment in Swedish bilingual children: A comparison between bilingual and monolingual children in Malmö. *Acta Paediatrica*, 91, 229–34.

Schiff-Meyers, N. (1992). Considering arrested language development and language loss in the assessment of second language learners. *Language, Speech and Hearing Services in Schools*, 23, 28–33.

17 Cross-Linguistic Perspectives on the Syntax and Semantics of Language Disorders

MARTHA CRAGO, JOHANNE PARADIS, AND LISE MENN

17.1 Introduction

Comparative study across languages provides a useful and fascinating means of understanding language impairment in both children and adults. This is because symptoms that are prominent in one language may have no counterpart in another language. Speakers of Chinese, Thai or Vietnamese may make errors in the choice of tone for a word, an error type which cannot occur in non-tone languages. Languages that have grammatical noun gender (e.g. French table, *la table*, feminine; coat, *le manteau*, masculine) afford the possibility of gender errors, and furthermore of gender agreement errors, because in these languages, the forms of adjectives (e.g. *blanc/blanche* 'white') must agree in gender with the noun they modify (*la table blanche, le manteau blanc*). French speakers with language disorders may have difficulty choosing the adjective form that has the correct gender, but English, Chinese, and Japanese have no grammatical gender, and therefore no gender agreement, so no comparable symptom can emerge. Using these similarities and differences between languages, the comparative study of language impairment can tease apart the universal from the variable aspects of language deficits. This, in turn, helps to determine which theories of language disorders can best explain the nature of the deficit.

There have been cross-linguistic studies of childhood developmental language disorders as well as of adult-acquired language disorders. The majority of these studies have focused on the language deficits of individuals who have one of two particular disorders, childhood-specific language impairment (SLI) and adult-acquired aphasia. Each of these two populations is described in turn; then follows a summary of the cross-linguistic findings pertinent to the nature of each of these populations' language deficits. Since the cross-linguistic studies of SLI are predominantly focused on morphosyntax, these studies will be reported according to various groups of languages. On the other hand, research on adult-acquired aphasia is usually based on various syndromes of aphasia, and, hence, the results of cross-linguistic studies are more appropriately reported on when based on the specific nature of the deficit displayed in various syndromes.

17.2   Specific Language Impairment

SLI is a developmental language-learning disorder whose effects can extend across the lifespan. Children with SLI exhibit language delay in the early years, and once language emerges they show deficits in the areas of pragmatics, the lexicon and morphosyntax when compared to same-aged, typically developing peers. The relative difficulty individual children with SLI have in each of these domains is subject to variation, making them a fairly heterogeneous population. The diagnostics for this disorder involve both inclusionary and exclusionary criteria. The latter consist of ruling out other possible etiologies of language disorder, such as mental retardation, or hearing impairment, and inclusionary criteria include below-age expectations in performance on omnibus standardized tests of language development and/or in performance with targeted structures such as finite verb morphology or mean length of utterance. See also chapters 10 (Clahsen), 12 (Marinis), 13 (Penke), 16 (de Jong), and 18 (Black & Chiat) in this volume for further discussion of SLI.

For some languages other than English, appropriate tools for diagnosis are often not widely available, which restricts the ability of researchers to conduct cross-linguistic comparisons of clinical groups with confidence. However, there has been a recent interest in establishing diagnostic criteria for SLI across different languages, and this research indicates that the presence of key symptoms in the lexical and morphosyntactic domains seems to hold across languages (Bortolini, Caselli, Deevy, & Leonard, 2002; Klee, Stokes, Wong, Fletcher, & Gavin, 2004).

17.3   Adult-Acquired Aphasia

Aphasia is defined as language damage due to relatively localized brain damage. This definition excludes the language problems associated with massive head trauma, general dementia and other forms of widespread damage to the brain and cognition. Adult acquired aphasia, affecting a fully developed and relatively stable language system, has clinical symptoms different from those associated with impairment in a young child's rapidly developing slanguage. Adults with aphasia are typically survivors of strokes, but they also include people with localized brain tumors (pre- and post-surgery), localized brain trauma, and a rare degenerative disorder, primary progressive aphasia. Certain recurrent and traditionally recognized constellations of aphasia symptoms are called aphasia syndromes. Aphasia syndromes are divided into fluent and nonfluent aphasias. The fluent aphasias include anomia and Wernicke's aphasia; the principal nonfluent aphasia syndrome of interest is agrammatic Broca's aphasia.

17.4   Cross-Linguistic Research on SLI

There is no consensus among researchers on the precise deficits that underlie SLI. Researchers disagree on whether the language difficulties displayed by children with SLI are caused by specific deficits in linguistic representation/ knowledge or by more general cognitive deficits in information processing that impact most noticeably on language. There is also no consensus on which linguistic characteristics of SLI are merely delayed in acquisition with respect to same-aged children with typical language development (TLD), and which display deviant or disrupted development, i.e., where affected children show distinct or uneven profiles compared to younger, language-matched children who are typically developing (see Leonard, 1998, 2003, and Rice, 2003 for further discussion). Cross-linguistic comparative research is essential for elucidating both the underlying cause of SLI and the delay vs. deviance or disruption issues because, presumably, the nature of this disorder should be the same regardless of which and how many languages are spoken by the child. Thus, SLI cannot be a processing-based deficit in one language but not in another, or show only delay manifestations in one language but deviant manifestations in another.

Most linguistically based studies of SLI across languages have concentrated on the search for clinical markers, defined briefly as linguistic characteristics or profiles that distinguish the clinical from the non-clinical population (see Rice, 2003 for elaboration). The degree to which clinical markers are language-specific or display tendencies across languages has been a key focus of this research. Thus, clinical markers research has direct relevance both to applied interests such as developing sound cross-linguistic diagnostic criteria, and to addressing the theoretical questions just mentioned. Studies focusing on syntactic constructions or semantic knowledge have been underrepresented in cross-linguistic research on SLI, as most studies focus on grammatical morphology. As will be demonstrated in the following sections related to various groups of languages, most of the cross-linguistic research on SLI has been focused on morphosyntactic deficits. However, recently, some research has emerged on lexical semantics in Hebrew SLI (Ravid, Levie, & Avivi Ben-Zvi, 2003), *wh*-questions in Cantonese SLI (Wong, Leonard, Fletcher, & Stokes, 2004) and relative clauses in Hebrew and Swedish SLI (Friedmann & Novogrodsky, 2004; Håkansson & Hansson, 2000).

17.4.1   *SLI in Germanic languages*

The greatest amount of research on SLI has been conducted on Germanic languages, notably English. Children with SLI who speak English have more pronounced difficulties with finite-verb morphology, such as verb inflections, auxiliaries and copulas, than they do with grammatical morphemes in the nominal domain, such as plural [-s], and intermittently omit finite verb morphology morphemes well into the school-age years (Bedore & Leonard, 1998; Rice, 2003; Rice & Wexler, 1996). Research on Dutch, German and Swedish confirms that difficulty with finite-verb morphology is characteristic of SLI across Germanic languages (de Jong, 2003; Hansson, 1997; Rice, Ruff Noll, & Grimm, 1997; Roberts & Leonard, 1997). In Swedish, the verb-second phenomenon, a word-order rule related to finiteness, also causes difficulty for children with SLI (Håkansson, 2001; Hansson, Nettelbladt, & Leonard, 2000). In contrast to English, German- and Dutch-speaking children make substitution errors in number and person agreement (Clahsen, Bartke, & Göllner, 1997; de Jong, 2003). Even though difficulties with verb morphology and verb placement are highly prominent, researchers have found that children with SLI acquiring Germanic languages also make errors with articles, and, in Swedish, with other aspects of nominal morphology (Leonard, Salameh, & Hansson, 2001; Rice & Wexler, 1996; Roberts & Leonard, 1997).

17.4.2   *SLI in Romance languages*

Studies of children with SLI acquiring French, Italian and Spanish have shown that these children produce nonfinite verb forms, such as bare past participles, infinitives and null copulas like their peers learning Germanic languages, and as well they make substitution errors with verb morphology marking person, number and tense (Bedore & Leonard, 2001; Bortolini, Caselli, Deevy, & Leonard, 2002; Bortolini, Caselli, & Leonard, 1997; Jakubowicz & Nash, 2001; Paradis & Crago, 2000, 2001). However, errors with verb morphology are a much less prominent feature of Spanish than of Italian and French SLI. On the other hand, Spanish- and Italian-speaking children with SLI both have difficulties with articles (Anderson & Souto, 2005; Bedore & Leonard, 2001, 2005; Bortolini, Caselli, & Leonard, 1997; Bortolini, Caselli, Deevy, & Leonard, 2002; Bottari, Cipriani, Chilosi, & Pfanner, 2001; Restrepo & Gutiérrez-Clellen, 2001), but difficulty with articles is not characteristic of French SLI (Jakubowicz, Nash, Rigaut, & Gérard, 1998; Le Normand, Leonard, & McGregor, 1993; Paradis & Crago, 2004; Paradis, Crago, & Genesee, 2007). The target structure that consistently causes difficulty for Romance-learning children with SLI is object pronouns, which take the form of preverbal clitics in these languages (Bedore & Leonard, 2001; Bortolini, Caselli, Deevy, & Leonard, 2002; Grüter, 2005; Hamann, 2004; Jacobson, & Schwartz, 2002; Jakubowicz, Nash, Rigaut, & Gérard, 1998; Leonard, Bortolini, Caselli, McGregor, & Sabbadini, 1992; J. Paradis, 2004). Children tend to make mainly omission errors with object clitics in French and Italian, while substitution errors are common in Spanish.

17.4.3   SLI in other languages

Among non-European languages, the best-studied with respect to impaired acquisition is Hebrew. Hebrew-speaking children with SLI exhibit inaccuracies with person, number and gender in the production of past-tense morphology, for which there are complex paradigms with person, number and gender marked (Dromi, Leonard, & Shteiman, 1993; Dromi, Leonard, Adam, & Zadunaisky-Ehrlich, 1999; Leonard, Dromi, Adam, & Zadunaisky-Ehrlich, 2000). They also have difficulties with derivational morphology, for example producing denominal adjectives accurately (Ravid, Levie, & Avivi Ben-Zvi, 2003). Turning to East Asian languages, Cantonese does not mark features such as tense, person or number morphologically, but there is a set of verbal aspect morphemes, and children with SLI have prominent difficulties in producing these aspect markers (Fletcher, Leonard, Stokes, & Wong, 2005; Stokes & Fletcher, 2003). In contrast to Cantonese, Japanese has a rich verbal inflectional system, although person and number agreement are not marked, and it also has case-marking particles. Japanese children with SLI make some errors in the choice of case particles, but have more prominent difficulties with the accurate use of verb morphology marking passives and causatives (Tanaka-Welty, Watanabe, & Menn, 2002).

17.4.4   Bilingual children with SLI

Studies of bilingual children with SLI can provide interesting information on how strongly language-specific effects operate on the nature of children's language impairment. There are very few studies of children who are simultaneous bilinguals with SLI. One study by J. Paradis, Crago, and Genesee (2007) has shown that French-English bilingual children with SLI omit object pronominals in their French but not in their English. This illustrates that problems with this structure are specific to Romance languages. Moreover, French-English bilinguals with SLI have difficulties with tense in both languages, and very little trouble with certain non-tense nominal-domain morphemes in either language, mirroring the monolingual SLI patterns (Paradis, Crago, & Genesee, 2007; Paradis, Crago, Genesee, & Rice, 2003). In addition, the degree of difficulty is similar between monolingual and bilingual children with SLI. These results with seven-year-old children with SLI demonstrate that acquiring two languages simultaneously under conditions of impairment does not disrupt language-specific patterns or exacerbate the effects of impairment. See also De Jong, chapter 16 in this volume, for further discussion of bilingual SLI.

17.4.5   Conclusions drawn from cross-linguistic research on SLI

There are no universal cross-linguistic characteristics of SLI, indicating that the underlying deficit causing this disorder interacts with features of the target-language input. However, there are characteristic tendencies, particularly within language families where a number of languages have been compared. Overall, one can expect some grammatical morphemes, either bound or free, to be a locus of difficulty in affected children. Importantly, where multiple morphemes have been examined in one language, children with SLI do not have equal difficulties with all of them, but instead certain morphemes tend to be highly problematic, and constitute clinical markers. In a majority of the languages surveyed, children with SLI displayed mild to severe difficulties with verb-related morphemes marking person, number, tense, aspect, direct objects or voice. There is also a tendency for omission to be more frequent than substitution errors where inflectional paradigms are impoverished, as in English, as opposed to more richly inflected languages like Italian and Hebrew. Furthermore, substitution errors are typically systematic, for instance, errors may consist of just one feature being different from the target, or the least morphophonologically complex form may be substituted more often, acting as a 'default' or 'elsewhere' form (see Dromi, Leonard, Adam, & Zadunaisky-Ehrlich, 1999, 2000; and Paradis & Crago, 2001, for further discussion of substitution patterns and defaults). Finally, whether children with SLI show delay or deviant/disrupted profiles, the problematic morphemes and the errors they make tend not to be unique, but to be present also in the acquisition of children with typical language development (but see Crago & Allen, 2001). In spite of the growing number of cross-linguistic studies, there is still an insufficient number of systematic comparisons of the same morpheme type using the same methodology across languages to enable firm cross-linguistic generalizations, although the work of Laurence Leonard and colleagues is a notable exception.

While no theoretical account to date can explain all documented clinical markers cross-linguistically, continued research into the underlying representational and processing-related properties of these structures is vital to building generalizations of cross-linguistic deficits in SLI and, in turn, to addressing the broader theoretical issues surrounding the nature of this disorder.

17.5   Cross-Linguistic Research on Adult-Acquired Aphasia

17.5.1   Comprehension

17.5.1.1   Syntax studies

Across languages, researchers investigating adult-acquired aphasia have usually found that comprehension of less common sentence patterns is relatively difficult. Clearly, people with aphasia rely on multiple cues for sentence comprehension, including morphological markings and the order of the noun phrases; when these conflict, as in the passive voice, it is not clear what governs their understanding, although much attention has been paid to this problem, especially for agrammatism (Burchert & De Bleser, 2004; Caramazza, Capasso, Capitani, & Miceli, 2005; Hagiwara, 1995; Grodzinsky, 1990; O'Grady & Kim, 2005). Studies of syntax across certain languages have been set up to examine the claims of two major explanatory hypotheses. As with SLI, one major theoretical position is that people with aphasia have a representational deficit. Another theoretical position, also similar to theories of SLI, is that the nature of the deficit is best explained by incapacities for processing of language. For instance, Lee, Hung, Tse, et al. (2005) studied the comprehension of Chinese compound words by speakers with aphasia. Their work supported a psycholinguistic processing-deficit approach to the aphasic comprehension of these words. Jakubowicz and Goldblum (1995) and Nicol, Jakubowicz and Goldblum (1996) studied French- and English-speaking people with aphasia to see whether a representation-based or a construction-based theory would best account for gender/number agreement errors. Their studies suggest that agreement markings within a noun phrase are better preserved than ones in which agreement information has to cross the boundary between a sentence's subject noun phrase and its main verb phrase. This pattern cannot be due simply to a representational deficit, nor to a static problem with agreement *per se*; the difficulty with computing agreement must be compounded either with a problem in working memory or with a limited construction-based computational capacity. Thus, both types of theoretical approaches were partly supported by their data.

17.5.1.2   Word-string interpretation studies

Many comparative experimental studies have used a non-natural but informative comprehension task developed by the late Elizabeth Bates and her international team of co-workers in which participants were presented with a possibly nonsensical string of two nouns and a transitive verb (e.g. 'The cows the pencil kick'). They were then asked to decide which one of the two nouns was the agent of the action described. Each string of words was presented in all possible orders, whether they were grammatical or not in the language in question. Normal speakers of different languages, when they heard one of these odd sequences, differed in the way that they preferred to interpret it; for example, English speakers relied more on word order, but Italian speakers relied more on the noun properties of animate vs. inanimate. The key finding with this method (Bates, Wulfeck, & MacWhinney, 1991; MacWhinney, Bates, & Kliegl, 1984) has been that both people without neurological impairment and people with aphasia show the same language-specific preferences for interpreting these strings; for example, in English, both groups relied more on word order but in Italian they relied more on agreement.

While these results demonstrated that people with agrammatic aphasia could use morphological information such as grammatical suffixes, the Bates group has also shown, across several languages, that morphological cues are the ones most likely to be underutilized by speakers with all forms of aphasia.

17.5.2   Production

Comparative studies of production are difficult to design, because the materials must contain comparable levels of difficulty across languages and cultures, and the details of the elicitation procedure must match. Drawings that are culturally appropriate in one country, for example showing blonde people in bathing suits, may be strange or offensive to people in another culture; words may have no exact translation equivalents, or they may be common in one language but rare in another.

Among the earliest and most important cross-linguistic studies of aphasic narratives were those showing that aphasia in a signed language (American Sign Language) strongly resembles aphasia in spoken language, in spite of very different grammars and totally different production and perception modalities (Bellugi, Poizner, & Klima, 1989). An international team focusing on morphosyntax in agrammatic narratives (Menn & Obler, 1988, 1990a) created a standard elicitation protocol and collected data from two speakers with agrammatic aphasia and two matched control speakers in each of fourteen languages: the non-Indo-European languages Mandarin Chinese, Finnish, Hebrew, and Japanese, and the Indo-European languages Dutch, English, French, German, Hindi, Icelandic, Polish, Serbo-Croatian, and Swedish. Studies of agrammatism in Farsi (Nilipour, 2000) and Korean (Halliwell, 2000) are available in the same format. More focused comparative studies include Ahlsén, Nespoulos, Dordain, et al.'s (1996) research on the noun phrase and Jarema's (1998) work on morphology.

17.5.2.1   Morphology, functors, and clause-level morphosyntax

A variety of production studies, including the narrative-based ones cited above, have supported the following general claims about what is likely to be preserved or impaired in aphasic language. First, grammatical morphemes such as plural endings, past-tense endings, and auxiliary verbs are in general prone to errors. Free grammatical morphemes (those not attached to other words such as auxiliary verbs) tend to be omitted by speakers with nonfluent aphasias, especially agrammatic aphasia. In English, people with agrammatic aphasia tend to omit word endings (plurals, past tense, verb 3rd person singular -s). However, in languages like Italian where virtually every form of a noun, verb, or adjective has an ending, people with agrammatism make substitution errors, not omission errors. These contradictory-sounding findings can be reconciled because, in English, leaving off an ending is indistinguishable from substituting a form without an ending, e.g., the singular of a noun, the 1st person singular present tense of a verb. The older literature, heavily influenced by English, described agrammatic aphasia as dominated by omission of endings and function words, and Wernicke's aphasia as dominated by substitution errors. However, cross-linguistic work (e.g. Halliwell, 2000; Slobin, 1991) indicates that both types of aphasia are dominated by substitution errors in grammatical endings, although omission of function words is, indeed, common. The substitution errors do differ qualitatively across syndromes: agrammatic aphasic substitution errors in morphology and syntax tend to be only one semantic feature away from the target (an error in gender, number, case or tense), while Wernicke's substitution errors are scattered more randomly across the paradigm of a word's forms (Menn & Obler, 1990b; Slobin, 1991).

Another major conclusion from this body of research is that the greater the semantic importance of a morpheme, the more likely it is to be produced. For example, negation is almost never omitted (Menn & Obler, 1990b). The larger the paradigm of choices for a given form, the more likely it is that substitution errors will be made; for example, many more errors are made in German definite articles, which have three genders, singular and plural and four cases, than in French where definite articles have only three forms, masculine, feminine, and plural (Bates, Wulfeck, & MacWhinney, 1991; M. Paradis, 2001). The direction of errors is variable. Sometimes masculine is substituted for feminine, and sometimes the reverse. However, the more frequent forms of a given word are more likely to be produced correctly (Dressler, 1991). For example, if plural is more frequent than singular for a particular word, plural endings may be added erroneously. Commonly, the present tense is used where past is required, but at least some people with agrammatism in Korean (Halliwell, 2000) and Arabic (Mimouni & Jarema, 1997) show a preference for the past tense.

Most substitution errors, especially those made by people with nonfluent aphasia, are mis-selections from existing paradigms. However, a few substitutions involve the creation of non-existent forms from existing morphemes, notably some instances in Basque (Laka & Erriondo Korostola, 2001), or the production of non-existent stem forms, for example in Swedish (Månsson & Ahlsén, 2001).

17.5.2.2   *Syntactic structures*

People with severe nonfluent aphasia may have very few words that appear in phrases, except for idioms and extremely frequent phrases such as 'I don't know'. However, when they use isolated words such as 'tired', they actually express predications as in 'She's tired', 'I'm tired', 'At that time, I was always tired'. To interpret such single-word utterances properly, their interlocutors must rely on pragmatic context and the person's gestures and intonation contours.

People with aphasia who can put words into phrases tend to rely on the basic word order of the language they speak, e.g. Subject–Verb–Object or Subject–Object–Verb. However, nonfluent speakers who can put words into simple sentences often still lack prenominal modifiers ('the red car') except for numbers, and they often have particular difficulties with expressions describing spatial location. The same may be true for fluent speakers, but fewer data are available for them. Definite and indefinite articles may be omitted by agrammatic speakers; the postposed definite article in Swedish (and other Scandinavian languages) may be easier than the prenominal articles of other Germanic and Romance languages (Månsson & Ahlsén, 2001; Havik & Bastiaanse, 2004).

Nonfluent speakers of a number of different languages have been shown to attempt few complex constructions. They are most likely to use the simple direct quotation ('she said', 'I think') and the chaining of main clauses with 'and then . . . and then'. If they do produce an embedded clause, they rarely succeed in returning to and completing the main clause. Bates et al. (1999) pointed out, however, that people with aphasia are more likely to attempt and produce non-canonical word order in languages that use such an order more often, e.g. Italian, as compared to English.

17.5.3 Bilingual aphasia

Bilingualism and multiple dialect use are present in most of the world's population. M. Paradis (2001) includes contributions on non-Indo-European Basque and Hungarian, and on the Indo-European languages Afrikaans, Catalan, Czech, Farsi (Persian), Friulian, Greek, and Spanish, as well as material on African American English, Finnish, Polish, Hebrew, and Swedish.

Bilingual people with aphasia may recover one of their languages better than another; sometimes it is the person's recently most-used language, sometimes the first language, sometimes neither. A few cases have been reported in which a bilingual person's aphasic symptoms in one of their languages seemed quite different from those in another of their languages, but this is rare (M. Paradis, 1983). Experimental studies of bilinguals, such as the work of de Diego Balaguer, Costa, Sebastián-Galles, Juncadella and Caramazza (2004) on the Spanish-Catalan regular and irregular verb morphology in agrammatism, has provided valuable insights into issues of where language is represented and processed in the bilingual brain. (See chapter 16 in this volume for additional information on bilingual impairment.)

17.5.4 Bi-dialectal aphasia and aphasia in second-language speakers

The usages of a non-standard dialect and the patterns of aphasic speech may be similar in certain cases, e.g. omission of 3rd person singular '-s' or an auxiliary verb ('he go' or 'he going' instead of 'he goes' or 'he is going'). Careful testing, a good personal history of the individual, and information on pre-stroke language forms are required to avoid inappropriate diagnoses. For example, it would be inappropriate to consider omission of articles ('the', 'a') as a consequence of aphasia if the client had been a native speaker of a language without articles, such as Chinese or Russian, and had learned English as an adult.

17.6 Conclusion

The comparative study of language impairment across languages has provided critical insights into the nature of deficits in both children and adults. It has also helped to establish appropriate language-specific diagnostic measures and informed theoretical explanations. Such research capitalizes on one of mankind's greatest treasures, the diversity of spoken languages, and is important in preserving such languages and rehabilitating the individuals who speak them.

REFERENCES

Ahlsén, E., Nespoulous, J.-L., Dordain, M., Stark, J., Jarema, G., Kadzielawa, D., Obler, L. K., and Fitzpatrick, P. M. (1996). Noun-phrase production by agrammatic patients: A cross-linguistic approach. *Aphasiology*, 10, 543–60.

Anderson, R. and Souto, S. (2005). The use of articles by monolingual Puerto Rican Spanish-speaking children with specific language impairment. *Applied Psycholinguistics*, 26, 621–48.

Bates, E., Wulfeck, B., and MacWhinney, B. (1991). Cross-linguistic studies of aphasia: An overview. Special issue on cross-linguistic studies of aphasia (E. Bates, ed.). *Brain and Language*, 41(2), 123–48.

Bedore, L. and Leonard, L. (1998). Specific language impairment and grammatical morphology: A discriminant function analysis. *Journal of Speech, Language and Hearing Research*, 41, 1185–92.

Bedore, L. and Leonard, L. (2001). Grammatical morphology deficits in Spanish-speaking children with specific language impairment. *Journal of Speech, Language and Hearing Research*, 44, 905–24.

Bedore, L. and Leonard, L. (2005). Verb inflections and noun phrase morphology in the spontaneous speech of Spanish-speaking children with specific language impairment. *Applied Psycholinguistics*, 26, 195–226.

Bellugi, U., Poizner, H., and Klima, E. S. (1989). Language, modality, and the brain. *Trends in Neurosciences*, 10, 380–8.

Bortolini, U., Caselli, M.-C., Deevy, P., and Leonard, L. (2002). Specific language impairment in Italian: The first steps in the search for a clinical marker. *International Journal of Language and Communication Disorders*, 37, 77–93.

Bortolini, U., Caselli, M.-C., and Leonard, L. (1997). Grammatical deficits in Italian speaking children with specific language impairment. *Journal of Speech, Language and Hearing Research*, 40, 809–20.

Bottari, P., Cipriani, P., Chilosi, A.-M., and Pfanner, L. (2001). The Italian determiner system in normal acquisition, specific language impairment, and childhood aphasia. *Brain and Language*, 77, 283–93.

Burchert, F. and De Bleser, R. (2004). Passives in agrammatic sentence comprehension: A German study. *Aphasiology*, 18, 29–45.

Caramazza, A., Capasso, R., Capitani, E., and Miceli, G. (2005). Patterns of comprehension performance in agrammatic Broca's aphasia: A test of the Trace Deletion Hypothesis. *Brain and Language*, 94, 43–53.

Clahsen, H., Bartke, S., and Göllner, S. (1997). Formal features in impaired grammars: A comparison of English and German SLI children. *Journal of Neurolinguistics*, 10, 151–71.

Crago, M. and Allen, S. (2001). Early finiteness in Inuktitut: The role of language structure and input. *Language Acquisition*, 9, 59–111.

de Diego Balaguer, R., Costa, A., Sebastián-Galles, N., Juncadella, M., and Caramazza, A. (2004). Regular and irregular morphology and its relationship with agrammatism: Evidence from two Spanish–Catalan bilinguals. *Brain and Language*, 91, 212–22.

de Jong, J. (2003). Specific language impairment and linguistic explanation. In Y. Levy and J. Schaeffer (eds.), *Language Competence across Populations: Toward a Definition of Specific Language Impairment* (pp. 151–70). Mahwah, NJ: Erlbaum.

Dressler, W. U. (1991). The sociolinguistic and patholinguistic attrition of Breton phonology, morphology, and morphonology. In H. W. Seliger and R. M. Vago (eds.), *First Language Attrition* (pp. 99–112). Cambridge: Cambridge University Press.

Dromi, E., Leonard, L., and Shteiman, M. (1993). The grammatical morphology of Hebrew-speaking children with specific language impairment: Some competing hypotheses. *Journal of Speech, Language and Hearing Research*, 36, 760–71.

Dromi, E., Leonard, L., Adam, G., and Zadunaisky-Ehrlich, S. (1999). Verb agreement morphology in Hebrew-speaking children with specific language impairment. *Journal of Speech, Language and Hearing Research*, 42, 1414–31.

Fletcher, P., Leonard, L., Stokes, S., and Wong, A. M.-Y. (2005). The expression of aspect in Cantonese-speaking children with specific language impairment. *Journal of Speech, Language and Hearing Research*, 48, 621–34.

Friedmann, N. and Novogrodsky, R. (2004). The acquisition of relative clause comprehension in Hebrew: A study of SLI and normal development. *Journal of Child Language*, 31, 661–81.

Grodzinsky, Y. (1990). *Theoretical Perspectives on Language Deficits*. Cambridge, MA: MIT Press.

Grüter, T. (2005). Comprehension and production of French object clitics by child second language learners and children specific language impairment. *Applied Psycholinguistics*, 26(3), 363–92.

Hagiwara, H. (1995). The breakdown of functional categories and the economy of derivation. *Brain and Language*, 50, 92–116.

Håkansson, G. (2001). Tense morphology and verb-second in Swedish L1 chidlren, L2 children and children with SLI. *Bilingualism: Language and Cognition*, 4, 85–99.

Håkansson, G. and Hansson, K. (2000). Comprehension and production of relative clauses: A comparison between Swedish impaired and unimpaired children. *Journal of Child Language*, 27, 313–33.

Halliwell, John F. (2000). Korean agrammatic production. *Aphasiology*, 14, 1187–1204.

Hamann, C. (2004). Comparing the development of the nominal and the verbal functional domain in French language impairment. In P. Prévost and J. Paradis (eds.), *The Acquisition of French in Different Contexts: Focus on Functional Categories* (pp. 109–46). Amsterdam: Benjamins.

Hansson, K. (1997). Patterns of verb usage in Swedish children with SLI: An application of recent theories. *First Language*, 17, 195–217.

Hansson, K., Nettelbladt, U., and Leonard, L. (2000). Specific language impairment in Swedish: The status of verb morphology and word order. *Journal of Speech, Language and Hearing Research*, 43, 848–64.

Havik, E. and Bastiaanse, R. (2004). Omission of definite and indefinite articles in the spontaneous speech of agrammatic speakers with Broca's aphasia. *Aphasiology*, 18, 1093–1102.

Jakubowicz, C. and Goldblum, M.-C. (1995). Processing of number and gender inflections by French-speaking aphasics. *Brain and Language*, 51, 242–68.

Jakubowicz, C. and Nash, L. (2001). Functional categories and syntactic operations in (ab)normal language acquisition. *Brain and Language*, 77, 321–39.

Jakubowicz, C., Nash, L., Rigaut, C., and Gérard, Ch.-L. (1998). Determiners and clitic pronouns in French-speaking children with SLI. *Language Acquisition*, 7, 113–60.

Jacobson, P. and Schwartz, R. (2002). Morphology in incipient bilingual Spanish-speaking preschool children with specific language impairment. *Applied Psycholinguistics*, 23, 416–33.

Jarema, G. (1998). The breakdown of morphology in aphasia: a cross-linguistic perspective. In B. Stemmer and H. Whitaker (eds.), *Handbook of Neurolinguistics* (pp. 221–34). Orlando, FL: Academic Press.

Klee, T., Stokes, S., Wong, A., Fletcher, P., and Gavin, W. (2004). Utterance length and lexical diversity in Cantonese-speaking children with and without specific language impairment. *Journal of Speech, Language and Hearing Research*, 47, 1396–1410.

Laka, I. and Erriondo Korostola, L. (2001). Aphasia manifestations in Basque. In M. Paradis (ed.), *Manifestations of Aphasia Symptoms in Different Languages* (pp. 49–73). Amsterdam: Pergamon.

Lee, C.-L., Hung, D. L., Tse, J. K.-P., Lee, C.-Y., Tsai, J.-L., and Tzeng, O. J.-L. (2005). Processing of disyllabic compound words in Chinese aphasia: Evidence for the processing limitations account. *Brain and Language*, 92,168–84.

Le Normand, M.-T., Leonard, L., and McGregor, K. (1993). A cross-linguistic study of article use by children with specific language impairment. *European Journal of Disorders of Communication*, 28, 153–63.

Leonard, L. (1998). *Children with Specific Language Impairment*. Cambridge, MA: MIT Press.

Leonard, L. (2000). SLI across languages. In D. V. M. Bishop and L. Leonard (eds.), *Speech and Language Impairments in Children: Causes, Characteristics, Intervention and Outcome* (pp. 115–29). Hove, Sussex: Psychology Press.

Leonard, L. (2003). Specific language impairment: Characterizing the deficits. In Y. Levy and J. Schaeffer (eds.), *Language Competence across Populations: Toward a Definition of Specific Language Impairment* (pp. 209–32). Mahwah, NJ: Erlbaum.

Leonard, L., Bortolini, U., Caselli, M.-C., McGregor, K., and Sabbadini, L. (1992). Morphological deficits in children with specific language impairment: The status of features in the underlying grammar. *Language Acquisition*, 2, 151–79.

Leonard, L., Dromi, E., Adam, G., and Zadunaisky-Ehrlich, S. (2000). Tense and finiteness in the speech of children with specific language impairment acquiring Hebrew. *International Journal of Language and Communication Disorders*, 35, 319–35.

Leonard, L., Salameh, E.-K., and Hansson, K. (2001). Noun phrase morphology in Swedish-speaking children with specific language impairment. *Applied Psycholinguistics*, 22, 619–39.

MacWhinney, B., Bates, E., and Kliegl, R. (1984). Cue validity and sentence interpretation in English, German and Italian. *Journal of Verbal Learning and Verbal Behaviour*, 23, 127–50.

Månsson, A.-C. and Ahlsén, E. (2001). Grammatical features of aphasia in Swedish. In M. Paradis (ed.), *Manifestations of Aphasia Symptoms in Different Languages* (pp. 281–96). Amsterdam: Pergamon.

Menn, L. and Obler, L. K. (1988). Findings of the cross-language aphasia study. Phase I: Agrammatic narrative. *Aphasiology*, 2, 347–50.

Menn, L. and Obler, L. K. (1990a). *Agrammatic Aphasia: A Cross-Language Narrative Sourcebook*. Amsterdam: John Benjamins.

Menn, L. and Obler, L. K. (1990b). Conclusion: Cross-language data and theories of agrammatism. In L. Menn and L. K. Obler. (eds.), *Agrammatic Aphasia*, vol. II (pp. 1369–89). Amsterdam: John Benjamins.

Mimouni, Z. and Jarema, G. (1997). Agrammatic aphasia in Arabic. *Aphasiology*, 11, 125–44.

Nicol, J. L., Jakubowicz, C., and Goldblum, M. C. (1996). Sensitivity to grammatical marking in English-speaking and French-speaking non-fluent aphasics. *Aphasiology*, 10, 593–622.

Nilipour, R. (2000). Agrammatic language: Two cases from Farsi. *Aphasiology*, 14, 1205–42.

O'Grady, W. and Kim, M. (2005). A mapping theory of agrammatic comprehension deficits. *Brain and Language*, 92, 91–100.

Paradis, J. (2004). The relevance of specific language impairment in understanding the role of transfer in second language acquisition. *Applied Psycholinguistics*, 25, 67–82.

Paradis, J. and Crago, M. (2000). Tense and temporality: Similarities and differences between language-impaired and second-language children. *Journal of Speech, Language and Hearing Research*, 43, 834–48.

Paradis, J. and Crago, M. (2001). The morphosyntax of specific language impairment in French: Evidence for an Extended Optional Default Account. *Language Acquisition*, 9, 269–300.

Paradis, J. and Crago, M. (2004). Comparing L2 and SLI grammars in French: Focus on DP. In P. Prévost and J. Paradis (eds.), *The Acquisition of French in Different Contexts: Focus on Functional Categories* (pp. 89–108). Amsterdam: Benjamins.

Paradis, J., Crago, M., and Genesee, F. (2007). Domain-specific versus domain-general theories of the deficit in SLI: Object pronoun acquisition by French-English bilingual children. *Language Acquisition*, 13, 33–62.

Paradis, J., Crago, M., Genesee, F., and Rice, M. (2003). Bilingual children with specific language impairment: How do they compare with their monolingual peers? *Journal of Speech, Language and Hearing Research*, 46, 1–15.

Paradis, M. (ed.) (1983). *Readings on Aphasia in Bilinguals and Polyglots*. Quebec: Didier.

Paradis, M. (2001). By way of a preface: The need for awareness of aphasia syndromes in different languages. In M. Paradis (ed.) *Manifestations of Aphasia Symptoms in Different Languages* (pp. 1–7). Amsterdam: Pergamon.

Ravid, D., Levie, R., and Avivi Ben-Zvi, G. (2003). The role of language typology in linguistic development: Implications for the study of language disorders. In Y. Levy and J. Schaeffer (eds.), *Language Competence across Populations: Toward a Definition of Specific Language Impairment* (pp. 171–96). Mahwah, NJ: Erlbaum.

Restrepo, M. and Gutiérrez-Clellen, V. (2001). Article use in Spanish-speaking children with specific language impairment. *Journal of Child Language*, 28, 433–53.

Rice, M. (2003). A unified model of specific and general language delay: Grammatical tense as a clinical marker of unexpected variation. In Y. Levy and J. Schaeffer (eds.), *Language Competence across Populations: Toward a Definition of Specific Language Impairment* (pp. 63–94). Mahwah, NJ: Erlbaum.

Rice, M., Ruff Noll, K., and Grimm, H. (1997). An Extended Optional Infinitive Stage in German-speaking children with specific language impairment. *Language Acquisition* 6(4), 255–96.

Rice, R. and Wexler, K. (1996). Toward tense as a clinical marker of specific language impairment. *Journal of Speech, Language and Hearing Research*, 39, 1236–57.

Roberts, S. and Leonard, L. (1997). Grammatical deficits in German and English: A crosslinguistic study of children with specific language impairment. *First Language*, 17, 131–50.

Slobin, D. (1991). Aphasia in Turkish: Speech production in Broca's and Wernicke's patients. *Brain and Language*, 41, 149–64.

Stokes, S. and Fletcher, P. (2003). Aspectual forms in Cantonese children with specific language impairment. *Linguistics*, 41, 381–406.

Tanaka-Welty, Y., Watanabe, J., and Menn, L. (2002). Language production in Japanese preschoolers with SLI: Testing theories. In E. Fava (ed.), *Clinical Linguistics: Theory and Applications in Speech Pathology and Therapy* (pp. 175–93). Amsterdam: Benjamins.

Wong, A. M.-Y., Leonard, L., Fletcher, P., and Stokes, S. (2004). Questions without movement: A study of Cantonese-speaking children with and without specific language impairment. *Journal of Speech, Language and Hearing Research*, 1440–53.

18 Interfaces between Cognition, Semantics, and Syntax

MARIA BLACK AND SHULA CHIAT

18.1 Introduction

Language enables us to talk about an infinite range of situations. To do this, we draw from an open-ended set of verbs and a very limited set of syntactic structures. Linguists have sought to analyze how different situations are filtered into a limited set of semantic types that map onto the limited set of syntactic structures. This chapter focuses on the application of linguistic analyses to the production of verb-argument structure in SLI and in aphasia. We start with brief descriptions of deficits observed in children and adults with language impairments. We then review the main linguistic analysis that has been applied to the data – thematic role analysis – and evaluate its contribution to the analysis of both linguistic and clinical linguistic data. The limitations of thematic role analysis identified by linguists have led to more recent analyses of event structure. We argue that event structure analysis may provide insights into patterns of verb-argument production which defy thematic role analysis.

18.2 Impairments in Acquiring the System

Verbs and verb-argument structure have been noted as a particular area of difficulty for children with SLI (Leonard, 1998). Studies of spontaneous production of verbs in language-impaired preschoolers have revealed limitations in verb production compared with age- and language-matched controls, as reflected in lower type–token ratios for verbs but not for overall vocabulary (Watkins, Rice, & Moltz, 1993), or in use of fewer verb tokens and verb types (Conti-Ramsden & Jones, 1997). Children with SLI have also been observed to omit verbs in some utterances, for example

*I my flowers back (want).
*Let me that (do) (Rice & Bode, 1993).

In a single case study of a six-year-old with language impairment which elicited description of 127 events (Chiat, 2000; Evelyn, 1996), the child omitted the verb in 22 of his 127 event descriptions. In contrast, there was only one instance of verb omission in the 381 event descriptions produced by three vocabulary-matched controls. Compare descriptions produced by controls of the researcher dropping apples:

> You dropped them.
> They dropped out.

with the description produced by Travis, the language-impaired child:

> Fruit on floor.

and controls' descriptions of the researcher emptying her pockets:

> Taking the things out.
> Getting things out.

with Travis's:

> Thing out.

Studies have also observed some verb substitutions that are inappropriate for the event, though semantically related to the target, as in the following examples from Rice and Bode (1993):

> *Birds *live* to California (go).
> *You *get* in that guy and it'll work (push).

When the child in the Evelyn study was asked to describe pictures using a given verb, he made inappropriate substitutions for more than a quarter of the pictures. These substitutions often involved a 'multi-verb' response, as in his description of a panda buying a pear from a monkey:

> Monkey / panda want a pear / monkey want money.

which he broke up into two events (see Chiat, 2000 for further examples). In contrast, substitutions by the controls were almost always appropriate and they never produced multi-verb responses like those above.

So, there is considerable consensus that children with SLI have less diverse verb vocabularies and are liable to omit verbs or use inappropriate substitutions.

There is also consensus that these limitations do not fall neatly into semantic or syntactic categories. Rice and Bode (1993) and Evelyn (1996) both observe that children made verb omissions and substitutions in contexts where they could have used verbs they used successfully in other contexts. For example, Travis used the verb *tip* to describe one emptying event, but omitted the verb in his description of four other emptying events for which the verb *tip* would have served just as well. Such examples provide evidence that children have sufficient knowledge of the semantics and syntax of verbs which they nevertheless fail to produce. Watkins, Rice, and Moltz (1993, p. 141) comment that the children's verbs "cut across semantic categories (e.g., *go* and *play* can be action verbs, *get* and *put* are generally locative action verbs, and *know*, *see* and *want* are state verbs . . .) and transitivity distinctions (e.g., *put* is always a transitive form, *go* is always an intransitive form, several of the other verbs can be used as either transitive or intransitive forms)". Their evidence, they suggest, points to limited 'semantic mapping'. Conti-Ramsden and Jones (1997) focus on the semantic characteristics of verbs as possible sources of difficulty, for example that verbs refer to relational concepts which show more variability in how they map onto the world, or that many actions "can only be observed for a brief period" (p. 1310). Interestingly, these tentative explanations for verb deficits in SLI all invoke the semantic properties of verbs, a point to which we will return in our own analysis.

Turning to argument structure, language-impaired children are also more likely to omit arguments than controls, e.g.

> *Give me (Give me that).
> *Me hit (Me hit him). (Rice & Bode, 1993)

The child in the Evelyn study occasionally omitted an object which was clearly required, e.g. 'Tip in there' (for emptying a jar). In addition, he frequently described events with a bare verb and no arguments, e.g. 'Break', 'Cut', 'Melt', 'Dry'.

Two studies reveal more specific limitations in the use of argument structure. Thordardottir and Weismer's study (2002) was based on spontaneous samples produced by preschoolers who had relatively mild deficits. These children included obligatory arguments as reliably as MLU controls, but used significantly fewer types of three-place argument structures, and differed in their use of the ditransitive structure, tending "not to include the *beneficiary* argument" (p. 243). They also demonstrated fewer instances of argument structure alternations in their samples than their age-matched controls. In Ebbels's (2005) study of verb-argument structure, 11–15 year olds with SLI were shown events on video and asked to say what was happening using a given verb. These children omitted obligatory object arguments more frequently than age-matched and vocabulary-matched children, though only in three-argument structures, e.g. 'She's been covering with a cloth'. They produced fewer correct responses for change-of-state verbs, using these incorrectly in change-of-location constructions, e.g.

The lady is filling the bricks into the jar.
The lady is covering the scarf on her head.

and were more likely to use a verb in the wrong construction consistently. Finally, the SLI group used the double object construction significantly less than the controls.

The picture emerging from these investigations is surprisingly consistent. They find no evidence of absolute semantic or syntactic gaps in the production of argument structure by children of widely varying ages. Nor is there any report of systematic mismapping, such as reversing syntactic positions of agent and theme roles. What they reveal is restricted, less flexible and sometimes erroneous use of verb-argument structures, particularly with three-argument structures and double-object structures which express caused change of possession or change of state.

18.3   Impairments to the Acquired System

Problems with the spoken and/or written production of verbs and verb-argument structures have been documented for adults with acquired aphasias, especially, though not exclusively, those with 'nonfluent' or 'agrammatic' aphasias (Berndt, Haendiges, Mitchum, & Sandson, 1997; Berndt, Mitchum, Haendiges, & Sandson, 1997; Laiacona & Caramazza, 2004; Webster, Morris, & Franklin, 2005; Zingeser & Berndt, 1990). Verbs are omitted more frequently than other content words in tasks such as picture description, constrained or cued elicitation and narrative production, e.g.

ROX: the man is sack of potatoes (*carrying* omitted; McCarthy & Warrington, 1985)
JG: the iron (for a picture of woman ironing; Byng, 1988)
AER: Cinderella shoe (Nickels, Byng, & Black, 1991)
EM: the hoover (for a picture of woman hoovering; Marshall, Pring, & Chiat, 1998)
SS: Eyes, chair, chair (*looking* omitted; Breedin, Saffran, & Schwartz, 1998).

Verbs are also more likely to be substituted by other verbs or categories such as nouns, e.g.

ML: The grandmother was kissing the boy. (target: *hugging*; Mitchum & Berndt, 1994)
PB: The girl is hoovering the towels. (target: *ironing*; Marshall, Chiat, & Pring, 1997)
ROX: The daughter was chairing. (target: *sitting*; McCarthy & Warrington, 1985)
EM: The man is globing the world. (Marshall, Pring, & Chiat, 1998).

As studies have tended to focus on the greater difficulty of verbs relative to nouns, there has been little systematic analysis of whether semantically different classes of verbs are less likely to be produced. As in the case of SLI, adults with verb problems seem to produce verbs from a range of semantic categories. Substitutions often involve cognitively or semantically related items but the relationships involved seem to depend on the type and level of impairment and no generally valid patterns have been isolated so far. In some cases, the ability to produce verbs varies with the type of task and its processing demands (Dean & Black, 2005; Kim, Kim, & Song, 2003).

The most clearly and consistently documented trend is that three-argument verbs tend to be more difficult than one- or two-argument verbs. Thompson, Lange, Schneider, and Shapiro (1997) found that both in picture description and in elicited description using a lead-in sentence, people with agrammatic aphasia had more difficulty in producing three-argument verbs. Verbs requiring fewer arguments were significantly easier for the agrammatic subjects reported by Kim and Thompson (2000), who conclude that "verb production is influenced by the syntactically relevant argument taking properties of verbs" (p. 152). What is not clear, however, is whether this well-documented tendency should be interpreted in syntactic or semantic terms, as we discuss in section 18.5 below. As in the case of SLI, some people with aphasia appear to have fewer problems with three-argument verbs when the verbs describe a caused change of location where only one of the participants is animate (e.g. 'The girl put the book on the table') than with three-argument verbs expressing a caused change of possession where two of the participants are animate. Sacchett (2005), who investigated the drawing of videoed events by seven aphasic people with very limited language output, found that their drawing patterns were closer to those of non-aphasic controls when they were drawing caused change-of-location than change-of-possession events. This suggests that the cognitive-semantic nature of the event and its participants may influence communication, even when language is not involved.

Problems in producing verbs often co-occur with problems in sentence production (Berndt, Haendiges, Mitchum, & Sandson, 1997), although problems with sentence production have also been documented in people who do not have verb-specific problems. People with verb problems typically produce 'structurally impoverished' utterances, consisting of single words or phrases and with frequent argument omissions. For instance, EM (Dean & Black, 2005) described a composite picture (Comprehensive Aphasia Test: Swinburn, Porter, & Howard, 2004) as follows:

> Man is sleeping . . . playing boy cars . . . and um sitting room. . . . And um shelves . . . and um CD . . . and um books and flowers . . . fishes . . . and table . . . coffee . . . armchair and books [prompted for more information] sleeping . . . and um over and ouch . . . and shock.   (Dean & Black, 2005, p. 528)

Omissions of arguments have been attested in most studies. For instance, the eight adults with aphasia described by Thompson (2003) all made argument omissions in picture-description and narrative tasks. In the narrative samples, only 35 percent of verbs produced occurred with the required arguments, while non-aphasic controls produced 94 percent of verbs in appropriate argument structures. Argument phrases are also realized in inappropriate positions, especially when the situation to be described involves participants who are equally plausible in different roles in that situation ('reversible' situations), or a picture presents a situation from a more unusual perspective. For instance, PW (Linebarger, Schwartz, & Saffran, 1983) made 'reversal' errors in picture description, e.g.

> PW: The man is running the girl. (target: a girl running to a man)
> PW: The boy . . . or a man is bumping the ball. (target: a ball hitting a man on the head)

Reversal errors of these kinds, however, seem to appear primarily in picture description, as opposed to narrative or conversation. For example, only two of the six people with aphasia documented in Byng and Black (1989) made reversal errors, and they did so only in picture description.

The picture emerging from the studies of acquired aphasia is more varied than for SLI. As with the children with SLI, three-argument verbs seem particularly vulnerable, but the lack of semantic analysis makes it harder to draw conclusions about whether semantic or syntactic factors, or both, influence verb retrieval and argument production.

18.4   Linguistic Concepts

Clinical analyses of verb deficits, both developmental and acquired, have generally adopted the thematic role analyses developed within linguistics between the 1970s and the 1990s. These analyses identified an exhaustive list of thematic roles (typically including Agent or Actor, Patient or Theme, Goal or Recipient, Source, Location, Experiencer and Stimulus) and the syntactic position(s) each might occupy (Subject, Direct Object, Indirect Object, Prepositional Object). Each verb then had a specified thematic structure which was paired with its syntactic subcategorization frame. This approach made it possible to capture regularities in mapping between thematic and syntactic roles across semantically diverse verbs. For example, *touch* and *break* would be similarly represented in terms of the mapping of the Actor/Agent role onto the Subject or external argument position, while the Patient/Theme role would map onto the Object or internal argument position, as in

> Sue_{Agent} touched the $glass_{Theme}$.
> Sue_{Agent} broke the $glass_{Theme}$.

This accounted for the apparent similarities between these verbs. Observed regularities in mapping gave rise to a proposed hierarchy of thematic roles:

where verbs entailed two or more thematic roles, the highest role in the thematic hierarchy would occupy the Subject or external argument position; lower roles in the hierarchy would occupy internal argument positions, the lowest being prepositional objects.

A considerable range of verbs could be specified semantically and syntactically in this way. However, application of thematic role analyses rapidly revealed a number of problems (Butt & Geuder, 1998; Dowty, 1991; Jackendoff, 1990). First, there was little consensus on how some of the main roles should be defined and differentiated from one another. For example, a problem arises with verbs of transfer such as *load* or *send* which allow alternations in their argument structure:

(1)   (a)   She loaded the cart with hay.
      (b)   She loaded hay onto the cart.

(2)   (a)   She sent Mary the parcel.
      (b)   She sent the parcel to Mary.

Should *Mary* and *the cart* be assigned the role of Goal in both (a) and (b) sentences? If so, how do we account for the 'goal' appearing more 'affected' when it is a Direct Object, as in the (a) sentences? How do we account for the impossibility of the double object in (3):

(3)   (a)   She sent the parcel to London.
      (b)   *She sent London the parcel?

If the Goal or Recipient was most 'affected', should we not assign it the thematic role of Patient rather than Goal/Recipient since Patient was defined as 'the entity affected by the action of the Actor/Agent'? As many linguists have pointed out, such interpretations of greater affectedness or 'holistic involvement' arise irrespective of the particular thematic role realized in the direct object position. Some linguists concluded that meaning effects could come from different sources: from the thematic roles themselves but also from the meaning of the construction in which a verb and its complements occurred. It was misguided to make thematic roles alone bear the whole semantic burden (Goldberg, 1995). For instance, phrases in the direct object position in the double NP construction would appear as more affected or holistically involved irrespective of whether a Goal or a Recipient were placed in them. If the meaning of the phrase was incompatible with the meaning of the construction in which it was placed, then that argument realization would be blocked, as it is for (3b) above.

A second problem arose with verbs that share thematic structures yet behave very differently with respect to the range of syntactic contexts in which they can appear, as illustrated by the different patterns in (4) and (5) below:

(4) *Sue touched.
     Sue and Mary touched.
     ?? Sue and the glass touched.
     *The glass touched.

(5) *Sue broke.
     *Sue and Mary broke.
     *Sue and the glass broke.
     The glass broke.

As the analysis of verb meaning developed, it became clear that these syntactic differences were largely due to semantic differences which were not revealed by a simple listing of thematic roles. For instance, *touch* expresses a simple action that involves contact between the Actor and the other participant in the event but it does not entail any change in that participant, unlike *break* which in its transitive or causative frame expresses a complex event involving a causal act that triggers a change in the other participant. These differences in the type of situation each verb expresses are clearly at the root of their differences in syntactic possibilities (see Levin & Rappaport Hovav, 2005).

Finally, attempts to characterize regularities in mapping relations through thematic hierarchies foundered. In their attempt to order the whole set of roles with respect to one another, even though some roles never co-occur, thematic hierarchies mixed "roles from incompatible event types" (Croft, 1998, p. 30). It is pointless, for example, to worry about the relative ordering of Actor/Agent and Experiencer, or Goal/Recipient and Location, since each of them occurs in different types of situations.

In conclusion, thematic role analysis opened up the semantic-syntactic interface and highlighted regularities in the links between semantics and syntax. But attempts to characterize these regularities exposed patterns that challenged the very basis of the analysis.

18.5   Clinical Linguistic Applications

Thematic roles and the notion of predicate argument structure have undoubtedly played an important role in clinical analysis of both developmental and acquired impairments. They provided clinical linguists with tools to analyze relational meanings and talk about the mapping between semantic and syntactic structure, at a time when most aspects of sentence meaning were treated as purely syntactic. For example, in the earliest analyses of agrammatism, verb and verb-argument problems were seen as yet another symptom of a general syntactic problem. The introduction of the notion of thematic roles and thematic structure made it possible to argue that some verb and sentence production problems, such as agrammatic reversal errors and the omission of arguments, reflected a deficit "in the translation between descriptions of sentence form and descriptions of sentence meaning" (Schwartz, Linebarger, & Saffran, 1985,

p. 121), rather than a syntactic problem. This "mapping hypothesis", first put forward by Linebarger, Schwartz, and Saffran (1983) and pursued by several investigators (Byng, 1988; Byng, Nickels, & Black, 1994; Jones, 1986; Marshall, Chiat, & Pring, 1997), also influenced therapy, as Marshall (2002, p. 360) points out: "The mapping hypothesis had clear implications for therapy. Rather than training surface sentence forms, therapy should aim to clarify connections between meaning and structure."

This influence is also evident in therapy with children, exemplified by interventions such as "colourful semantics" (Bryan, 1997), which color-codes thematic roles to help the child identify and use them to create sentences. However, thematic role analysis did very little clinical work in these therapies; its key contribution was to give a semantic gloss to the syntactic positions of Subject, Direct Object, and Prepositional Object.

Thematic role analysis provided semantic tools, but these tools were too limited to throw any new light on the patterns of impairment in production of verb-argument structures (see sections 18.2 and 18.3). Like children with SLI, people with agrammatic aphasia did not seem to have particular problems with specific thematic roles or the syntactic mapping of particular roles. For instance, Byng and Black (1989, p. 255) conclude from their detailed analysis of the narrative samples of six clients with aphasia that "the type of thematic role played by an argument, however, does not seem to influence its realization; in our data, omitted arguments have a variety of thematic roles, and external arguments expressing the Agent are not more likely to be realized than external arguments expressing other thematic roles."

With respect to reversal errors, what seemed to matter most was the relative prominence of two participants/arguments with respect to one another, independently of their particular thematic roles. For instance, PW (Schwartz, Linebarger, & Saffran, 1985; see section 18.3 above) made reversal errors in describing pictures when Agent and Patient were involved ('The boy ... or a man is bumping the ball') or when an Agent/Theme was paired with a Goal ('The man is running the girl'). Because thematic role analysis did not provide the relevant concepts, researchers had to fall back on a perceptually based, general notion of "salience" (Schwartz, Linebarger, & Saffran, 1985), which could not be defined in terms of thematic roles. As cognitive linguistics has shown, relative prominence can only be defined in relation to particular event types (see section 18.4).

As the semantic content of the roles was downplayed, what became most important was the number, rather than the type, of arguments, especially given the robustness of the finding that verbs with three arguments were most difficult across subjects and tasks. Devoid of much semantic content, argument structure was reasserted as a primarily syntactic level of representation, as in the work of Thompson and her colleagues (Thompson, Lange, Schneider, & Shapiro, 1997; Kim & Thompson, 2000; Thompson, 2003). According to Kim and Thompson (2000, p. 153), "As the number of syntactic arguments increases, so too does verb selection difficulty."

The 'argument complexity hypothesis' did not keep its elegantly simple form for very long. Although the evidence that one- or two-argument verbs tended to be significantly easier than three-argument verbs was strong, there was also evidence from Thompson's own work, as well as that of other researchers (Kegl, 1995), that verbs with the same number of arguments were not equally difficult (e.g. one-argument verbs such as *laugh* were easier than one-argument verbs such as *fall*). Furthermore, some two argument verbs (e.g. *kiss*) were easier than some one-argument verbs such as *fall*, and easier than two-argument verbs such as non-causative *break*. To account for these differences, Thompson (2003) reformulated the 'argument complexity hypothesis', incorporating into it the linguistic distinction between unergative verbs (e.g. *laugh*) and unaccusative verbs (e.g. *fall*, and non-causative *break*). Unaccusative verbs are said to be more difficult because they have only one internal (Theme) argument which must be moved before it can be mapped onto the Subject position, to meet various theoretical constraints. Unergative verbs, on the other hand, undergo the more typical mapping of an external (Agent) role onto the Subject position (Levin and Rappaport Hovav, 1996). Thompson therefore restates the argument complexity hypothesis as "verbs with a greater number of arguments or with argument structures that trigger movement operations render them more complex" (2003, p. 163). In the following section, we argue that more semantically oriented theories of complexity, based on the notion of event structure, give a more revealing account of these differences and point to further insights.

18.6   New Directions

As we have argued in previous sections, thematic roles are linguistically inadequate in a number of ways. Recent linguistic analyses, from a variety of theoretical approaches, have all arrived at a similar conclusion: situations and their properties are what is important in analyzing how language expresses situations. Thematic roles, therefore, are increasingly treated as no more than convenient labels identifying the participants in different types of situations. As Levin and Rappaport Hovav (2005, p. 238) say in their review of the linguistic literature, "what is necessary is a lexical semantic representation that explicitly encodes properties of events, including their 'subeventual' structure – a desideratum recognized by the now common use of the term 'event structure' to refer to such representations".

Although there is no consensus about the best way of specifying 'event structure', there is agreement as to the most important properties of situations that such event structures should include:

1   the aspectual type of the situation (e.g. whether it is dynamic or static, bounded by an end point or unbounded);
2   the causal structure of situations, indicating how different 'subevents' are causally and temporally related;

3　some indication of the properties of participants that affect their linguistic mapping (e.g. sentience and animacy).

Consider the sentence

(6)　The apples are on the floor.

which expresses a static situation. The sentence only tells us where the apples are – a locational state. Nothing is mentioned about the process that got them there. But we could include some information about how the apples got there by changing the main verb to one that expresses a process (a change of position), e.g.

(7)　The apples fell on the floor.

Although there may be a cause to the apple's fall, some act that triggered their motion, the sentence gives no information about that aspect of the causal chain. This additional information, or 'subevent' in a longer causal chain, could be introduced by, again, changing the verb, e.g.

(8)　Bill dropped the apples on the floor.

Each of these sentences can be treated as corresponding to a particular situation type; that is, each corresponds to a particular 'event structure'. The meaning of their main verbs (*be, fall, drop*) links to that event structure, which is the conceptual 'frame' for the meaning of the verb. For instance, verbs of static spatial relations like *be, lie, sit*, can be linked to the same event structure (they are all locational states) but each of them will pick out, or "profile" (Croft & Cruse, 2004) a specific aspect of that static relationship. Similarly, the verb *fall* will be linked to an event structure shared with other verbs of change but will profile a particular path of the motion, one of a small set of English verbs that link to that event structure and profile a specific path (e.g. *rise, cross*). The verb *drop*, however, will link to a more complex event structure, with an initial act by one participant (Bill in (8) above) that triggers a process of change in another participant (the apples). So the verb *drop* will link to an event structure with a more complex 'subeventual' structure in that what is schematized in that event structure is a longer causal chain where an act has been combined with a process. Other verbs of caused motion will link to the same event structure but may profile different kinds of causal acts (e.g. *throw*) or different types of motion (*spin*) or path of motion (*lift*) (Black & Chiat, 2003; Talmy, 2003).

　　We can already see, even from this highly simplified sketch, how *touch* and *break* (see section 18.4) differ in terms of their event structures and the consequences of this difference for argument realization. The verb *touch* will correspond to a simple event involving an act carried out by one participant with respect to another. The act is "simple" in the sense that nothing but that act is profiled by the verb meaning. It does not entail a change in the other participant (the act is not combined with another 'subevent'). The verb *break*, on the other hand, has a more complex event structure in that a process leading to a specific state is implied; furthermore, it can be linked to another event structure which is more complex still, similar to that we discussed above for *drop*. From the different event structures these two verbs are linked to, we can predict their different possibilities for argument realization: The verb *break* has both transitive and intransitive possibilities because the event structures it is linked to can motivate these two syntactic structures. What it profiles, however, remains constant in the sense that its meaning directs attention only to the process+state subcomponents, irrespective of which of the two event structures it is linked to. When it is linked to the longer act+process+state structure, the act subcomponent is supplied by the event structure, but the 'lexical' meaning of the verb gives no specific information about that act. The verb *touch*, on the other hand, is only linked to the simple, one-component act structure, and all the information its meaning includes has to do with that act (the particular gesture) and the fact that contact between the participants in the act is made. Their different syntactic possibilities follow from these semantic differences.

The distinction between simple and complex event structures, which we have drawn in terms of one- vs. two- or three-event components (see also Levin & Rappaport Hovav, 2005; Pustejovsky, 1995), can be used as a descriptive alternative to Thompson's (2003) revised 'argument complexity hypothesis' (section 18.5), which involved two distinct, and possibly conflicting, syntactic characterizations of difficulty. Using a single distinction, drawn in conceptual-semantic terms but with syntactic consequences, we can predict that simple verbs (those that link to single-component event structures) are less difficult for people with agrammatic aphasia to produce than those verbs linked to complex structures (more than one component).

This alternative works for all the verbs used in the studies by Thompson and her colleagues. All the one-place predicates listed by Thompson, Lange, Schneider, and Shapiro (1997) are simple in our event-structure sense, and so are all the unergative verbs listed in Thompson (2003) (one-place: *sleep, skate, smile, run, listen, ski, snore, laugh, pray*; unergative: *crawl, cry, jump, laugh, pray, run, sit, sneeze, snore, swim, wink*). All the verbs that are systematically and significantly more difficult in these studies are complex in our terms (three-place: *lean, put, feed, give, stick, glue, nail, mail, read, teach, bake, throw, write, pour*; unaccusative: *bounce, break, crack, crash, drop, flat, melt, roll, sink, tear*), except for two of the 10 unaccusative verbs (*fall, flow*). The two-place verbs listed in Thompson, Lange, Schneider, and Shapiro (1997) fall into both simple (six verbs) and complex categories (10 verbs), which would explain why the one-place vs. two-place verb comparisons reported in the literature have yielded less clear and consistent results. Of course, post hoc reinterpretations of other studies' results can only be suggestive and we have to wait for more stringent empirical tests of the two descriptive alternatives. But for clinical linguists the really interesting question is whether each way of describing the data opens up new inroads as to *why* such differences in relative difficulty come about. We would argue that explanation can only come from an integration of linguistic concepts with psycholinguistic models of the tasks used to elicit language output. From a clinical point of view, the main advantage of an approach based on event structures, in comparison to one based on thematic roles or syntactic argument structure, is that it facilitates such an integration and, therefore, opens the way towards explanation.

If we ask a person to describe a pictured or filmed situation, as we do in many clinical assessments, their descriptions may be affected by a number of perceptual features of the situation. However, eye fixation and other psycho-linguistic measures reveal that scene processing involves the interaction of bottom-up perceptual factors and top-down cognitive, communicative and linguistic factors (Henderson & Ferreira, 2004; Zacks & Tversky, 2001). For instance, what people attend to first in a scene depends on the task, so that people who are asked to simply inspect a pictured scene direct their gaze to different areas of the picture from people who are asked to describe that scene (Griffin & Bock, 2000; Henderson & Ferreira, 2004).

Perceptual 'salience' of the kind mentioned in section 18.5 only exerts its influence directly and determines what is said first, if other cognitive, communicative and linguistic constraints that determine relative prominence cannot be accessed. Consider the three pictures in figure 18.1. In terms of the relative perceptual salience of their human participants, the three scenes are pretty equal, although their position on the left of the picture may privilege the women in (a) and (b) and the woman with black hair in (c) (see Sacchett, 2005). However, some crucial differences emerge as we plan and execute a description in English. In (a), the most appropriate event schema to interpret the picture is that of a simple action involving someone acting with respect to another participant. This event structure activates a number of individual verbs

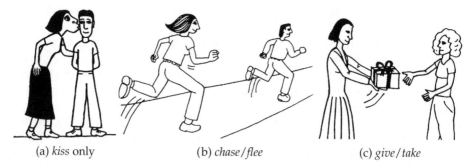

(a) *kiss* only   (b) *chase/flee*   (c) *give/take*

Figure 18.1   Three scenes: (a) *kiss* only, (b) *chase/flee*, (c) *give/take*. Pictures (a–c) are by Eldad Druks. (Picture (a) is from unpublished materials made available by Jane Marshall. Pictures (b) and (c) are reproduced with permission from *The Sentence Processing Resource Pack* (Marshall, Black, Byng, Chiat, & Pring, 1999). We are grateful to Eldad Druks and Jane Marshall for the use of their pictures.)

expressing physical gestures, with and without contact between the actor and the other participant. But all of the verbs linked to this event structure express variations of meaning that have to do with the actor's body, the manner or intensity of her action and whether or not the actor makes contact with the other participant. Thus, the meanings of this class of verbs focus attention on one participant, who may already have been identified as more prominent on cognitive grounds as the initiator and executor of the action. In this case cognitive and linguistic constraints converge to single out one more prominent participant who is maximally differentiated and is mapped onto a position of communicative prominence – the Subject. With this kind of situation, English does not give us any other choice but to describe the situation from the kisser's perspective, since there is no (active) verb that describes the situation from the point of view of the 'kissee'.

On the other hand, the event schema for scene (b) activates different subclasses of verbs all linked to the same event schema. One subclass focuses attention on one participant (the 'chaser') and her motion towards a destination, and another subclass directs attention to the 'fleer' and his motion away from the other participant. The scene can be described from either perspective. A choice between the two perspectives must be made to single out a more prominent participant, which is mapped onto the subject. A similar argument can be applied to scene (c), where different verbs direct attention to the temporal and causal beginning of the transfer event (*give*-type verbs) or its end point (*take*-type verbs), with the further complication that a secondary relative prominence judgment must be made with respect to the third participant (the present), so that we can decide whether to map it onto Direct or Prepositional Object position.

So, at different points in the complex chain of interactions that characterizes scene description, there will be choices determined by: the features of the perceptual input; the availability of event structures that allow us to construe the scene in particular ways; the (successful) activation of verbs linked to a particular event structure; and the patterns of attention defined by those verbs' meanings (Dipper, Black, & Bryan, 2005). We would predict that, all other things being equal, the more convergence there is between perceptual, cognitive and linguistic constraints, the easier it is to describe a scene. Describing scenes like (c) requires reconciling and integrating multiple constraints – another reason why these scenes are so often difficult for people with agrammatic aphasia.

We would argue that language learning, like language production, should be seen as a process of multiple-constraint satisfaction. Perceptual concepts and cognitive event schemas serve as the initial scaffolding which is reshaped and enriched to take into account communicative, linguistic and language-specific factors that cannot be derived straightforwardly from the perceptual and cognitive scaffolding. Given the variety of event types that children with SLI are able to produce (see section 18.2), they must have developed a basic set of event structures to which they can link the verbs of the language they are learning. Furthermore, as they do produce mostly appropriate syntactic realizations for arguments, they must have learned to map event structures onto syntactic representations. If certain aspects of events are privileged by non-linguistic as well as linguistic biases, this convergence will result in earlier and easier production for both typical and atypical learners. However, if the non-linguistic biases work against the linguistic distinctions to be learned, we would expect children who have problems in processing, holding and storing linguistic forms (Chiat, 2000, 2001) to show particular difficulties with these aspects of events. As Gentner and Ratterman (1991, p. 260) point out, "a word can function as a promissory note, signaling subtle commonalities that the child does not yet perceive." Difficulties with words would make it harder to discover such commonalities.

To illustrate this point, it has been shown that children have a "non-linguistic conceptual bias" in favor of Goal Paths and end states (Lakusta & Landau, 2005; Regier, 1996), as opposed to Source Paths and initial configurations. Regier argues that "the child has more of a chance to absorb the result of an event than its starting configuration. By the time the child's attention has been captured by the motion, the starting configuration is no longer available – only the motion itself is, followed by the resultant end-state" (p. 202). Although language also has a bias in favor of Goal Paths and end states, many languages have verbs and closed-class items that focus on the Source Path (e.g. English verbs of motion such as *leave*, of transfer such as *remove* or *empty*, and prepositions such as *from, off, away*). A child learning a language like English will have to pay close attention to these forms and the contexts in which she hears linguistic expressions that go against the Goal Path cognitive bias. Consider the contexts where Travis produces some arguments while omitting the verb (see section 18.2), e.g.

> Fruit on floor. (for dropping apples)
> Thing out. (for emptying a pocket)

The majority of his verb omissions occurred in similar situations which, in terms of event structure, involve a complex combination of subevents (act+change+state) and Travis includes only the end point of the motion. This could reflect the non-linguistic bias towards Goal Paths and end states in preference to other aspects of events. It is not the case that Travis can *only* express Goal Paths. When he is describing a scene that corresponds to a simpler situation, where only one 'subevent' is involved, Travis can express information about different aspects of that subevent. Indeed, he uses a wide range of verbs expressing the manner of the motion (e.g. *roll, spin*) in situations where the Goal Path bias does not come into play. Nevertheless, when the situation corresponds to a complex combination of more than one subevent, his ability to hold to the specifics of each subevent is severely taxed and he tends to just express the most salient aspect or subevent – the Goal Path or end state.

The examples we have given indicate how event structure analysis may be applied to clinical data and the kind of insights that can be gained from a shift in linguistic perspective.

REFERENCES

Berndt, R. S., Haendiges, A., Mitchum, C., and Sandson, J. (1997). Verb retrieval in aphasia. 2. Relationship to sentence processing. *Brain and Language*, 56, 107–37.

Berndt, R. S., Mitchum, C., Haendiges, A., and Sandson, J. (1997). Verb retrieval in aphasia. 1. Characterising single word impairments. *Brain and Language*, 56, 68–106.

Black, M. and Chiat, S. (2000). Putting thoughts into verbs: Developmental and acquired impairments. In W. Best, K. Bryan, and J. Maxim (eds.), *Semantic Processing: Theory and Practice* (pp. 52–79). London: Whurr Publishers.

Black, M. and Chiat, S. (2003). *Linguistics for Clinicians*. London: Arnold.

Breedin, S. D., Saffran, E. M., and Schwartz, M. F. (1998). Semantic factors in verb retrieval: An effect of complexity. *Brain and Language*, 63, 1–31.

Bryan, A. (1997). Colourful semantics: Thematic role therapy. In S. Chiat, J. Law, and J. Marshall (eds.), *Language Disorders in Children and Adults* (pp. 143–61). London: Whurr Publishers.

Butt, M. and Geuder, W. (1998). *The Projection of Arguments: Lexical and Compositional Factors*. Stanford, CA: CSLI Publications.

Byng, S. (1988). Sentence processing deficits: Theory and therapy. *Cognitive Neuropsychology*, 5, 629–76.

Byng, S. and Black, M. (1989). Some aspects of sentence production in aphasia. *Aphasiology*, 3, 241–63.

Byng, S., Nickels, L., and Black, M. (1994). Replicating therapy for mapping deficits in agrammatism: Remapping the deficit? *Aphasiology*, 8, 315–41.

Chiat, S. (2000). *Understanding Children with Language Problems*. Cambridge: Cambridge University Press.

Chiat, S. (2001). Mapping theories of developmental language impairment: Premises, predictions and evidence. *Language and Cognitive Processes*, 16, 113–42.

Conti-Ramsden, G. and Jones, M. (1997). Verb use in specific language impairment. *Journal of Speech, Language, and Hearing Research*, 40, 1298–1313.

Croft, W. (1998). Event structure and argument linking. In M. Butt and W. Geuder (eds.), pp. 21–63.

Croft, W. and Cruse, D. A. (2004). *Cognitive Linguistics*. Cambridge: Cambridge University Press.

Dean, M. P. and Black, M. (2005). Exploring event processing and description in aphasia. *Aphasiology*, 19, 521–44.

Dowty, D. R. (1991). Thematic proto-roles and argument selection. *Language*, 67, 547–619.

Ebbels, S. H. (2005). Argument structure in specific language impairment: From theory to therapy. Unpublished PhD thesis, University College London.

Evelyn, M. (1996). An investigation of verb processing in a child with a specific language impairment. Unpublished MPhil thesis, City University, London.

Gentner, D. and Ratterman, M. J. (1991). Language and the career of sentimentality. In S. A. Gelman and J. P. Byrnes (eds.), *Perspectives on Language and Thought: Interrelations in Development*. Cambridge: Cambridge University Press.

Goldberg, A. E. (1995). *Constructions: A Construction Grammar Approach to Argument Structure*. Chicago and London: University of Chicago Press.

Griffin, Z. M. and Bock, K. (2000). What the eyes say about speaking. *Psychological Science*, 11, 274–9.

Henderson, J. M. and Ferreira, F. (2004). *The Interface of Language, Vision, and Action: Eye Movements and the Visual World*. New York: Psychology Press.

Jackendoff, R. (1990). *Semantic Structures*. Cambridge, MA: MIT Press.

Jones, E. (1986). Building the foundation for sentence production in a non-fluent aphasic. *British Journal of Disorders of Communication*, 21, 63–82.

Kegl, J. (1995). Levels of representation and units of access relevant to agrammatism. *Brain and Language*, 50, 151–200.

Kim, Y-J., Kim, H., and Song, H-K. (2003). Argument structure distribution of predicates in Korean agrammatic speech. *Applied Psycholinguistics*, 24, 343–67.

Kim, M. and Thompson, C. K. (2000). Patterns of comprehension and production of nouns and verbs in agrammatism: Implications for lexical organization. *Brain and Language*, 74, 1–25.

Laiacona, M. and Caramazza, A. (2004). The noun/verb dissociation in language production: Varieties of causes. *Cognitive Neuropsychology*, 21, 103–23.

Lakusta, L. and Landau, B. (2005). Starting at the end: The importance of goals in spatial language. *Cognition*, 96, 1–33.

Leonard, L. B. (1998). *Children with Specific Language Impairment*. Cambridge, MA: MIT Press.

Levin, B. and Rappaport Hovav, H. (1996). *Unaccusativity: At the Syntax–Lexical Semantics Interface*. Cambridge, MA: MIT Press.

Levin, B. and Rappaport Hovav, M. (2005). *Argument Realization*. Cambridge: Cambridge University Press.

Linebarger, M., Schwartz, M. F., and Saffran, E. M. (1983). Sensitivity to grammatical structure in so-called agrammatic aphasics. *Cognition*, 13, 361–92.

Marshall, J. (2002). Assessment and treatment of sentence processing disorders: A review of the literature. In A. E. Hillis (ed.), *The Handbook of Language Disorders* (pp. 351–72). New York: Psychology Press.

Marshall, J., Black, M., Byng, S., Chiat, S., and Pring, T. (1999). *The Sentence Processing Resource Pack*. Bicester: Winslow Press.

Marshall, J., Chiat, S., and Pring, T. (1997). An impairment in processing verbs' thematic roles: A therapy study. *Aphasiology*, 11, 855–76.

Marshall, J., Pring, T., and Chiat, S. (1993). Sentence processing therapy: Working at the level of the event. *Aphasiology*, 7, 177–99.

Marshall, J., Pring, T., and Chiat, S. (1998). Verb retrieval and sentence production in aphasia. *Brain and Language*, 63, 159–83.

McCarthy, R. A. and Warrington, E. K. (1985). Category-specificity in an agrammatic patient: The relative impairment of verb retrieval and comprehension. *Neuropsychologia*, 23, 709–23.

Mitchum, C. C. and Berndt, R. S. (1994). Verb retrieval and sentence construction: Effects of targeted intervention. In M. J. Riddock and G. W. Humphreys (eds.), *Cognitive Neuropsychology and Cognitive Rehabilitation*. Hove, Sussex: Lawrence Erlbaum Associates.

Nickels, L., Byng, S., and Black, M. (1991). Sentence processing deficits: A replication of therapy. *British Journal of Disorders of Communication*, 26, 175–99.

Pustejovsky, J. (1995). *The Generative Lexicon*. Cambridge, MA: MIT Press.

Regier, T. (1996). *The Human Semantic Potential: Spatial Language and Constrained Connectionism*. Cambridge, MA: MIT Press.

Rice, M. L. and Bode, J. V. (1993). GAPS in the verb lexicons of children with specific language impairment. *First Language*, 113, 1–31.

Sacchett, C. L. M. (2005). An investigation of the relationship between conceptualisation and non-linguistic communication: Evidence from drawing production in severe aphasia. Unpublished PhD thesis, University College London.

Schwartz, M., Linebarger, M., and Saffran, E. M. (1985). The status of the syntactic deficit theory of agrammatism. In M. L. Kean (ed.), *Agrammatism*. Orlando, FL: Academic Press.

Swinburn, C., Porter, G., and Howard, D. (2004). *The Comprehensive Aphasia Test*. Hove, Sussex: Psychology Press.

Talmy, L. (2003). *Toward a Cognitive Semantics. Volume 1: Concept Structuring Systems*. Cambridge, MA: MIT Press.

Thompson, C. K. (2003). Unaccusative verb production in agrammatic aphasia: The argument structure complexity hypothesis. *Journal of Neurolinguistics*, 16, 151–67.

Thompson, C. K., Lange, K. L., Schneider, S. L., and Shapiro, L. P. (1997). Agrammatic and non-brain damaged subjects' verb and verb argument structure production. *Aphasiology*, 11, 473–90.

Thordardottir, E. T. and Weismer, S. E. (2002). Verb argument structure weakness in specific language impairment in relation to age and utterance length. *Clinical Linguistics and Phonetics*, 16, 233–50.

Watkins, R. V., Rice, M. L., and Moltz, C. C. (1993). Verb use by language-impaired and normally developing children. *First Language*, 13, 133–43.

Webster, J., Morris, J., and Franklin, S. (2005). Effects of therapy targeted at verb retrieval and the realisation of the predicate argument structure: A case study. *Aphasiology*, 19, 748–64.

Zacks, J. and Tversky, B. (2001). Event structure in perception and conception. *Psychological Bulletin*, 127, 3–21.

Zingeser, L. and Berndt, R. S. (1990). Retrieval of nouns and verbs in agrammatism and anomia. *Brain and Language*, 39, 14–32.

Part III Phonetics and
          Phonology

19 Instrumental Analysis of Articulation in Speech Impairment

FIONA E. GIBBON

19.1 Introduction

An instrumental approach offers researchers and clinicians the opportunity to measure directly articulator activity during speech. This has some advantages over other approaches, such as acoustic or perceptual analysis, where articulator activity can only be inferred from recorded data. Direct measures make it possible to identify motor impairments and articulation abnormalities as well as to quantify objectively changes in behavior due to factors such as maturation, disease progression or the effects of therapeutic intervention. Another benefit of direct physiological measures in the field of clinical linguistics and phonetics is that the data contribute to current debates in the discipline, for example the precise role of motor control in normal and abnormal speech production. A final reason for using instruments is that some of them have the facility to provide visual feedback, which can be used in a therapy program to modify abnormal articulator behavior. Despite the advantages, measuring articulation is a challenging task. Some instruments are not widely available in speech laboratories or clinics because they are expensive and have high maintenance and operational costs. This restricts their use to specialized laboratories or medical facilities. Some techniques are invasive or uncomfortable for the speaker and so are not well suited for gathering naturalistic speech samples or large data sets. The procedural demands of using some techniques makes them unsuitable for use with certain clinical populations, such as infants, young children or those in poor health. Finally, analysis of instrumental data can be a technically complex and time-consuming task and often involves processing large quantities of data.

This chapter illustrates, with examples from the literature, how instruments have been used to measure articulator position and movement during speech in children and adults with articulation disorders. The articulators to be discussed are the main moving parts of the oral cavity, namely the tongue, lips and lower jaw. These articulators vary widely in terms of their speed and complexity of movement and also in their structural composition, shape and location. These differences mean that instruments that are well suited to measuring one articulator may not be suitable for measuring another. Some of the advantages and disadvantages of the techniques will be discussed in the sections that follow. Detailed technical descriptions of the techniques are not provided in this chapter – there are many excellent surveys available that give comprehensive coverage for the interested reader (e.g., Baken & Orlikoff, 2000; Ball & Code, 1997; Hiiemae & Palmer, 2003; Stone, 1997; Thompson-Ward & Murdoch, 1998; Wood & Hardcastle, 2000).

Techniques used for measuring tongue activity are prominent in this review. Instrumental measurement of the tongue poses particular challenges due to its inaccessible location within the mouth, its sensitivity, the unique properties of its internal structure, and the speed and complexity of its movements. The clinical usefulness of some techniques for measuring tongue activity is greatly enhanced by having a real-time visual feedback facility. This facility is especially useful because it provides a visual display of speakers' own tongue position or movement, details of which they are unaware under normal circumstances. Visual feedback can be incorporated into a speech therapy program so that individuals with speech disorders can learn normal patterns of tongue movements and thus improve their speech intelligibility.

19.2   Electropalatography

The chapter begins with electropalatography (EPG) because of its widespread use for clinical and research purposes. EPG (also termed palatometry and dynamic palatometry) was developed for the purpose of recording an important aspect of articulation, namely the timing and location of the tongue's contact with the hard palate. A component of all EPG systems is a custom-made artificial plate molded to fit the speaker's hard palate. Embedded in the artificial plate are electrodes exposed to the lingual surface that detect when the tongue is touching them. Three different EPG systems have dominated in research and clinical use over the past 40 years. A British system – the EPG3 system developed at the University of Reading – has been used in the majority of studies conducted by researchers in Europe and Hong Kong (Hardcastle, Gibbon, & Jones, 1991; Hardcastle & Gibbon, 1997). A new Windows® version of the Reading EPG has recently been developed at Queen Margaret University, Edinburgh (Wrench, Gibbon, McNeill, & Wood, 2002). The Kay Palatometer has been used most widely in research carried out in the United States (Fletcher, 1983) and the Rion EPG has been most widely used in Japan (Fujimura, Tatsumi, & Kagaya, 1973; Hiki & Itoh, 1986). All EPG systems share some common general features, but differ in details such as the construction of the plates, the number and configuration of electrodes, and hardware/software specifications (Gibbon & Nicolaidis, 1999; Hardcastle & Gibbon, 1997).

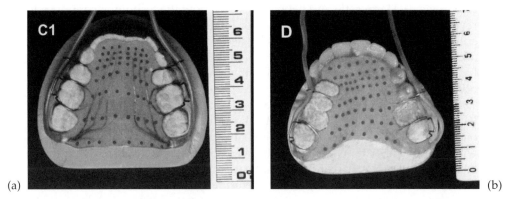

(a)

(b)

Figure 19.1   Photograph of artificial plate placed on top of the plaster impression of the upper palate and teeth. The plates are those used in the Reading EPG system and are from an adult with normal craniofacial anatomy (a) and an adult with a repaired cleft palate and a partial denture (b). Notice that the electrodes on the alveolar ridge are more closely spaced than those further back so that details such as tongue grooving for /s/ and /ʃ/ can be recorded.

The Reading plates are made from a relatively rigid acrylic, and are held in place by metal clasps that fit over the upper teeth. There are 62 sensors placed according to identifiable anatomical landmarks. Although it is relatively expensive to construct EPG plates, one advantage of the fact that they are custom-made is that they can be tailored to fit individuals with abnormally shaped hard palates (e.g., cleft palate) or dental anomalies, as well as those who wear dental braces or dentures. Figure 19.1 shows two Reading plates, one for an adult speaker with a normal palatal arch and one for an adult with a repaired cleft palate. EPG records movements of the tongue tip/blade and the front of the tongue body as they touch the hard palate and records characteristic patterns in normal speakers for all English lingual phoneme targets /t/, /d/, /k/, /g/, /s/, /z/, /ʃ/, /ʒ/, /tʃ/, /dʒ/, the palatal approximant /j/, nasals /n/, /ŋ/, and the lateral /l/. Varying amounts of contact are registered during bunched and retroflex varieties of /r/, relatively close vowels such as /i/, /ɪ/, /e/, /u/, /ʊ/, and rising diphthongs such as /eɪ/, /aɪ/, /ɔɪ/, /aʊ/ and /əʊ/. There is, however, usually minimal contact during open vowels, such as /ɑ/, /æ/ and /ɒ/ and consonants that have their primary constriction either further forward than the most anterior row of electrodes (e.g., dentals or bilabials) or further back than the most posterior row of electrodes (e.g., velars in the context of open vowels, uvular, pharyngeal and glottal sounds). Some EPG contact will be present during these categories of sounds where they occur in the context of relatively close vowels or rising diphthongs, however (Gibbon, Lee, & Yuen, 2007).

There is now a substantial literature on EPG as a diagnostic and therapy tool for speech disorders in children and adults (see Hardcastle & Gibbon, 2005, for a review). Hardcastle and Gibbon describe how the technique continues to reveal previously undescribed details of lingual dynamics, such as undifferentiated gestures (Gibbon, 1999), misdirected articulatory gestures (Wood, 1997) and labial-lingual double articulations (Gibbon & Crampin, 2002). EPG data have led researchers to propose a possible motor-based explanation for phenomena that have previously been interpreted as having linguistic origins. These include phonological processes and Smith's (1973) *puzzle* phenomenon (Gibbon, 2002). A recent bibliography showed more than 150 research papers on the clinical applications of EPG, with half of the studies investigating children with cleft palate or functional articulation disorders, and a substantial number focusing on neurogenic disorders and hearing impairment (Gibbon, 2003). EPG studies of disorders reported in the literature include: functional articulation disorders (Carter & Edwards, 2004; Dagenais, Critz-Crosby, & Adams, 1994; Gibbon, 1999); cleft palate (Gibbon, 2004; Gibbon & Crampin, 2002; Hardcastle, Morgan Barry, & Nunn, 1989; Howard, 2004; Michi, Suzuki, Yamashita, & Imai, 1986; Whitehill, Stokes, & Man, 1996; Yamashita, Michi, Imai, Suzuki, & Yoshida, 1992); neurogenic disorders (Edwards & Miller, 1989; Goozée, Murdoch, & Theodoros, 2003; Hardcastle, Morgan Barry, & Clark, 1985; Wood, 1997); hearing impairment (Dagenais & Critz-Crosby, 1991; Nicolaidis, 2004); malocclusion and osteotomy (Wakumoto, Isaacson, Friel, et al., 1996); glossectomy (Barry & Timmermann, 1985; Imai & Michi, 1992; Suzuki, 1989); stuttering (Wood, 1995); and Down's syndrome (Gibbon, McNeill, Wood, & Watson, 2003).

Hardcastle and Gibbon (1997) suggested that the EPG patterns produced by speakers with articulation disorders could be classified in terms of those that have abnormal spatial configurations of tongue–palate contact (e.g., complete tongue–palate contact), those that have abnormal timing (e.g., long durations) and those that are normal in terms of spatial configuration and timing but occur in an abnormal location (e.g., substitutions). Dynamic EPG data illustrating abnormal spatial patterns from children with articulation disorders are shown in figure 19.2. These examples are from four children aged 8–15 years; three have articulation disorders and one has normal speech. The patterns are for the /ʃ/ target in the phrase *a shop*. All /ʃ/ targets are produced by the children with disorders as distortions and transcribed in a perceptual analysis as lateral fricatives. The figure shows that the child with normal speech produces /ʃ/ with lateral contact and an anterior groove configuration. These two features (lateral contact and anterior groove) are absent from the patterns produced by the children with speech disorders. Each of the speech-disordered children had rather different EPG patterns for the /ʃ/ target, although these differences were not detected in a perceptual analysis. For example, one child (see figure 19.2b) raised her tongue to make extensive contact across most of the palate during the production of this sound. This form of articulation is typical of the undifferentiated gesture described by Gibbon (1999). Another child had a pattern rather like that of an alveolar stop (figure 19.2c), but with some asymmetry and incomplete lateral seal on the right side. This incomplete seal could indicate where air was escaping into the buccal cavity during the

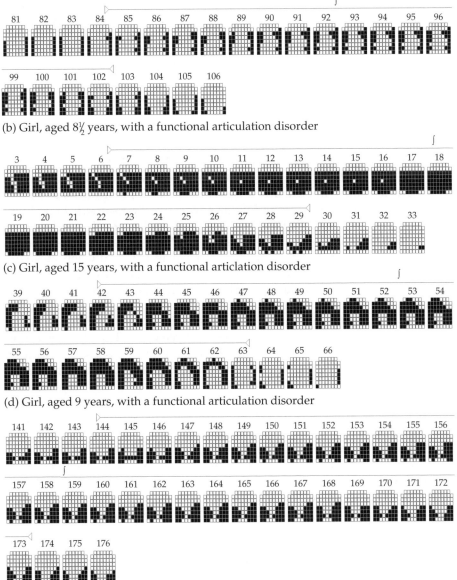

Figure 19.2 EPG printouts for four children's productions of /ʃ/ in the phrase *a shop*. These are full EPG printouts, where the top of individual palatograms represents the alveolar region and the bottom is the velar region located at the junction between the hard and soft palates. The sampling interval is 10 ms. Of note is that the typically developing child's tongue–palate contact patterns shown in (a) display lateral contact and a groove configuration in the anterior region of the palate. The three children with articulation disorders shown in (b), (c), and (d) show different EPG patterns, although all were heard by listeners as lateral fricatives [ɬ].

lateral fricative. The third child had contact predominantly in the palatal and velar regions of the palate (figure 19.2d). Here there is evidence of a posterior groove configuration, which could indicate that air was escaping centrally as well as laterally during these productions of lateral fricatives. Identifying the exact tongue–palate contact patterns is considered important because visual feedback therapy aims to modify existing patterns so that they more closely resemble normal patterns (Gibbon, 1999).

An important advantage of EPG is that it is safe and convenient to use, which means that it is a suitable tool for use with clinical populations. Another plus is that it has a high sampling rate (usually 100–200 Hz), which allows it to record in detail the activities of the fast-moving tongue tip. It also provides detailed articulatory information on a wide range of phonemes that are frequently produced as errors in individuals with speech disorders. In addition, EPG is one of the few techniques that can record the lateral margins of the tongue. Fletcher (1992) emphasized the importance of contact between the lateral borders of the tongue and the hard palate for production of lingual stops, lingual fricatives and high vowels. Another particularly attractive property of EPG to speech-language pathologists is that the data are intuitive. This means that when EPG is used to provide visual feedback in therapy, it is possible even for young children to understand how different sounds are articulated and displayed on the computer screen. A relatively recent innovation has been the use of EPG portable training units (Jones & Hardcastle, 1995). The major design features of these units are that they are small, lightweight units, making them portable, relatively inexpensive, and simple to operate. The portable units allow visual feedback therapy to take place close to a child's home, so increasing opportunities for practice and avoiding the need to travel long distances for therapy sessions.

Like all instruments, EPG has limitations. Individuals need a specially constructed artificial plate, which takes time to construct, is relatively costly and is invasive to the extent that an intraoral device such as this might interfere with natural speech production. Adults with normal speech can usually adapt in a short period to wearing the plate, allowing them to speak naturally with it in place (McLeod & Searl, 2006). However, EPG is not widely used with very young children, toddlers or infants due to the procedural demands of wearing the EPG plate. Furthermore, some individuals find wearing the plate uncomfortable and do not easily adapt to its presence in the mouth. Another limitation is that EPG records only when the tongue is raised to touch the plate, making it less useful when the tongue is lowered away from the plate because in this situation there is minimal EPG contact. EPG is therefore not informative when investigating some consonants (e.g., bilabials, glottals and pharyngeals) or low vowels. A final limitation is that there is no way of inferring from EPG data alone which part of the tongue is producing a particular contact pattern; this must be deduced from the shape of the person's palate and knowledge of the anatomy and physiology of the tongue (Hardcastle & Gibbon, 1997).

19.3   Imaging Techniques

The following section covers three techniques: X-ray, ultrasound and magnetic resonance imaging (MRI). Imaging techniques such as these have developed to create images of the human body primarily for clinical purposes and medical science, and have subsequently been used to record the movement and position of the articulators. Collectively, these techniques have the advantages of minimum disruption to the natural process of speech production and the capability of providing a much more extensive view of the vocal tract than other techniques. There have been significant advances in the development of ultrasound and MRI techniques in recent years, although X-ray is no longer used for nonessential purposes due to the well-recognized health hazards associated with radiation exposure.

19.3.1   X-ray

X-ray uses ionizing radiation to obtain images, which are created by exposing an object to X-rays and capturing the resultant shadow on photographic film. X-ray provides clear images and it is possible to view most of the vocal tract, including the moving articulators (e.g., tongue, lips) contrasted against the fixed structures (e.g., hard palate). Images may be still or cine, with static X-ray images of a single posture or vocal tract configuration usually taken from the side of the head in speech research to create a lateral image. Serial or cineradiography can record dynamic events; it was a widely used imaging technique for investigating articulator motion until the early 1970s (Hiiemae & Palmer, 2003).

Fluoroscopic and fluorographic techniques consist of an X-ray image intensifier linked to photographic and video cameras. Videofluorography became widely used in the late 1980s for diagnostic radiological purposes and had the advantage of having lower radiation levels. A number of previous studies have used X-ray to investigate tongue behavior in articulation disorders including dysarthria (Kent & Netsell, 1975), hearing impairment (Tye-Murray, 1987), stuttering (Zimmermann, 1980), and cleft palate (Brooks, Shelton, & Youngstrom, 1965; Powers, 1962; Tanimoto, Henningsson, Isberg, & Ren, 1994). A specialized X-ray system has been used at the University of Tokyo (Fujimura, Kiritani, & Ishida, 1973), and the University of Wisconsin-Madison (Westbury, 1994). In this system, the X-ray beam is sharply focused and controlled to track markers placed on the articulators. The advantage of this system is that it can collect large amounts of data with relatively little radiation exposure to the speaker. A number of studies have used the X-ray microbeam technique to investigate tongue and lip movements in speech disorders such as dysarthria (Weismer, Yunusova, & Westbury, 2003) and hearing impairment (Tye-Murray, 1991).

X-ray is still used routinely in clinical contexts for imaging velum and pharyngeal activity during speech in individuals who may have to undergo surgery to improve velopharyngeal function. Although the primary purpose is to view velum movements, it is possible to view at the same time the actions of the tongue, lips and jaw and to observe abnormal behavior, such as compensatory movements of the tongue. One such compensatory action is the maneuver known as *lingual assistance* (Brooks, Shelton, & Youngstrom, 1965). Brooks and colleagues used cineradiography to investigate tongue position, mobility and compensatory movements in children with cleft palate and normal controls. These authors observed that a small number of children with cleft palate "appeared to elevate the palate by means of the tongue during speech" (p. 170). This phenomenon was not observed in any control children. Figure 19.3 shows an image from a videofluoroscopy clip illustrating lingual assistance. The image shows the midpoint of a voiced bilabial plosive (/b/) produced by a teenager with Pierre-Robin syndrome and velopharyngeal

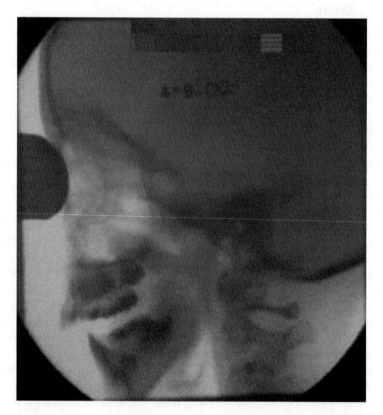

Figure 19.3 X-ray image of a child with velopharyngeal dysfunction, who is using an abnormal tongue maneuver known as *lingual assistance*, whereby the back of the tongue pushes upwards and backwards in an attempt to achieve velopharyngeal closure. The image is from the /b/ in the word *boy.*

dysfunction. The dynamic sequence, from which this static image was extracted, showed the back of the tongue pushing upwards and backwards in the speaker's attempt to achieve velopharyngeal closure during the production of this sound.

X-ray has some limitations in addition to the obvious health hazard. X-ray presents a composite two-dimensional image of a three-dimensional structure, namely the head. This can make identifying the soft tissues of the tongue difficult because the bony structures of the jaw and teeth may obscure the view (Stone, 1997). Another problem with this technique for imaging the tongue is identifying which part of the tongue (lateral or midline) is being imaged unless a contrast medium is used to mark the midline (ibid.).

19.3.2   Ultrasound

The past 20 years have seen a rapid rise in the number of studies using ultrasound to investigate tongue movements in speech and swallowing in children and adults (Ball, Gracco, & Stone, 2001; Bressmann, Uy, & Irish, 2005; Chi-Fishman, 2005; Stone, 1991; 1997; 2005). The use of ultrasound for imaging the tongue in speech has been pioneered by Maureen Stone and colleagues over the past 15 years and the reader is directed to Stone (2005) for a description of the technical details and principles of ultrasound. Ultrasound imaging creates images of body tissue using sound waves of ultra high frequency, revealing distinct tongue shapes and movements for alveolar and velar articulations and also for vowels (Lundberg & Stone, 1999; Sonies, Shawker, Hall, Gerber, & Leighton, 1981; Stone, 2005; Stone & Lundberg, 1996). To image the tongue, a probe that emits and receives ultrasound waves is placed below the chin and the beam angled upwards. The sound waves travel up through the tongue, and when they reach the boundary between soft tissue and air at the tongue surface, some of the sound waves, or echoes, are reflected back to the probe and are picked up by it. The reflected sound waves are recorded and displayed as real-time visual images of lengthwise (sagittal) or cross-sectional (coronal) views of the tongue. Traditionally, ultrasound makes two-dimensional images but it is possible to produce three-dimensional images by making multiple scans and then combining them using computer software (Bressmann, Heng, & Irish, 2005; Lundberg & Stone, 1999).

Figure 19.4 depicts ultrasound images of the sagittal and coronal tongue during the /a/ in the word *cap*. It is possible to view much of the tongue's length in the sagittal plane (figure 19.4a). This figure shows the characteristic bright white line of the tongue, which is the reflection caused by the ultrasound waves from the probe under the chin hitting the air at the tongue surface. The dark area underneath the bright white line is the tongue body. In the sagittal image the mandible and the hyoid bone create a shadow (black region) at both edges of the image, obscuring parts of the tongue tip and root. Figure 19.4b is an ultrasound image in the coronal plane, and shows the raised lateral edges of the tongue as well as medial compression.

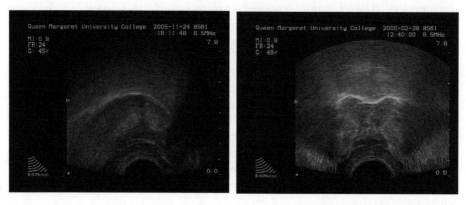

(a) (b)

Figure 19.4   An example of a sagittal ultrasound image of the tongue is shown in (a), with the anterior tongue towards the right side of the image. An example of a coronal section is shown in (b). The images are from the middle of the vowel /a/ in the word *cap*.

Ultrasound has advantages that make it an attractive technique for using with clinical populations, and recently it has been used as a diagnostic tool to investigate tongue movements in individuals with hearing impairment (Bernhardt, Gick, Bacsfalvi, & Adler-Bock, 2005; Bernhardt, Gick, Bacsfalvi, & Ashdown, 2003), glossectomy (Bressmann, Uy, & Irish, 2005) and residual articulation difficulties (Shawker & Sonies, 1985). The technique is safe and noninvasive, which means that it is possible to gather extensive speech material from clinical populations. The fact that it is noninvasive means that it interferes minimally with natural speech and can be used with young children and infants as well as adults. It can visualize the tongue in real time with relatively inexpensive and portable equipment (Ball, Gracco, & Stone, 2001; Bressmann, Heng, & Irish, 2005). Its portability, the ease with which data can be collected, and its ready availability in hospitals and clinics mean that this technique has potential for routine use in clinical contexts. Temporal and spatial resolutions are relatively good, although frame rates for the dynamic images that are usually exported to video are limited to 25–30 frames per second. One disadvantage of ultrasound is that it provides only a partial view of the tongue. For example, it is not always possible to image the tongue tip and tongue root, because the tip can be obscured by the air beneath it and the root can be obscured by the hyoid bone shadow. A second difficulty is that it is not possible to image vocal-tract structures beyond the surface of the tongue, making it difficult to know its position in relation to the hard and soft palates or the pharynx.

Apart from the practical advantages already outlined, an important feature of ultrasound of relevance to its development as a clinical tool is that, like EPG, it can display images of the tongue in real time and the ultrasound images that appear on the computer screen are intuitive and relatively easy to interpret. These features mean that this technique can be used to provide visual feedback of tongue surface shape with children and adults with speech disorders. Ultrasound has so far been underutilized for therapy purposes, but it is now beginning to be used more frequently (Bernhardt, Gick, Bacsfalvi, & Adler-Bock, 2005; Bernhardt, Gick, Bacsfalvi, & Ashdown, 2003; Shawker & Sonies, 1985). Bernhardt, Gick, Bacsfalvi, and Adler-Bock (2005), using a series of studies of adolescents and adults with hearing impairment, residual speech impairment or accented speech, have developed ultrasound treatment techniques based on visual feedback of tongue shape features for English lingual stops, vowels, sibilants and liquids. This is a promising new approach to therapy, but requires further controlled research based on larger groups of individuals with speech disorders.

19.3.3   *Magnetic resonance imaging (MRI)*

MRI is a noninvasive technique that can produce high quality images of the soft and hard tissues of the vocal tract from the lips to the larynx (Baer, Gore, Gracco, & Nye, 1991; Stone, 1991). MRI uses radiofrequency waves with scanners consisting of electromagnets that surround the body to create a magnetic field. MRI scanning detects the presence of hydrogen atoms; the images highlight differences in the water content and distribution in body tissues. The visual result is that tissue with fewer hydrogen atoms, such as bones and air, is dark, whereas tissue with many hydrogen atoms, such as muscle, is lighter. Like ultrasound, MRI scans generate two-dimensional images, which can be combined to produce three-dimensional images.

   Although MRI is being used increasingly to investigate speech movement in normal speakers, in the past its use to investigate impaired articulation focused on identifying abnormal tongue mass, shape and position as opposed to movement (Cha & Patten, 1989; Wein, Drobnitzky, Klajman, & Angerstein, 1991). The technique's limited use to investigate movement has been due largely to its slow temporal resolution, making it unsuitable for investigating dynamic aspects of speech or speech disorders. However, recent improvements in temporal resolution mean that it is now possible to examine these dynamic aspects of speech, including segment durations, articulator positions, and interarticulator timing (Narayanan, Nayak, Lee, Sethy, & Byrd, 2004).

   The advantages of MRI are that the images provide a higher level of detail than other imaging techniques such as ultrasound, and that, unlike X-ray, the technique is safe to use. Furthermore, the technique allows imaging of the whole of the vocal tract, which is advantageous when it is not known prior to making a recording which articulators are implicated in a speech disorder. These benefits mean that the technique has potential for research purposes to investigate articulation impairments in a wide range of clinical populations. There are practical limitations, however. MRI scanners are costly and require specialists to operate and maintain them. They are also in high demand for medical diagnostic purposes so access for speech-recording purposes may be limited. A final disadvantage is that the procedure involves the person lying inside a large cylinder, which could cause distress to individuals who suffer from claustrophobia, and the supine position can also alter articulator relationships during speech.

19.4   Motion Tracking

Motion-tracking instruments are most widely used to investigate articulatory kinematics, which involves measuring aspects of motion, such as displacement, velocity, acceleration, duration and amplitude. The so-called point-tracking systems track movement of discrete fleshpoints at high sampling rates and have proved one of the most useful methods for directly measuring speech motor control in normal speakers and those with impaired articulation.

19.4.1   *Magnetic systems*

The most commonly used magnetic motion-capture system in speech research is electromagnetic articulography (EMA) or electromagnetic midsagittal articulography (EMMA). The two most widely used systems have been developed in Germany (Schönle, Gräbe, Wenig, et al., 1987) and the United States (Perkell, Cohen, Svirsky, et al., 1992). These systems record two-dimensional movement trajectories for selected fleshpoints on the tongue, lips and jaw in the midsagittal plane. Transmitter coils mounted on a specially constructed helmet form an equilateral triangle in front of the chin, in front of the forehead, and behind the neck. The transmitters produce an alternating magnetic field at different frequencies, making it possible to track movement at discrete points in the vocal tract during speech production. Sensors are glued to various locations on the vocal tract – typically on the bridge of the nose, the maxillary gum ridge (to monitor head movement) on the upper and lower lips, the mandibular gum ridge, and three or four points on the tongue. A recently developed three-dimensional system is now available which allows for measurement outside the midsagittal plane (Zierdt, Hoole, & Tillmann, 1999).

There is now a substantial literature using EMA to investigate speech motor control in clinical populations, focusing mainly on stuttering (Max, Caruso, & Gracco, 2003; Story, Alfonso, & Harris, 1996), neurogenic disorders (Jaeger, Hertrich, Stattrop, Schönle, & Ackermann, 2000; Murdoch & Goozée, 2003; Nijland, Maassen, Hulstijn, & Peters, 2001) and to a lesser extent children with cleft lip (van Lieshout, Rutjens, & Spauwen, 2002). Nijland, Maassen, Hulstijn and Peters (2001) used EMA to study the phenomenon of *articulator coupling* in children with developmental apraxia of speech. This phenomenon involves sets of articulators producing gestures in a largely synchronous manner. Synchronous gestures are interpreted as reflecting a motor constraint, insofar as the basic control mechanism that allows the different articulators to operate relatively independently has not yet developed. An example of coupling is the undifferentiated gesture, whereby the tongue apex, lateral margins and tongue

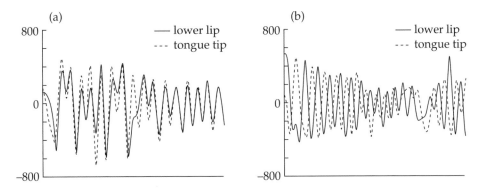

Figure 19.5   Lower lip and tongue-tip movement recorded using electromagnetic articulography (EMA) from two children aged nine years. The traces are from one child with developmental apraxia of speech (a) and one with typical speech development (b) during productions of /pata/ sequences. From Nijland, Maassen, Hulstijn and Peters (2001, p. 219, figs. 3 & 4).

body appear to move together in a synchronous way (Gibbon, 1999). In Nijland and colleagues' EMA study, they found differences in coupling between children with developmental apraxia of speech and typically developing children. Figure 19.5 shows the lower lip and tongue tip movement signal during the nonsense sequence /pata/ for a child with apraxia (left) and a typically developing child (right). The figure shows that for the typically developing child, the peaks of the lower lip and tongue tip movement alternate. This is in contrast to the child with apraxia, whose lower lip and tongue tip movements are coupled, so appearing to move simultaneously and with equivalent amplitudes.

One of the advantages of EMA is that due to the high sampling rate, the output data contain precise information about the location of discrete points. This factor makes EMA well suited for measuring speech motor control of the lips, jaw and tongue, and the timing relationships between them. This capability, combined with the fact that it is safe, makes EMA ideal for investigating speech impairments associated with known or suspected motor origin. EMA has also been used as a therapy tool in a small number of studies. Katz, Bharadwaj and Carstens (1999) explored the use of EMA to provide visual feedback for articulation deficits in adults with apraxia of speech. Although the findings from this study suggest that feedback of tongue-tip position with EMA could be used to treat abnormal speech motor behavior, its use for this purpose is not currently widespread in research or clinical practice. Its limited use as a therapy tool may be due to the procedural demands of the technique combined with the fact that the visual display of EMA data is perhaps not as easy to interpret as the more intuitive data provided by other techniques, such as EPG and ultrasound.

The disadvantages of EMA are that it is relatively expensive to buy and invasive to the extent that it involves gluing magnetic coils directly onto the articulators, which can interfere with normal speech. Also, the experimental set-up is restrictive and may be uncomfortable because it involves the speaker wearing a helmet, although new developments in the German EMA system mean that the helmet is no longer fixed to the head, allowing free head movement for the speaker. The procedural restrictions of earlier versions of EMA have meant that it has not been used with young children or infants. Another limitation is that the technique only records data at discrete points in the vocal tract, unlike the imaging techniques already described. This limitation means that it does not provide information about the rest of the vocal tract, nor about what is occurring between fleshpoints. Lack of information about what is occurring between discrete points is more of a problem for speech segments that involve complex tongue configurations, such as retroflexed sounds, than for less complex vowel shapes.

19.4.2   Optoelectronic systems

An ordinary cine/video camera can be used to investigate the coordinated actions of the visually accessible articulators, namely the lips and jaw (Baken, 1987). More sophisticated optical motion systems, such as Optotrak (Guiard-Marigny & Ostry, 1997), Selspot (Kelso, Vatikiotis-Bateson, Saltzman, & Kay, 1985) and VICON (Gibert, Bailly, Beautemps, Elisei, & Brun, 2005), can record movement at discrete points located on the lips and jaw in three dimensions. These systems collect movement data with a video camera by attaching small, infrared, light-emitting diodes or reflective markers to the articulators. The camera tracks the markers attached to the jaw and lips and the use of several cameras makes it possible to measure the movements of each marker. A number of studies have used optical devices to study abnormal lip and jaw movements in clinical populations, such as individuals with dysarthria (Ackermann, Hertrich, Daum, Scharf, & Spieker, 1997; Svensson, Henningson, & Karlsson, 1993) and stuttering (Jäncke, Bauer, Kaiser, & Kalveram, 1997). Although the markers used in systems such as VICON may interfere with natural speech to some extent, an important advantage is that it is one of the few techniques that can record orofacial movements in young children, infants and even newborn babies (Green, Moore, & Reilly, 2002). The limitation of these techniques is that they can measure movements of external structures only and cannot be used to investigate articulators within the vocal tract.

19.4.3   Glossometry

Glossometry is a technique that uses light-emitting diodes and phototransistor pairs mounted on an artificial plate molded to fit against the hard palate in a way similar to the EPG plate (Flege, 1989). The phototransistor pairs are located in the midline of the plate. Infrared light emitted from the diodes is scattered by the tongue and the light is reflected back from the surface of the tongue to the photosensors. The distance between the sensors and the tongue is computed and displayed on a computer screen. Glossometry has not been used widely to investigate speech disorders, although one study has used it to provide visual feedback of tongue position. Fletcher, Dagenais and Critz-Crosby (1991) used glossometry to teach selected vowels to school-aged children with hearing impairment. Therapy involved displaying model tongue positions on a computer screen and a dynamic display providing real-time feedback of the child's own tongue's position in the oral cavity. The results of this study showed that glossometry was beneficial in enabling some children with hearing impairment to produce more intelligible vowels and to use an expanded vowel space.

19.5   Conclusion

There have been significant advances over the past two decades in the instruments available to investigate articulation. For example, the capability of the standard EPG technique to record tongue–palate contact has been extended recently with the development of a prototype system that can detect dynamic tongue–palate pressures (Murdoch, Goozée, Veidt, Scott, & Meyers, 2004). A further advance has been a multi-channel approach to investigating speech production (Engwall, 2003), which entails recording data from a number of techniques simultaneously. Multi-channel approaches overcome the general limitation inherent in most techniques, which is that they record a specific aspect of articulation in a particular part of the vocal tract. Such new developments offer exciting possibilities for conducting basic research into the articulatory processes underlying speech disorders, particularly for directly measuring speech motor control.

Despite the progress in the technical specifications of the instruments, many remain underutilized, particularly in clinical settings. It may be that the technical, practical and procedural challenges involved in using instruments, which were outlined at the beginning of this chapter, have limited their use. Another possible explanation for their underutilization is that, in clinical practice, essential medical decisions (e.g., the need for surgery) are rarely reliant on instrumental data about the functioning of the tongue, jaw or lips during speech. In contrast, instrumental investigations of the actions of the vocal folds or velum during speech play a central role in the decision as to whether an individual undergoes palatal or laryngeal surgery. As a result, instruments for investigating velum and laryngeal function are used routinely in specialist cleft palate and voice clinics. Furthermore, studies have not yet demonstrated conclusively that clinical decisions taken by the speech-language pathologist, such as making a differential diagnosis or proceeding with a particular type of intervention, depend on results from instrumental investigations. These may be some of the reasons why instruments are not currently used more widely for investigating articulation impairments.

A feature of some techniques (e.g., EPG and ultrasound) that is promoting their more widespread use in clinical contexts is the facility to provide visual feedback. The growing literature showing the effectiveness of using visual feedback as part of a speech therapy program to improve intelligibility is likely to further promote their clinical use. Although there is now a relatively large number of studies documenting therapy using visual feedback, the quality of the evidence needs to improve. For example, the number of individuals reported in treatment studies is small; most studies investigate single cases or small groups. Furthermore, studies with adequate control groups are lacking. There is therefore a need for large, controlled group studies to establish the effectiveness of using visual feedback to improve speech intelligibility in children and adults with articulation disorders.

REFERENCES

Ackermann, H., Hertrich, I., Daum, I., Scharf, G., and Spieker, S. (1997). Kinematic analysis of articulatory movements in central motor disorders. *Movement Disorders*, 12, 1019–27.

Baer, T., Gore, J. C., Gracco, L. C., and Nye, P. W. (1991). Analysis of vocal tract shape and dimensions using magnetic resonance imaging: Vowels. *Journal of the Acoustical Society of America*, 90, 799–828.

Baken, R. J. (1987). *Clinical Measurement of Speech and Voice*. Boston, MA: College Hill.

Baken, R. J. and Orlikoff, R. F. (2000). *Clinical Measurement of Speech and Voice*. 2nd ed. San Diego, CA: Singular.

Ball, M. J. and Code, C. (1997). *Instrumental Clinical Phonetics*. London: Whurr Publishers.

Ball, M., Gracco, V., and Stone, M. (2001). A comparison of imaging techniques for the investigation of normal and disordered speech production. *Advances in Speech-Language Pathology*, 3, 13–24.

Barry, W. J. and Timmermann, G. (1985). Mispronunciations and compensatory movements of tongue operated patients. *British Journal of Disorders of Communication*, 20, 81–90.

Bernhardt, B., Gick, B., Bacsfalvi, P., and Adler-Bock, M. (2005). Ultrasound in speech therapy with adolescents and adults. *Clinical Linguistics and Phonetics*, 19, 605–17.

Bernhardt, B., Gick, B., Bacsfalvi, P., and Ashdown, J. (2003). Speech habilitation of hard of hearing adolescents using electropalatography and ultrasound as evaluated by trained listeners. *Clinical Linguistics and Phonetics*, 17, 199–216.

Bressmann, T., Heng, C. L., and Irish, J. C. (2005). Applications of 2D and 3D ultrasound imaging in speech-language pathology. *Journal of Speech-Language Pathology and Audiology*, 29, 158–68.

Bressmann, T., Uy, C., and Irish, J. C. (2005). Analysing normal and partial glossectomee tongues using ultrasound. *Clinical Linguistics and Phonetics*, 19, 35–52.

Brooks, A. R., Shelton, R. L., and Youngstrom, K. A. (1965). Compensatory tongue-palate-posterior pharyngeal wall relationships in cleft palate. *Journal of Speech and Hearing Disorders*, 30, 166–73.

Carter, P. and Edwards, S. (2004). EPG therapy for children with long-standing speech disorders: Predictions and outcomes. *Clinical Linguistics and Phonetics*, 18, 359–72.

Cha, C. H. and Patten, B. M. (1989). Amyotrophic lateral sclerosis: Abnormalities of the tongue on magnetic resonance imaging. *Annals of Neurology*, 25, 468–72.

Chi-Fishman, G. (2005). Quantitative lingual, pharyngeal and laryngeal ultrasonography in swallowing research: A technical review. *Clinical Linguistics and Phonetics*, 19, 589–604.

Dagenais, P. A. and Critz-Crosby, P. (1991). Consonant lingual-palatal contacts produced by normal-hearing and hearing impaired children. *Journal of Speech and Hearing Research*, 34, 1423–35.

Dagenais, P. A., Critz-Crosby, P., and Adams, J. B. (1994). Defining and remediating persistent lateral lisps in children using electropalatography: Preliminary findings. *American Journal of Speech-Language Pathology*, 3, 67–76.

Edwards, S. and Miller, N. (1989). Using EPG to investigate speech errors and motor agility in a dyspraxic patient. *Clinical Linguistics and Phonetics*, 3, 111–26.

Engwall, O. (2003). Combining MRI, EMA and EPG measurements in a three-dimensional tongue model. *Speech Communication*, 41, 303–29.

Flege, J. E. (1989). Differences in inventory size affect the location but not the precision of tongue positioning in vowel production. *Language and Speech*, 32, 123–47.

Fletcher, S. (1983). New prospects for speech by the hearing impaired. In N. Lass (ed.), *Speech and Language: Advances in Basic Research and Practice* (pp. 1–42). New York: Academic Press.

Fletcher, S. G. (1992). *Articulation: A Physiological Approach*. San Diego, CA: Singular Publishing Group.

Fletcher, S. G., Dagenais, P. A., and Critz-Crosby, P. (1991). Teaching vowels to profoundly hearing-impaired speakers using glossometry. *Journal of Speech and Hearing Research*, 34, 943–56.

Fujimura, O., Kiritani, S., and Ishida, H. (1973). Computer controlled radiography for observation of movements of articulatory and other human organs. *Computers in Biology and Medicine*, 3, 371–84.

Fujimura, O., Tatsumi, I. F., and Kagaya, R. (1973). Computational processing of palatographic patterns. *Journal of Phonetics*, 1, 47–54.

Gibbon, F. E. (1999). Undifferentiated lingual gestures in children with articulation/phonological disorders. *Journal of Speech, Language, and Hearing Research*, 42, 382–97.

Gibbon, F. E. (2002). Features of impaired tongue control in children with phonological disorder. In F. Windsor, N. Hewlett, and M. L. Kelly (eds.), *Investigations in Clinical Phonetics and Linguistics* (pp. 299–309). London: Lawrence Erlbaum.

Gibbon, F. E. (2003). Using articulatory data to inform speech pathology theory and clinical practice. In M. J. Solé, D. Recasens, and J. Romero (eds.), *Proceedings of the 15th International Congress of Phonetic Sciences, Barcelona, 3–9 August 2003* (pp. 261–4). Rundle Mall, Adelaide: Causal Productions.

Gibbon, F. E. (2004). Abnormal patterns of tongue–palate contact in the speech of individuals with cleft palate. *Clinical Linguistics and Phonetics*, 18, 285–311.

Gibbon, F. and Crampin, L. (2002). Labial-lingual double articulations in cleft palate speech. *Cleft Palate-Craniofacial Journal*, 39, 40–9.

Gibbon, F., Lee, A., and Yuen, I. (2007). Tongue palate contact during bilabials in normal speech. *Cleft Palate-Craniofacial Journal*, 44, 87–91.

Gibbon, F. E., McNeill, A. M., Wood, S. E., and Watson, J. M. M. (2003). Changes in linguapalatal contact patterns during therapy for velar fronting in a 10-year-old with Down's syndrome. *International Journal of Language and Communication Disorders*, 38, 47–64.

Gibbon, F. and Nicolaidis, K. (1999). Palatography. In W. J. Hardcastle and N. Hewlett (eds.), *Coarticulation in Speech Production: Theory, Data, and Techniques* (pp. 229–45). Cambridge: Cambridge University Press.

Gibert, G., Bailly, G., Beautemps, D., Elisei, F., and Brun R. (2005). Analysis and synthesis of the three-dimensional movements of the head, face and hand of a speaker using cued speech. *Journal of the Acoustical Society of America*, 118, 1144–53.

Goozée, J. V., Murdoch, B. E., and Theodoros, D. G. (2003). Electropalatographic assessment of tongue-to-palate contacts exhibited in dysarthria following traumatic brain injury: Spatial characteristics. *Journal of Medical Speech-Language Pathology*, 11, 115–29.

Green, J. R., Moore, C. A., and Reilly, K. J. (2002). The sequential development of jaw and lip control for speech. *Journal of Speech, Language, and Hearing Research*, 45, 66–79.

Guiard-Marigny, T. and Ostry, D. J. (1997). A system for three-dimensional visualization of human jaw motion in speech. *Journal of Speech, Language, and Hearing Research*, 40, 1118–1121.

Hardcastle, W. J. and Gibbon, F. (1997). Electropalatography and its clinical applications. In M. J. Ball and C. Code (eds.), *Instrumental Clinical Phonetics* (pp. 149–93). London: Whurr Publishers.

Hardcastle, W. J. and Gibbon, F. (2005). EPG as a research and clinical tool: 30 years on. In W. J. Hardcastle and J. Mackenzie Beck (eds.), *A Figure of Speech: A Festschrift for John Laver* (pp. 39–60). Mahwah, NJ: Lawrence Erlbaum Associates.

Hardcastle, W. J., Gibbon, F. E., and Jones, W. (1991). Visual display of tongue–palate contact: Electropalatography in the assessment and remediation of speech disorders. *British Journal of Disorders of Communication*, 26, 41–74.

Hardcastle, W. J., Morgan Barry, R., and Clark, C. (1985). Articulatory and voicing characteristics of adult dysarthric and verbal dyspraxic speakers: An instrumental study. *British Journal of Disorders of Communication*, 20, 249–70.

Hardcastle, W., Morgan Barry, R., and Nunn, M. (1989). Instrumental articulatory phonetics in assessment and remediation: Case studies with the electropalatograph. In J. Stengelhofen (ed.), *Cleft Palate: The Nature and Remediation of Communication Problems*, pp. 136–64. Edinburgh: Churchill Livingstone.

Hiiemae, K. M. and Palmer, J. B. (2003). Tongue movements in feeding and speech. *Critical Reviews in Oral Biology and Medicine*, 14, 413–29.

Hiki, S. and Itoh, H. (1986). Influence of palate shape on lingual articulation. *Speech Communication*, 5, 141–58.

Howard, S. (2004). Compensatory articulatory behaviours in adolescents with cleft palate: comparing the perceptual and instrumental evidence. *Clinical Linguistics and Phonetics*, 18, 313–40.

Imai, S. and Michi, K. (1992). Articulatory function after resection of the tongue and floor of the mouth: Palatometric and perceptual evaluation. *Journal of Speech and Hearing Research*, 35, 68–78.

Jaeger, M., Hertrich, I., Stattrop, U., Schönle, P. W., and Ackermann, H. (2000). Speech disorders following severe traumatic brain injury: Kinematic analysis of syllable repetitions using electromagnetic articulography. *Folia Phoniatrica et Logopaedica*, 52, 187–96.

Jäncke, L., Bauer, A., Kaiser, P., and Kalveram, K. (1997). Timing and stiffness in speech motor control of stuttering and nonstuttering adults. *Journal of Fluency Disorders*, 22, 309–21.

Jones, W. and Hardcastle, W. J. (1995). New developments in EPG3 software. *European Journal of Disorders of Communication*, 30, 183–92.

Katz, W. F., Bharadwaj, S. V., and Carstens, B. (1999). Electromagnetic articulography treatment for an adult with Broca's aphasia and apraxia of speech. *Journal of Speech, Language, and Hearing Research*, 42, 1355–66.

Kelso, J. A. S., Vatikiotis-Bateson, E., Saltzman, E. L., and Kay, B. (1985). A qualitative dynamic analysis of reiterant speech production: Phase portraits, kinematics, and dynamic modeling. *Journal of the Acoustical Society of America*, 77, 266–80.

Kent, R. and Netsell, R. (1975). A case study of an ataxic dysarthric: Cineradiographic and spectrographic observations. *Journal of Speech and Hearing Disorders*, 40, 115–34.

Lundberg, A. and Stone, M. (1999). Three-dimensional tongue surface reconstruction: practical considerations for ultrasound data. *Journal of the Acoustical Society of America*, 106, 2858–67.

Max, L., Caruso, A. J., and Gracco, V. L. (2003). Kinematic analyses of speech, orofacial nonspeech, and finger movements in stuttering and nonstuttering adults. *Journal of Speech, Language, and Hearing Research*, 46, 215–32.

McLeod, S. and Searl, J. (2006). Adaptation to an electropalatography palate: Acoustic, impressionistic, and perceptual data. *American Journal of Speech-Language Pathology*, 15, 192–206.

Michi, K., Suzuki, N., Yamashita, Y., and Imai, S. (1986). Visual training and correction of articulation disorders by use of dynamic palatography: Serial observation in a case of cleft palate. *Journal of Speech and Hearing Disorders*, 51, 226–38.

Murdoch, B. E. and Goozée, J. V. (2003). EMA analysis of tongue function in children with dysarthria following traumatic brain injury. *Brain Injury*, 17, 79–93.

Murdoch, B. E., Goozée, J. V., Veidt, M., Scott, D. H., and Meyers, I. A. (2004). Introducing the pressure-sensing palatograph: The next frontier in electropalatography. *Clinical Linguistics and Phonetics*, 18, 433–45.

Narayanan, S., Nayak, K., Lee, S., Sethy, A., and Byrd, D. (2004). An approach to real-time magnetic resonance imaging for speech production. *Journal of the Acoustical Society of America*, 115, 1771–6.

Nicolaidis, K. (2004). Articulatory variability during consonant production by Greek speakers with hearing impairment: an electropalatographic study. *Clinical Linguistics and Phonetics*, 18(6–8), 419–32.

Nijland, L., Maassen, B., Hulstijn, W., and Peters, H. (2001). Articulatory coupling in children with DAS studied with EMMA. In B. Maassen, W. Hulstijn, R. Kent, H. Peters, and P. van Lieshout (eds.), *Speech Motor Control in Normal and Disordered Speech* (pp. 216–19). Nijmegen: Uitgeverij Vantilt.

Perkell, J. S., Cohen, M. H., Svirsky, M. A., Matthies, M. L., Garabieta, I., and Jackson, M. T. T. (1992). Electromagnetic midsagittal articulometer systems for transducing speech articulatory movements. *Journal of the Acoustical Society of America*, 92, 3078–96.

Powers, G. R. (1962). Cinefluorographic investigation of articulatory movements of selected individuals with cleft palates. *Journal of Speech and Hearing Research*, 5, 59–69.

Schönle, P. W., Gräbe, K., Wenig, P., Hohne, J., Schrader, J., and Conrad, B. (1987). Electromagnetic articulography: Use of alternating magnetic fields for tracking movements of multiple points inside and outside the vocal tract. *Brain and Language*, 31, 26–35.

Shawker, T. H. and Sonies, B. C. (1985). Ultrasound biofeedback for speech training: instrumentation and preliminary results. *Investigative Radiology*, 20, 90–3.

Smith, N. V. (1973). *The Acquisition of Phonology: A Case Study*. Cambridge: Cambridge University Press.

Sonies, B. C., Shawker, T. H., Hall, T. E., Gerber, L. H., and Leighton, S. B. (1981). Ultrasonic visualization of tongue motion during speech. *Journal of the Acoustical Society of America*, 70, 683–6.

Stone, M. (1991). Towards a model of three-dimensional tongue movement. *Journal of Phonetics*, 19, 309–20.

Stone, M. (1997). Laboratory techniques for investigating speech articulation. In W. J. Hardcastle and J. Laver (eds.), *The Handbook of Phonetic Sciences* (pp. 11–32). Oxford: Blackwell.

Stone, M. (2005). A guide to analysing tongue motion from ultrasound images. *Clinical Linguistics and Phonetics*, 19, 455–501.

Stone, M. and Lundberg, A. (1996). Three-dimensional tongue surface shapes of English consonants and vowels. *Journal of the Acoustical Society of America*, 99, 3728–37.

Story, R. S., Alfonso, P. J., and Harris, K. S. (1996). Pre- and posttreatment comparison of the kinematics of the fluent speech of persons who stutter. *Journal of Speech and Hearing Research*, 39, 991–1005.

Suzuki, N. (1989). Clinical applications of EPG to Japanese cleft palate and glossectomy patients. *Clinical Linguistics and Phonetics*, 3, 127–36.

Svensson, P., Henningson, C., and Karlsson, S. (1993). Speech motor control in Parkinson's disease: A comparison between a clinical assessment protocol and a quantitative analysis of mandibular movements. *Folia Phoniatrica*, 45, 157–64.

Tanimoto, K., Henningsson, G., Isberg, A., and Ren, Y. F. (1994). Comparison of tongue position during speech before and after pharyngeal flap surgery in hypernasal speakers. *Cleft Palate-Craniofacial Journal*, 31, 280–6.

Thompson-Ward, E. C. and Murdoch, B. E. (1998). Instrumental assessment of the speech mechanism. In B. E. Murdoch (ed.), *Dysarthria: A Physiological Approach* (pp. 68–101). Cheltenham, Glos.: Stanley Thornes.

Tye-Murray, N. (1987). Effects of vowel context on the articulatory closure postures of deaf speakers. *Journal of Speech and Hearing Research*, 30, 99–104.

Tye-Murray, N. (1991). The establishment of open articulatory postures by deaf and hearing talkers. *Journal of Speech and Hearing Research*, 34, 453–9.

van Lieshout, P. H., Rutjens, C. A., and Spauwen, P. H. (2002). The dynamics of interlip coupling in speakers with a repaired unilateral cleft-lip history. *Journal of Speech, Language, and Hearing Research*, 45, 5–19.

Wakumoto, M., Isaacson, K. G., Friel, S., Suzuki, N., Gibbon, F., Nixon, F., Hardcastle, W. J., and Michi, K-I. (1996). Preliminary study of articulatory reorganisation of fricative consonants following osteotomy. *Folia Phoniatrica et Logopaedica*, 48, 275–89.

Wein, B. B., Drobnitzky, M., Klajman, S., and Angerstein, W. (1991). Evaluation of functional positions of tongue and soft palate with MR imaging: Initial clinical results. *Journal of Magnetic Resonance Imaging*, 1, 381–3.

Weismer, G., Yunusova, Y., and Westbury, J. R. (2003). Interarticulator coordination in dysarthria: An X-ray microbeam study. *Journal of Speech, Language, and Hearing Research*, 46, 1247–61.

Westbury, J. (1994). *X-ray Microbeam Speech Production Database: User's Handbook*, version 1.0. Madison: University of Wisconsin.

Whitehill, T. L., Stokes, S. F., and Man, Y. H. Y. (1996). Electropalatography treatment in an adult with late repair of cleft palate. *Cleft Palate-Craniofacial Journal*, 33, 160–8.

Wood, S. (1995). An electropalatographic analysis of stutterers' speech. *European Journal of Disorders of Communication*, 30, 226–36.

Wood, S. (1997). Electropalatographic study of speech sound errors in adults with acquired aphasia. Unpublished PhD dissertation, Queen Margaret College, Edinburgh.

Wood, S. and Hardcastle, W. J. (2000). Instrumentation in the assessment and therapy of motor-speech disorders: A survey of techniques and case studies with EPG. In I. Papathanasiou (ed.), *Acquired Neurogenic Communication Disorders: A Clinical Perspective*. London: Whurr Publishers.

Wrench, A. A., Gibbon, F. E., McNeill, A. M., and Wood, S. E. (2002). An EPG therapy protocol for remediation and assessment of articulation disorders. In J. H. L. Hansen and B. Pellom (eds.), *Proceedings of ICSLP-2002* (pp. 965–8).

Yamashita, Y., Michi, K., Imai, S., Suzuki, N., and Yoshida, H. (1992). Electropalatographic investigation of abnormal lingual-palatal contact patterns in cleft palate patients. *Clinical Linguistics and Phonetics*, 6, 201–17.

Zierdt, A., Hoole, P., and Tillmann, H. G. (1999). Development of a system for three-dimensional fleshpoint measurements of speech movements. In *Proceedings of the XIVth International Congress of Phonetic Sciences, Stockholm*, vol. 1 (pp. 73–6).

Zimmermann, G. (1980). Articulatory behaviors associated with stuttering: A cinefluorographic analysis. *Journal of Speech and Hearing Research*, 23, 108–21.

20 Instrumental Analysis of Resonance in Speech Impairment

TARA L. WHITEHILL AND ALICE S.-Y. LEE

20.1 Resonance and Resonance Disorders

Resonance, a term derived from the physics of sound, is used in acoustic phonetics to refer to the vibratory response of air in the vocal tract set in motion by a source of phonation (Crystal, 2003). The balance of oral and nasal resonance of speech is regulated by the velopharyngeal port, which includes the velum, the lateral pharyngeal walls and the posterior pharyngeal wall. In principle, velopharyngeal closure occurs during the production of vowels and oral consonants; the velopharyngeal port opens during production of nasal sounds. Any disturbance to velopharyngeal structures or function will affect the balance of oral and nasal resonance, and may lead to resonance disorders.

Resonance disorders include hypernasality, hyponasality, and mixed resonance disorder. Hypernasality refers to the perception of excessive nasal resonance when producing vowels, voiced oral consonants or both (Kent, 1999). It is observed in speakers with velopharyngeal dysfunction (VPD) due to anatomical or physiological deficiencies, but may also be seen as a learned behavior. Hyponasality refers to reduced normal nasal resonance during speech, particularly during the production of nasal consonants (Kummer, 2001). Although hyponasality is usually associated with blockage in the nasopharynx or nasal cavity, it is also demonstrated in speakers with VPD due to neurological impairment. Mixed resonance disorder is a combination of hypernasality and hyponasality which occurs when there is a velopharyngeal dysfunction as well as a blockage at the nasal airway (Kummer, 2001). It may also occur in individuals with inappropriate timing of velopharyngeal movement during speech due to oral-motor disorders (Kummer, 2001; Netsell, 1969).

Nasal emission is characterized by an inappropriate release of air pressure through the nares during consonant production. Although both nasal emission and hypernasality are associated with VPD, nasal emission is considered an articulation disorder, rather than a resonance disorder. Phoneme-specific nasal emission, where speakers show nasal emission for certain pressure consonants but can achieve adequate velopharyngeal closure when producing other consonants and vowels, is considered a learned disorder (not associated with VPD).

There have been inconsistencies in the use of the terms velopharyngeal insufficiency, velopharyngeal incompetence, velopharyngeal inadequacy and velopharyngeal dysfunction to refer to disorders of the velopharyngeal valve. Some authors use the terms interchangeably, while others use them differentially to specify etiology. In this chapter, we use the generic term velopharyngeal dysfunction (VPD).

It is important to have methods of assessing resonance disorders which are both reliable and valid, in order to document severity and change over time. Perceptual judgment of resonance disorders is considered the gold standard, as resonance disorders are by definition perceptual qualities. However, perceptual judgment has been associated with poor reliability, and does not provide insight into the cause of the problem. Hence, researchers have sought to develop instrumental measures to evaluate velopharyngeal structure and movement, as well as the consequences of velopharyngeal dysfunction. Although instrumental measures do not measure hypernasality resonance disorder *per se*, they can supplement the perceptual evaluation of resonance disorders.

20.2   Instrumentation for Evaluating Velopharyngeal Dysfunction

Instrumental procedures for evaluating VPD can be divided into direct and indirect measures. Direct measures allow direct visual inspection of velopharyngeal structure and movement during speech production, and include nasendoscopy, videofluoroscopy and ultrasound. Indirect measures evaluate the sequelae of velopharyngeal dysfunction. These include acoustic analyses (including nasometry), accelerometry, aerodynamic measures, and photo-detection. The following sections review the most widely used instrumental measures.

20.2.1   *Videofluoroscopy and nasendoscopy*

Videofluoroscopy is a radiographic procedure that records images of internal body parts on videotape. Velopharyngeal movements during speech are examined from multiple views (usually the lateral, frontal and base views) so that the three-dimensional structures can be evaluated. Speech materials for evaluating velopharyngeal movement in speakers with hypernasality include sentences loaded with pressure-sensitive consonants, repetition of syllables, and rote speech such as counting. When hyponasality is suspected, nasal-loaded sentences and nasal syllables are used.

Multiview videofluoroscopy is widely used in the study of cleft palate populations for diagnosing velopharyngeal dysfunction and for evaluating the effect of surgery on speech. It has also been used with speakers with dysarthria and speakers with hearing impairment. The value of this technique is that it allows diagnosis of the cause of VPD, based on examination of the relative contributions of the velum and the pharyngeal walls. This information is important in deciding which treatment options would be suitable for a specific individual.

Although the radiation dosage is fairly limited, the major drawback of videofluoroscopy is the exposure to radiation. In order to reduce exposure, the frequency of videofluoroscopy examinations and the duration of each examination must be limited. There is an additional drawback to using video-fluoroscopy with speakers with cleft palate who have had surgery to insert a pharyngeal flap. In such cases it is typically difficult to evaluate the placement and function of the flap using videofluoroscopy. In the investigation of speakers with a pharyngeal flap, therefore, endoscopic techniques are more suitable.

Nasendoscopy, also known as nasopharyngoscopy, is an endoscopic technique that involves a flexible fiberoptic tube being inserted into a speaker's nostril to allow the velopharyngeal port to be viewed from above. The view obtained is similar to the base view of videofluoroscopy, but rotated 180 degrees.

Nasendoscopy has been used mainly in the study of speakers with cleft palate or with VPD due to other anatomical defects, but has also been used in speakers with dysarthria and speakers with hearing impairment. Like video-fluoroscopy, endoscopy allows direct visual inspection of the relative contribution of palatal and pharyngeal movements during speech production. Its advantages over videofluoroscopy are that it allows examination of anatomical defects on the nasal surface of the palate, and the closure of the lateral portals in individuals who were fitted with a pharyngeal flap. In addition, it does not involve radiation exposure, which means there are fewer limitations on the frequency and duration of the procedure.

One disadvantage of nasendoscopy is that the procedure is invasive. The insertion of a fiberoptic tube into the nasal cavity could cause discomfort, particularly in individuals with nasal blockage due to anatomical defects. Furthermore, since nasendoscopy cannot give a lateral view of the velopharynx, the location of maximal palatal-pharyngeal wall contact, and the length and thickness of the palate, cannot be appreciated with this technique. This information is considered important to decisions regarding location of operating site where surgical treatment is being considered. Therefore, both multiview videofluoroscopy and nasendoscopy are recommended for use in clinical settings and research studies for the assessment of velopharyngeal structure and movement. Guidelines on the use of and reporting techniques for multi-view videofluoroscopy and nasendoscopy are reported in Golding-Kushner, Argamaso, Cotton, et al. (1990) and Karnell (1994).

There have been few studies of the reliability of videofluoroscopy and nasendoscopy measurements or judgments (but see Karnell, Ibuki, Morris, & Van Demark, 1983, and D'Antonio, Marsh, Province, Muntz, & Philips, 1989, both of which found moderate to high reliability for experienced judges). There have also been few studies of the correlation between direct measures of velopharyngeal function and perceptual judgment of hypernasality. However, a recent study by Kummer, Briggs, and Lee (2003) found that velopharyngeal gap size could be predicted by perceptual variables for 70 percent of subjects with cleft palate.

20.2.2 *Nasometry*

The Nasometer (Kay Pentax, Lincoln Park, NJ) is a computer-based device which provides data on the acoustic results of velopharyngeal function. The Nasometer picks up oral and nasal signals through two microphones attached to either side of a sound separator. The device provides a nasalance score, which is a ratio of nasal acoustic energy to the sum of nasal and oral acoustic energy multiplied by 100. In principle, the higher the nasalance score, the higher the degree of nasality.

The Nasometer has been used to evaluate individuals with hypernasality and hyponasality due to various etiologies such as cleft palate, hearing impairment, dysarthria, and nasal airway impairment. In addition, there have been several studies providing normative data for different languages and dialects (for review, see Dalston, 2004). Standard speech materials developed for nasometry include oral materials (containing no nasal consonants), nasal materials (heavily loaded with nasal consonants), and phonetically balanced materials.

Various cut-off scores have been suggested to differentiate normal resonance and hypernasality (for example, 32 percent in Dalston, Warren, & Dalston, 1991; 26 percent in Hardin, Van Demark, Morris, & Payne, 1992), but there is no consensus, particularly as nasalance scores may vary according to language, dialect, racial group, age and gender. Factors such as mixed nasality and the co-occurrence of nasal emission, breathy voice and articulation errors have also been found to influence nasalance scores.

The majority of studies investigating the relationship between nasalance scores and listener judgment of hypernasality have found correlations between 0.5 and 0.7, although a few studies have found correlations below 0.5, and a few above 0.8 (see Keuning, Wieneke, & Dejonckere, 2004, for a review). A few studies have examined the sensitivity and specificity of nasalance scores (Dalston, Warren, & Dalston, 1991; Hardin, Van Demark, Morris, & Payne, 1992; McHenry, 1999). Discrepancies in the correlations and sensitivity/specificity scores may be due to several factors, including the use of different perceptual rating scales (equal-appearing interval [EAI], visual analogue, and direct magnitude estimation), differing numbers of scale points on the EAI scale, different speech materials, differing numbers of listeners and experience of listeners, and combining vs. separating hypernasality and hyponasality scales.

There are also controversial findings regarding the relationship between nasalance scores and other instrumental measures. Dalston, Warren, and Dalston (1991) investigated the relationship between nasalance scores and aerodynamic measures and found high sensitivity and specificity (above 0.7). In contrast, McHenry (2002) found no significant correlation between nasalance and aerodynamic measures in 22 speakers with dysarthria. Rah, Ko, Lee, and Kim (2001) found low correlations (ranging from 0.49 to 0.58) between nasalance and an acoustic measure involving linear predictive coding (LPC). A higher correlation (0.84) was obtained when including only data points with nasalance scores of 35 or higher.

A new, digital version of the Nasometer, the Nasometer II (Model 6400), was released recently by Kay Pentax. Watterson, Lewis, and Brancamp (2005) showed a small but significant difference in the nasalance scores between the two versions of Nasometer. Hence, users should be cautious when comparing nasalance scores collected by the two instruments.

Other instruments for measuring the ratio of nasal and oral acoustic energy have been developed, namely the NasalView (Tiger Electronics Inc., Seattle, WA) and the OroNasal System (Glottal Enterprises Inc., Syracuse, NY). Bressmann (2005) found significant differences between the three systems, and cautioned that scores from the different devices are not interchangeable.

20.2.3   *Spectrography*

Acoustic analysis of nasalization is based on the principle that the addition of nasal resonance to oral resonance brings about changes in the acoustic properties of speech sounds. These changes consist primarily of the presence of additional resonance–antiresonance pairs. Nasalization can be identified acoustically from some combination of the presence of nasal formants and anti-formants, an upward shift in the first formant (F1) and downward shifts of the second (F2) and third (F3) formants, increased bandwidths of formants, and reduced overall energy (Kent & Read, 2002).

A number of studies have attempted to identify the spectral properties which characterize nasalization of speech sounds. The speech materials analyzed have included vowels produced by speakers with hypernasality, speech materials loaded with and without nasal phonemes produced by normal speakers, vowels produced by normal speakers simulating hypernasality, and synthesized vowels.

Until recently, most acoustic studies of nasalization in speakers with cleft palate and dysarthria involved qualitative descriptions of the presence of nasalization, due to the difficulty in quantifying the degree of nasalization of speech signals by spectrography. However, there have been several recent attempts at quantification. These have included LPC analysis, formant analysis, and spectral analysis.

LPC analysis estimates the vocal tract resonances in terms of a set of 'predictor' coefficients, based on a small duration of the preceding acoustic waveform

(Johnson, 2003). Plante, Berger-Vachon, and Kauffmann (1993) found a significant difference between children with VPD and normal controls for specific cepstral coefficients, and discriminant analysis differentiated the two groups with few misclassifications. However, both measures were found to be vowel-dependent. Rah, Ko, Lee, and Kim (2001) used both low-order and high-order linear predictive models. They found low correlations (below 0.58) between nasalance values and the distance for high orders. However, a correlation of 0.84 was obtained when nasalance scores below 35 were not included.

Chen and colleagues used *formant analysis* to evaluate hypernasality in speakers with a variety of etiologies (Chen, 1995, 1997; Chen & Metson, 1997). Two acoustic correlates were employed, A1-P1 and A1-P0, where A1 refers to F1 amplitude, P1 represents the amplitude of the extra nasal peak in the vicinity of F1, and P0 is the amplitude of a nasal peak at low frequencies. These measures were reportedly useful in differentiating speakers with VPD from control speakers, and speakers before and after sinus surgery. Perceptual judgments were reportedly consistent with acoustic findings, although correlations were not reported. Kataoka, Warren, Zajac, Mayo, and Lutz (2001) criticized the measures suggested by Chen and colleagues, claiming that the nasal peaks P0 and P1 were difficult to identify when they appeared near F1, that there is variability in the frequency and amplitude of the nasal peak when the fundamental frequency is high (as in children's speech), that A1-P1 was vowel-dependent, and that A1-P0 could be affected by breathiness of voice.

One-third-octave spectral analysis is a measurement of the average energy level for each consecutive frequency band, where the bandwidth is one-third of an octave, within a frequency range. Kataoka and colleagues applied this method to children and young adults with cleft palate or VPD (Kataoka, Michi, Okabe, Miura, & Yoshida, 1996; Kataoka, Warren, Zajac, Mayo, & Lutz, 2001) and in adults after maxillectomy (Yoshida, Furuya, Shimodaira, et al., 2000). The earlier two studies (1996 and 2000) showed some variability in terms of which one-third-octave bands distinguished hypernasality and normal resonance, and which bands showed statistically significant correlations with listener judgment. However, both studies concluded that hypernasality was indicated by a rise in the amplitude between F1 and F2, in the region of about 1000 Hz, and by a decrease in the amplitude above F2. The 2001 study showed that the spectral characteristics associated with hypernasality of vowel /i/ in children with cleft palate were an increase in the amplitude of F1, an increase in the amplitude between F1 and F2, and a reduction in the amplitude of the F2 and F3 regions. There was a significant correlation (0.84) between listener ratings of the hypernasality of synthesized vowel /i/ and acoustic measures. Lee, Ciocca, and Whitehill (2003) applied one-third-octave analysis to vowel /i/ segmented from real words. The results were similar to previous findings in that the speakers with hypernasality showed significantly higher amplitude for the one-third-octave bands centered at 630, 800, and 1000 Hz than the normal controls, and significantly lower amplitude for the band centered at 2500 Hz. Lee, Ciocca, and Whitehill (2004) examined four vowels, and concluded that one-third-octave spectral analysis is a vowel-dependent measure. Given that one-third-octave analysis can be performed in real time, Kataoka, Warren, Zajac, Mayo, and Lutz (2001) suggested that this method might be suitable for use in clinical settings.

20.2.4   *Accelerometry*

Accelerometry involves the use of a lightweight device attached to the surface of the nose, to transduce the nasal vibration that is caused by acoustic energy being resonated in the nasal cavity. The output level of the accelerometer, expressed in decibels, is expected to increase during the production of nasal consonants and nasalized vowels.

Accelerometry has been employed to study the normal production of nasal and non-nasal speech materials, simulated hypernasality by normal speakers, speech produced by speakers with hypernasality due to VPD or after repaired cleft palate, by speakers with hyponasality, by individuals with hearing impairment, and by persons with acquired dysarthria after traumatic brain injury (TBI) or cerebral vascular accident (CVA).

Horii (1980) proposed the Horii Oral-Nasal Coupling (HONC) index, a logarithmic ratio of nasal amplitude to voice amplitude scaled to each speaker's maximal nasal production of [m] by means of a constant. Several subsequent studies have investigated speech-sample and speaker effects. Mra, Sussman, and Fenwick (1998) found no significant difference in the HONC indices across age groups and gender groups. Larson and Hamlet (1987) showed that the amplitudes of nasal-to-voice ratio were significantly larger for vowels preceding a nasal consonant (anticipatory coarticulation) than for postnasal vowels (carryover coarticulation). Jones (2000) found more dramatic differences between normal speakers and speakers with hypernasality when using sentences rather than syllable or word tasks, and recommended the use of connected speech samples.

Intra-listener and inter-listener reliability measures for accelerometry are reportedly high. However, there have been no published reports of test–retest reliability, involving removing and reattaching the nasal accelerometer. Correlations between accelerometric measures and perceptual judgments of hypernasality are reportedly moderate to strong, ranging from 0.52 to 0.91, for non-nasal stimuli (for review, see Laczi, Sussman, & Stathopoulos, Huber, 2005). However, a low correspondence between accelerometric measures and perceptual diagnosis of resonance problems in speakers with acquired dysarthria has been reported, possibly related to concomitant speech and voice problems (Thompson & Murdoch, 1995). Further studies on the correspondence between accelerometry and other acoustic and aerodynamic measures are warranted. In addition, Krakow and Huffman (1993) warned that changes in oral output may alter the oral-nasal ratio, even when nasal output remains constant, thus potentially giving a false picture of velopharyngeal or resonance status or changes. The final limitation of this technique is that the equipment is not commercially available as a preassembled package. As a result, the technique is underused compared to other noninvasive instrumental analysis, and has been used almost exclusively in research studies.

20.2.5 Aerodynamics

Warren and DuBois (1964) proposed a pressure-flow technique for assessing individuals with VPD due to anatomical defects. The technique is based on the assumption that the cross-sectional area of an orifice can be calculated if the pressure difference across the orifice and the rate of airflow are measured at the same time. Many studies have subsequently applied the pressure-flow technique for evaluating velopharyngeal function in speakers with VPD due to anatomical deficits or neurological impairment, and in speakers with normal velopharyngeal function. Aerodynamic procedures and data interpretation are readily available (for example, Warren, 2004; Zajac, 2002).

Aerodynamic measures are objective and noninvasive. Measures can distinguish individuals with VPD from speakers with normal velopharyngeal function (for review, see Zajac, 2002). However, a significant decrease in the accuracy of velopharyngeal orifice-size estimations has been reported for velopharyngeal openings of 0.8 cm^2 or above (Warren, 2004). Although cut-off scores for mild, moderate and severe hypernasality have been suggested (see Warren, 2004), the measurements vary greatly among speakers. Furthermore, contrasting findings have been reported regarding the extent to which aerodynamic measures correspond to perceptual judgments of hypernasality. McHenry (1999) studied 31 individuals following traumatic brain injury and found a low specificity of velopharyngeal airway resistance (0.59) and estimated velopharyngeal area (0.40). Dotevall, Lohmander-Agerskov, Enjell, and Bake (2002) studied 14 children with cleft palate and 15 normal controls. Using a five-point EAI scale for rating hypernasality and a perceptual cut-off score of ≥ 2, there was high specificity for four aerodynamic measures (ranging from 0.81 to 0.96). The contrasting findings between these two studies are possibly related to the different study populations (the later study included speakers with normal velopharyngeal function, while the former did not) and different aerodynamic variables.

20.3 Conclusions

There are a variety of instrumental methods for the evaluation of resonance and resonance disorders. These include both direct methods, which allow visualization of the velopharyngeal port, and indirect measures, which permit evaluation of the consequences of velopharyngeal status.

Instrumental measures have been used to evaluate resonance in a number of clinical populations, including both congenital and acquired disorders. The most common population has been speakers with cleft palate, a population with a relatively high incidence of resonance disorders. Other populations have included speakers with neurological damage (such as follows stroke or head injury), with hearing impairment, and following oral surgery.

A key consideration in evaluating instrumental methods is the correlation between instrumental measures and perceptual judgments of resonance. Poor correspondence between the two may be due to limitations with the instrumental method, but may also be due to limitations associated with perceptual judgment. Although not a focus of this chapter, there are a number of factors which can influence the perceptual judgment of resonance. These include the number of listeners and experience of the listeners, the speech materials used, and the rating scale employed. Inter-rater and intra-rater reliability for perceptual judgment of hypernasality is notoriously low. There have been few attempts to systematically train listeners to rate hypernasality reliably (but see Lee, 2005). In addition to offering objective measures which correspond to perceptual judgments, instrumental measures may complement perceptual judgments and offer diagnostic information not available through perceptual ratings. For example, videofluoroscopy can offer insights into velopharyngeal functioning which may assist our understanding of velopharyngeal disorder and its possible relationship with resonance disorders.

While several instrumental methods, such as nasometry, have sought to establish cut-off scores to distinguish normal and abnormal resonance patterns, at the current time the most reliable application of instrumental measures appears to be for the purpose of comparing individual speakers pre- and post-treatment (surgical, prosthetic or behavioral). While instrumental methods for evaluating resonance disorders seem to offer objectivity, users need to be aware that several of the methods require subjective judgments (for example, judgment of velopharyngeal gap size from videofluoroscopy). Users also need to be aware of factors such as test–retest reliability, which may influence the accuracy of instrumental measures.

Well-equipped laboratories which are involved with the study of individuals with resonance disorders will have most, if not all, of the instrumental measures described in this chapter. A goal for the future is to make instrumental methods more available in clinical settings. One method for doing so is to ensure that students of speech and hearing sciences are exposed to these methods, both theoretically and in practice.

REFERENCES

Bressmann, T. (2005). Comparison of nasalance scores obtained with the Nasometer, the NasalView, and the OroNasal System. *Cleft Palate-Craniofacial Journal*, 42, 423–33.

Chen, M. Y. (1995). Acoustic parameters of nasalized vowels in hearing-impaired and normal-hearing speakers. *Journal of the Acoustical Society of America*, 98(5 Pt 1), 2443–53.

Chen, M. Y. (1997). Acoustic correlates of English and French nasalized vowels. *Journal of the Acoustical Society of America*, 102, 2360–70.

Chen, M. Y. and Metson, R. (1997). Effects of sinus surgery on speech. *Archives of Otolaryngology – Head and Neck Surgery*, 123, 845–52.

Crystal, D. (2003). *A Dictionary of Linguistics and Phonetics*. Oxford: Blackwell.

Dalston, R. M. (2004). The use of nasometry in the assessment and remediation of velopharyngeal inadequacy. In K. R. Bzoch (ed.), *Communicative Disorders Related to Cleft Lip and Palate*. 5th ed. (pp. 493–516). Austin, TX: Pro-Ed.

Dalston, R. M., Warren, D. W., and Dalston, E. T. (1991). Use of nasometry as a diagnostic tool for identifying patients with velopharyngeal impairment. *Cleft Palate-Craniofacial Journal*, 28, 184–8; discussion 188–9. (Erratum published 28(4), 446, 1991.)

D'Antonio, L. L., Marsh, J. L., Province, M. A., Muntz, H. R., and Philips, C. J. (1989). Reliability of flexible fiberoptic nasopharyngoscopy for evaluation of velopharyngeal function in a clinical population. *Cleft Palate Journal*, 26, 217–25.

Dotevall, H., Lohmander-Agerskov, A., Enjell, H., and Bake, B. (2002). Perceptual evaluation of speech and velopharyngeal function in children with and without cleft palate and the relationship to nasal airflow patterns. *Cleft Palate-Craniofacial Journal*, 39, 409–24.

Golding-Kushner, K. J., Argamaso, R. V., Cotton, R. T., Grames, L. M., Henningsson, G., Jones, D. L., Karnell, M. P., Klaiman, P. G., Lewin, M. L., Marsh, J. L., McCall, G. N., McGrath, C. O., Muntz, H. R., Nevdahl, M. T., Rakoof, S. J., Shprintzen, R. J., Sidoti, E. J., Vallino, L. D., Volk, M., Williams, W. N., Witzel, M. A., Dixon Wood, V. L., Ysunza, A., D'Antonio, L., Isberg, A., Pigott, R. W., and Skolnick, L. (1990). Standardization for the reporting of nasopharyngoscopy and multiview videofluoroscopy: A report from an international working group. *Cleft Palate Journal*, 27, 337–48.

Hardin, M. A., Van Demark, D. R., Morris, H. L., and Payne, M. M. (1992). Correspondence between nasalance scores and listener judgments of hypernasality and hyponasality. *Cleft Palate-Craniofacial Journal*, 29, 346–51.

Horii, Y. (1980). An accelerometric approach to nasality measurement: A preliminary report. *Cleft Palate Journal*, 17, 254–61.

Johnson, K. (2003). *Acoustic and Auditory Phonetics*. 2nd ed. Oxford: Blackwell.

Jones, D. L. (2000). The relationship between temporal aspects of oral-nasal balance and classification of velopharyngeal status in speakers with cleft palate. *Cleft Palate-Craniofacial Journal*, 37, 363–9.

Karnell, M. P. (1994). *Videoendoscopy: From Velopharynx to Larynx*. San Diego, CA: Singular.

Karnell, M. P., Ibuki, K., Morris, H. L., and Van Demark, D. R. (1983). Reliability of the nasopharyngeal fiberscope (NPF) for assessing velopharyngeal function: Analysis by judgment. *Cleft Palate Journal*, 20, 199–208.

Kataoka, R., Michi, K., Okabe, K., Miura, T., and Yoshida, H. (1996). Spectral properties and quantitative evaluation of hypernasality in vowels. *Cleft Palate-Craniofacial Journal*, 33, 43–50.

Kataoka, R., Warren, D. W., Zajac, D. J., Mayo, R., and Lutz, R. W. (2001). The relationship between spectral characteristics and perceived hypernasality in children. *Journal of the Acoustical Society of America*, 109(5 Pt 1), 2181–9.

Kent, R. D. (1999). Improving the sensitivity and reliability of auditory-perceptual assessment. *American Speech-Language-Hearing Association: Special Interest Division*, 5, 9(1), 12–15.

Kent, R. D. and Read, C. (2002). *The Acoustic Analysis of Speech*. 2nd ed. New York: Singular.

Keuning, K. H. D. M., Wieneke, G. H., and Dejonckere, P. H. (2004). Correlation between the perceptual rating of speech in Dutch patients with velopharyngeal insufficiency and composite measures derived from mean nasalance scores. *Folia Phoniatrica et Logopaedica*, 56, 157–64.

Krakow, R. A. and Huffman, M. K. (1993). Instruments and techniques for investigating nasalization and velopharyngeal function in the laboratory: An introduction. In M. K. Huffman and R. A. Krakow (eds.), *Phonetics and Phonology. Volume 5: Nasals, Nasalization, and the Velum* (pp. 3–69). San Diego, CA: Academic Press.

Kummer, A. W. (2001). *Cleft Palate and Craniofacial Anomalies: The Effects on Speech and Resonance*. San Diego, CA: Singular.

Kummer, A. W., Briggs, M., and Lee, L. (2003). The relationship between the characteristics of speech and velopharyngeal gap size. *Cleft Palate-Craniofacial Journal*, 40, 590–6.

Laczi, E., Sussman, J. E., Stathopoulos, E. T., and Huber, J. (2005). Perceptual evaluation of hypernasality compared to HONC measures: The role of experience. *Cleft Palate-Craniofacial Journal*, 42, 202–11.

Larson, P. L. and Hamlet, S. L. (1987). Coarticulation effects on the nasalization of vowels using nasal/voice amplitude ratio instrumentation. *Cleft Palate Journal*, 24, 286–90.

Lee, S. Y. A. (2005). Perceptual and instrumental analysis of hypernasality. Unpublished doctoral dissertation, University of Hong Kong.

Lee, S. Y. A., Ciocca, V., and Whitehill, T. L. (2003). Acoustic correlates of hypernasality. *Clinical Linguistics and Phonetics*, 17, 259–64.

Lee, S. Y. A., Ciocca, V., and Whitehill, T. L. (2004). Spectral analysis of hypernasality. *Journal of Medical Speech-Language Pathology*, 12, 173–7.

McHenry, M. A. (1999). Aerodynamic, acoustic, and perceptual measures of nasality following traumatic brain injury. *Brain Injury*, 13, 281–90.

McHenry, M. A. (2002). A comparison of nasalance and velopharyngeal orifice area in dysarthria. *Journal of Medical Speech-Language Pathology*, 10, 299–305.

Mra, Z., Sussman, J. E., and Fenwick, J. (1998). HONC measures in 4- to 6-year-old children. *Cleft Palate-Craniofacial Journal*, 35, 408–14.

Netsell, R. (1969). Evaluation of velopharyngeal function in dysarthria. *Journal of Speech and Hearing Disorders*, 34, 113–22.

Plante, F., Berger-Vachon, C., and Kauffmann, I. (1993). Acoustic discrimination of velar impairment in children. *Folia Phoniatrica*, 45, 112–19.

Rah, D. K., Ko, Y. I., Lee, C., and Kim, D. W. (2001). A noninvasive estimation of hypernasality using a linear predictive model. *Annals of Biomedical Engineering*, 29, 587–94.

Thompson, E. C. and Murdoch, B. E. (1995). Disorders of nasality in subjects with upper motor neuron type dysarthria following cerebrovascular accident. *Journal of Communication Disorders*, 28, 261–76.

Warren, D. W. (2004). Aerodynamic assessments and procedures to determine extent of velopharyngeal inadequacy. In K. R. Bzoch (ed.), *Communicative Disorders Related to Cleft Lip and Palate*. 5th ed. (pp. 595–628). Austin, TX: Pro-Ed.

Warren, D. W. and DuBois, A. B. (1964). A pressure-flow technique for measuring velopharyngeal orifice area during continuous speech. *Cleft Palate Journal*, 1, 52–71.

Watterson, T., Lewis, K., and Brancamp, T. (2005). Comparison of nasalance scores obtained with the Nasometer 6200 and the Nasometer II 6400. *Cleft Palate-Craniofacial Journal*, 42, 574–9.

Yoshida, H., Furuya, Y., Shimodaira, K., Kanazawa, T., Kataoka, R., and Takahashi, K. (2000). Spectral characteristics of hypernasality in maxillectomy patients. *Journal of Oral Rehabilitation*, 27, 723–30.

Zajac, D. J. (2002). Speech aerodynamics of cleft palate. In A. W. Kummer (ed.), *Cleft Palate and Craniofacial Anomalies: The Effects on Speech and Resonance* (pp. 331–58). San Diego, CA: Singular.

21 Instrumental Analysis of Phonation

SHAHEEN N. AWAN

21.1 Introduction

The perceptual evaluation of voice is considered to be an essential aspect of the conventional voice diagnostic that is of primary relevance to most voice-disordered patients and provides a global measure of vocal performance readily available to all clinicians (Orlikoff, Dejonckere, Dembowski, et al., 1999). Though perceptual evaluation of voice has obvious importance, there are several limitations associated with this method of assessment that clearly affect its clinical utility. These limitations include problems with scale validity and reliability, particularly for mid-scale (i.e., mild to moderate) pathological voices, lack of credibility for medical-legal purposes, poorly defined and/or shifting definitions of severity, and the intrusive effects of voice and speech characteristics other than the quality dimension that is meant to be judged (de Krom, 1994; Kreiman, Gerratt, Kempster, Erman, & Berke, 1993; Orlikoff, Dejonckere, Dembowski, et al., 1999). Many of these limitations stem from the attempt to describe the voice via a temporary auditory impression of the acoustic signal.

   As a response to many of the aforementioned difficulties, voice clinicians and researchers have added to the perceptual assessment of voice quality with other methods that provide a permanent record of the vocal behavior and allow for a more objective analysis of the patient's voice quality. In particular, these methods have taken two forms: *indirect and direct methods of phonatory analysis*. Indirect methods allow for inferences regarding normal vs. abnormal function by assessing byproducts of phonatory function rather than via descriptions of phonatory function itself. A prime example of an indirect method of describing phonation is the acoustic analysis of the voice signal. Acoustic methods of voice evaluation have been particularly useful in both clinical and research situations since they are noninvasive, available at low cost compared with other methods of voice analysis, applicable to treatment as well as diagnosis, and supported by a substantial body of literature. In addition, acoustic evaluation methods have the benefit that (1) the algorithms will analyze voice signals in a similar manner every time (no shift in analysis definition), and (2) the results are provided in numerical format, allowing for built-in scaling and ease of communication. In contrast, direct methods provide information regarding structure and/or function derived from first-hand observation of the structure itself. In voice analysis, laryngoscopic/endoscopic methods and those derived from laryngoscopy (e.g. videostroboscopy) provide a direct, visual description of the laryngeal mechanism. It is important to note that indirect and direct methodologies are complementary in nature; the use of one does not render the other redundant. While the laryngoscopic/endoscopic evaluation is a primary tool for arriving at the specific medical diagnosis of vocal fold pathology, it is not necessarily an accurate gauge of vocal dysfunction. It is quite possible that a relatively severe dysphonia may be observed in a patient with healthy-looking vocal folds and surrounding structures, while a less severe dysphonia may be observed in a patient with quite obvious structural and functional abnormalities; the relationship between pathology and a resulting dysphonia is not necessarily obvious. In contrast, vocal dysfunction may be best gauged via the methods that assess the byproducts of phonation (perceptions, acoustics, and aerodynamics) (Wuyts, De Bodt, Molenberghs, et al., 2000).

It is the purpose of this chapter to review a number of advances in both indirect (acoustic) and direct (laryngeal-imaging) methods of voice analysis that aid in documenting and understanding the disordered voice. While many of the methods described in this chapter have been described primarily via the research literature, it is hoped that these methods will find their place in the clinical realm within the near future.

21.2   Indirect Phonatory Analysis: Multidimensional Acoustic Methods

Acoustic methods of voice analysis have been primary tools of both the clinician and researcher for many years. These methods have become widely used in both research and clinical situations since the advent of relatively low-cost personal computers and analogue-to-digital acquisition hardware in the early 1990s. Acoustic methods used to quantify characteristics such as the severity of dysphonia have frequently been based on the assumption that many voice-quality disturbances (breathiness, hoarseness, roughness) affect, in one way or another, the periodicity of the voice signal. The normal human voice is highly periodic (quasi-periodic), with relatively little variation from cycle to cycle in terms of period and/or amplitude during sustained voicing. On the other hand, phonatory disturbances (e.g., unilateral or bilateral organized lesions or distributed tissue change, organic pathology affecting the ability to effectively approximate the folds during phonation) often result in disturbances in the periodicity of phonation and its accompanying acoustic waveform. Many of the frequently used methods of measuring voice quality attempt to quantify these disturbances (i.e., perturbations) by identifying (1) cycle boundaries (i.e., where each cycle of vibration begins and ends), followed by (2) cycle-to-cycle comparisons of characteristics such as period/frequency, amplitude, and profile (waveform shape). Techniques that focus on the identification of individual cycles of vibration may be referred to as *time-based* analysis methods, since the cycle boundaries are identified on the time axis of the acoustic waveform. Commonly used time-based perturbation methods include jitter and shimmer (measures of cycle-to-cycle variations in frequency and amplitude, respectively) and the harmonics-to-noise ratio (HNR).

While a number of investigations have shown reasonable relationships between the aforementioned perturbation measures and voice-quality categories, two key issues with traditional forms of acoustic analysis of the voice need to be addressed. First, how can we address the inherent difficulties in time-based analysis of severely disturbed voice signals? As previously mentioned, traditional perturbation measures depend on the accurate identification of cycle boundaries, and it has become increasingly evident that the increased aperiodicity in the voice signal makes it more difficult to accurately locate these cycle onsets/offsets. This problem introduces errors in tracking the periodic vibration of the voice signal, and thus contributes to inaccuracy in perturbation measurements. As a result, the validity and clinical usefulness of certain perturbation measures (such as jitter and shimmer) have been questioned, especially when applied to moderately or severely disordered voices.

Secondly, how can we address and quantify the multidimensional nature of the voice signal? It has been recognized that voice (both normal and disordered) varies in a multidimensional manner (i.e., a vocal disruption affects the patient's ability to control pitch/frequency, loudness/intensity, and/or quality, as well as aerodynamic aspects of voice production in many different ways), which cannot be adequately captured using isolated, univariate methods of voice analysis. In addition, Wuyts, De Bodt, Molenberghs, et al. (2000) have pointed out that the typically large variation found in individual test procedures can make it difficult to determine that a specific case is truly abnormal. As a way of circumventing these problems, multivariate approaches that combine the results of several test variables may be applied. Multivariate approaches have the benefit of (1) using more information in determining normal/abnormal behavior than univariate approaches, and (2) of producing an optimal combination of variables regardless of their individual strength. Finally, multivariate approaches should provide a much better reflection of the multidimensional character of the voice signal than individual, isolated voice-assessment procedures.

Several studies have described methods of voice analysis that attempt to address both of the aforementioned issues. The concern surrounding the validity of traditional methods of perturbation analysis has prompted researchers to consider other methods of quantifying noise components in the voice signal. Several investigators have reported that measures derived from spectral analysis of the voice signal may be strong predictors of additive noise in the voice signal, perceived severity of dysphonia, and type of voice disorder (Dejonckere & Wieneke, 1996; de Krom, 1995; Hillenbrand, Cleveland, & Erickson, 1994; Hillenbrand & Houde, 1996). The principal advantage of spectral analysis methods (i.e., frequency-based analysis) is the capacity to produce estimates of aperiodicity and/or additive noise without the identification of individual cycle boundaries. Therefore, the identification of these variables should not be affected by errors in detecting cycle boundaries, as is the case with traditional methods of perturbation analysis such as jitter, shimmer, and HNR.

One method that holds promise as a means of quantifying dysphonia is *cepstral analysis*. Cepstral analysis was originally described by Noll (1964) as a procedure for extracting the fundamental frequency from the spectrum of a sound wave. The cepstrum, a Fourier transform of the power spectrum of the voice signal, graphically displays the extent to which the spectral harmonics, and in particular the vocal fundamental frequency, are individualized and emerge out of the background noise level (see figure 21.1). A periodic signal will show a well-defined harmonic structure and fundamental, corresponding to a more prominent (i.e., distinct, high-amplitude) cepstral peak. It is the dominance of the cepstral peak in relation to extraneous vocal frequencies which, theoretically, provides a more efficient and effective method of quantification for the disordered voice (Hillenbrand, Cleveland, & Erickson, 1994).

Spectral/cepstral-based analysis methods have been incorporated into a number of recent studies which have used multivariate analyses to describe normal vs. dysphonic voice quality. Callan, Kent, Roy, and Tasko (1999)

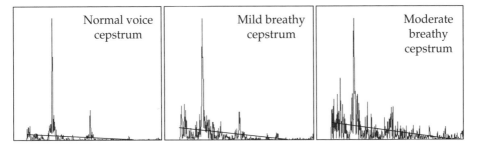

Figure 21.1 Cepstral analysis results for normal, mild breathy, and moderate breathy sustained vowel samples. In the normal sample, the dominant cepstral peak corresponds to the fundamental period and is substantially greater than the average cepstral amplitude. In the disordered samples, the overall amplitude of other spectral components is increased. A regression line used to quantify the relative height of the cepstral peak is shown overlaid on the cepstra (x-axis: frequency; y-axis: amplitude in arbitrary units). (Courtesy of the author)

achieved a 76 percent success rate in classifying normal and disordered voice types via the use of a self-organizing map (SOM). SOMs are used to visualize data through the use of self-organizing neural networks. In particular, SOMs are used to visualize and reduce multidimensional data by producing a map (generally one- or two-dimensional) which plots similarities in data and groups similar data items together. The SOM was 'trained' by using various time-based and spectral/cepstral-based measures of the acoustic signal. A low degree of amplitude and fundamental frequency variability, as well as a high degree of harmonic energy as observed via the cepstrum, characterized non-pathologic voice. Studies by Awan and Roy (2005, 2006) have also demonstrated the effectiveness of multivariate models incorporating automatic cepstral analysis in the prediction of both severity of dysphonia and vocal quality type (normal, breathy, hoarse, rough). In the Awan and Roy (2005) study, discriminant analysis produced a multivariate model that correctly classified voice type with 79.9 percent accuracy in a diverse set of normal and disordered voice. In a second study (Awan & Roy, 2006), stepwise multiple regression analysis indicated that a similar multivariate model was able to strongly predict perceived severity of dysphonia (mean R = 0.88). In both studies, a cepstral-based measure was determined to be the most significant contributor to the prediction of dysphonia severity and type, though it was clear that the addition of other acoustic measures (pitch sigma, shimmer (dB), and a measure of low- vs. high-frequency spectral energy) added substantially to the accuracy of the results.

An alternative spectral-based measure used in the description of vocal quality and designed to assess the amount of additive noise in a speech signal is the glottal-to-noise excitation ratio (GNE) (Michaelis, Gramss, & Strube, 1997). The GNE is based on the assumption that different bands of spectral energy (e.g. bands with 500, 1500, and 2500 Hz center frequencies, and 1000 Hz bandwidth) will be excited in a similar fashion (and therefore be highly correlated) by periodic glottal pulses. On the other hand, the addition of turbulent noise (as found in breathy voice signals) will lead to poor interband correlations (particularly between lower- and higher-frequency bands). The GNE has been used for the objective description of voice quality, indicating whether a particular voice signal originates from vocal-fold vibrations or from turbulent noise generated in the vocal tract. In addition, the GNE has been incorporated into a multivariate approach to voice analysis referred to as the *Hoarseness Diagram* (Fröhlich, Michaelis, Strube, & Kruse, 2000). In the Hoarseness Diagram, the X- and Y-axes are labeled 'roughness' and 'breathiness' respectively. The breathiness coordinate is calculated using the GNE, while the roughness component is determined via a measure of irregularity (a weighted product of jitter, shimmer, and period correlation). By combining the GNE with other measures of the acoustic signal, an attempt is made to account for the multidimensional nature of the voice signal. A complete description of the GNE and its incorporation into the Hoarseness Diagram is available at www.physik3.gwdg.de/~micha/english/hd_background.html.

21.3 Direct Methods: Strobovideolaryngoscopy, High-Speed Imaging and Videokymography

While the aforementioned indirect acoustic methods show great promise as ways of documenting the multidimensional nature of the voice and the patient's degree of voice dysfunction, to date, acoustic methods have not been effective in specifying the precise nature of the underlying structural and/or physiological disturbance. In voice disorders, the underlying laryngeal structures may appear relatively normal (as in many functional disorders), show the presence of discrete or distributed benign lesions (e.g., nodules, polyps), or be affected by conditions that have significant, even life-threatening, effects on the patient's overall health (e.g., progressive neurological disease, carcinoma). Unfortunately, these conditions may have quite similar perceptual and acoustic characteristics, with hoarseness, increased perturbation levels, and increased spectral noise observed as common perceptual and acoustic signs. While perceptual and acoustic signs must be interpreted in light of case-history and medical-history information, it is clear that the voice clinician (particularly one with relatively little experience) could easily mistake a potentially life-threatening voice problem for one that is functional in nature. It is therefore essential that direct visualization of the vocal folds and surrounding structures be added to the information gathered from indirect methods of voice analysis.

Traditionally, some form of laryngoscopy (mirror laryngoscopy, flexible nasendoscopy) has been used to visualize the laryngeal structures. While laryngoscopy is useful for describing the structure of the vocal folds and surrounding tissues, it is not particularly useful for the description of phonation. During phonation, the vocal folds are expected to vibrate at a high rate (approximately 80–300 times per second during speech production in adult males, females, and children). Due to this high rate of vibration, the vibratory characteristics of the vocal folds are relatively unobservable. Fortunately, a commonly used method by which phonatory activity may be observed is *stroboscopy* (also referred to as laryngeal stroboscopy, videostroboscopy, strobovideo-laryngoscopy; see figure 21.2). In stroboscopy, the examiner views the larynx via a rigid or flexible endoscope. The use of a stroboscope provides the examiner with the illusion of slow motion, in which the vibratory activity of the vocal folds may be examined in detail. If the strobe light is used to illuminate the vibrating vocal folds at a frequency identical to the rate of phonatory vibration, the illusion of stop motion will be produced. On the other hand, if the strobe frequency differs slightly from the phonatory frequency (e.g. 2–3 Hz difference), the illusion of slow motion will be produced. When stroboscopic images are recorded, they provide the examiner with a visual replication of vocal-fold activity for review at any time post-examination, and with an opportunity to make observations regarding structure, movement, vibratory pattern, and timing relationships during phonation. Stroboscopy has been determined

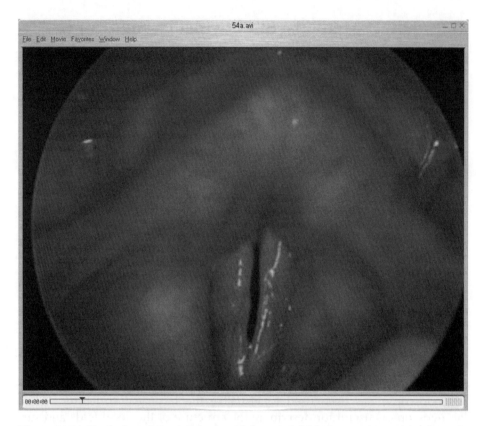

Figure 21.2 Typical stroboscopic image of the vocal folds in a patient with bilateral edema, erythema, and asymmetry of vibration. (Courtesy of the author)

to be a valuable tool in diagnosing vocal pathologies that may otherwise be overlooked; it provides the capability to describe several key characteristics of vocal-fold vibration such as amplitude, phase symmetry, presence and movement of the mucosal cover, periodicity of vibration, and degree of glottal closure during the closed phase of phonation.

While stroboscopic assessment has become commonplace in the clinical assessment of voice-disordered patients, this method shares a disadvantage previously discussed for the acoustic methodology, in that interpretations of stroboscopy are primarily valid for those patients who show periodic oscillation of the vocal folds. In those patients who have more severe quality disturbances, intermittent disturbances, or who have instability of pitch, the stroboscopic image may not accurately reflect the true vibratory nature of the folds, since the stroboscopic image is actually an average of many cycles of vibration. Even for patients with relatively mild difficulties, the stroboscopic method may 'average out' occurrences of instability that underlie the voice problem. This limitation can be addressed through the use of high-speed cameras, capable of over 1000 images per second, thereby providing multiple, high-detail images per cycle of vibration at modal register; unfortunately, the high cost of this method has made it prohibitive in the past. However, in recent years, high-speed digital imaging systems (High Speed Video; HSV) and analysis software have been developed (see, for example, www.kayelemetrics.com) which have image-acquisition rates of approximately 2000–4000 frames per second, allowing for detailed examination of pathologic vibration which is not possible with the stroboscopic method. Granqvist (2003) and Hertegard, Larsson, and Wittenberg (2003) describe several applications of digital high-speed imaging such as measurements of glottal area, vibrational amplitude of each vocal fold, mucosal wave movements, and quantification of vocal tremor. To date, color images are problematic for high-speed imaging systems, limiting the method somewhat in the description of certain laryngeal pathologies such as inflammation. In addition, the huge amount of information provided via the method is itself a limitation since the examiner may be restricted in his or her ability to focus on the most pertinent details of the analysis. Table 21.1 provides a comparison of stroboscopy and high-speed video on several key parameters, and figure 21.3 provides an example of the instrumentation required for HSV acquisition.

An alternative method of high-speed analysis is videokymography. Videokymography was developed as a low-cost alternative to high-speed video that

Table 21.1   Comparison of stroboscopy and high-speed video (HSV) laryngeal imaging techniques (incorporates information from Crump, 1999).

	Stroboscopy	*High-speed video (HSV)*
Field of view	Offers a full view of the vocal folds and surrounding structures.	Uses only a small section of the CCD camera element, resulting in a limited field of view (only 7–12% of the field of view of stroboscopy).
Color vs. gray-scale image	Offers a full palette of colors (24-bit).	In its most practical configuration, HSV is gray-scale (8 bits). Color is possible, but with accompanying reductions in characteristics such as brightness and resolution.
Brightness and heat	Uses all of the light power of the typical 150-watt xenon pulse. The available light power allows for stroboscopy via flexible endoscopy.	Because of the high shutter speed used, HSV uses a small fraction of the light available in stroboscopy. This results in the need for a more powerful light source (typically, a 300-watt bulb) which generates more heat. HSV via flexible endoscopy is currently not available.

Table 21.1   (*Continued*)

	Stroboscopy	High-speed video (HSV)
Real-time display	Images can be viewed and interpreted during acquisition (i.e., in real time), allowing for rapid clinical decision-making.	HSV captures images in 2-second blocks which cannot be interpreted during real time. HSV images are played out at slower rates (e.g., 15 frames/sec.) after capture, requiring approx. 5 minutes to review the 2 second capture.
Audio	Simultaneous audio can be played back while visualizing images.	During playback of HSV, the audio for that segment cannot readily be played, making the relationship between auditory impressions and observed images difficult.
Phonatory 'lock-on'	Requires a few seconds to lock to the pitch/frequency of the voice. In addition, the voice must be quasi-periodic for lock-on to occur. Short duration and/or aperiodic productions may not be analyzed.	No lock-on time, as required in stroboscopy. HSV can record *any* behavior, even extremely short duration voicing, aperiodic productions, coughs, and spasms. In addition, initiation of vocal fold vibration may be analyzed.
Phonatory analysis	Images are assembled from many cycles to 'represent' intra-cycle behavior. Observation of the actual intra-cycle behavior of any single vibratory cycle is not possible.	Due to its high rate of image acquisition, HSV has the potential to visualize intra-cycle voicing behavior as well as any type of aperiodic or periodic laryngeal behavior.
Cost analysis	May be implemented at a substantially lower cost than HSV.	If it could replace stroboscopy, an HSV system would cost about $5–10K more than a digital stroboscopy system. If used as option to stroboscopy, HSV adds approx. 50% to the cost of a digital stroboscope system.

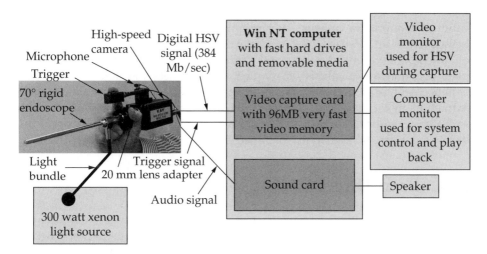

Figure 21.3 Components of a High-Speed Video (HSV) system for high-speed laryngeal/phonatory analysis. (Courtesy of J. Crump and KayPentax)

utilizes a specially modified CCD camera functioning in both standard (50–60 fields/sec) and high-speed modes (7812.5 line images/sec) (Švec, 2000). In high-speed mode, data from a single line/field of the CCD chip is acquired. The successive lines are displayed successively to create a videokymogram (i.e., a spatio-temporal image showing a fixed horizontal line from an image as it varies over time; see figure 21.4). Kymography has been extended to the

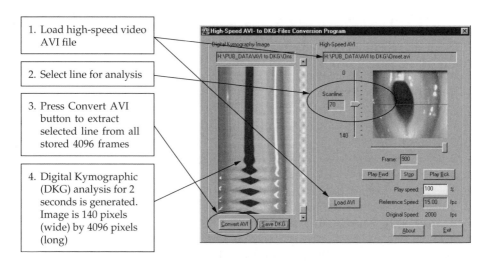

Figure 21.4 An example of the KayPentax utility program to convert HSV to Digital Kymographic (DKG) images. The DKG image represents vocal-fold movement at a user-selected analysis line. (Courtesy of J. Crump and KayPentax)

digital realm (digital kymography – DKG) which provides several seconds of continuous vibratory images with minimum variation in light-source brightness. Deliyski and Petrushev (2003) have described the simultaneous recording of high-speed videoendoscopy and digital kymography, as well as accompanying phonatory analysis techniques. Image-processing methods for edge enhancement, noise removal, mucosal wave recognition, and dynamic feature extraction methods which automatically provide estimates of glottal width and area waveforms make possible phonatory analysis that far surpasses the depth of information currently obtained from strobovideolaryngoscopy.

21.4   Semi-Direct Methods

It is clear that, to achieve a comprehensive description of the disordered voice, multiple procedures that address both dysfunction and pathology are necessary. The clinical evaluation of the voice is always initiated by the perceptual nature of the voice itself. It is this characteristic which has the most meaning to the patient and family and is the most meaningful gauge of vocal change. However, the indeterminate nature of perceptual evaluation requires the addition of other methods of analysis to provide a complete characterization of the voice problem at hand. Indirect voice-analysis methods such as the acoustic methods described in this chapter may provide effective gauges of vocal dysfunction, while direct methods derived from laryngoscopy (strobovideolaryngoscopy, high-speed digital analysis, and kymography) allow for specification of disorder type and associated physiological disruption. When direct and indirect methods are organized and analyzed in light of the patient's case-history information, a highly comprehensive analysis of the dysphonic voice may be achieved.

While the focus of this chapter has been on issues dealing with acoustic (indirect) vs. laryngoscopic (direct) methods of phonatory assessment, insight into phonatory behavior may be expanded by using what may be termed *semi-direct* methods. These methods fall into an area between the aforementioned measurement techniques, providing information somewhat closer to the actual source of vibration than that obtained via acoustic analysis methods, but without direct laryngeal visualization. These methods provide information regarding vocal-fold physiology and include electromyography, inverse filtering, subglottal pressure estimates, and electroglottography (Colton & Casper, 1996). Originally described by Fabre (1957) and advanced by the work of researchers such as Abberton and Fourcin (1997), Abberton, Fourcin, and Howard (1989), Fourcin and Abberton (1971), Fourcin, Abberton, Miller, and Howells (1995) and Rothenberg (1992), electroglottography (EGG; alternatively electrolaryngography – ELG) is an attractive adjunct to voice profiling due to its noninvasive nature and relative ease of administration. In EGG, a physiologically safe, high-frequency electrical current is passed between two electrodes placed on opposite sides of the neck at the level of the thyroid lamina (i.e., the alae of the thyroid cartilage). Resistance to this current will vary as the vocal folds separate during the open phase of vocal-fold closure (increased resistance) and approximate during the closed phase (decreased resistance). The graphical display of these variations in electrical resistance (an *electroglottogram*) may be used to provide measures of vocal-fold contact area over time (Titze, 1994). In particular, the relative durations of the closed vs. open phases of the glottal cycle have been used in the computation of measures such as the closed quotient (CQ – the time that the vocal folds are closed as a percentage of the complete glottal cycle), open quotient (OQ – the time that the vocal folds are open as a percentage of the complete glottal cycle), and the speed quotient (SQ – the ratio of closing and opening times within the closed phase). The identification of the various phases of the glottal cycle may be achieved using techniques such as the time-differentiated EGG (DEGG – see figure 21.5) or by applying a set baseline at 25 to 50 percent of the peak-to-peak amplitude

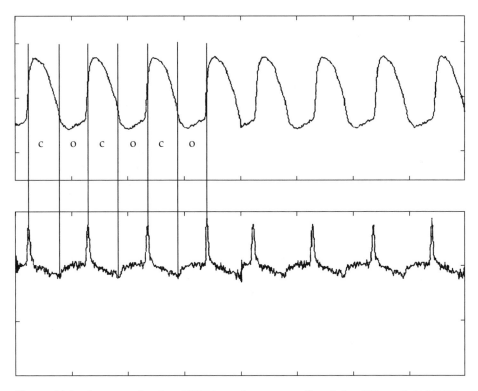

Figure 21.5   An example of an EGG trace (upper panel) and the differentiated EGG (DEGG – lower panel). The positive peaks in the DEGG are used as indicators of glottal closure, while the negative peaks are used as indicators of glottal openings. The letter C indicates the closed phase of the glottal cycle; the letter O indicates the open phase. Vocal-fold contact area increases as the EGG trace moves upward. (Courtesy of the author)

(Higgins & Saxman, 1993; Orlikoff, 1991; Rothenberg & Mahshie, 1988). The EGG has had a variety of applications in the voice literature, including use in the diagnostic characterization of non-pathological and pathological voice (Fourcin, 2000; Heinrich, d'Alessandro, Doval, & Castellengo, 2004), application to the assessment of treatment adequacy (Carding, Horsley, & Docherty, 1999; Elliot, Sundberg, & Gramming, 1997); and use in the categorization of the trained vs. untrained singing voice (Howard, 1995). It should be noted that there are some important limitations in the use of EGG. The quality of the EGG signal is dependent upon adequate vocal-fold contact, and therefore the signal and information derived from it are weakened in patients with more severe forms of hypoadduction. In addition, weak signals may be obtained in subjects who present with thicker or larger necks which result in poor transmission of the electrical current being passed between the electrode pair. An excellent over-view of EGG and its application to voice analysis is presented by Dr. K. Marasek at www.ims.uni-stuttgart.de/phonetik/EGG/.

21.5   Conclusion

Future additions to complete the profile of the dysphonic voice should move towards expanded analysis of the continuous speaking voice. Most methods of phonatory analysis that have some relation to the quality of the voice, including those discussed in this chapter, are generally applied to sustained vowel productions. However, measures obtained from continuous speech samples may have more relation to the 'real-world' judgment of vocal character-istics (Parsa & Jamieson, 2001). Acoustic methods that can provide a gauge of dysphonic severity which will not be adversely affected by the expected pitch, loudness, and phonetic changes found in continuous speech would be valu-able additions to current voice assessment protocols. In addition, alternative methods for encompassing the multidimensional nature of the voice signal which include other aspects of voice production such as respiratory control (e.g. The Dysphonia Severity Index (DSI) – Wuyts, De Bodt, Molenberghs, et al., 2000) hold promise for the further documentation of dysphonia. Whatever future developments may occur, it is essential that we strive to incorporate these methods into the everyday clinical environment and not leave them as tools solely for the research lab. Further reading in this area can be found in Awan (2001), Baken and Orlikoff (2000), Kent and Ball (2000), and Woo (2006).

ACKNOWLEDGMENT

The author would like to express his gratitude to J. Crump at KayPentax (Lincoln Park, NJ) for his help in preparing the sections of this chapter that deal with high-speed video and videokymography.

REFERENCES

Abberton, E. and Fourcin, A. (1997). Electrolaryngography. In M. J. Ball and C. Code (eds.), *Instrumental Clinical Phonetics*. London: Whurr, pp. 119–48.

Abberton, E., Fourcin, A., and Howard, D. (1989). Laryngographic assessment of normal voice: A tutorial. *Clinical Linguistics and Phonetics*, 3, 281–96.

Awan, S. N. (2001). *The Voice Diagnostic Protocol: A Practical Guide to the Diagnosis of Voice Disorders*. Austin, TX: Pro-Ed.

Awan, S. N. and Roy, N. (2005). Acoustic prediction of voice type in adult females with functional dysphonia. *Journal of Voice*, 19, 268–82.

Awan, S. N. and Roy, N. (2006). Toward the development of an objective index of dysphonia severity: A four-factor model. *Clinical Linguistics and Phonetics*, 20, 35–49.

Baken, R. J. and Orlikoff, R. F. (2000). *Clinical Measurement of Speech and Voice*. 2nd ed. San Diego, CA: Singular Publishing Group.

Callan, D. E., Kent, R. D., Roy, N., and Tasko, S. M. (1999). Self-organizing maps for the classification of normal and disordered female voices. *Journal of Speech and Hearing Research*, 42, 355–66.

Carding, P. N., Horsley, I. A., and Docherty, G. J. (1999). A study of the effectiveness of voice therapy in the treatment of 45 patients with nonorganic dysphonia. *Journal of Voice*, 13, 72–104.

Colton, R. H. and Casper, J. K. (1996). *Understanding Voice Problems: A Physiological Perspective for Diagnosis and Treatment*. 2nd ed. Baltimore, MD: Lippincott, Williams and Wilkins.

Crump, J. (1999). Technical analysis of high-speed video for applications to laryngeal examinations. Paper presented at the Twenty-fourth Annual Meeting of the Collegium Medicorum Theatri, Aspen, CO.

Dejonckere, P. H. and Wieneke, G. H. (1996). Cepstra of normal and pathological voices: Correlation with acoustic, aerodynamic and perceptual data. In M. J. Ball and M. Duckworth (eds.), *Advances in Clinical Phonetics* (pp. 217–26). Amsterdam: John Benjamins.

de Krom, G. (1994). Consistency and reliability of voice quality ratings for different types of speech fragments. *Journal of Speech and Hearing Research*, 37, 985–1000.

de Krom, G. (1995). Some spectral correlates of pathological breathy and rough voice quality for different types of vowel fragments. *Journal of Speech and Hearing Research*, 38, 794–811.

Deliyski, D. and Petrushev, P. (2003). Methods for objective assessment of high-speed videoendoscopy. In *Proceedings: 6th International Conference: Advances in Quantitative Laryngology, Voice and Speech Research (AQL 2003), Hamburg, Germany* (pp. 28–43).

Elliot, N., Sundberg, J., and Gramming, P. (1997). Physiological aspects of a vocal exercise. *Journal of Voice*, 11, 171–7.

Fabre, P. (1957). Un procédé électrique percutané d'inscription de l'accolement glottique au cours de la phonation: Glottographie de haute fréquence. Premiers résultats. *Bulletin de l'Académie Nationale de Médecine*, 141, 66.

Fourcin, A. (2000). Precision stroboscopy, voice quality and electrolaryngography. In R. D. Kent and M. J. Ball (eds.), *Voice Quality Measurement*. San Diego, CA: Singular Publishing Group.

Fourcin, A. J. and Abberton, E. (1971). First applications of a new laryngograph. *Medical and Biological Illustration*, 21, 172–82.

Fourcin, A., Abberton, E., Miller, D., and Howells, D. (1995). Laryngograph: Speech pattern element tools for therapy, training and assessment. *European Journal of Disorders of Communication*, 30, 101–15.

Fröhlich, M., Michaelis, D., Strube, H. W., and Kruse, E. (2000). Acoustic voice analysis by means of the Hoarseness Diagram. *Journal of Speech and Hearing Research*, 43, 706–20.

Granqvist, S. (2003). Computer methods for voice analysis. Doctoral dissertation, Kungl. Tekniska Högskolan, Stockholm.

Heinrich, N., d'Alessandro, C., Doval, B., and Castellengo, M. (2004). On the use of the derivative of electroglottographic signals for characterization of nonpathological phonation. *Journal of the Acoustical Society of America*, 115, 1321–32.

Hertegard, S., Larsson, H., and Wittenberg, T. (2003). High-speed imaging: Applications and development. *Logopedics Phoniatrics and Vocology*, 28, 133–9.

Higgins, M. B. and Saxman, J. H. (1993). Inverse-filtered air flow and EGG measures for sustained vowels and syllables. *Journal of Voice*, 7(1), 47–53.

Hillenbrand, J., Cleveland, R. A., and Erickson, R. L. (1994). Acoustic correlates of breathy vocal quality. *Journal of Speech and Hearing Research*, 37, 769–78.

Hillenbrand, J. and Houde, R. A. (1996). Acoustic correlates of breathy vocal quality: dysphonic voices and continuous speech. *Journal of Speech and Hearing Research*, 39, 311–21.

Howard, D. M. (1995). Variation of electrolaryngographically derived closed quotient for trained and untrained adult singers. *Journal of Voice*, 9, 163–72.

Kent, R. D. and Ball, M. J. (eds.) (2000). *Voice Quality Measurement*. San Diego, CA: Singular Publishing Group.

Kreiman, J., Gerratt, B., Kempster, G. B., Erman, A., and Berke, G. S. (1993). Perceptual evaluation of voice quality: Review, tutorial, and a framework for future research. *Journal of Speech and Hearing Research*, 36, 21–40.

Michaelis, D., Gramss, T., and Strube, H. W. (1997). Glottal-to-noise excitation ratio: A new measure for describing pathological voices. *Acustica/Acta Acustica*, 83, 700–6.

Noll, A. M. (1964). Short-term spectrum and 'cepstrum' techniques for vocal pitch detection. *Journal of the Acoustical Society of America*, 41, 293–309.

Orlikoff, R. F. (1991). Assessment of the dynamics of vocal fold contact from the electroglottogram: data from normal male subjects. *Journal of Speech and Hearing Research*, 34, 1066–72.

Orlikoff, R. F., Dejonckere, P. H., Dembowski, J., Fitch, J., Gelfer, M. P., Gerratt, B. R., Haskell, J. A., Kreiman, J., Metz, D. E., Schiavetti, N., Watson, B. C., and Wolfe, V. (1999). The perceived role of voice perception in clinical practice. *Phonoscope*, 2, 89–104.

Parsa, V. and Jamieson, D. G. (2001). Acoustic discrimination of pathologic voice: Sustained vowels versus continuous speech. *Journal of Speech and Hearing Research*, 44, 327–39.

Rothenberg, M. (1992). A multichannel electroglottograph. *Journal of Voice*, 6, 36–43.

Rothenberg, M. and Mahshie, J. J. (1988). Monitoring vocal fold abduction through vocal fold contact area. *Journal of Speech and Hearing Research*, 31, 338–51.

Švec, J. G. (2000). On vibration properties of human vocal folds: Voice registers, bifurcations, resonance characteristics, development and application of videokymography. Doctoral dissertation, University of Groningen, The Netherlands.

Titze, I. R. (1994). *Principles of Voice Production*. Englewood Cliffs, NJ: Prentice-Hall.

Woo, P. (2006). *Stroboscopy*. San Diego, CA: Plural Publishing.

Wuyts, F. L., De Bodt, M. S., Molenberghs, G., Remacle, M., Heylen, L., Millet, B., Van Lierde, K., Raes, J., and Van de Heyning, P. H. (2000). The dysphonia severity index: An objective measure of vocal quality based on a multiparameter approach. *Journal of Speech, Language, and Hearing Research, 43,* 796–809.

22 Acoustic Analysis of Speech

RAY D. KENT AND YUNJUNG KIM

22.1 Introduction

Acoustic analysis is attractive for the study of speech for several reasons, but one of the most important is that the acoustic signal bridges the acts of speech production and speech perception. Therefore, acoustic analysis is informative about both a talker's behavior and a listener's perception of the signal that is so generated. Acoustic analysis is also appealing because of the relative ease with which it can be accomplished. Modern digital processing techniques have greatly increased the speed and power of acoustic analyses, to the point that even a modest budget is sufficient to enable sophisticated analyses. Underpinning these analyses is the availability of quantitative theories that permit the interpretation of acoustic data with respect to speech production and perception. Acoustic analysis is a natural complement to studies of speech physiology, just as it is a natural complement to studies of speech perception. Theory and technology may usher in a new era in the clinical application of acoustics, and this chapter takes a brief look at progress and potential. Although progress is notable, there is considerable potential for a greatly enlarged acoustic database on a variety of speech and language disorders. This database could support improvements in both the assessment and the management of these disorders. Table 22.1 gives some recent examples of the use of acoustics for the description and analysis of speech-language disorders in children and adults. This table is both a summary of progress and a blueprint for some aspects of future research.

The literature on acoustic analysis easily overwhelms even a lengthy book chapter, so the effort here is to offer a condensed and selective overview of what can be accomplished through acoustic analysis for the deeper understanding of communicative disorders. We begin with a brief introduction to the theory of speech acoustics.

Table 22.1 Recent acoustic studies on speech-language disorders in children or adults

		Childhood motor speech disorders	Adult dysarthria	Adult apraxia of speech	Aphasia
Spectral measures	Vowel space (F1–F2)	Higgins & Hodge (2002)	Tjaden et al. (2005) Tjaden & Wilding (2004) Bunton & Weismer (2001) Turner & Tjaden (2000) Weismer et al. (2000) Roy et al. (2001)	Haley et al. (2001)	Haley et al. (2001)
	Moment analysis (consonant spectra)		Chen & Stevens (2001) Tjaden & Turner (1997) McRae et al. (2002) Tjaden & Wilding (2004)	Haley (2002, 2004)	Haley (2002, 2004)
	Formant trajectories	Nijland, Maassen, & van der Meulen (2003), Nijland et al. (2003), Sussman et al. (2000)	Tjaden (2003) Ansel & Kent (1992) Weismer et al. (1992)	Tjaden (1999)	
Temporal measures	VOT	Munson et al. (2003)	Wang et al. (2004) Hertrich & Ackermann (1994)	Wambaugh et al. (2004), Rogers (1997)	Misiurski et al. (2005), McHenry (2004) Baum et al. (1990)
	Segment duration (fricative noise, pause, vowel)	Nijland et al. (2003) Skinder et al. (2000)	Patel (2004) Patel (2003) Rosen et al. (2003) Chen & Stevens (2001) Bunton & Weismer (2001)	Haley (2002, 2004) Haley et al. (2001) Van Putten et al. (2003) Strand & McNeil (1996) Seddoh et al. (1996)	Haley (2002, 2004), Kurowski et al. (2003), Baum & Boyczuk (1999), Hanlong & Edmondson (1996) Seddoh et al. (1996), Baum (1996)

Table 22.1 *(Continued)*

		Childhood motor speech disorders	Adult dysarthria	Adult apraxia of speech	Aphasia
Prosody	F0	Munson et al. (2003) Skinder et al. (2000)	Patel (2004) Patel (2003) Le Dorze et al. (1992) Bunton et al. (2001) Bunton et al. (2000)	Van Putten et al. (2003)	
	Rate	Thoonen et al. (1999)	Schalling & Hartelius (2004) Ozawa et al. (2001) Le Dorze et al. (1994) Wang et al. (2004, 2005) Tjaden & Watling (2003) Whitehill & Tsang (2002) Ziegler (2002) Wang et al. (2005)	Ziegler (2002)	
	Pairwise variability index				

Note: Rate category includes speaking rate, articulation rate, and DDK

22.2   Acoustical Theory of Speech Production

The acoustics of speech can be understood to a considerable degree through a parsimonious model known as the source-filter model. This model, illustrated in figure 22.1 for vowel sounds, essentially states that speech sounds are produced by the combination of a filter that operates on a source of sound energy. For a typical vowel sound, the source of energy is the vibration of the vocal folds, and the filter is the combined effect of the vocal tract resonances (formants). If the assumptions of linearity and time-invariance are granted, this model can be implemented with powerful and well-known mathematics, such as Fourier analysis. In short, this model means that the laryngeal source spectrum (voice) is modified by the filtering effects of the vocal tract. These filtering effects include the formants and the radiation characteristic, which together comprise the transfer function that relates source energy to radiated acoustic energy (figure 22.2). The model for non-nasal vowels is relatively simple in that (1) it is commonly assumed that the source is independent of

Vocal tract = filter

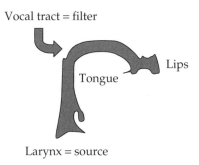

Larynx = source

Figure 22.1   Source-filter theory applied to the vocal tract. For voiced vowels, the vibrating vocal folds are the energy source, and the resonances of the vocal tract comprise the filter or transfer function.

Transfer function =
Resonances (formants) + Radiation Characteristic

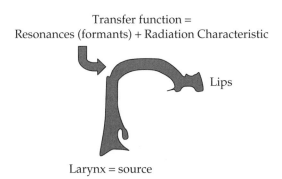

Larynx = source

Figure 22.2   Elaboration of the source-filter theory to show that the transfer function includes the formant pattern and the radiation characteristic.

the filter (i.e., source and filter are non-interactive), (2) only formants (resonances or poles) are involved in the transfer function, and (3) both source and radiation characteristics can be considered as constants (i.e., unchanging across vowels). Things become more complicated with other classes of sounds, but the basic model of source + filter can be extended to any class of speech sounds with some additional assumptions and adjustments. The following discussion considers various classes of sounds with regard to the source + filter analysis. First, various types of sources are considered, and then attention is given to the filtering performed by the vocal tract.

22.2.1   Sources

The main energy sources of speech include the following (for each source type, a listing is given in parentheses of the types of sounds associated with it):

Quasi-periodic glottal pulses (voiced vowels and voiced consonants)
Turbulence noise (fricatives)
Noise burst (stop release release)
Silence (stop and affricate gaps)

In general, a given source type can be identified with a particular site in the vocal tract. Voicing is associated with vibration of the vocal folds, and turbulence noise and noise bursts are associated with a constriction somewhere in the vocal tract. It may seem unusual to classify silence as a source type, but silent intervals are part of the acoustic pattern of speech and carry information relevant to phonetic interpretation. For example, stop consonants are produced with a complete obstruction of the vocal tract, and this obstruction is signaled by silence (especially for voiceless stops). For certain speech sounds, sources are combined. For instance, voiced fricatives require two sources, glottal pulses and fricative noise, which are essentially simultaneous.

This chapter does not cover the acoustic analysis of voice, a topic that is considered elsewhere in this book. But it should be emphasized that voice is integral to speech production and the role of vocal function is implicit in much of what follows.

22.2.2   Filtering (transfer function)

Acoustic energy from one of the sources previously discussed is subjected to filtering by the vocal tract resonances and the radiation characteristic. Assuming that the latter is constant across sounds, we need to specify only the pattern of formants and antiformants. This pattern will be abbreviated to $T(f)$ for transfer function (input/output ratio as a function of frequency, fs) in the following discussion.

$T(f)$ is determined by the resonating cavities of the vocal tract. For the production of vowels, it is typically assumed that only the supralaryngeal

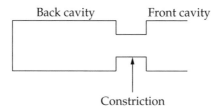

Figure 22.3 Simplified model of fricative production in terms of a back and front cavity separated by an articulatory constriction. As the place and length of the constriction change, the lengths of the back and front cavities change as well.

cavities need to be taken into account. This assumption works to a reasonable first approximation, but a finely detailed analysis must recognize that the infralaryngeal structures (tracheobronchial tree) exert an influence on $T(f)$. Most discussions of $T(f)$ for non-nasal voiced vowels neglect these infralaryngeal effects, on the assumption that the voicing source has infinite impedance, and is therefore not influenced by variations in $T(f)$. For other classes of sounds, such as fricatives, it is essential to take account of cavities on either side of the constriction (figure 22.3). Under certain conditions, both the front and back cavity resonances shape the sound output. Under other conditions, the front cavity is the primary influence.

22.3 Vowels

22.3.1 *Voiced non-nasal vowels*

A simple but effective illustration used by legions of phonetics or speech science instructors goes as follows: The instructor shapes her vocal tract for a given vowel (let us say the vowel in *we*) and then, as she taps her head sharply, she asks the class to identify the vowel. For speakers who have fairly resonant heads, the demonstration works well. Each time the instructor positions her vocal tract for a given vowel and taps her head, a distinctive vowel sound can be heard. The point of the demonstration is simply that vowels are identified by their resonance patterns (formant patterns) and these are determined by the length and shape of the vocal tract. The tap is the source of sound energy that activates the resonances. A voiced vowel is similar insofar as the vocal–fold pulses, each one similar to a tap, provide a continuous activation of the resonances of the vocal tract.

Formant patterns are not the only way of describing vowels, and for certain purposes, other acoustic representations may be better than formants (de Wet, Weber, Boves, et al., 2004; Molis, 2005; Zahorian & Jagharghi, 1993). But formant specification is useful as a low-dimensional description of vowels, in that only two or three formants are sufficient to describe the vowels in most languages.

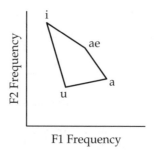

Figure 22.4   The classic F1–F2 chart for vowels. The labeled vowels are the corner vowels of the acoustic vowel quadrilateral.

Another advantage to formant specification is that the relationships of formants (including their frequencies and amplitudes) to vowel articulation are fairly well understood. Let us consider the classic F1–F2 formant plot (figure 22.4) as an example. This is probably the most commonly used graph in speech acoustics. It depicts a fundamental articulatory-acoustic relationship in which the F1 and F2 frequencies are related principally to tongue height and advancement, respectively. The relationship can also be expressed this way: the F2–F1 difference can be interpreted as tongue advancement/retraction, and the F1 value can be taken as an index of tongue height.

The simple relationships just described are extremely useful, but they understate the challenges in formant descriptions. A major challenge is the variation of formant frequencies with vocal-tract length (which is to say, speaker sex and age, which are the primary determinants of vocal-tract length). The vowel formant patterns for any given vowel produced by a man, a woman, and a child are not identical. Attempts to classify tokens of vowel sounds from different speakers as having the same phonetic identity in spite of formant-frequency differences are obstructed by the problem of vowel (or speaker) normalization, and the most popular attempts at a solution rely on relational computations such as logarithms or ratios. The dependence of vowel formant frequencies on the age and gender of the speaker is a hindrance to comparisons of formant data from speakers who represent different age–sex combinations.

The acoustic vowel quadrilateral is not only a way of describing individual vowels, which appear as points on or within the quadrilateral; it can be used for other purposes as well. One of these is an index of the vowel working space. The index is the F1–F2 planar area that can be computed with the following formula for the area of an irregular quadrilateral:

Area = 0.5*{(/i/F2*/ae/F1 + /ae/F2*/a/F1 + /a/F2*/u/F1 + /u/F2*/i/F1) −
   (/i/F1*/ae/F2 + /ae/F1*/a/F2 + /a/F1*/u/F2 + /u/F1*/i/F2)}

where Fn = the formant number for the vowel symbol shown in the preceding slashes; e.g., /i/F2 is the second formant for vowel /i/.

22.3.2   *Clinical example 1: Acoustic vowel space*

Several characteristics of vowels have been used in studies of speech, language, and hearing disorders, but the two main categories of data are formant frequencies (a spectral property) and duration (a temporal property). With respect to formant frequencies, the size of the vowel space has potential value for the study of several types of disorder, and this topic is the first example of clinical application in this chapter. The vowel space size is reduced in certain speech disorders in adults (Turner, Tjaden, & Weismer, 1995; Ziegler & von Cramon, 1983) and in children (Higgins & Hodge, 2001; Kent, Osberger, Netsell, & Hustedde, 1987; Liu, Tsao, & Kuhl, 2005; Rvachew, Slawinski, Williams, & Green, 1996). Presumably, reduced acoustic space reflects a constricted articulatory space; that is a reduced range of tongue, jaw, and/or lip movement. Vowel space size is one factor that relates to the capacity for intelligible speech, given that larger spaces ensure a high degree of acoustic contrastivity.

22.4   Consonants

Consonants are a complex group of sounds, best considered in major classes defined by their articulatory and acoustic characteristics. In the following discussion, statistics on frequency of occurrence are integrated with comments on articulatory-acoustic properties for classes of consonants.

22.4.1   *Sonorant consonants*

Sonorant consonants are defined by a resonant pattern consisting of formants and/or antiformants. These sounds are less intense than vowels. Unlike the obstruents, sonorant consonants are nearly free of noise components, such as bursts or sustained frication. Acoustically, then, these sounds are described primarily in respect to patterns of resonance.

22.4.1.1   *Glides (semi-vowels)*

There are only two or three glides in American English. Just about all phoneticians agree that the phonemes /w/ and /j/ should be numbered as glides, and some also maintain that /h/ should be treated as a glide. For present purposes, only /w/ and /j/ are considered as glides. These sounds share the acoustic property of a relatively gradual (glide-like) change in formant frequency. This gradual transition in formant frequencies contrasts with the rapid transition in stop consonants, which are considered later. The main point to be made here is that glides have a well-defined formant pattern characterized by a relatively long duration of formant-frequency shift.

22.4.1.2   *Nasal consonants*

Nasal consonants are ordinarily voiced and they can be classified phonetically as sonorants. But their acoustic properties are easily distinguished from oral vowels, first by their characteristic low intensity, and secondly by a dense pattern of resonances and anti-resonances. Fujimura (1962) noted three common properties of the nasal consonants: (1) all of them have a first formant of about 300 Hz that is clearly separated from higher formants, (2) the formants tend to be highly damped (i.e., they have large bandwidths), and (3) they have a high density of formants combined with antiformants. These basic principles certainly help to characterize nasal consonants, but the detailed acoustic properties of these sounds are not so easily described. For a more detailed discussion, see Kent and Read (2002).

Nasal segments occur with considerable frequency. In English, the three nasals /m/, /n/ and /ŋ/ account for nearly one-fifth (18.45 percent) of all consonants produced in initial, medial, and final positions (Mines, Hanson, & Shoup, 1978). This statistic is even more impressive when we realize that /ŋ/ does not occur in syllable-initial position. The alveolar nasal /n/ is the most frequently occurring of all consonants in American English. Other alveolars that occur with high frequency include the stop /t/, fricative /s/, lateral /l/, and stop /d/, all of which rank in the top six of the most frequently occurring consonants. Because vowels adjacent to nasal consonants are themselves usually nasalized to some degree, nasalization is a frequently encountered property of speech.

22.4.1.3   Liquid consonants

Liquid is a cover term for the consonant phonemes /l/ and /r/. The lateral /l/ is acoustically similar to the nasal consonants. This similarity is rooted in the shared production factor of a bifurcated vocal tract that introduces antiformants into the transfer function. For nasal consonants, the bifurcation relates to the oral and nasal cavities. For laterals, the bifurcation results from the midline obstruction with lateral openings for sound transmission. The rhotic /r/ is one of the most complex and variable sounds in American English. It can be produced in various ways, including a retroflex articulation and a bunched articulation. Acoustically, /r/ is associated with a low F3 frequency or a small F3–F2 difference.

The /l/ and /r/ sounds occur with nearly the same frequency in American English – just over 6 percent of all consonant sounds in adult speech (Mines, Hanson, & Shoup, 1978). Their combined percentage of over 12 percent gives them considerable importance.

22.4.2   Non-sonorant consonants

22.4.2.1   Stop consonants

Stop or plosive consonants are made with a complete obstruction of the vocal tract. If the resulting overpressure is abruptly released, a burst is produced. Stops therefore are sometimes taken to be consonants par excellence, that is, the ultimate contrast with vowels. Vowels are resonant, but stops are a combination of silence and noise burst. Vowels are made with an open vocal tract, but stops are made with a complete closure and a rapid opening. When stops are produced in association with a vowel, as in CV and VC syllables, formant transitions are created as the vocal tract opens from stop constriction to vowel (CV transition) or as the vocal tract closes from vowel to stop constriction (VC). Taking the formant transitions into account, we see that stop consonants are really a sequence of acoustic segments, including stop gap (corresponding to the interval of oral constriction), noise burst (signaling release of the constriction), and formant transition (associated with the transition into or out of a more open vocal tract). The exact appearance of these segments varies with the position of a stop in a syllable.

Stops are among the earliest sounds to appear in infant babbling (especially the labials and alveolars) and they also appear in early words. Virtually all languages draw on stops as part of their phonetic repertoires. Stops play a major role in English, as they account for nearly one-third (29.21 percent) of all consonants appearing in initial, medial, and final positions of words produced by adults (Mines, Hanson, & Shoup, 1978). As mentioned earlier, nasals account for nearly 20 percent of consonants, so stops and nasals together make up almost half of all consonant productions. Anything that reduces the stop vs. nasal distinction is a major threat to speech intelligibility, and this is one reason why velopharyngeal dysfunction can have devastating effects on intelligibility.

Stop consonants have been studied fairly extensively in both normal and disordered speech. Several different acoustic features are of interest: the stop gap, stop burst, formant transitions and voice onset time. As an example of clinical application, we consider the last of these, which is one of the most frequently investigated aspects of the production and perception of stops.

22.4.2.2 *Clinical example 2: Voice onset time (VOT)*

Among various acoustic features of consonants, voice onset time (VOT) has been the focus of numerous investigations of both normal and disordered speech, largely on the assumption that this acoustic interval between the burst and the onset of periodic energy corresponds to the physiological interval between the release of the consonantal constriction and the onset of vocal–fold vibration (see Auzou, Ozsancak, Morris, et al., 2000 for a review). Therefore, VOT is a possible index of intersystem coordination or timing. Distribution of VOT values has been reported for speakers with various disorders, including aphasia (Baum, Blumstein, Naeser, & Palumbo, 1990; Blumstein & Baum, 1987; Blumstein, Cooper, Goodglass, Statlender, & Gottlieb, 1980), apraxia of speech (Kent & McNeil, 1987; Wambaugh, West, & Doyle, 1997), and dysarthria (Kent, Netsell, & Abbs, 1979; Caruso & Burton, 1987; Morris, 1989).

For the most part, VOT has been used for the purpose of identifying the prominent features of specific types of disorders. In studies of aphasia, VOT differences have been reported to be generally more variable for speakers with a reduced distinction between voiced and voiceless pairs, compared to results for healthy speakers. In particular, more overlapped VOT distributions for voiced and voiceless cognates are observed for Broca's aphasia, while overall intact VOT categories are observed for Wernicke's aphasia.

A few studies have shown that apraxic speakers also exhibit an overlap in VOT distribution between voiced and voiceless cognate (Freeman, Sands, & Harris, 1978; Itoh, Sasanuma, Tatsumi, et al., 1982). These results have been interpreted as representing different levels of deficits; that is, the phonetic level versus the phonemic/phonological level (Blumstein, Cooper, Goodglass, Statlender, & Gottlieb, 1980). Numerous studies of different languages have basically replicated the results of Blumstein et al. (1980), such as Thai (Gandour & Dardarananda, 1984; Gandour, Ponglorpisit, Khunadorn, et al., 1992), and Japanese (Itoh, Sasanuma, Tatsumi, et al., 1982).

A considerable amount of data has been published on VOT in dysarthric speech as an index of subsystem coordination deficits. VOT has been used both for identifying subtypes of dysarthria and for investigating the relationship between VOT values and speech intelligibility. The features of VOT of dysarthric speakers have been reported to depend on the type or etiology of the dysarthria. For example, longer VOT values than healthy speakers have been reported for ataxic dysarthria (Kent, Netsell, & Abbs, 1979), shorter for spastic dysarthria (Hardcastle, Morgan Barry, & Clark, 1985; Morris, 1989), and no abnormalities in patients with mixed spastic-flaccid dysarthria in amyotrophic lateral sclerosis (Caruso & Burton, 1987). In spite of the abnormality of VOT values, the relationship between VOT values and speech intelligibility has not been well established. While Ansel and Kent (1992) reported that VOT was not significantly related to intelligibility scores in speakers with cerebral palsy, another study of similar methodology but in a different language (Mandarin) showed that VOT variation was one of the major factors in predicting the intelligibility of Mandarin speakers with cerebral palsy (Liu, Tseng, & Tsao, 2000). More data across different languages and substantial number of subjects are needed in future studies.

Recently, several caveats of VOT regarding its measurement and the interpretation of the data, particularly in disordered speech, have been raised (see Weismer, forthcoming). Alternative measurements such as duration of stop gap, voiceless interval, or aspiration are recommended. VOT is an attractive measure because of its relative simplicity, but its value in clinical applications can be enhanced by considering it in the context of other measures.

22.4.2.3   *Fricative consonants*

A fricative (noise) sound is made by a combination of a narrow constriction somewhere in the vocal tract and an appropriate flow of air through this constriction. Several fricative classes are defined with respect to the position of the narrow constriction. English has four classes of supraglottal fricatives: labiodental /f, v/, (inter)dental /θ, ð/, alveolar /s, z/, and palato-alveolar /ʃ, ʒ/ (see Jongman, Wayland, & Wong, 2000). In addition, a glottal fricative / h/ is recognized by many phoneticians.

Previous studies of fricatives have tended to concentrate on the alveolar fricative /s/ in normal and disordered speech, because of its well-defined spectral pattern and its high frequency of occurrence in many languages. In American English, /s/ is reported as the third most frequently occurring phoneme in normal conversation (Mines, Hanson, & Shoup, 1978).

Since a relatively precise articulation process is required to produce a fricative sound, primarily due to the narrow constriction in the oral cavity, it is expected that speakers with diverse speech-language disorders might exhibit errors for fricative consonants. Several studies have reported on the possibility that fricatives might have a role in categorizing disorder types based on the acoustic properties of /s/ in speakers with specific deficits, including speakers with nonfluent aphasia, with or without apraxia of speech (Baum, 1996; Haley, 2002; Haley, Ohde, & Wertz, 2000; Harmes, Daniloff, Hoffman, et al., 1984; Kurowski, Hazen, & Blumstein, 2003), and speakers with diverse dysarthrias (Chen & Stevens, 2001).

Similar to VOT distributions, patients with aphasia were reported to be unable to consistently differentiate voiced and voiceless fricatives in terms of duration-to-signal voicing contrasts (e.g., Baum, Blumstein, Naeser, & Palumbo, 1990). In particular, fricatives have been a key interest in dysarthria studies in that the articulation process requires fine motor control in speech, which is lacking in persons with dysarthria. Speech intelligibility of speakers with dysarthria has been related to several attributes of fricatives (see Chen & Stevens, 2001).

Several acoustic analyses can be conducted from fricatives, such as amplitude of the frication noise, duration of the noise, and patterning of glottal excitation. Moment analysis has recently been of particular focus and this topic is considered in more detail as an example of clinical application.

22.4.2.4 *Clinical example 3: First moment analysis*

Spectral moment analyses have been used to explore the precision of articulatory positioning for /s/ and /ʃ/. Most spectral energy peaks in normal speakers are reported to occur between 2.5 and 3.5 kHz for /ʃ/ and between 3.5 kHz and 5 kHz for /s/, due to a more anterior place of articulation and smaller magnitude of constriction for /s/ (Behrens & Blumstein, 1988). However, the comparison of frication spectra is complicated in that no single measure has the sensitivity and reliability suited to clinical application.

Moments analysis, first described for speech by Forrest, Weismer, Milenkovic, and Dougall (1988), has been used in several recent clinical studies of fricative production. Haley, Ohde, and Wertz (2000) reported that speakers who have aphasia with and without apraxia of speech have substantial spectral variability and overlap between targets. The authors interpreted this result as evidence of impaired phonetic-motor control in the spatial domain of speech sproduction much as deviations in frication duration reflect motor control abnormalities in the temporal domain. Speakers with dysarthria also exhibit a reduced distinction between /s/ and /ʃ/ compared with healthy speakers (Kim, Weismer, Kent, & Duffy, 2006; Tjaden, & Turner, 1997). Differing results have been reported on the relationship between the first moment coefficient of /s/ and /ʃ/ and speech intelligibility. Tjaden and Wilding (2004) reported a significant relationship, while McRae, Tjaden, and Schoonings (2002) did not find a strong relationship between them.

22.4.2.5   *Affricate consonants*

Affricates are complex sounds that include aspects of both stop and fricative. Like a stop, the affricate involves a sequence of stop (complete obstruction of the vocal tract) followed by a noise segment that is intermediate in duration between the burst for stops and the frication interval for fricatives (Kent & Read, 2002). In American English, only two affricates, [tʃ] and [dʒ], exist.

Although several instrumental and perceptual studies have reported that production of affricates is vulnerable across a wide range of speech-language disorders and that affricates appear late in language development, very few acoustic analyses have been reported on characteristics of affricates in both normal and disordered speech.

22.5   Prosody

The term prosody is not easily defined in a straightforward way that represents the complicated literature on this topic. It is even more difficult to describe and to explain aberrant prosodic patterns of disordered speech, given potential factors that may affect prosodic features, such as speech task (reading, repetition, conversation), utterance units (word, sentence, paragraph), and the type and severity of disorders. For present purposes, prosody is defined as the suprasegmental features of speech that are conveyed by the parameters of fundamental frequency, intensity, and duration (Kent & Read, 2002; Lowit-Leuschel & Docherty, 2000). These acoustic properties relate to linguistic features such as stress, intonation, tone, and rhythm (see Awan, chapter 21 in this volume, for a discussion of the acoustic characteristics of voice quality, and Wells and Whiteside, chapter 34 in this volume, for more on prosodic impairments).

Prosodic disturbances have been described in speakers with various speech-language disorders, including hearing impairment (Friedman, 1985; O'Halpin, 2001), right-hemisphere damage (Gandour, Larsen, Dechongkit, Ponglorpisit, & Khunadorn, 1995; van Lancker & Sidtis, 1992), left-hemisphere damage (Blumstein & Baum, 1987; Ryalls, 1982; van Lancker & Sidtis, 1992), apraxia of speech (Kent & Rosenbek, 1983; Odell, McNeil, Rosenbek, & Hunter, 1991) and dysarthria (Bunton, Kent, Kent, & Rosenbek, 2000; Patel, 2002; Schlenck, Bettrich, & Willmes, 1993). These studies reflect the manifold nature of prosody and its disorders. For example, while studies of left-hemisphere damage have been associated especially with deficits in linguistic prosody (e.g., Baum, Pell, Leonard, & Gordon, 1997), studies of right-hemisphere-damaged speakers have focused more on deficits in emotional prosody (Gandour et al., 1995). The motor speech disorders (apraxia of speech and dysarthria) have often been characterized by several perceptual prosodic disturbances, such as 'monopitch', 'monoloudness', and 'abnormal speaking rate'. In other words, impairments in range and flexibility of control of f_0, intensity, and excessively fast or slow rate have been noted across motor speech disorders, although specific effects depend on the type and/or severity of a disorder.

Apraxia of speech is regarded as a disorder having a prominent pattern of impaired prosody (Kent & Rosenbek, 1983; Rosenbek, 1980; Square-Storer, Dadley, & Sommers, 1988). A number of studies have revealed acoustic properties corresponding to perceptual aspects of dysprosody of apraxia of speech, including slow speaking rate with prolongations of utterance units, reduced intensity variation across syllables, and equalized vowel durations within utterances (Kent & Rosenbek, 1983; Kim, Kent, & Duffy, 2004). Interestingly, f_0 patterns seemed to be less reliably affected despite the large intersubject variability in these patterns (Kent & Rosenbek, 1983).

Especially since the classic research of Darley et al. (1969a, 1969b), efforts have been made to explore prosodic disturbances in dysarthric speech. Acoustic analyses have investigated the salient features of acoustic variables in order to address perceptual dysprosody of different types of dysarthria. Prosody has also been the focus of studies for the purpose of identifying prosodic features that have a strong influence on perceptual abnormality. This question has not been fully answered yet. Several studies have revealed that f_0 range (Bunton, Kent, Kent, & Duffy, 2001; Jeng, Weismer, & Kent, 2006; Le Dorze et al., 1994; Patel, 2003) and intensity range (Tjaden & Wilding, 2004) covaried with speech severity of dysarthria, while the relationship between rate and severity is more variable (Le Dorze et al., 1994; Tjaden & Wilding, 2004).

A cross-language approach also has been launched, using tonal languages such as Mandarin (Jeng, Weismer, & Kent, 2006; Whitehill, Ciocca, & Lam, 2001). Language-unique prosodic features may be a key to understanding the motoric disturbances in aphasic, apraxic, or dysarthric speech.

But it has to be acknowledged that the analysis of prosodic disorders is fraught with complications. First, the speech materials that are most appropriate to the study of prosody (e.g., conversation) are also the most difficult to analyze acoustically. Second, we lack a consensus on perceptual, acoustic, physiologic, or linguistic systems that are most suited to the analysis of prosody and its disorders. Third, the nature of prosodic disturbances appears to vary with the type and severity of speech disorder, and even the emotional state of the speaker. Despite this rather discouraging assessment of the potential for analysis, prospects for progress are notable. In the next section, we consider an index that appears to be useful for characterizing the temporal structure of multisyllabic utterances.

22.5.1   *Pairwise variability index (PVI)*

The pairwise variability index (PVI) was originally introduced in a dialectal study by Low, Grabe, and Nolan (2000), who compared a syllable-timed dialect

(Singapore English) and a stress-timed dialect (British English) in conversational samples. More recently, PVI has been used to quantify the rhythmic properties of speech production as a potential index of abnormalities such as scanning speech in ataxic dysarthria. The PVI value is derived from vowel or syllable durations, using the formula

$$PVI = 100 \times [\Sigma | (d_k - d_{k-1}) / d_k + d_{k-1}) / 2 | / (m - 1)] \text{ (Low, Grabe, \& Nolan, 2000)}$$

where m equals the number of vowels (syllables) in an utterance and d is the duration of the kth vowel (syllable).

PVI has been used to investigate prosodic properties of motor speech disorders such as ataxic dysarthria and apraxia of speech. It has been reported that these clinical groups had significantly lower PVI values than control groups, a result which agrees with perceptual descriptions such as staccato style or scanning speech (Kim, Kent, & Duffy, 2004; Stuntebeck, 2002; Wang, Kent, Duffy, Thomas, & Fredericks, 2006).

22.6   Conclusion

With advances in techniques, acoustic analyses provide many opportunities to describe the core features of speech-language disorders and to explain the mechanisms of speech production in both normal and disordered speech. However, it is not surprising that abnormal acoustic patterns are identified for most dimensions of disordered speech. A primary interest is to determine which acoustic variables are selectively or commonly vulnerable to diverse speech-language deficits and how efficiently those explain underlying breakdowns in a speech-production model constructed from normal speech data.

REFERENCES

Ansel, B. M. and Kent, R. D. (1992). Acoustic-phonetic contrasts and intelligibility in the dysarthria associated with mixed cerebral palsy. *Journal of Speech and Hearing Research*, 35, 296–308.

Auzou, P., Ozsancak, C., Morris, R. J., Jan, M., Eustache, F., and Hannequin, D. (2000). Voice onset time in aphasia, apraxia of speech and dysarthria: review. *Clinical Linguistics and Phonetics*, 14, 131–50.

Baum, S. R. (1996). Fricative production in aphasia: Effects of speaking rate. *Brain and Language*, 52, 328–41.

Baum, S. R., Blumstein, S. E., Naeser, M., and Palumbo, C. (1990). Temporal dimensions of consonant and vowel production: An acoustic and CT scan analysis of aphasic speech. *Brain and Language*, 39, 33–56.

Baum, S. and Boyczuk, J. (1999). Speech timing subsequent to brain damage: Effects of utterance length and complexity. *Brain and Language*, 67, 30–45.

Baum, S., Pell, M., Leonard, C., and Gordon, J. (1997). The ability of right- and left-hemisphere-damaged individuals to produce and interpret prosodic cues marking phrasal boundaries. *Language and Speech*, 40, 313–30.

Behrens, S. and Blumstein, S. E. (1988). Acoustic characteristics of English voiceless fricatives: A descriptive analysis. *Journal of Phonetics*, 16, 295–8.

Blumstein, S. E. (1980). Speech perception: An overview. In G. Yeni-Komshian, J. Kavanaugh, and C. Ferguson (eds.), *Child Phonology: Perception and Production*. New York: Academic Press.

Blumstein, S. E. and Baum, S. (1987). Consonant production deficits in aphasia. In J. Ryalls (ed.), *Phonetic Approaches to Speech Production in Aphasia and Related Disorders*. Boston: College-Hill.

Blumstein, S. E., Cooper, W. E., Goodglass, H., Statlender, S., and Gottlieb, J. (1980). Production deficits in aphasia: A voice-onset time analysis. *Brain and Language*, 9, 153–70.

Bunton, K., Kent, R. D., Kent, J. F., and Duffy, J. R. (2001). The effects of flattening fundamental frequency contours on sentence intelligibility in speakers with dysarthria. *Clinical Linguistics and Phonetics*, 15(3), 181–93.

Bunton, K., Kent, R. D., Kent, J. F., and Rosenbek, J. C. (2000). Perceptuo-acoustic assessment of prosodic impairment in dysarthria. *Clinical Linguistics and Phonetics*, 14, 13–24.

Bunton, K. and Weismer, G. (2001). The relationship between perception and acoustic for a high–low vowel contrast produced by speakers with dysarthria. *Journal of Speech, Language and Hearing Research*, 44, 1215–28.

Caruso, A. J. and Burton, E. K. (1987). Temporal acoustic measures of dysarthria associated with amyotrophic lateral sclerosis. *Journal of Speech and Hearing Research*, 30, 80–7.

Chen, H. and Stevens, K. N. (2001). An acoustical study of the fricative /s/ in the speech of individuals with dysarthria. *Journal of Speech, Language, and Hearing Research*, 44, 1300–14.

Darley, F. L., Aronson, A. E., and Brown, J. R. (1969a). Differential diagnostic patterns of dysarthria. *Journal of Speech and Hearing Research*, 12, 246–69.

Darley, F. L., Aronson, A. E., and Brown, J. R. (1969b). Clusters of deviant speech dimensions in the dysarthrias. *Journal of Speech and Hearing Research*, 12, 462–96.

Darley, F. L., Aronson, A. E., and Brown, J. R. (1975). *Motor Speech Disorders*. Philadelphia, PA: W. B. Saunders.

De Wet, F., Weber, K., Boves, L., Cranen, B., Bengio, S., and Burlard, H. (2004). Evaluation of formant-like features in an automatic vowel classification task. *Journal of the Acoustical Society of America*, 116, 1781–92.

Forrest, K., Weismer, G., Milenkovic, P., and Dougall, R. N. (1988). Statistical analysis of word-initial voiceless obstruents: Preliminary data. *Journal of Acoustical Society of America*, 84, 115–23.

Freeman, F., Sands, E. S., and Harris, K. (1978). Temporal coordination of phonation and articulation in a case of verbal apraxia: A voice onset time study. *Brain and Language*, 6, 106–11.

Friedman, M. (1985). Remediation of intonation contours of hearing-impaired students. *Journal of Communication Disorders*, 18, 259–72.

Fujimura, O. (1962). Analysis of nasal consonants. *Journal of the Acoustical Society of America*, 34(12), 1865–75.

Gandour, J. and Dardarananda, R. (1984). Voice onset time in aphasia: Thai. II. Production. *Brain and Language*, 23, 177–205.

Gandour, J., Larsen, J., Dechongkit, S., Ponglorpisit, S., and Khunadorn, F. (1995). Speech prosody in affective contexts in Thai patients with right hemisphere lesions. *Brain and Language*, 51, 422–43.

Gandour, J., Ponglorpisit, S., Khunadorn, F., Dechongkit, S., Boongird, P., and Boonklam, R. (1992). Timing characteristics of speech after brain damage: Stop voicing in Thai. *Nopparat Rajathanee General Hospital Medical Journal* (Thailand), 3, 41–56.

Haley, K. L. (2002). Temporal and spectral properties of voiceless fricatives in aphasia and apraxia of speech. *Aphasiology*, 16, 595–607.

Haley, K. L. (2004). Vowel duration as a cue to postvocalic stop voicing in aphasia and apraxia of speech. *Aphasiology*, 18, 443–56.

Haley, K. L., Ohde, R. N., and Wertz, R. T. (2000). Precision of fricative production in aphasia and apraxia of speech: A perceptual and acoustic study. *Aphasiology*, 14, 619–34.

Haley, K. L., Ohde, R. N., and Wertz, R. T. (2001). Vowel quality in aphasia and apraxia of speech: Phonetic transcription and formant analyses. *Aphasiology*, 12, 1107–23.

Hanlon, R. E. and Edmondson, J. A. (1996). Disconnected phonology: A linguistic analysis of phonemic jargon aphasia. *Brain and Language*, 55, 199–212.

Hardcastle, W. J., Morgan Barry, R. A., and Clark, C. J. (1985). Articulatory and voicing characteristics of adult dysarthric and verbal dyspraxic speakers: An instrumental study. *British Journal of Disorders of Communication*, 20, 249–70.

Harmes, S., Daniloff, R., Hoffman, P., Lewis, J., Kramer, M., and Absher, R. (1984). Temporal and articulatory control of fricative articulation by speakers with Broca's aphasia. *Journal of Phonetics*, 12, 367–85.

Hertrich, I. and Ackermann, H. (1994). Acoustic analysis of speech timing in Huntington's disease. *Brain and Language*, 47, 182–96.

Higgins, C. M. and Hodge, M. M. (2001). F2/F1 vowel quadrilateral area in young children with and without dysarthria. *Canadian Acoustics*, 29(3), 66–7.

Higgins, C. and Hodge, M. (2002). Vowel area and intelligibility in children with and without dysarthria. *Journal of Medical Speech-Language Pathology*, 10, 271–4.

Itoh, M., Sasanuma, S., Tatsumi, I. F., Murakami, S., Fukusako, Y., and Suzuki, T. (1982). Voice onset time characteristics in apraxia of speech. *Brain and Language*, 17, 193–210.

Jeng, J.-Y., Weismer, G., and Kent, R. D. (2006). Production and perception of mandarin tone in adults with cerebral palsy. *Clinical Linguistics and Phonetics*, 20 (1), 67–87.

Jongman, A., Wayland, R., and Wong, S. (2000). Acoustic characteristics of English fricatives. *Journal of Acoustical Society of America*, 108(3), 1252–63.

Kent, R. D. and McNeil, M. R. (1987). Relative timing of sentence repetition in apraxia of speech and conduction aphasia. In J. H. Ryalls (eds.), *Phonetic Approaches to Speech Production in Aphasia and Related Disorders* (pp. 181–220). Boston, MA: College-Hill Press.

Kent, R. D., Netsell, R., and Abbs, J. H. (1979). Acoustic characteristics of dysarthria associated with cerebellar disease. *Journal of Speech and Hearing Research*, 22, 627–48.

Kent, R. D., Osberger, M. J., Netsell, R., and Hustedde, C. G. (1987). Phonetic development in identical twins differing in auditory function. *Journal of Speech and Hearing Disorders*, 52, 64–75.

Kent, R. D. and Read, C. (2002). *The Acoustic Analysis of Speech*. San Diego, CA: Singular Publishing.

Kent, R. D. and Rosenbek, J. C. (1983). Acoustic patterns of apraxia of speech. *Journal of Speech and Hearing Research*, 26, 231–49.

Kim, Y.-J., Kent, R. D., and Duffy, J. (2004). Temporal-spectral aspects of apraxic and ataxic dysarthric speech. Philadelphia, PA: ASHA convention.

Kim, Y.-J., Weismer, G., Kent, R. D., and J. Duffy (2006). Effects of severity of speech involvement on acoustic measures in diverse dysarthric types. Paper presented at the 2006 Conference on Motor Speech: Motor Speech Disorders, Austin, TX.

Kurowski, K., Hazen, E., and Blumstein, S. E. (2003). The nature of speech production impairments in anterior aphasics: An acoustic analysis of voicing in fricative consonants. *Brain and Language*, 353–71.

Le Dorze, G., Dionne, L., Ryalls, J., Julien, M., and Ouellet, L. (1992). The effects of speech and language therapy for a case of dysarthria associated with Parkinson's disease. *European Journal of Communication Disorders*, 27(4), 313–24.

Le Dorze, G., Ouellet, L., and Ryalls, J. (1994). Intonation and speech rate in dysarthric speech. *Journal of Communication Disorders*, 27, 1–18.

Liu, H. M., Tsao, F. M., and Kuhl, P. K. (2005). The effect of reduced vowel working space on speech intelligibility in Mandarin-speaking young adults with cerebral palsy. *Journal of Acoustical Society of America*, 117, 3879–89.

Liu, H. M., Tseng, C. H., and Tsao, F. M. (2000). Perceptual and acoustic analysis of speech intelligibility in Mandarin-speaking young adults with cerebral palsy. *Clinical Linguistics and Phonetics*, 14(6), 447–64.

Low, E. L., Grabe, E., and Nolan, F. (2000). Quantitative characterisations of speech rhythm: 'Syllable-timing' in Singapore English. *Language and Speech*, 43, 377–401.

Lowit-Leuschel, A. and Docherty, G. J. (2000). Dysprosody. In R. D. Kent and M. J. Ball (eds.), *Voice Quality Measurement* (pp. 59–72). San Diego, CA: Singular.

McHenry, M. A. (2004). Variability within and across physiological systems in dysarthria: A comparison of STI and VOT. *Journal of Medical Speech-Language Pathology*, 12, 179–82.

McRae, P. A., Tjaden, K., and Schoonings, B. (2002). Acoustic and perceptual consequences of articulatory rate change in Parkinson disease. *Journal of Speech, Language, and Hearing Research*, 45(1), 35–50.

Mines, M. A., Hanson, B. F., and Shoup, J. E. (1978). Frequency of occurrence of phonemes in conversational English. *Language and Speech*, 21(3), 221–41.

Misiurski, C., Blumstein, S. E., Rissman, J., and Berman, D. (2005). The role of lexical competition and acoustic-phonetic structure in lexical processing: Evidence from normal subjects and aphasic patients. *Brain and Language*, 93, 64–78.

Molis, M. R. (2005). Evaluating models of vowel perception. *Journal of Acoustical Society of America*, 118, 1062–71.

Morris, R. J. (1989). VOT and dysarthria: A descriptive study. *Journal of Communication Disorders*, 22, 23–33.

Munson, B., Bjorum, E. M., and Windsor, J. (2003). Acoustic and perceptual correlates of stress in nonwords produced by children with suspected developmental apraxia of speech and children with phonological disorder. *Journal of Speech, Language and Hearing Research*, 46, 189–202.

Nijland, L., Maassen, B., and van der Meulen, S. (2003). Evidence of motor programming deficits in children diagnosed with DAS. *Journal of Speech, Language and Hearing Research*, 46, 437–50.

Odell, K., McNeil, M. R., Rosenbek, J. C., and Hunter, L. (1991). Perceptual characteristics of vowel and prosody production in apraxic, aphasic, and dysarthric speakers. *Journal of Speech and Hearing Research*, 34, 67–80.

O'Halpin, R. (2001). Intonation issues in the speech of hearing impaired children: Analysis, transcription and remediation. *Clinical Linguistics and Phonetics*, 15, 529–50.

Ozawa, Y., Shiromoto, O., Ishizaki, F., and Watamori, T. (2001). Symptomatic differences in decreased alternating motion rates between individuals with spastic and with ataxic dysarthria: An acoustic analysis. *Folia Phoniatrica et Logopaedica*, 53, 67–72.

Patel, R. (2002). Prosodic control in severe dysarthria: Preserved ability to mark the question–statement contrast. *Journal of Speech, Language and Hearing Research*, 45, 858–70.

Patel, R. (2003). Acoustic characteristics of the question–statement contrast in severe dysarthria due to cerebral palsy. *Journal of Speech, Language and Hearing Research*, 46, 1401–15.

Patel, R. (2004). The acoustics of contrastive prosody in adults with cerebral palsy. *Journal of Medical Speech-Language Pathology*, 12, 189–93.

Rogers, M. A. (1997). The vowel lengthening exaggeration effect in speakers with apraxia of speech: Compensation, artifact, or primary deficit? *Aphasiology*, 11, 433–45.

Rosen, K., Kent, R. D., and Duffy, J. R. (2003). Lognormal distribution of pause length in ataxic dysarthria. *Clinical Linguistics and Phonetics*, 17, 469–86.

Rosenbek, J. C. (1980). Apraxia of speech: Relationship to stuttering. *Journal of Fluency Disorders*, 5, 55–68.

Roy, N., Leeper, H. A., Blomgren, M., and Cameron, R. M. (2001). Description of phonetic, acoustic, and physiological changes associated with improved intelligibility in a speaker with spastic dysarthria. *American Journal of Speech-Language Pathology*, 10, 274–90.

Rvachew, S., Slawinski, E. B., Williams, M., and Green, C. (1996). Formant frequencies of vowels produced by infants with and without early onset otitis media. *Canadian Acoustics*, 24, 19–28.

Ryalls, J. H. (1982). Intonation in Broca's aphasia. *Neuropsychologia*, 20, 355–60.

Schalling, E. and Hartelius, L. (2004). Acoustic analysis of speech tasks performed by three individuals with spinocerebellar ataxia. *Folia Phoniatrica et Logopaedica*, 56, 367–80.

Schlenck, K.-J., Bettrich, R., and Willmes, Z. K. (1993). Aspects of disturbed prosody in dysarthria. *Clinical Linguistics and Phonetics*, 7, 119–28.

Seddoh, S. A. K., Robin, D. A., Sim, H.-S., Hageman, C., Moon, J. B., and Folkins, J. W. (1996). Speech timing in apraxia of speech versus conduction aphasia. *Journal of Speech and Hearing Research*, 39, 590–603.

Skinder, A., Connaghan, K., Strand, E., and Betz, S. (2000). Acoustic correlates of perceived lexical stress errors in children with developmental apraxia of speech. *Journal of Medical Speech-Language Pathology*, 8, 279–84.

Square-Storer, P., Dadley, F., and Sommers, R. (1988). Nonspeech and speech processing skills in patients with aphasia and apraxia of speech. *Brain and Language*, 33, 65–85.

Strand, E. A. and McNeil, M. R. (1996). Effects of length and linguistic complexity on temporal acoustic measures in apraxia of speech. *Journal of Speech and Hearing Research*, 39, 1018–33.

Stuntebeck, S. (2002). Acoustic analysis of the prosodic properties of ataxic speech. Unpublished master's thesis, University of Wisconsin, Madison.

Sussman, H. M., Marquardt, T. P., and Doyle, J. (2000). An acoustic analysis of phonemic integrity and contrastiveness in developmental apraxia of speech. *Journal of Medical Speech-Language Pathology*, 8, 301–13.

Thoonen, G., Maassen, B., Gabreels, F., and Schreuder, R. (1999). Validity of maximum performance tasks to diagnose motor speech disorders in children. *Clinical Linguistics and Phonetics*, 13, 1–23.

Tjaden, K. (1999). Can a model of overlapping gestures account for scanning speech patterns? *Journal of Speech, Language and Hearing Research*, 42, 604–17.

Tjaden, T. (2003). Anticipatory coarticulation in multiple sclerosis and Parkinson's disease. *Journal of Speech, Language and Hearing Research*, 46, 990–1008.

Tjaden, K., Rivera, D., Wilding, G., and Turner, G. S. (2005). Characteristics of the lax vowel space in dysarthria. *Journal of Speech, Language and Hearing Research*, 48, 554–66.

Tjaden, K. and Turner, G. S. (1997). Spectral properties of fricatives in amyotrophic lateral sclerosis. *Journal of Speech, Language and Hearing Research*, 40, 1358–72.

Tjaden, K. and Turner, G. (2000). Segmental timing in amyotrophic lateral sclerosis. *Journal of Language and Hearing Research*, 43(3), 686–96.

Tjaden, K. and Watling, E. (2003). Characteristics of diadochokinesis in multiple sclerosis and Parkinson's disease. *Folia Phoniatrica et Logopaedica*, 55, 241–59.

Tjaden, K. and Wilding, G. E. (2004). Rate and loudness manipulations in dysarthria: acoustic and perceptual findings. *Journal of Speech, Language and Hearing Research*, 47(4), 766–83.

Turner, G. S. and Tjaden, K. (2000). Acoustic differences between content and function words in amyotrophic lateral sclerosis. *Journal of Speech, Language and Hearing Research*, 43, 769–81.

Turner, G., Tjaden, K., and Weismer, G. (1995). The influence of speaking rate on vowel space and speech intelligibility for individuals with amyotrophic lateral sclerosis. *Journal of Speech and Hearing Research*, 38, 1001–13.

van Lancker, D. and Sidtis, J. J. (1992). The identification of affective prosodic stimuli by left and right hemisphere damaged subjects: All errors are not created equal. *Journal of Speech and Hearing Research*, 35, 963–70.

van Putten, S. M. and Walker, J. P. (2003). The production of emotional prosody in varying degrees of severity of apraxia of speech. *Journal of Communication Disorders*, 36, 77–95.

Wambaugh, J. L., Nessler, C., Bennett, J., and Mauszycki, S. C. (2004). Variability in apraxia of speech: A perceptual and VOT analysis of stop consonants. *Journal of Medical Speech-Language Pathology*, 12, 221–7.

Wambaugh, J. L., West, J. E., and Doyle, P. J. (1997). A VOT analysis of apraxic/aphasic voicing errors. *Aphasiology*, 11, 521–32.

Wang, Y.-T., Kent, R. D., Duffy, J. R., Thomas, J. E., and Fredericks, G. V. (2006). Dysarthria following cerebellar mutism secondary to resection of a fourth ventricle medulloblastoma: A case study. *Journal of Medical Speech-Language Pathology*, 14, 109–22.

Wang, Y.-T., Kent, R. D., Duffy, J. R., Thomas, J. E., and Weismer, G. (2004). Alternating motion rate as an index of speech motor disorder in traumatic brain injury. *Clinical Linguistics and Phonetics*, 18, 57–84.

Wang, Y.-T., Kent, R. D., Duffy, J. R., Thomas, J. E., and Weismer, G. (2005). Dysarthria associated with traumatic brain injury: Speaking rate and emphatic stress. *Journal of Communication Disorders*, 38, 231–60.

Weismer, G. (forthcoming). Speech disorders. In M. Gernsbacher and M. Traxler (eds.), *Handbook of Psycholinguistics*. Oxford: Blackwell.

Whitehill, T. L., Ciocca, V., and Lam, S. L.-M. (2001). Fundamental frequency control in connected speech in Cantonese speakers with dysarthria. In B. Maassen, W. Hulstijn, R. Kent, H. F. M. Peters, and P. H. M. M. van Lieshout (eds.), *Speech Motor Control in Normal and Disordered Speech* (pp. 228–31). Nijmegen: University of Nijmegen Press.

Whitehill, T. L. and Tsang, E. S.-L. (2002). Relationship between speech and DDK measures in hypokinetic speech. *Journal of Medical Speech-Language Pathology*, 10, 333–8.

Zahorian, S. A. and Jagharghi, A. J. (1993). Spectral-shape features versus formants as acoustic correlates for vowels. *Journal of the Acoustical Society of America*, 94, 1966–82.

Ziegler, W. (2002). Task-related factors in oral motor control: Speech and oral diadochokinesis in dysarthria and apraxia of speech. *Brain and Language*, 80, 556–75.

Ziegler, W. and von Cramon, D. (1983). Vowel distortion in traumatic dysarthria: A formant study. *Phonetica*, 40, 63–78.

23 Clinical Phonetic Transcription

BARRY HESELWOOD AND
SARA HOWARD

Phonetic transcription records not an utterance but an analysis of an utterance.
(Abercrombie, 1967, p. 127)

23.1 The Purposes of Clinical Phonetic Transcription

In the phonetic and phonological analysis of atypical speech production the ultimate goal of subjecting an individual's speech to scrutiny is to identify where, and understand how, it differs from the norms of the relevant language variety. A phonological analysis is therefore required which shows how the speaker's systematic use of consonants, vowels, phonation, voice pitch, etc. maps onto the language's phonological structure. Before that can be done, however, we need as accurate a picture as possible of the kinds of consonants, vowels, pitch movements, and so on, that the individual produces when speaking. To obtain that picture, the speech must be observed, not as a lay-person might observe it, but in a manner informed by knowledge of how speech is structured – informed, that is, by phonetic theory. In this chapter we are concerned with the tools and procedures that go into making phonetic transcriptions as the first stage in the process of understanding the pronunciation systems and communication behaviors of speakers with impaired speech.

Phonetic transcription of atypical speech data is fraught with challenges and pitfalls (Howard & Heselwood, 2002a, 2002b; Kent, 1996; Powell, 2001), so it is important, and something of a reassurance, to take the view that a transcription need not be a *final* phonetic analysis but can be changed: "the process of producing any transcription is a cyclic one. There is no 'perfect' final transcription" (Ball & Local, 1996, p. 70). Indeed, because of the difficulties associated with transcription for clinical purposes, arguments are sometimes advanced against using transcription at all. Such objections tend to emphasize one or more of the following:

- Phonetic transcription is based on perceptual analysis which is inherently subjective, unreliable and limited by the constraints of perception;
- Instrumental techniques provide more objective measures which are nowadays widely available;
- Phonetic transcription perpetuates the misleading view that speech comprises a linear sequence of discrete sounds;
- The time it takes to transcribe could be better spent.

The first of these objections, if taken to its logical conclusion, is an argument against listening to impaired speech at all. But it is *only* by listening that we can experience the effect an individual's speech impairment has on his or her spoken communication and intelligibility. By bringing phonetic knowledge to the act of listening we begin the process of analysis which leads us towards phonetic explanations for the abnormalities that we hear. Transcription is a way of recording the results of our moment-by-moment analytic listening which, when laid out before us on paper, enable us to see recurring patterns. The phonetic analysis embodied in a transcription is thus the starting point for the phonological analysis of the data.

However, the charges of subjectivity, unreliability and perceptual limitations do have to be acknowledged and faced. Subjectivity and reliability can be addressed to some extent through controlling the conditions under which transcriptions are made (see section 23.4 below), but we are undeniably constrained by the biological and cognitive limitations of our perceptual abilities. That being so, it is important to remember that spoken communication takes place within precisely those limitations. We therefore have a perceptual tool exactly tailored to the natural conditions of the phenomena we wish to investigate. As we have said elsewhere, "[w]e don't speak palatograms or hear spectrograms" (Howard & Heselwood, 2002b, p. 47). Whatever is beyond perception can have no separate communicative function in speech. That is not to say, of course, that we should not explore beyond the limits of our senses by means of instruments in order to more fully understand what a speaker is doing, but phonetic transcriptions help us to better target what to explore instrumentally. As Ladefoged (2003, p. 27) observes, "instrumental aids can often illuminate particular points, acting like a magnifying glass" but "the ultimate authority in all phonetic questions is the human ear".

The third objection raises a serious issue. Throughout all transcription activity it must be appreciated that speech is certainly not a linear sequence of discrete sound segments. Phoneticians have stressed this point repeatedly over many years (Abercrombie, 1967, p. 42; Ashby & Maidment, 2005, pp. 15–16; Laver, 1994, pp. 566–70), and much phonetic research has focused on events that last over more than one identifiable sound. Local (2003, pp. 328–33) draws attention to 'long domain' components and discusses examples that suggest that phonologically useful information is distributed considerably beyond notional segment boundaries in ways that cannot be easily explained as physiological accommodation. The introduction of the 'labeled braces' convention in the Voice Quality Symbols system (Ball, Esling, & Dickson, 1995) provides a means of representing some long-domain features in a segmental transcription. The problems of segmental analysis notwithstanding, treating speech *as if* it is a linear sequence of segments is, as Laver (1994, p. 568) observes, a "convenient way of organising our initial analytic thinking about speech."

The amount of time taken to make a good transcription is often a pressing issue not only in the clinical context, but also in research work where time is increasingly tightly constrained. In response, it has frequently been argued that a good transcription, i.e. a good initial analytic record, saves time at later stages by identifying and prioritizing those aspects of an individual's speech most in need of the clinician's or researcher's attention (Crystal, 1984; Perkins & Howard, 1995; Shriberg & Lof, 1991). Shriberg, Kwiatkowski and Hoffmann (1984, p. 456) claim that "valid and reliable phonetic transcription is *central* to the study and management of persons with communicative disorders" (our italics). This sentiment is echoed by Sell (2005) in a discussion of speech assessment in cleft palate. (It is, therefore, dispiriting to note that Lohmander and Olsson, 2004, in a review of 88 articles on speech production in cleft palate, found that phonetic transcription was used in only eight of them.)

23.2 Types of Transcription

A general distinction between 'broad' and 'narrow' transcription has been made at least since the time of Henry Sweet in the nineteenth century (Jones, 1972, pp. 332–3). It is based on the relative amount of phonetic detail represented in a transcription and is therefore a continuum (Howard & Heselwood, 2002a, p. 390). Cutting somewhat across this distinction is the one between 'systematic' and 'impressionistic' transcription. If the transcriber knows the phonological system that the speaker is employing, then much of the phonetic detail is predictable and need not be represented in a transcription. The broadest systematic transcription is a phonemic transcription, where the symbols stand for phonemes. Information about the occurrence of the various allophones of a phoneme is absent and is assumed to be recoverable from the realization rules of the speaker's phonological system. A narrower systematic transcription might be preferred in cases of so-called 'free variation' if the transcriber wishes to record which phonetic variant a speaker uses. While the broadness of systematic transcriptions will vary according to the purposes for which the transcription is being made, it is usual for an impressionistic transcription to aim to be as narrow as possible. If the transcriber does not know anything about the speaker's phonological system then he or she should not start out with any assumptions about which phonetic details will and will not be important. This point is obvious if we are talking about fieldwork on a hitherto undocumented language (Abercrombie, 1967, p. 128; Jones, 1972, p. 349; Kelly & Local, 1989, p. 5; Laver, 1994, p. 556). Until we know whether a feature such as aspiration or nasalization is distinctive, we cannot safely omit it from our transcription. But when dealing with impaired speech in a language with which we are familiar, the point, though equally important, may not be quite so obvious. Faced with a new sample of impaired English speech, we cannot predict *what* will be impaired, nor *how* it will be impaired, which puts us in much the same position as the fieldworker. For this reason, it is recognized that the most appropriate type of transcription in clinical contexts is impressionistic (Abercrombie, 1967, p. 128; Ball & Local, 1996, pp. 51–2; Buckingham & Yule, 1987, p. 123; Grunwell, 1987, pp. 34–5; IPA, 1999, p. 29). As a general principle, the less we can predict about someone's speech, the narrower and more impressionistic our transcription has to be. Knowledge of the etiology of a patient's condition gives us no privileged position from which to predict phonetic behavior, and may introduce preconceptions that could influence the transcriber in ways that are unhelpful.

23.3 Types of Speech Sample

In clinical phonetic analysis there are important methodological questions to ask about the size and the kind of speech sample to be gathered. Grunwell (1987) argues, for example, that at least 200–250 words should be collected, and Lambert (1989, p. 108) suggests "75–100 utterances", whereas Crary (1983) suggests that 50 may suffice. Grunwell (1987) and Peterson-Falzone, Trost-Cardamone, Karnell, and Hardin-Jones (2006) are amongst those who stress the need to sample connected speech, and Grunwell advocates collecting real spontaneous speech, but with the requirement that any sample should be 'glossable': unless we know what a speaker is trying to say we cannot judge how well or badly they are succeeding. Often the speech impairment prevents the glossability of spontaneous speech, in which case Grunwell advises recourse to elicited material.

Two related points arise here. Firstly, differences between spontaneous and elicited speech mean that, just as clinical intervention may not generalize to spontaneous speech, there are severe limits on how much the analyst can generalize from elicited speech. Single-word picture-naming is probably the most glossable kind of elicited speech after repetition, and is widely used in clinical assessment. But it completely lacks the junctural phenomena of connected speech and gives no opportunity to observe rhythmic and intonational organization over more than a few syllables at best (Howard, 2004, 2007; Howard, Wells, & Local, chapter 36 in this volume; Wells, 1994). Furthermore, it does not offer the opportunity to explore phonetic details at specific points in conversational interaction in order to investigate how phonetic features may correlate with such conversational behaviors as turn-taking, repair and topic management. Dobbinson, Perkins, and Boucher (2003) and Damico and Nelson (2005), for example, note cases of individuals with autistic spectrum disorders where creaky phonation relates to specific interactional and discourse behaviors, and Local and Wootton (1995) and Tarplee and Barrow

(1999) use narrow transcription, including interlinear pitch contours, to capture significant interactional behaviors in their analyses of conversational interaction between mothers and their autistic children.

The second point concerns the requirement of glossability. Ideally, for transcription and phonetic analysis, the transcriber should not know the speaker's lexical targets; otherwise his or her own internal phonetic/phonological representations of those words will become active, 'echoing' in the mind, and may bias the judgment as to what sounds are being heard (Oller & Eilers, 1975). The practice of eliciting target words in phonological assessments means that in much clinical work the transcriber cannot but have a good idea of what the speaker is trying to say. Even where speech cannot confidently be glossed it is probably impossible to completely suppress the instinct to guess a speaker's lexical targets and by so doing to activate one's own representations: as Laver (1994, p. 557) points out, the hardest language to transcribe impressionistically is one's own. The paradox is that glossing is an obstacle to phonetic analysis but a prerequisite for phonological analysis and for rating intelligibility.

23.4 Methods of Transcription

The problems of subjectivity and unreliability can be tackled to a significant extent by controlling the conditions under which a transcription is made. The first necessity is to record the speech sample on a good-quality recording system so that the transcription can be made from listening to, and preferably looking at, a high-quality recording. (For advice on making recordings, see Ladefoged, 2003, pp. 16–26, and Shriberg, McSweeny, Anderson, et al., 2005; portable solid-state digital recorders are probably the best convenient recorders to use.)

Transcription of live speech is notoriously unreliable because, first, it is impossible to write the symbols and diacritics down at the speed at which the speaker produces sounds (Amorosa, von Benda, Wagner, & Keck, 1985). Normal speech rate is about five syllables per second (Laver, 1994, p. 541) with often up to five or six segments per syllable in English. There is no time for analytic listening, or for trying to reproduce the sounds oneself as an aid to analysis. Secondly, there is no second bite at the cherry. Asking the speaker to repeat something is no guarantee that they will pronounce it the same way the second time. Indeed, in the clinical context, asking a speaker to repeat a lexical item is often undertaken with the specific objective of observing intra-speaker variability. A third point is that in live situations it is much harder to ignore the linguistic aspects of the speech and to concentrate solely on the sounds (Amorosa, von Benda, Wagner, & Keck; Oller & Eilers, 1975).

Is it enough to have a good-quality audio recording, or should we have a synchronized video recording as well? Abercrombie (1958, p. 232) speaks for most of us in saying that when transcribing we use our eyes and not just our ears, a point that Kelly and Local (1989, p. 35) emphasize: "in doing phonetic transcription it is important to pay attention to at least part of what a speaker can be *seen* to be doing" (our italics). Silent articulation (mouthing) is potentially an important phonetic behavior in impaired speech which will not be evident on audio recordings, but there are other features as well that can only be reliably captured on video or film (Daniloff, Wilcox, & Stephens, 1980). Ball, Code, Rahilly, & Hazlett (1994, p. 80) advocate provision of conventions for the non-linguistic facial activity that sometimes accompanies dysfluency and may also occur in speech production in cleft palate; clearly, they could not be accurately used without video recordings. Once a recording is made, the next consideration is how best to listen to it. Modern technology and computer software have increased the range of recording, storing and listening conditions for transcription (Shriberg, McSweeny, Anderson, et al., 2005). As well as having the choice between free-field listening and listening through headphones (the latter also presenting a choice between earbuds and various designs of earphone), we can now choose to listen at different speeds without a change of pitch, and even to listen to speech backwards. Ladefoged (2003, pp. 26–7) recommends using headphones, listening to vowels at half speed, and using a reverse-play function "to focus more easily on off-glides, which will have been made to sound like onsets". Transcribers should experiment with these procedures, but with the awareness that the speech is not being listened to in its natural state. The reason for choosing to change the playback speed, and/or reverse the direction, is much the same as the reason for using instrumentation, i.e. to get a more accurate picture of the phonetic structure of the speaker's output. This leads to a fundamental division of perspectives which has been referred to as the difference between listener-oriented analysis and speaker-oriented analysis (Hewlett, 1985; IPA, 1999, pp. 36–7). Is one's aim to record one's own perception of the speech, as implied by the term 'impressionistic transcription', or to record the speaker's articulatory behavior? If it is the former, and only the former, it would make more sense to listen without modifying the playback. If the aim is to use the speech sample as a window into the speaker's vocal tract then all possible means should be used, including slow and reverse playback, spectrographic analysis, and so on. Attempting to capture inaudible speaker behaviors in a transcription may subsequently require transcription conventions which signal such differences. Thus, for example, Sell, Harding and Grunwell (1999, p. 22), in a discussion of the transcription of speech production associated with cleft palate, advocate the use of different symbols for active and passive nasal fricatives, stating that the two articulations may be "perceptually indistinguishable . . . but they are distinguishable by the manner in which they are articulated".

Comparing listener-oriented and speaker-oriented transcriptions can reveal interesting instances of non-correspondence where something sounded like *x* but seems to have been produced as *y*. For example, in speech production associated with glossectomy, a convincing impression of an alveolar articulation may be achieved even in a speaker where the tongue has been largely excised (Morrish, 1988). Valuable insights into the relationship between a client's intelligibility, articulation strategies and underlying phonological system are to be gained by studying such non-correspondences closely. Furthermore, they are often intrinsically interesting from a phonetic point of view. The practice of using instrumental analysis to validate perceptual analysis runs the risk of obscuring such insights if, in the case of any conflict, the former is taken as evidence that the latter is 'wrong'. The two types of analysis should not be seen as competitors but as complementary.

How many times one should listen to an item is another choice the transcriber has to make. Shriberg, Kwiatkowski and Hoffmann (1984, p. 459) are wary of too much sensory exposure and advise listening no more than three times to items about which different transcribers have disagreed. More than this and the ear may start to play tricks. By contrast, the technique of analytic listening (see, for example, Ashby, Maidment and Abberton, 1996) is likely in practice to dictate that one listens to an item many times. For example, one may wish to focus on some aspect of a particular consonant or vowel and then, having made a decision on that, shift attention to another aspect, or another sound in the same word or phrase, or to prosodic features such as stress. It may nonetheless be wise to take note of Shriberg and colleagues' advice and not listen too many times when focusing on a particular aspect or feature.

We have already mentioned attempting to mimic the speech to be transcribed. Compared to the fieldworker who can copy an informant's productions and then ask if they are acceptable, the clinical transcriber is at a disadvantage. Nevertheless, where one can reasonably make the assumption that the transcriber's vocal tract is not too different from the speaker's, making use of one's own articulatory-auditory feedback loop is a very useful strategy for trying to pinpoint precise lip and tongue configurations, amount of nasality, phonatory quality, pitch movement, etc. It must of course not be forgotten that different articulatory activities can produce remarkably similar acoustic output (Maurer, Gröne, Landis, Hoch, & Schönle, 1993; Perkell, 1997), but if a transcription is taken primarily as a listener-oriented analysis then this is no great problem.

A further choice for the transcriber is whether to rely solely on his or her own judgments or to ask other phonetically competent listeners to make transcriptions of the same data. The various transcriptions can then be compared for level of agreement, normally expressed in percentage terms. Shriberg, Kwiatkowski, and Hoffmann (1984) suggest four 'consensus procedures' and seventeen 'consensus rules' for such a situation. Although some of these are potentially problematic (for example, opting for a compromise phonetically midway between the variants, quite apart from 'midway' being somewhat vague in multidimensional phonetic space, results in a transcription that none of the listeners actually heard), many are helpful in resolving disagreements.

The authors importantly draw attention to the possibility of 'functionally equivalent' transcriptions. Use of different symbols and diacritics by different transcribers to represent the same analysis is something all experienced transcribers will be familiar with. It emphasizes the fact that a transcription has to be made, and interpreted, within a framework of phonetic theory. Sometimes two or more pieces of transcription are susceptible to the same interpretation. For example, [jʷ] in many if not all instances is unlikely to be interpreted significantly differently from [ɥ] or [wʲ]. Similarly, [kɬ] and [k(̥] say much the same thing about the relationship of phonatory and articulatory gestures. For these reasons, Cucchiarini (1996) discusses the problem of aligning transcriptions for meaningful comparison and wisely warns against a simplistic symbol agreement count, arguing convincingly that this latter method of calculating transcription agreement is dangerously misleading.

23.5   Transcription Systems and Conventions

The commonest system of transcription in use for clinical and research purposes is the roman-alphabet-based notation of the International Phonetic Alphabet (IPA) which began its long development with the founding of the International Phonetic Association in 1886. The most recent revision of the system was in 2005, including the addition of a symbol for a labiodental flap (see appendix). A set of symbols for use especially in the transcription of impaired speech, officially adopted by the International Clinical Phonetics and Linguistics Association (ICPLA) in 1994, is known as ExtIPA (extensions to the IPA). It first appeared in Duckworth, Allen, Hardcastle, and Ball (1990); some additions and changes were made in Bernhardt and Ball (1993). ExtIPA provides a set of symbols which can capture unusual places of articulation (produced, for example, by speakers with unusual dentition and occlusion), as well as a range of unusual phonatory, resonatory and airstream behaviors. For particularly challenging speech data, it usefully includes an asterisk to denote 'sound with no available symbol' (which can be augmented by accompanying notes), and various bracketing devices to represent sounds for which only certain features can be identified (e.g. (C̄) – indeterminate consonant; (Pl. vls) – an indeterminate voiceless plosive) and also silent articulations, where there is visual evidence of articulatory behavior which has no auditory accompaniment (e.g. (ʃ)). Transcription of non-segmental aspects of speech such as pauses, stress, intonation, speech rate and loudness using IPA and ExtIPA symbols is discussed and exemplified in Ball and Rahilly (2002) and in Ball, Code, Rahilly, and Hazlett (1994:75), where the authors caution that the IPA intonation conventions "may be more of a hindrance than a help". To denote the long-domain features of airstream type, phonation type and supralaryngeal setting, Ball, Esling, and Dickson (1995) draw on Laver (1980) to establish the VoQS (Voice Quality Symbols, cf. Latin *vox* 'voice') conventions. (Suggestions for redefining some of the phonation categories are presented in Esling and Harris, 2005.) The VoQS are included in the ExtIPA set to which IPA numbers are assigned in the 1999 IPA *Handbook* (pp. 188–92). Taken together, the standard IPA chart, ExtIPA and VoQS provide a rich set of conventions for clinical transcription (see the appendix to this chapter for charts of these symbols). It is worth noting, however, that the symbols they provide have not been universally adopted. For example, conventions in the USA for the transcription of speech production associated with cleft palate differ markedly at times from standard IPA usage. Thus Peterson-Falzone, Trost-Cardamone, Karnell, and Hardin-Jones (2006) use [ʕ] for the voiceless pharyngeal fricative, compared with IPA [ħ], and [Δ] for a velopharyngeal fricative compared with ExtIPA [[fŋ]. The ToBI ('tone break and indices') system (Beckman, Hirschberg, & Shattuck-Hufnagel, 2005) is available for intonational transcription, but because it represents phonological categories it is a language-specific system and not suitable for clinical work, although O'Halpin (2001, pp. 537–8) suggests it could be adapted for impaired speech. More in keeping with the principles of impressionistic transcription, and therefore useful for the clinician, is the interlinear tonetic representation of pitch movements as used, for example, by Cruttenden (1997). Snow (2001) also provides a useful overview of the transcription of prosodic information for clinical purposes.

The IPA, ExtIPA and VoQS have been developed with the speech production of children and adults in mind, but increasing attention has been paid recently to the vocalizations and babbling of prelingual infants. Child language specialists have been keen to explore the nature of the relationship between these behaviors and the development of first language pronunciation (Ingram, 1989; Kent & Miolo, 1995; Oller, 2000; Vihman, 1996). Furthermore, and of significance here, their diagnostic and prognostic value in speech impairment has been noted (Menyuk, Liebergott & Schultz, 1986; Oller, 2000, pp. 143–50). The suitability of IPA-type symbols for the transcription of infant vocalizations has been questioned by several researchers (Holmgren, Lindblom, Aurelius, Jalling, & Zetterström, 1986; Oller, 2000; Stoel-Gammon, 2001), particularly given the differences between infants and adults in vocal-tract structure and dimensions (Kent & Miolo, 1995, p. 327). Categories unique to infants have been proposed, e.g. 'saliva constrictive', 'subharmonic break' (Stark, 1986), 'squeal', 'growl', 'goo', 'quasi-resonant nucleus' (Oller, 1980) which can be incorporated into transcriptions as [SQ], [GR], [QRN], etc. However, there is no reason why Oller's suggested conventions could not be used alongside IPA and ExtIPA conventions where this is felt to be useful. If we take a listener-oriented stance, then using IPA and ExtIPA symbols is a way of expressing that a squeal or growl had the 'flavor' of a particular adult category about it as in 1, and brace notation can be used to specify their quasi-resonant nature:

(1)   ʔ SQ ʔː GR
    {QRN [ɪ]   [ʒ]   QRN}

23.6   The Content of Transcriptions

To ask what should be in a transcription is to ask what aspects of the speech sample should be analyzed. The simple answer is 'everything' but it might not

Table 23.1   Aspects of speech and resources available for their narrow transcription

Functional component	Phenomena	Relevant transcription conventions
Initiation	Airstream	IPA pulmonic and non-pulmonic symbols; VoQS symbols for airstream types; VoQS labeled braces
	Breathing patterns	VoQS 'down full arrow' [↓] and 'up full arrow' [↑]
Phonation	Vocal fold activity and glottal states	IPA diacritics; ExtIPA voicing diacritics; VoQS diacritics; VoQS labeled braces
	Ventricular fold activity	VoQS diacritics; VoQS labeled braces
Articulation Resonance	Nasality	IPA and ExtIPA nasal consonant symbols; IPA nasalized and nasal release diacritics, ExtIPA denasal, nasal escape and velopharyngeal friction diacritics; VoQS labeled braces
	Pharynx and mouth chamber resonance	IPA vowel and approximant symbols; ExtIPA approximant symbols; VoQS supralaryngeal setting diacritics; VoQS labeled braces
Articulation	Primary articulations	IPA vowel symbols; IPA and ExtIPA consonant symbols; IPA and ExtIPA diacritics
	Double articulations	IPA 'other symbols'; use of tie bar with IPA and ExtIPA symbols
	Secondary articulations	IPA, ExtIPA and VoQS diacritics
	Silent articulation	ExtIPA ( ) parentheses
	Articulation strength	ExtIPA diacritics
Prosodic phenomena	Syllable structure	IPA syllable break 'dot'
	Rhythm and intonation	IPA suprasegmental symbols/ diacritics and boundary markers; interlinear tonetic transcription
	Tempo and loudness	ExtIPA connected speech symbols in conjunction with VoQS labeled braces
	Fluency	ExtIPA reiterated diacritic, sliding articulation diacritic, pause symbols and length marks
	Length	IPA suprasegmental length and shortness diacritics
	Key and register	interlinear tonetic transcription

always be the appropriate answer. Analyzing and transcribing 'everything' is certainly going to be difficult and labor-intensive and may, frankly, be impossible. We would do well to heed Clark (1996, p. 337), who cautions in this regard that "[t]he problem is that transcripts are like footprints in the sand. They are merely the inert traces of the activities that produced them, and impoverished traces at that." However, we need not be too downhearted about this. In dealing with an individual's atypical speech production, whether as a clinician or as a researcher, we will already have formed a professional opinion about what aspects of it we think we should most attend to. That opinion may of course have to be revised as we engage more deeply with the data, and we should heed the warning by Dinnsen (1999) that even correct productions may have clinical implications. We should be prepared to include analysis relating to any aspects of speech as set out and grouped into the functional components and phonetic phenomena in table 23.1 which also identifies the kinds of conventions available for their impressionistic transcription (the table is indicative rather than exhaustive).

In principle, a transcription should aim to balance segmental and non-segmental representations. It should identify, as far as is possible, rhythm-group and intonation-group boundaries, speech rate, pauses, and long-domain resonance and voice quality features as well as details about phonation, and articulation. The effects that boundaries are known to have in normal speech production, such as lengthening (Gussenhoven & Rietveld, 1992), cannot be assessed in clinical samples if they are not included in the analysis. Vaissière (2005, p. 254) calls for prosodic transcriptions to include the perceived strength of such boundaries. Ultimately, it is the transcriber's sensitivity to the data together with his or her experience and phonetic knowledge that will determine what is included in a given transcription. Also, of course, because every sample of impaired speech potentially contains rare or even new phonetic phenomena, we have to be ready to deal with things for which there are as yet no transcription conventions. Crystal (1987, p. 16) proffers useful guidance when he suggests that "if we have made a transcription at the right level for our purposes, it should be unnecessary to have to refer back to the tape in carrying out our analyses later."

23.7   Transcription Layout

How a transcription is laid out will depend on whether it is intended to be 'private' or 'public'. Ball and Local (1996, pp. 69–71) distinguish between "working records" and "presentation transcriptions", the former being as all-inclusive as possible and rather 'messy', and the latter being structured for particular purposes of exemplification. If the record is only for the eyes of the transcriber then it only matters that he or she can read and interpret it. But if it is to be published or made accessible to other professionals, the 'messiness' of private transcriptions needs to be cleaned up to make sure they are legible and interpretable, and things are in the right order. It may be useful with some speakers to use or adapt the pro forma in Poyatos (2002, p. 140) for making what he calls a "total transcription of interactive discourse", which includes, besides phonetic transcription, transcription of facial expression, gesture and proxemics (see also Müller, 2006).

Turning a private into a public transcription will also involve decisions about who is likely to read it and what we want to tell them about the speaker. Where a transcription includes the utterances of two or more speakers, even if the utterances of one of them, e.g. a speech and language pathologist or other conversational partner, are only transcribed orthographically, the social relations implied by the layout should be borne in mind. Bucholtz (2000, p. 1462) cites Ochs (1979) regarding the tendency to give primacy to the speaker whose speech is presented first and to see the other speaker/s as passive respondents. She also makes the point that the very practice of representing one speaker's speech using IPA symbols while another's is represented orthographically may have undesirable implications (Bucholtz, 2000, p. 1453). It has the effect of identifying the phonetically transcribed speech as 'other' and laying the blame for any communication difficulties exclusively at the door of the speaker whose speech has been transcribed phonetically. By using narrow phonetic transcription to document the utterances of both the speech-language pathologist and the child with impaired speech in a clinical context, Gardner (1997) is able to pinpoint breakdowns in interaction and communication which can be ascribed to the speech-language pathologist's failure to notice or respond to fine phonetic details in the child's speech which nevertheless have phonologically contrastive value. Indeed, recent perspectives on intelligibility and communication breakdown locate the problem not squarely with one of the speakers but in the interactional space between them (Perkins, in press).

23.8   Conclusion

We note elsewhere (Howard & Heselwood, 2002b, p. 395) that "while narrow phonetic transcription of clinical speech data is difficult, and teaching and learning it is difficult, both are rich and valuable activities." This is a view which is widely shared (Ball & Rahilly, 2002; Buckingham and Yule, 1987; Kelly & Local, 1989; Kent, 1996; Powell, 2001; Sell, 2005; Shriberg & Lof, 1991). Not only can narrow phonetic transcription offer insights in the clinical context into the ways in which an individual's spoken output differs from what might reasonably be expected for a speaker of a particular accent and language variety, but it also facilitates theoretical insights into the nature of impaired speech production.

REFERENCES

Abercrombie, D. (1958). The recording of dialect material. *Orbis*, 111, 232–5.

Abercrombie, D. (1967). *Elements of General Phonetics*. Edinburgh: Edinburgh University Press.

Amorosa, H., von Benda, U., Wagner, E., and Keck, A. (1985). Transcribing detail in the speech of unintelligible children: a comparison of procedures. *British Journal of Disorders of Communication*, 20, 281–87.

Ashby, M. and Maidment, J. (2005). *Introducing Phonetic Science*. Cambridge: Cambridge University Press.

Ashby, M., Maidment, J., and Abberton, E. (1996). Analytic listening: a new approach to ear-training. *Speech, Hearing and Language*, 9, 1–10.

Ball, M. J., Code, C., Rahilly, J., and Hazlett, D. (1994). Non-segmental aspects of disordered speech: developments in transcription. *Clinical Linguistics and Phonetics*, 8, 67–83.

Ball, M. J., Esling, J. H., and Dickson, G. (1995). The VoQS system for the transcription of voice quality. *Journal of the International Phonetic Association*, 25, 61–70.

Ball, M. J. and Local, J. (1996). Current developments in transcription. In M. J. Ball and M. Duckworth (eds.), *Advances in Clinical Phonetics*. Amsterdam: John Benjamins, pp. 51–89.

Ball, M. J. and Rahilly, J. (2002). Transcribing disordered speech: the segmental and prosodic layers. *Clinical Linguistics and Phonetics*, 16(5), 329–44.

Beckman, M. E., Hirschberg, J., and Shattuck-Hufnagel, S. (2005). The original ToBI system and the evolution of the ToBI framework. In S-A. Jun (ed.), *Prosodic Typology: The Phonology of Intonation and Phrasing*. Oxford: Oxford University Press.

Bernhardt, B. and Ball, M. J. (1993). Characteristics of atypical speech currently not included in the Extensions to the IPA. *Journal of the International Phonetic Association*, 23, 35–8.

Bucholtz, M. (2000). The politics of transcription. *Journal of Pragmatics*, 32, 1439–65.

Buckingham, H. and Yule, G. (1987). Phonemic false evaluation: theoretical and clinical aspects. *Clinical Linguistics and Phonetics*, 1, 113–25.

Clark, H. H. (1996). *Using Language*. Cambridge: Cambridge University Press.

Crary, M. A. (1983). Phonological process analysis from spontaneous speech: the influence of sample size. *Journal of Communication Disorders*, 16, 133–41.

Cruttenden, A. (1997). *Intonation*. 2nd ed. Cambridge: Cambridge University Press.

Crystal, D. (1984). *Linguistic Encounters with Language Handicap*. London: Edward Arnold.

Crystal, D. (1987). *Clinical Linguistics*. London: Edward Arnold.

Cucchiarini, C. (1996). Assessing transcription agreement: methodological aspects. *Clinical Linguistics and Phonetics*, 10. 131–56.

Damico, J. and Nelson, R. (2005). Interpreting problematic behaviour: Systematic compensatory adaptations as emergent phenomena in autism. *Clinical Linguistics and Phonetics*, 19(5), 405–17.

Daniloff, R. G., Wilcox, K., and Stephens, M. I. (1980). An acoustic-articulatory description of children's defective /s/ productions. *Journal of Communication Disorders*, 13, 347–63.

Dinnsen, D. A. (1999). Some empirical and theoretical issues in disordered child phonology. In W. C. Ritchie and T. K. Bhatia (eds.), *Handbook of Child Language Acquisition*. San Diego, CA: Academic Press, pp. 647–74.

Dobbinson, S. J., Perkins, M. R. and Boucher, J. (2003). The interactional significance of formulas in autistic language. *Clinical Linguistics and Phonetics*, 17(4/5), 299–307.

Duckworth, M., Allen, G., Hardcastle, W. and Ball, M. J. (1990). Extensions to the International Phonetic Alphabet for the transcription of atypical speech. *Clinical Linguistics and Phonetics*, 4, 273–80.

Esling, J. H. and Harris, J. G. (2005). States of the glottis: an articulatory phonetic model based on laryngoscopic observations. In W. J. Hardcastle and J. M. Beck (eds.), *Figures of Speech: A Festschrift for John Laver*. Mahwah, NJ: Lawrence Erlbaum Associates, pp. 347–83.

Gardner, H. (1997). Are your minimal pairs too neat? The dangers of phonemicisation in phonology therapy. *European Journal of Disorders of Communication*, 32(2), 167–75.

Grunwell, P. (1987). *Clinical Phonology*. 2nd ed. London: Croom Helm.

Gussenhoven, C. and Rietveld, A. C. M. (1992). Intonation contours, prosodic structure and preboundary lengthening. *Journal of Phonetics*, 20, 283–303.

Hewlett, N. (1985). Phonological versus phonetic disorders: some suggested modifications to the current use of the distinction. *British Journal of Disorders of Communication*, 20, 155–64.

Holmgren, K., Lindblom, B., Aurelius, G., Jalling, B., and Zetterström, R. (1986). On the phonetics of infant vocalisation. In B. Lindblom and R. Zetterström (eds.), *Precursors to Early Speech*. New York: Stockton Press.

Howard, S. J. (2004). Connected speech processes in developmental speech impairment: observations from an electropalatographic perspective. *Clinical Linguistics and Phonetics*, 18(6–8), 405–17.

Howard, S. J. (2007). The interplay between articulation and prosody in children with impaired speech: observations from electropalatographic and perceptual analysis. *Advances in Speech-Language Pathology*, 9(1), 20–35.

Howard, S. J. and Heselwood, B. (2002a). Learning and teaching phonetic transcription for clinical purposes. *Clinical Linguistics and Phonetics*, 16, 371–401.

Howard, S. J. and Heselwood, B. (2002b). The contribution of phonetics to the study of vowel development and disorders. In M. J. Ball and F. Gibbon (eds.), *Vowel Disorders*. New York: Butterworth-Heinemann, 37–82.

Ingram, D. (1989) *Phonological Disability in Children*. 2nd ed. London: Whurr.

IPA (1999). *Handbook of the International Phonetic Association*. Cambridge: Cambridge University Press.

Jones, D. (1972). *An Outline of English Phonetics*. 9th ed. Cambridge: Cambridge University Press.

Kelly, J. and Local, J. (1989). *Doing Phonology*. Manchester: Manchester University Press.

Kent, R. D. (1996). Hearing and believing: some limits to the auditory-perceptual assessment of speech and voice disorders. *American Journal of Speech-Language Pathology*, 5, 7–23.

Kent, R. D. and Miolo, G. (1995). Phonetic abilities in the first year of life. In P. Fletcher and B. MacWhinney (eds.), *The Handbook of Child Language*. Oxford: Blackwell.

Ladefoged, P. (2003). *Phonetic Data Analysis*. Oxford: Blackwell.

Lambert, J. (1989). Childhood phonological disorders. In M. M. Leahy (ed.), *Disorders of Communication: The Science of Intervention*. London: Taylor & Francis.

Laver, J. (1980). *The Phonetic Description of Voice Quality*. Cambridge: Cambridge University Press.

Laver, J. (1994). *Principles of Phonetics*. Cambridge: Cambridge University Press.

Local, J. (2003). Variable domains and variable relevance: interpreting phonetic exponents. *Journal of Phonetics*, 31, 321–39.

Local, J. and Wootton, T. (1995). Interactional and phonetic aspects of immediate echolalia in autism: a case study. *Clinical Linguistics and Phonetics*, 9, 155–84.

Lohmander, A. and Olsson, M. (2004). Methodology for perceptual assessment of speech in patients with cleft palate: a critical review of the literature. *Cleft Palate-Craniofacial Journal*, 41, 64–70.

Maurer, D., Gröne, B., Landis, T., Hoch, G. and Schönle, P. W. (1993). Re-examination of the relation between the vocal tract and the vowel sound with electro-magnetic articulography (EMA) in vocalizations. *Clinical Linguistics and Phonetics*, 7, 129–43.

Menyuk, P., Liebergott, J. and Schultz, M. (1986). Predicting phonological development. In B. Lindblom and R. Zetterström (eds.), *Precursors of Early Speech*. New York: Stockton Press, pp. 79–93.

Morrish, E. C. E. (1988). Compensatory articulation in a subject with total glossectomy. *British Journal of Disorders of Communication*, 23, 13–22.

Müller, N. (ed.) (2006). *Multi-layered Transcription*. San Diego, CA: Plural.

Ochs, E. (1979). Transcription as theory. In E. Ochs and B. Schiefflin (eds.), *Developmental Pragmatics*. New York: Academic Press.

O'Halpin, R. (2001). Intonation issues in the speech of hearing impaired children: analysis, transcription and remediation. *Clinical Linguistics and Phonetics*, 15, 529–50.

Oller, D. K. (1980). The emergence of speech sounds in infancy. In G. H. Yeni-Komshian, J. F. Kavanagh and C. A. Ferguson (eds.), *Child Phonology. Volume 1: Production*. New York: Academic Press.

Oller, D. K. (2000). *The Emergence of the Speech Capacity*. Mahwah, NJ: Lawrence Erlbaum Associates.

Oller, D. K. and Eilers, R. E. (1975). Phonetic expectation and transcription validity. *Phonetica*, 31, 288–304.

Perkell, J. S. (1997). Articulatory processes. In W. J. Hardcastle and J. Laver (eds.), *The Handbook of Phonetic Sciences*. London: Blackwell, pp. 333–70.

Perkins, M. R. (in press). *Pragmatic Impairment*. Cambridge: Cambridge University Press.

Perkins, M. R. and Howard, S. J. (1995). Principles of clinical linguistics. In M. R. Perkins and S. J. Howard (eds.), *Case Studies in Clinical Linguistics*. London: Whurr, pp. 10–35.

Peterson-Falzone, S. J., Trost-Cardamone, J. E., Karnell, M. P., and Hardin-Jones, M. A. (2006). *The Clinician's Guide to Treating Cleft Palate Speech*. St. Louis, MO: Mosby Elsevier.

Powell, T. W. (2001). Phonetic transcription of disordered speech. *Topics in Language Disorders*, 21, 52–72.

Poyatos, F. (2002). *Nonverbal Communication across Disciplines. Volume 1: Culture, Sensory Interaction, Speech Conversation*. Amsterdam: John Benjamins.

Sell, D. (2005). Issues in perceptual speech analysis in cleft palate and related disorders: a review. *International Journal of Language and Communication Disorders*, 40: 103–21.

Sell, D., Harding, A. and Grunwell, P. (1999). GOS.SP.ASS.'98: an assessment for speech disorders associated with cleft palate and/or velopharyngeal dysfunction (revised). *International Journal of Language and Communication Disorders*, 34(1), 17–33.

Shriberg, L. D., Kwiatkowski, J. and Hoffmann, K. (1984). A procedure for phonetic transcription by consensus. *Journal of Speech and Hearing Research*, 27, 456–65.

Shriberg, L. D. and Lof, G. L. (1991). Reliability studies in broad and narrow phonetic transcription. *Clinical Linguistics and Phonetics*, 5, 225–79.

Shriberg, L. D., McSweeny, J. L., Anderson, B. E., Campbell, T. F., Chial, M. R., Green, J. R., Hauner, K. K., Moore, C. A., Rusiewicz, H. L., and Wilson, D. L. (2005). Transitioning from analog to digital audio recording in childhood speech sound disorders. *Clinical Linguistics and Phonetics*, 19, 335–59.

Snow, D. (2001). Transcription of suprasegmentals. *Topics in Language Disorders*, 21, 41–51.

Stark, R. (1986). Prespeech segmental feature development. In P. Fletcher and M. Garman (eds.), *Language Acquisition*. 2nd ed. Cambridge: Cambridge University Press, 149–173.

Stoel-Gammon, C. (2001). Transcribing the speech of young children. *Topics in Language Disorders*, 21, 12–21.

Tarplee, C. and Barrow, E. (1999). Delayed echoing as an interactional resource: a case study of a 3-year-old child on the autistic spectrum. *Clinical Linguistics and Phonetics*, 13, 449–82.

Vaissière, J. (2005). Perception of intonation. In D. B. Pisoni and R. E. Remez (eds.), *The Handbook of Speech Perception*. Malden, MA: Blackwell, 236–63.

Vihman, M. M. (1996). *Phonological Development*. Oxford: Blackwell.

Wells, B. (1994). Junction in developmental speech disorder: a case study. *Clinical Linguistics and Phonetics*, 8(1), 1–25.

Appendix: IPA, ExtIPA, and VoQS Charts

THE INTERNATIONAL PHONETIC ALPHABET(revised to 2005)

CONSONANTS (PULMONIC)

© 2005 IPA

	Bilabial	Labiodental	Dental	Alveolar	Postalveolar	Retroflex	Palatal	Velar	Uvular	Pharyngeal	Glottal
Plosive	p b			t d		ʈ ɖ	c ɟ	k ɡ	q ɢ		ʔ
Nasal	m	ɱ		n		ɳ	ɲ	ŋ	N		
Trill	B			r					R		
Tap or Flap		ⱱ		ɾ		ɽ					
Fricative	ɸ β	f v	θ ð	s z	ʃ ʒ	ʂ ʐ	ç ʝ	x ɣ	χ ʁ	ħ ʕ	h ɦ
Lateral fricative				ɬ ɮ							
Approximant		ʋ		ɹ		ɻ	j	ɰ			
Lateral approximant				l		ɭ	ʎ	L			

Where symbols appear in pairs, the one to the right represents a voiced consonant. Shaded areas denote articulations judged impossible.

CONSONANTS (NON-PULMONIC)

Clicks	Voiced implosives	Ejectives
ʘ Bilabial	ɓ Bilabial	ʼ Examples:
ǀ Dental	ɗ Dental/alveolar	pʼ Bilabial
ǃ (Post)alveolar	ʄ Palatal	tʼ Dental/alveolar
ǂ Palatoalveolar	ɠ Velar	kʼ Velar
ǁ Alveolar lateral	ʛ Uvular	sʼ Alveolar fricative

OTHER SYMBOLS

ʍ Voiceless labial-velar fricative   ɕ ʑ Alveolo-palatal fricatives

w Voiced labial-velar approximant   ɺ Voiced alveolar lateral flap

ɥ Voiced labial-palatal approximant   ɧ Simultaneous ʃ and x

ʜ Voiceless epiglottal fricative

ʢ Voiced epiglottal fricative

ʡ Epiglottal plosive

Affricates and double articulations can be represented by two symbols joined by a tie bar if necessary.   k͡p t͡s

VOWELS

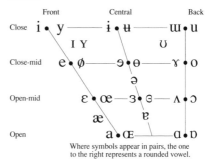

Where symbols appear in pairs, the one to the right represents a rounded vowel.

SUPRASEGMENTALS

ˈ	Primary stress
ˌ	Secondary stress
	ˌfoʊnəˈtɪʃən
ː	Long	eː
ˑ	Half-long	eˑ
˘	Extra-short	ĕ
ǀ	Minor (foot) group
‖	Major (intonation) group
.	Syllable break	ɹi.ækt
‿	Linking (absence of a break)

DIACRITICS   Diacritics may be placed above a symbol with a descender, e.g. ŋ̊

̥	Voiceless	n̥ d̥	̤	Breathy voiced	b̤ a̤	̪	Dental	t̪ d̪
̬	Voiced	s̬ t̬	̰	Creaky voiced	b̰ a̰	̺	Apical	t̺ d̺
ʰ	Aspirated	tʰ dʰ	̼	Linguolabial	t̼ d̼	̻	Laminal	t̻ d̻
̹	More rounded	ɔ̹	ʷ	Labialized	tʷ dʷ	̃	Nasalized	ẽ
̜	Less rounded	ɔ̜	ʲ	Palatalized	tʲ dʲ	ⁿ	Nasal release	dⁿ
̟	Advanced	u̟	ˠ	Velarized	tˠ dˠ	ˡ	Lateral release	dˡ
̠	Retracted	e̠	ˤ	Pharyngealized	tˤ dˤ	̚	No audible release	d̚
̈	Centralized	ë	̴	Velarized or pharyngealized	ɫ			
̽	Mid-centralized	e̽	̝	Raised	e̝	(ɹ̝ = voiced alveolar fricative)		
̩	Syllabic	n̩	̞	Lowered	e̞	(β̞ = voiced bilabial approximant)		
̯	Non-syllabic	e̯	̘	Advanced Tongue Root	e̘			
˞	Rhoticity	ɚ a˞	̙	Retracted Tongue Root	e̙			

TONES AND WORD ACCENTS

LEVEL			CONTOUR		
e̋ or	˥	Extra high	ě or	˩˥	Rising
é	˦	High	ê	˥˩	Falling
ē	˧	Mid	e᷄	˧˥	High rising
è	˨	Low	e᷅	˩˧	Low rising
ȅ	˩	Extra low	e᷈	˧˩˧	Rising-falling
↓	Downstep		↗	Global rise	
↑	Upstep		↘	Global fall	

ExtIPA SYMBOLS FOR DISORDERED SPEECH
(Revised to 2002)

CONSONANTS (other than on the IPA Chart)

	bilabial	labiodental	dentolabial	labioalv	linguolabial	interdental	bidental	alveolar	velar	velophar
Plosive		p̪ b̪	p͆ b͆	p͇ b͇	t̼ d̼	t̪͆ d̪͆				
Nasal			m͆	m͇	n̼	n̪͆				
Trill					r̼	r̪͆				
Fricative median			f͆ v͆	f͇ v͇	θ̼ ð̼	θ̪͆ ð̪͆	h̪͆ ɦ̪͆			ʩ
Fricative lateral+median								ʪ ʫ		
Fricative nareal	m͋							n͋	ŋ͋	
Percussive	ʬ						ʭ			
Approximant lateral					l̼	l̪͆				

Where symbols appear in pairs, the one to the right represents a voiced consonant. Shaded areas denote articulations judged impossible.

DIACRITICS

͍	labial spreading	s͍	͈	strong articulation	f͈	͊	denasal	m͊
͆	dentolabial	v͆	͉	weak articulation	v͉	͋	nasal escape	v͋
̪͆	interdental/bidental	n̪͆	\	reiterated articulation	p\p\p	≈	velopharyngeal friction	s͌
͇	alveolar	t͇	͎	whistled articulation	s͎	↓	ingressive airflow	p↓
̼	linguolabial	d̼	→	sliding articulation	θ͢s	↑	egressive airflow	!↑

CONNECTED SPEECH

(.)	short pause
(..)	medium pause
(...)	long pause
f	loud speech [{$_f$ laʊd $_f$}]
ff	louder speech [{$_{ff}$ laʊdɚ $_{ff}$}]
p	quiet speech [{$_p$ kwaɪət $_p$}]
pp	quieter speech {{$_{pp}$ kwaiətɚ $_{pp}$}]
allegro	fast speech [{$_{allegro}$ fast $_{allegro}$}]
lento	slow speech [{$_{lento}$ sloʊ $_{lento}$}]
crescendo, ralentando, etc. may also be used	

VOICING

̬	pre-voicing	̬z
̬	post-voicing	z̬
(̥)	partial devoicing	(z̥)
(̥	initial partial devoicing	(z̥
̥)	final partial devoicing	z̥)
(̬)	partial voicing	(s̬)
(̬	initial partial voicing	(s̬
̬)	final partial voicing	s̬)
˭	unaspirated	p˭
ʰ	pre-aspiration	ʰp

OTHERS

(◌), (C̲)	indeterminate sound, consonant	(( ))	extraneous noise ((2 sylls))
(V̲), (P̲l̲.v̲l̲s̲)	indeterminate vowel, voiceless plosive, etc.	¡	sublaminal lower alveolar percussive click
(N̲), (v̲)	indeterminate nasal, probably [v], etc.	!¡	alveolar and sublaminal clicks (cluck-click)
( )	silent articulation (ʃ), (m)	*	sound with no available symbol

VoQs: Voice Quality Symbols

Airstream Types

Œ	œsophageal speech	И	electrolarynx speech
Ю	tracheo-œsophageal speech	↓	pulmonic ingressive speech

Phonation types

V	modal voice	F	falsetto
W	whisper	C	creak
V̰	whispery voice (murmur)	V̰	creaky voice
Vʰ	breathy voice	C̰	whispery creak
V!	harsh voice	V!!	ventricular phonation
V͈!!	diplophonia	V̰!!	whispery ventricular phonation
V̟	anterior or pressed phonation	W̲	posterior whisper

Supralaryngeal Settings

L̝	raised larynx	L̞	lowered larynx
Vᵚ	labialized voice (open round)	Vᵂ	labialized voice (close round)
V͍	spread-lip voice	Vᵛ	labio-dentalized voice
V̺	linguo-apicalized voice	V̻	linguo-laminalized voice
Vˆ	retroflex voice	V̪	dentalized voice
V̠	alveolarized voice	V̠ʲ	palatoalveolarized voice
Vʲ	palatalized voice	Vˠ	velarized voice
Vᴮ	uvularized voice	Vˤ	pharyngealized voice
V̴ˤ	laryngo-pharyngealized voice	Vᴴ	faucalized voice
Ṽ	nasalized voice	V̊	denasalized voice
J̞	open jaw voice	J̝	close jaw voice
J̪	right offset jaw voice	J̺	left offset jaw voice
J̟	protruded jaw voice	Θ	protruded tongue voice

USE OF LABELED BRACES & NUMERALS TO MARK STRETCHES OF SPEECH AND DEGREES AND COMBINATIONS OF VOICE QUALITY:

[ˈðɪs ɪz ˈnɔɹməl ˈvɔɪs {ʒV! ˈðɪs ɪz ˈveɹi ˈhaɹʃ ˈvɔɪs ʒV} ˈðɪs ɪz ˈnɔɹməl ˈvɔɪs wʌns ˈmɔɹ {L̝ ɪV! ˈðɪs ɪz ˈlɛs ˈhaɹʃ ˈvɔɪs wɪð ˈloʊɚd ˈlæɹɪŋks ɪV!L̞}]

24 Comparisons in Perception between Speech and Nonspeech Signals

TESSA BENT AND DAVID B. PISONI

24.1 Introduction

A long-standing debate in the field of speech perception concerns whether the processing of speech is different from the processing of other types of auditory signals and whether specialized neural mechanisms are necessary to perceive speech signals. The complex acoustic structure of speech sounds sets it apart from other auditory signals in the listener's environment (Stevens, 1980). Speech contains two channels of information: linguistic and indexical. Within the linguistic channel, the meaning of utterances is conveyed rapidly and effortlessly. The indexical channel includes information about regional dialect, social status, sex, age, emotional state, and physical state (Abercrombie, 1967). Lastly, speech differs from many other types of environmental sounds because humans produce speech sounds in addition to perceiving them, suggesting a close connection between sensory and motor neural systems. While speech signals and other auditory signals may differ, the question of how speech *perception* differs from general auditory perception is still a fundamental problem in the field of speech perception.

One of the critical issues regarding the perception of speech and nonspeech is whether there is an encapsulated processing module for phonetic perception (Fodor, 1983; Mattingly & Liberman, 1990). By definition, modular systems must meet four major criteria: domain specificity (the module only responds to specific types of stimuli), mandatoriness (the functions of the module are automatically computed), information encapsulation (only local information is available to the module), and speed (the processing in the module is very fast) (Fodor, 1983; Garfield, 1987).

The strong claim that speech perception is a modular system also entails that speech and nonspeech signals do not share cognitive processing resources.

The evidence reviewed in this chapter suggests that a strictly modular view of speech perception is probably incorrect because speech and nonspeech signals appear to share common neural mechanisms. Current evidence supports a weakly modular view in which speech and nonspeech perception share some processing areas. However, during the perception of speech specifically, these areas may show increased activation compared to similar nonspeech signals. Under this view, only two of the four major criteria for modularity would be met: mandatoriness and speed.

In this chapter, several findings from classic studies on speech and nonspeech sound perception are described. Following this section, we discuss recent studies on the perception of indexical information available during speech perception and the plasticity of phonemic categories. The chapter concludes with observations on current and future directions. Throughout the chapter, implications for clinical populations are discussed where applicable.

24.2   Classic Experimental Findings

The three experimental paradigms discussed in this section sought to identify perceptual patterns unique to speech perception; however, later results showed that nonspeech stimuli were perceived in ways similar to speech.

24.2.1   *Categorical perception*

One of the earliest findings cited as support for the existence of a specialized processing mode for speech perception was categorical perception in which continuous stimuli are perceived in a categorical fashion. Liberman, Harris, Hoffman, and Griffith (1957) presented listeners with stimuli from a synthetically generated continuum of stop consonants which varied in place of articulation (e.g. from /b/ to /d/ to /g/). The listeners were required to perform two tasks: a labeling-identification task and an ABX discrimination task. In the labeling task, listeners were presented with a single stimulus on each trial and were required to allocate it to one of the categories provided by the experimenter. In the discrimination task, listeners were presented with three stimuli on each trial in an ABX format, where A and B were always different, and listeners were asked to determine whether the third stimulus (X) was the same as the first or the second.

Two requirements need to be met for perception to be considered categorical (Lane, 1965; Studdert-Kennedy, Liberman, Harris, & Cooper, 1970). First, in the identification task the listeners have to show abrupt boundaries between the categories rather than responses that vary continuously with the acoustic changes of the stimuli. Second, in the discrimination task, the listeners need to exhibit better discrimination of pairs of stimuli selected from between categories than of pairs selected within categories as defined by their labeling functions. Moreover, within-category discrimination has to be close to chance performance.

Initially, findings of categorical perception in speech were cited as evidence for a specialized speech mode of processing (e.g. Liberman, Harris, Eimas, Lisker, & Bastian, 1961). However, later experiments demonstrated categorical perception of complex nonspeech signals (Miller, Wier, Pastore, Kely, & Dooling, 1976). Furthermore, non-human animals demonstrated categorical-like perception of human speech although no animal study has ever collected both labeling and discrimination functions or assessed the relations between these functions (Trout, 2001). Together these findings were interpreted as support for the proposal that categorical perception may be a general mechanism of cognition rather than a unique defining feature of speech perception.

Atypical phonological representations in dyslexics may lead to their difficulty in developing phoneme-to-grapheme correspondences. Categorical perception tests with dyslexic listeners have helped to determine what underlies their impairment and whether it is a speech-specific or general auditory deficit. Children with dyslexia are more accurate than others at discriminating within-category differences (Semiclaes, Sprenger-Charolles, Carre, & Demoney, 2001; Werker & Tees, 1987) but less consistent in their labeling performance (Godfrey et al., 1981; Werker & Tees, 1987). There is evidence for a speech-specific component of this deficit (Mody, Studdert-Kennedy, & Brady, 1997; Semiclaes & Sprenger-Charolles, 2003).

24.2.2   Rate and talker normalization

Listeners are faced with substantial variation in the speech signal yet they are able to recover the talker's intended utterance automatically without conscious awareness. The ability to handle speech variability declines with age and hearing impairment; older listeners are affected more by talker- and amplitude-variability than young listeners, and hearing-impaired elderly individuals are affected more by variations in speaking rate and talker variability than normally hearing elderly listeners (Gordon-Salant & Fitzgibbons, 2004; Sommers, 1997). Understanding the cause of this decline and whether it is specific to speech may help determine appropriate clinical intervention strategies.

Miller and Liberman (1979) demonstrated that the location of a phoneme boundary between [b] and [w] changes relationally depending on the duration of the following vowel. Infants also demonstrate relational processing of these same speech signals (Eimas & Miller, 1980). Rate normalization requires phonemic information to be integrated across widely distributed acoustic cues in the speech signal and has been proposed to be unique to speech processing.

However, both adults and infants have relational processing for nonspeech signals because listeners' placement of the boundary between two nonspeech sounds (gradual onset versus abrupt onset) is influenced by overall stimulus duration (Jusczyk, Pisoni, Reed, Ferald, & Myers, 1983; Pisoni, Carrell, & Gans, 1983). Therefore, nonspeech sounds can be processed in a relational and non-linear manner comparable to speech signals. The perceptual abilities used by adults and infants to handle variability in speech may draw on general-purpose auditory capabilities as well as specialized speech perception mechanisms.

24.2.3   Multimodal speech perception

Sumby and Pollack (1954) were the first researchers to systematically explore the contribution of visual information to speech intelligibility. Listeners were able to correctly perceive more words presented in noise when visual information was available. Therefore, listeners are able to integrate information from the two sensory modalities in order to recover the intended utterance. Listeners with hearing loss (Erber, 1975) and hearing-impaired individuals with cochlear implants (CI) (Tyler, Parkinson, Woodworth, Lowder, & Gantz, 1997) also show improved speech understanding with the addition of visual information (see also Bergeson & Pisoni, 2004). Furthermore, for deaf children, preimplantation scores on both lipreading and cross-modal speech perception are correlated with outcomes on speech perception and production tasks after several years of implant use, suggesting a close coupling in development between multimodal perception and language acquisition (Bergeson, Pisoni, & Davis, 2005).

The 'McGurk effect' (McGurk & MacDonald, 1976) is another well-known example of cross-modal integration. In this paradigm, listeners hear one syllable (i.e. /ga/) but see a face producing a different syllable (i.e. /ba/). Their final perception (/da/) reflects a fusion of the features from the audio and visual signals, leading to the perception of an element not present in either modality (i.e. the alveolar place of articulation for /da/). The McGurk effect is stronger in adults than children suggesting that this ability develops over time. The question of how these auditory-articulatory correspondences develop and whether a specialized perceptual mechanism is needed to account for cross-modal integration and fusion is still an open question (Calvert, Spence, & Stein, 2004) but recent work on cross-modal speech perception in children with cochlear implants suggests that there is a sensitive period for the development of cross-modal integration in speech. The likelihood of displaying cross-modal integration (as evidenced by the McGurk effect) is much stronger in deaf children who received cochlear implants before 2.5 years of age than children who were implanted later in life (Schorr, Fox, van Wassenhove, & Knudsen, 2005).

24.3   Indexical Properties of Speech and Malleability of Speech Categories

Two issues related to the specialization for speech perception are (1) whether indexical and linguistic information interact during speech perception; and (2) malleability of speech categories after some critical period in development.

24.3.1   Talker-contingent phonetic coding

One question in speech perception research is whether phonetic processing is independent of the indexical properties of speech, including idiosyncratic properties specific to a particular talker's voice. Evidence for interactions between phonetic, phonological and lexical representations of speech on the one hand and indexical properties of the signal on the other suggest that speech perception and spoken word recognition are typically carried out with reference to properties of the speaker's voice.

First, spoken-word recognition is affected by talker variability. Listeners are faster and more accurate at recognizing words when spoken by one talker than by many talkers (Mullennix, Pisoni, & Martin, 1989). Second, a talker's voice influences recognition memory for words. In recognition memory tasks, listeners are presented with lists of spoken words and then later required to determine whether they had heard the words before or not. Listeners are faster and more accurate at identifying 'old' words when they are presented in the same voice at test rather than in a different voice (Palmeri, Goldinger, & Pisoni, 1993). Third, prior familiarity and experience with a particular voice influences the intelligibility of words. Listeners who are trained to identify talkers' voices are more accurate at identifying words produced by familiar talkers than by talkers whom they have never heard before (Nygaard, Sommers, & Pisoni, 1994). Lastly, perception of a talker's gender and sexual orientation influences phoneme boundary placement (Johnson, Strand, & D'Imperio, 1999; Munson, Jefferson, & McDonald, 2006). Together these results suggest the operation of parallel streams of information in speech which interact during phoneme identification and lexical access.

Difficulties in encoding and processing indexical properties of speech may underlie some of the speech-perception problems clinical populations experience (see also Docherty & Khattab, chapter 37 in this volume). For example, Cleary, Pisoni, and Kirk (2005) reported strong correlations between the ability to discriminate between different talkers and keyword identification scores for children with CIs and normally hearing children. Incorporating variability from indexical speech properties into clinical assessment tests (e.g. use of multiple talkers of both genders from various dialect regions) may reveal speech perception difficulties that are not apparent in traditional assessment tests which typically use only a single talker producing utterances in isolation or highly constrained contexts. These types of tests will, thus, provide a broader and more accurate picture of listeners' speech perception abilities (Pisoni, 1998).

24.3.2   Plasticity and modification of phonetic categories

Two central issues in the field of speech perception are how linguistic experience influences adult phonetic categories and the extent to which these categories are subject to modification based on experience and learning. Infants are able to perceive the sound categories of any natural language but they develop native-language-specific categories within the first year of life (Werker & Tees, 1984). This language-specific tuning decreases the abilities of adults to discriminate many non-native phoneme contrasts (Best, 1995) and increases humans' abilities to perceive native categories (Kuhl, Stevens, Hayashi, et al., 2006).

While early attempts to train adult listeners to perceive new phonemic distinctions in the laboratory were consistently unsuccessful (Strange & Dittman, 1984), other training studies demonstrated that new phonemic categories can be trained and learned easily in the laboratory in a short period of time (McClaskey, Pisoni, & Carrell, 1983). Later studies showed that, for more difficult non-native contrasts (e.g. the distinction between English /r/ and /l/ for Japanese listeners), listeners could be trained using a novel high-variability training paradigm (Logan, Lively, & Pisoni, 1991). The key methodological innovations of this approach were the incorporation of stimulus variability (both in terms of talker variability and position within the word) and the emphasis on categorization and identification, which encourage listeners to make abstract generalizations about categories rather than discrimination, which focuses the listener's attention on fine details in the test signals. Through this high-variability training technique, Japanese listeners were shown to generalize their learning to new talkers and new words, to retain learning for three months after training, and to transfer perceptual learning to improvements in production of words containing /r/ and /l/ (Bradlow, Akahane-Yamada, Pisoni, & Tohkura, 1999; Bradlow, Pisoni, Yamada, & Tohkura, 1997). Thus, phonemic categories are robust and flexible and can be modified under well-defined experimental conditions.

Training techniques have also been successfully used to help children with auditory-based learning impairments, including dyslexia, improve their speech discrimination and language-processing skills (Hayes, Warrier, Nicol, Zecker, & Kraus, 2003; Merzenich, Jenkins, Johnston, et al., 1996; Tallal, Miller, Bedi, et al., 1996), but these perceptual improvements have not transferred to reading skills (Agnew, Dorn, & Eden, 2004). These training regimes have not used the high-variability training paradigm. Thus, bringing the key methodological innovations of high-variability training to other populations, including children with learning problems, elderly adults, and the hearing-impaired, may lead to more robust and widely transferable learning.

24.4   Current and Future Directions

24.4.1   Brain-imaging studies

Brain-imaging studies are providing new information regarding the extent to which the neural mechanisms that underlie the processing of speech and nonspeech sounds are shared (see Scott, 2005). Recent studies have generally found some areas of activation specific to speech stimuli, compared to none in analogous nonspeech stimuli (e.g. Benson, Whalen, Richardson, et al., 2001; Vouloumanos, Kiehl, Werker, & Liddle, 2001).

Another method used in neuroimaging research involves studies of the perception of speech or speech-like stimuli while varying listeners' expectations or language backgrounds. Gandour, Wong, and Hutchins (1998) and Jacquemot, Pallier, Lebihan, Dehaene, and Dupoux (2003) showed that there is increased activation for speech stimuli when the acoustic distinctions are phonologically or lexically relevant in a listener's native language compared to when the distinctions are not linguistically contrastive. In both of these studies, the regions of activation did not differ significantly but, rather, the amount of activation within the implicated regions was different depending on whether the signals were linguistically relevant.

Remez, Rubin, Pisoni, and Carrell (1981) were the first to demonstrate that listeners are able to perceive speech when all the traditional acoustic cues to speech are removed. They used sine-wave speech in which the first three formants are replaced with time-varying sinusoids that follow the peaks in the vocal-tract transfer function. The resulting sounds were perceived as speech although they had an unnatural sound quality.

Using fMRI, Mottonen, Calvert, Jaaskeleinen, et al. (2006) scanned listeners while they were listening to sine-wave speech. The listeners' expectations were manipulated by initially playing the stimuli without informing them that the sounds were speech, and then later training them to perceive the stimuli as speech. Compared to the nonspeech conditions, Mottonen and colleagues' results showed additional activation when the same stimuli were perceived as speech. The results from these studies provide support for specialized processing of speech signals which is modulated not by the acoustic characteristics of the stimuli themselves, but by the listeners' processing mode and perceptual interpretation of the signals.

Information about neural circuits may help researchers and clinicians understand more about the development and underlying deficits of various clinical populations. For example, the auditory brainstem response to speech signals but not nonspeech signals is impaired in children with language-based learning problems (Song, Banai, Russo, & Kraus, 2006). Furthermore, Sharma, Dorman, and Kral's (2005) tests of children with cochlear implants have provided evidence, through the use of cortical auditory evoked potentials, that there is a sensitive period for central auditory development. Children implanted before age 3.5 years showed very rapid development (within a week of implantation) of the P1 component in response to a speech syllable, whereas children implanted after seven years of age showed atypical responses 1 to 1.5 years after implantation.

24.4.2   Cross-linguistic studies

A number of cross-linguistic studies have sought to determine whether the language background of listeners can influence their perception of nonspeech stimuli. For example, Tanner and Rivette (1964) observed that the frequency discrimination thresholds of several tone-language (Punjabi) listeners were much higher than those of American listeners. In a follow-up study, Tanner and Sorkin (1972) showed that these listeners could be trained to improve their discrimination thresholds. More recent studies have also found that non-tone-language listeners are more accurate than tone language listeners at (1) discriminating pitch differences in pure-tones (Stagray & Downs, 1993), (2) discriminating frequency differences in nonspeech tone complexes that varied minimally from synthetic syllables (Francis & Ciocca, 2003), and (3) identifying some sine-wave pitch contours (Bent, Bradlow, & Wright, 2006). In contrast to these findings, several other studies have reported no differences between tone- and non-tone-language listeners' abilities to discriminate pure tones (Bent, Bradlow, & Wright, 2006; Burns & Sampat, 1980) or to discriminate lexical tone stimuli which had been low-pass filtered or presented as music (Burnham, Francis, Webster, et al., 1996).

The findings on the effects of linguistic experience on nonspeech perception suggest a moderate influence of linguistic experience on nonspeech perception which is modulated by stimuli and/or task requirements. Listeners from different language groups may not perform differently on simple nonspeech stimuli, which are very distinct from more complex naturally produced speech stimuli, in a discrimination task that requires attention to small acoustic differences. However, language groups may differ on tasks that require categorization or identification of stimuli which are more complex and speech-like and approximate the process of speech perception more closely.

24.5 Summary and Conclusions

Assessing differences in perception between speech and nonspeech sounds has been and continues to be an important area of research in the field of speech perception. The primary motivation for carrying out these kinds of studies is to determine the extent to which speech perception is unique and draws on specialized neural mechanisms for perception.

The recent use of neural imaging methods has provided speech scientists with new methodological techniques that can be used to answer several fundamental questions that were difficult or impossible to explore using traditional behavioral paradigms. While the experimental methods have evolved and become more refined, the issue of whether there is a specialized neural module for processing speech still remains an open research problem. Furthermore, how listeners' prior experiences and their past developmental history influence their processing of sounds in other domains is also an important area of research. While earlier research has shown that speech and nonspeech stimuli elicit many of the same behavioral responses and that experience in one domain can influence processing in the other domain, recent neuroimaging work has provided some new converging evidence to support the hypothesis that neural activation differs during the perception of highly familiar speech signals compared to nonspeech signals. These new findings will not only advance our basic knowledge of normal processes in speech and language but will also provide a solid foundation for understanding a wide range of clinical issues in speech and hearing.

ACKNOWLEDGMENTS

This work was supported by NIH NIDCD T32 Training Grant No. DC00012 and NIH NIDCD R01 Research Grant No. DC00111 to Indiana University. We thank Adam Buchwald, Chris Conway, Susanna Levi, Jeremy Loebach, and Steve Winters for their helpful suggestions.

REFERENCES

Abercrombie, D. (1967). *Elements of General Phonetics*. Edinburgh: Edinburgh University Press.

Agnew, J. A., Dorn, C., and Eden, G. V. (2004). Effects of intensive training on auditory processing and reading skills. *Brain and Cognition*, 88, 21–5.

Benson, R., Whalen, D. H., Richardson, M., Swainson, B., Clark, V., Lai, S., and Liberman, A. M. (2001). Parametrically dissociating speech and nonspeech perception in the brain using fMRI. *Brain and Language*, 78, 364–96.

Bent, T., Bradlow, A. R., and Wright, B. A. (2006). The influence of linguistic experience on the cognitive processing of pitch in speech and nonspeech sounds. *Journal of Experimental Psychology: Human Perception and Performance*, 32, 97–103.

Bergeson, T. R. and Pisoni, D. B. (2004). Audiovisual speech perception in deaf adults and children following cochlear implantation. In G. A. Calvert, C. Spence, and B. E. Stein (eds.), *The Handbook of Multisensory Processes* (pp. 749–71). Cambridge, MA: MIT Press.

Bergeson, T. R., Pisoni, D. B., and Davis, R. A. (2005). Development of audiovisual comprehension skills in prelingually deaf children with cochlear implants. *Ear and Hearing*, 26, 149–64.

Best, C. (1995). A direct realist view of cross-language speech perception. In W. Strange (ed.), *Speech Perception and Linguistic Experience: Issues in Cross-language Research* (pp. 171–204). Baltimore, MD: York.

Bradlow, A. R., Akahane-Yamada, R., Pisoni, D. B., and Tohkura, Y. (1999). Training Japanese listeners to identify English /r/ and /l/: Long-term retention of learning in perception and production. *Perception and Psychophysics*, 61, 977–85.

Bradlow, A. R., Pisoni, D. B., Yamada, R. A., and Tohkura, Y. (1997). Training Japanese listeners to identify English /r/ and /l/. IV: Some effects of perceptual learning on speech production. *Journal of the Acoustical Society of America*, 101, 2299–310.

Burnham, D., Francis, E., Webster, D., Luksaneeyanawin, S., Attapaiboon, C., Lacerda, F., and Keller, P. (1996). Perception of lexical tone across languages: Evidence for a linguistic mode of processing. In T. Bunnell and W. Idsardi (eds.), *Proceedings of the Fourth International Conference on Spoken Language Processing*, vol. I (pp. 2514–17).

Burns, E. M. and Sampat, K. S. (1980). A note on possible culture-bound effects in frequency discrimination. *Journal of the Acoustical Society of America*, 68, 1886–8.

Calvert, G. A., Spence, C., and Stein, B. E. (2004). *The Handbook of Multisensory Processes*. Cambridge, MA: MIT Press.

Cleary, M., Pisoni, D. B., and Kirk, K. I. (2005). Influence of voice similarity on talker discrimination in children with normal hearing and children with cochlear implants. *Journal of Speech, Language, and Hearing Research*, 48, 204–23.

Erber, N. P. (1975). Auditory-visual perception of speech. *Journal of Speech and Hearing Disorders*, 40, 481–92.

Eimas, P. D. and Miller, J. L. (1980). Contextual effects in infant speech perception. *Science*, 209, 1140–1.

Fodor, J. A. (1983). *The Modularity of Mind*. Cambridge, MA: MIT Press.

Francis, A. L. and Ciocca, V. (2003). Stimulus presentation order and the perception of lexical tones in Cantonese. *Journal of the Acoustical Society of America*, 114, 1611–21.

Gandour, J., Wong, D., and Hutchins, G. (1998). Pitch processing in the human brain is influenced by language experience. *Neuroreport*, 9, 2115–19.

Garfield, J. L. (1987). Introduction: Carving the mind at its joints. In J. L. Garfield (ed.) *Modularity in Knowledge Representation and Natural Language Understanding*. Cambridge, MA: MIT Press.

Godfrey, J., Syrdal-Lasky, A., Millay, K., and Knox, C. (1981). Performance of dyslexic children on speech perception tests. *Journal of Experimental Child Psychology*, 32, 401–24.

Gordon-Salant, S. and Fitzgibbons, P. J. (2004). Effects of stimulus and noise rate variability on speech perception by younger and older adults. *Journal of the Acoustical Society of America*, 115, 1808–17.

Hayes, E. A., Warrier, C. A., Nicol, T. G., Zecker, S. G., and Kraus, N. (2003). Neural plasticity following auditory training in children with learning problems. *Clinical Neurophysiology*, 114, 674–84.

Jacquemot, C., Pallier, C., Lebihan, D., Dehaene, S., and Dupoux, E. (2003). Phonological grammar shapes the auditory cortex: A functional Magnetic Resonance Imaging study. *Journal of Neuroscience*, 23, 9541–6.

Johnson, K., Strand, E. A., and D'Imperio, M. (1999). Auditory-visual integration of talker gender in vowel perception. *Journal of Phonetics*, 27, 359–84.

Jusczyk, P. W., Pisoni, D. B., Reed, M. A., Ferald, A., and Myers, M. (1983). Infants' discrimination of the duration of a rapid spectrum change in nonspeech signals. *Science*, 222, 175–7.

Kuhl, P. K., Stevens, E., Hayashi, A., Geguchi, T., Kiritani, S., and Iverson, P. (2006). Infants show a facilitation effect for native language phonetic perception between 6 and 12 months. *Developmental Science*, 9, F13–F21.

Lane, H. (1965). The motor theory of speech perception: A critical review. *Psychological Review*, 72, 275–309.

Liberman, A. M., Harris, K., Eimas, P., Lisker, L., and Bastian, J. (1961). An effect of learning on speech perception: The discrimination of durations of silence with and without phonemic significance. *Language and Speech*, 4, 175–95.

Liberman, A. M., Harris, K. S., Hoffman, H. S., and Griffith, B. C. (1957). The discrimination of speech sounds with and across phoneme boundaries. *Journal of Experimental Psychology*, 54, 358–68.

Logan, J. D., Lively, S. E., and Pisoni, D. B. (1991). Training Japanese listeners to perceive English /r/ and /l/: A first report. *Journal of the Acoustical Society of America*, 89, 874–86.

Mattingly, I. G. and Liberman, A. M. (1990). Speech and other auditory modules. In G. M. Edelman, W. E. Gall, and W. M. Cowan (eds.), *Signal and Sense: Local and Global Order in Perceptual Maps* (pp. 501–20). New York: Wiley.

McClaskey, C. L., Pisoni, D. B., and Carrell, T. D. (1983). Transfer of training of a new linguistic contrast in voicing. *Perception and Psychophysics*, 34, 323–30.

McGurk, H. and MacDonald, J. (1976). Hearing lips and seeing voices. *Nature*, 264, 746–8.

Merzenich, M. M., Jenkins, W. M., Johnston, P., Schreiner, C., Miller, S. L., and Tallal, P. (1996). Temporal processing deficits of language-learning impaired children ameliorated by training. *Science*, 271, 77–81.

Miller, J. L. and Liberman, A. M. (1979). Some effects of later-occurring information on the perception of stop consonant and semi-vowel. *Perception and Psychophysics*, 25, 457–65.

Miller, J. D., Wier, C. C., Pastore, R., Kely, W. J., and Dooling, R. J. (1976). Discrimination and labeling of noise-buzz sequences with varying noise-lead times: An example of categorical perception. *Journal of the Acoustical Society of America*, 60, 410–17.

Mody, M., Studdert-Kennedy, M., and Brady, S. (1997). Speech perception deficits in poor readers: Auditory processing or phonological coding? *Journal of Experimental Child Psychology*, 64, 199–231.

Mottonen, R., Calvert, G. A., Jaaskeleinen, I. P., Matthews, P. M., Thesen, T., Tuomainen, J., and Sams, M. (2006). Perceiving identical sounds as speech or nonspeech modulated activity in the left posterior superior temporal sulcus. *NeuroImage*, 30, 563–9.

Mullennix, J. W., Pisoni, D. B., and Martin, C. S. (1989). Some effects of talker variability on spoken word recognition. *Journal of the Acoustical Society of America*, 85, 365–78.

Munson, B., Jefferson, S. V., and McDonald, E. C. (2006). The influence of perceived sexual orientation on fricative identification. *Journal of the Acoustical Society of America*, 119, 2427–37.

Nygaard, L. C., Sommers, M. S., and Pisoni, D. B. (1994). Speech perception as a talker-contingent process. *Psychological Science*, 5, 42–5.

Palmeri, T. J., Goldinger, S. D., and Pisoni, D. B. (1993). Episodic encoding of voice attributes and recognition memory for spoken words. *Journal of Experimental Psychology: Learning, Memory and Cognition*, 19, 309–38.

Pisoni, D. B. (1998). Development of perceptually robust tests (PRT) of speech discrimination: research, theory and preliminary findings. Guest presentation for the American Academy of Audiology, Los Angeles.

Pisoni, D. B., Carrell, T. D., and Gans, S. J. (1983). Perception of the duration of rapid spectrum changes in speech and nonspeech signals. *Perception and Psychophysics*, 34, 314–22.

Remez, R. E., Rubin, P. E., Pisoni, D. B., and Carrell, T. D. (1981). Speech perception without traditional speech cues. *Science*, 212, 947–50.

Schorr, E. A., Fox, N. A., van Wassenhove, V., and Knudsen, E. I. (2005). Auditory-visual fusion in speech perception in children with cochlear implants. *Proceedings of the National Academy of Science*, 102(51), 18748–50.

Scott, S. K. (2005). The neurobiology of speech perception. In Ann Cutler (ed.), *Twenty-first Century Psycholinguistics: Four Cornerstones* (pp. 141–56). Mahwah, NJ: Lawrence Erlbaum.

Semiclaes, W. and Sprenger-Charolles, L. (2003). Categorical perception of speech sounds and dyslexia. *Current Psychology Letters: Behaviour, Brain and Cognition*, 10(1). http://cpl.revues.org/document379.html.

Semiclaes, W., Sprenger-Charolles, L., Carre, R., and Demoney, J.-F. (2001). Perceptual discrimination of speech sounds in developmental dyslexia. *Journal of Speech, Language, and Hearing Research*, 44, 384–99.

Sharma, A., Dorman, M. F., and Kral, A. (2005). The influence of a sensitive period on central auditory development in children with unilateral and bilateral cochlear implants. *Hearing Research*, 203, 134–43.

Sommers, M. S. (1997). Stimulus variability and spoken word recognition. II. The effects of age and hearing impairment. *Journal of the Acoustical Society of America*, 101, 2278–88.

Song, J. H., Banai, K., Russo, N. M., and Kraus, N. (2006). On the relationship between speech- and nonspeech-evoked auditory brainstem responses. *Audiology and Neurotology*, 11, 232–41.

Stagray, J. R. and Downs, D. (1993). Differential sensitivity for frequency among speakers of a tone and a non-tone language. *Journal of Chinese Linguistics*, 21, 144–63.

Stevens, K. N. (1980). Acoustic correlates of some phonetic categories. *Journal of the Acoustical Society of America*, 68, 836–42.

Strange, W. and Dittman, S. (1984). Effects of discrimination training on the perception of /r-l/ by Japanese adults learning English. *Perception and Psychophysics*, 36, 131–45.

Studdert-Kennedy, M., Liberman, A. L., Harris, K. S., and Cooper, F. S. (1970). Motor theory of speech perception: A reply to Lane's critical review. *Psychological Review*, 77, 234–49.

Sumby, W. H. and Pollack, I. (1954). Visual contributions to speech intelligibility in noise. *Journal of the Acoustical Society of America*, 26, 212–15.

Tallal, P., Miller, S. L., Bedi, G., Byma, G., Wang, X., Nagarajan, S. S., Schreiner, C., Jenkins, W. M., and Merzenich, M. M. (1996). Language comprehension in language-learning impaired children improved with acoustically modified speech. *Science*, 217, 81–4.

Tanner, W. P. and Rivette, C. L. (1964). Experimental study of 'tone deafness'. *Journal of the Acoustical Society of America*, 36, 1465–7.

Tanner, W. P. and Sorkin, R. D. (1972). The theory of signal detectability. In J. V. Tobias (ed.), *Foundations of Modern Auditory Theory*. New York: Academic.

Trout, J. D. (2001). The biological basis of speech: what to infer from talking to the animals. *Psychological Review*, 108, 523–49.

Tyler, R. F., Parkinson, A. J., Woodworth, G. G., Lowder, M. W., and Gantz, B. J. (1997). Performance over time of adult patients using the Ineraid or Nucleus cochlear implant. *Journal of the Acoustical Society of America*, 102, 508–22.

Vouloumanos, A., Kiehl, K. A., Werker, J. F., and Liddle, P. F. (2001). Detection of sounds in the auditory stream: event-related fMRI evidence for differential activation to speech and nonspeech. *Journal of Cognitive Neuroscience*, 13, 994–1005.

Werker, J. and Tees, R. (1984). Phonemic and phonetic factors in adult cross-language speech perception. *Journal of the Acoustical Society of America*, 75, 1866–78.

Werker, J. F. and Tees, R. C. (1987). Speech perception in severely disabled and average reading children. *Canadian Journal of Psychology*, 41, 48–61.

25 Phonological Analysis, Phonological Processes

ADELE W. MICCIO AND
SHELLEY E. SCARPINO

25.1 Introduction

Phonological process analysis has had considerable influence on the analysis of children's phonological systems and, to a lesser extent, on the methods that have been used to treat disordered phonological systems since the 1980s. This chapter provides a summary of the theoretical basis of this approach and discusses some of the clinical issues that have arisen through the application of phonological processes to the assessment and treatment of disordered phonological systems.

25.2 Theoretical Underpinnings

According to natural phonology theory (Donegan & Stampe, 1979; Stampe, 1979), phonological processes describe phonetically motivated and natural patterns of speech production. Supporting evidence for natural theory comes from examples of evolutionary language change and from descriptions of sound change in children's developing phonological systems. Stampe (1979) argued that the sound patterns of language are governed by the limitations of the human speech perception and production mechanisms and are thus both innate and natural. During development, phonological processes merge potential phonological oppositions into the member of the opposition that puts the least strain on a human's speech ability. A phonological process will, for example, merge the potential contrast between /t/ and /k/, resulting in production of [t], the unmarked member of the pair. A child whose language requires a contrast between /t/ and /k/ will learn from experience to suppress this process (velar fronting) and produce the contrast between /t/ and /k/. A phonological process may apply to a class of sounds or sound sequences (Stampe, 1979); for example, the process of stopping results in the production of stops where fricatives occur in the adult language. The reverse would not occur naturally because fricatives have the more difficult property. A sequence of consonants may reduce to a singleton, e.g., /pl/ may reduce to the simpler member of the cluster /p/, reflecting the physiological constraints of the speech mechanism. Phonological processes can co-occur, giving rise to more unique pronunciations. On the other hand, phonological processes that do not have a clear physiological basis are not natural and are considered deviant processes.

Natural phonology does not view a child's underlying mental representation as distinct from its surface form. The underlying representation (UR) is assumed to be correct even when production is incorrect. This is a major distinction between natural phonology and generative phonology, the primary alternative view at the time (Chomsky & Halle, 1968; Kenstowicz, 1994). The generative approach, as applied to children with phonological disorders, argues against assuming that children have adult-like URs (Dinnsen, 1984). Rather, the status of the UR must be determined for each child through evaluation. To determine the nature of a child's URs, morphophonemic alterations are observed. A child who omits the final consonant of the word *dog*, for example, but produces the /g/ in the diminutive *doggie* provides evidence of an adult-like UR for *dog* and a rule for deletion of final consonants. This is not the case, however, for the child who omits /g/ in both contexts because a final consonant cannot be deleted if it is not in the UR. The primary problem with the clinical application of this approach does not relate to its utility in describing phonological change or in predicting change that would result from treatment, but is rather that the approach requires an in-depth knowledge of phonology and an understanding of rule formulation (Edwards, 1997).

In natural phonology, on the other hand, there is no need to distinguish between competence and performance by writing phonological rules that change the UR to a simpler phonetic form because the URs are equivalent to the adult forms (with the exception of predictable phonetic details). Thus, the formalisms required to write phonological rules are avoided in natural phonology. These differences led researchers (Grunwell, 1982, 1985; Ingram, 1976, 1981) to describe patterns observed in the delayed or disordered speech of young children as phonological processes. As a result of their work, the concept of phonological processes was made accessible to speech-language pathologists.

The concept of identifying patterns of change was particularly appealing in cases with multiple speech sounds in error. To describe patterns without having to understand distinctive features or write formal phonological rules was also immensely appealing to clinicians. As a result, phonological process analysis continues to influence clinical practice.

25.3   Clinical Application of Phonological Processes

Historically, linguistic theory was not applied clinically; rather clinicians used standardized articulation tests that do not differentiate among error types.

Treatment concentrated on school-age populations with residual errors related to one or a few consonants, e.g., /s/, /r/, /l/. Speech errors were viewed individually and assumed to be peripheral in nature. Phonemes in error were taught one at a time, first in words, then in larger units, following a behaviorist framework (Hodson, 1997). As increased attention was paid to early intervention with preschool children, the unintelligible speech of children with multiple errors began to receive notice.

Describing errors as phonological processes met a need to describe multiple errors. With the publication of a number of phonological process analysis procedures, process analysis became more widely applied in clinical practice, especially during the 1980s and 1990s (Dean, Howell, Hill, & Waters, 1990; Grunwell, 1985; Hodson, 1980; Ingram, 1981; Shriberg & Kwiatkowski, 1980; Weiner, 1979). Unfortunately, these assessments utilized a number of different criteria for defining phonological processes and resulted in a wide variation in the number and types of processes used to describe children's speech patterns. Grunwell (1985), for example, described nine common natural processes and 13 less common processes. Shriberg and Kwiatkowski (1980), proposed eight processes. According to these authors, a process must result in the simplification of speech production and be widely attested in natural languages. The eight processes involved phoneme deletions and/or substitutions, but not distortions. Processes also had to occur frequently in the speech of children with delayed language development and had to be transcribed reliably. This resulted in the exclusion of context-sensitive voicing from the basic processes described in Grunwell. Alternatively, Hodson (1983) included 42 observed deficient patterns and grouped them into 10 categories.

Many of the analysis procedures do not distinguish between natural and deviant processes; others include processes that describe any observed patterns without attention to the theoretical underpinnings. In general, all approaches view processes as attempts by children to simplify the adult target. While each analysis procedure differs in the number and types of processes assessed, they all attempt to describe children's productions as patterns of error.

Common processes used clinically to describe children's error patterns are listed below, with an example of each. For a more complete discussion of types of phonological processes and examples, see Velleman (1998) or Vihman (2004).

25.3.1   *Word- and syllable-level processes*

These processes affect the shape of a word or a syllable.

Unstressed syllable deletion: deletion of a syllable that is present in the adult form, usually the weak syllable before a strong syllable. 'banana' [nana]
Final consonant deletion: deletion of a word-final consonant. 'boat' [bo]
Cluster reduction: reduction of the number of consonants in a cluster. 'play' [pe]

25.3.2   Assimilation processes

These processes occur when two elements become more alike, usually in terms of consonant place, manner or voicing. Vowel harmony may also occur but is not seen as frequently in children of preschool age or older. *Assimilation* refers to two adjacent segments becoming more alike, whereas *harmony* occurs across other segments. Clinically, a distinction is not always made between harmony and assimilation; assimilation is commonly used to describe both types of sound changes.

Consonant harmony: two or more segments become more alike. 'coat' [tot]
Reduplication: the co-occurrence of consonant and vowel harmony resulting in repetition of a syllable. 'water' [wawa]

25.3.3   Substitution processes

These processes describe the substitution of one segment for another. Typical substitutions are segments with a different place of articulation, a simplification of the manner of articulation or a voicing change.

Velar fronting: production of a coronal stop for a dorsal stop. 'car' [tar]
Stopping: production of a fricative (or affricate) as the homorganic stop. 'see' [ti]
Gliding: production of a glide for a liquid. 'rope' [wop]
Vowelization (vocalization): production of a vowel for a consonant; usually for a postvocalic liquid. 'call' [ka.o]
Context-sensitive voicing: voiceless obstruents produced as voiced, usually in the word-onset or intervocalic positions. 'top' [dap]. Voiced obstruents produced as their voiceless cognates, usually in word-final codas. 'bob' [bap]

25.3.4   Atypical processes

A number of different labels describe sound changes that are not considered natural processes. Two common ones are mentioned here.

Initial consonant deletion: deletion of the word-onset consonant. 'top' [ap]
Backing: producing a consonant further back in the oral cavity for a more anterior target. This process usually describes the production of a dorsal stop for a coronal stop. 'toe' [ko]

Phonological processes call attention to systematic relationships between the target adult production and the child's simplified production, and provide a framework for describing patterns of both typical and atypical phonological acquisition (cf. Grunwell, 1985; Stoel-Gammon & Dunn, 1985). In addition to describing segment-level simplifications, phonological processes provide a straightforward way to describe common nonlinear phenomena through syllable structure and word-level processes. Over the years, the theoretical bases of phonological processes have become virtually ignored in the clinical domain. This has not been without consequences. Some of these issues are discussed below.

25.4   Issues in the Clinical Application of Phonological Processes

25.4.1   *Lack of agreement on what constitutes a process*

Natural phonology theory is based on observations of 'normal' phonological acquisition, not the clinical observation of phonological disorders. Patterns observed in disordered systems cannot always be described by natural phonological processes. As a result, most clinicians use phonological processes to label the patterns observed in a child's speech production without regard to theoretical underpinnings. Subsequently, most clinical procedures now use the term phonological patterns to refer not only to natural phonological processes, but to any patterns observed in children's productions. Totally discarding the concepts put forth in natural phonology allows clinicians to label more patterns, but it results in a lack of distinction between patterns that occur in typical development and those that are atypical or unusual (Edwards, 1992). Determining the presence of typical patterns vs. unusual ones provides information on intelligibility, severity of disorder, prognosis and appropriate targets for intervention.

25.4.2   *Lack of agreement on labels*

The same pattern is not described uniformly across process analyses. Fronting, for example, may refer to velar fronting or to any phone produced more anterior to the target, for example, producing [p] for /k/. Some terms used to describe processes result in contradictory or redundant processes within an individual and lead to confusion when analyzing data.

25.4.2.1   *Conflicting processes*

Fronting and backing, for example, may be reported in the same child. Productions of [kap] for 'top' and [ti] for 'key' may be described as backing and fronting respectively. When this happens, a key pattern is ignored. A more likely explanation of this example, and a more helpful one with regard to treatment planning, is that both instances are the result of assimilation, with front vowels triggering a more anterior production and back vowels triggering the dorsal stop. Teaching this child to produce more words with /k/ or /t/ without consideration of vowel context would not be efficacious.

25.4.2.2   Redundant processes

Stridency deletion refers to the lack of a stridency contrast. Although this label is not common across all analysis programs, it is often used to refer to any pattern that results in the loss of a strident phoneme regardless of whether or not the two segments in question contrast in stridency. Producing 'sea' as [ti], for example, may be described as both stridency deletion and as stopping. The two opposing segments, /s/ and /t/, however, do not contrast in stridency. In English, the only non-redundant stridency contrasts are /s/ and voiceless /θ/ as in 'sink' and 'think' and the contrast between /z/ and /ð/. Ignoring this distinction prevents the understanding of what a child is doing. To produce 'sink' as 'think' is not the same process as producing 'sink' as 'tink'. Clearly distinguishing among patterns describes a child's system more accurately and yields more useful information regarding treatment priorities.

25.4.3   Lack of understanding of what a child can do

Process analyses describe each word in a sample and assign processes to that individual word without looking at the entire sample for commonalities in the actual productions. Velleman (1998, p. 125) described the process analysis of a hypothetical child's speech that revealed eight processes: fronting, backing, initial consonant devoicing, stopping of fricatives, stopping of liquids, cluster reduction, alveolar consonant harmony and reduplication. One process, alveolar consonant harmony, described the largest number of errors. There were, however, a number of errors that did not conform to this pattern. In addition, contradictory processes occurred, such as fronting and backing. A reanalysis of the data, with attention to the entire sample and using the most general possible description of the child's productions, revealed that the child's phonological system contained two singleton consonants, [d] and [n]. Typically, attention is paid to what a child cannot do in relation to the adult, but not to what a child can do. Understanding that a child's phonetic inventory is limited to two consonants explains the problem and provides the information needed to design an efficacious treatment. A process account does not allow for a description of a system of this type. Recent constraints-based theories show promise for facilitating more elegant descriptions of highly constrained phonological systems.

25.4.4   Cross-linguistic application of process analysis

With the rapidly increasing number of clinical referrals for children whose first language is not English (in anglophone countries), it is important to consider the cross-linguistic application of phonological processes. If phonological processes are innate and universal, they must be attested across languages. A study of Italian children (Bortolini & Leonard, 1991) found commonalities across languages in the developmental patterns of both typically developing and disordered phonological systems. Exceptions were attributed to differences in the sound classes that occur. The trilled Italian /r/, for example, was commonly replaced with [l], rather than glides, as commonly occurs for the English rhotic consonant. Yavas and Lamprecht (1988) observed cluster reduction and liquid gliding in Portuguese-speaking children, but stopping of fricatives, glottal replacement and obstruent devoicing did not occur. So and Dodd (1994) found common processes used by both Cantonese- and English-speaking children, but observed a low frequency of gliding as well as processes in Cantonese that are not typical in English (e.g., initial consonant deletion, backing of alveolars, and substitution of [h] for aspirated plosives and /s/). Although these investigators found phonological process analysis to be a useful means of describing speech patterns cross-linguistically, there were major differences in the frequency of usage of processes across languages. This suggests that the articulatory account of children's productions is not a complete explanation of the patterns (Ingram, 1997).

Other factors, such as functional load or frequency of occurrence, are also important (Pye, Ingram, & List, 1987; Vihman & Velleman, 2000). Pye and colleagues argue that sounds will be acquired early if they occur in a greater number of important words in the child's early expressive vocabulary. The fricative /v/, for example, occurs in the early vocabulary of Italian children, whereas it is a later-occurring fricative in English (see Ingram, 1997, for an extensive discussion of cross-linguistic evidence). Findings of cross-linguistic studies suggest that more information is needed to make appropriate clinical decisions than is provided by process analysis alone.

25.5   Phonological Processes and Treatment Decision Making

As phonological processes made inroads into clinical assessment procedures, the prevalent treatments were sound-by-sound approaches that taught one sound at a time, usually in a developmental order. Alternatively, minimal-pair approaches paired a child's target sound with its substitution. In both cases, behavioral modification strategies were used to teach the target sound.

According to natural phonology, learning to pronounce requires suppression of the innate phonological system (Stampe, 1979). Evidence for this claim is provided by the observation that children make across-the-board changes once they produce a segment that they did not use previously. This view is popular among many practitioners as it asserts that a child knows the sound; consequently, he or she simply needs to learn from experience to suppress the innate processes in question.

Treatment research has not always supported this conclusion (Miccio, 1995). McReynolds and Elbert (1981) found that in the case of cluster reduction, generalization was limited to the targeted cluster type. Children who were taught /s/-clusters did not learn /r/-clusters and vice versa. Elbert and

McReynolds (1985) found that when children with final consonant deletion were taught stop-ending words, they learned words ending in stops, but generalization did not extend to words ending in fricatives. A study by Saben and Costello Ingham (1991) provides an example of more issues that arose from the application of phonological processes to treatment. Based on a phonological process analysis, they administered a minimal-pairs treatment to two children with no direct teaching of the target sound. Participants were asked to produce a target sound paired with its substitution. For both children, modeling and phonetic placement cues had to be added before change occurred and generalization did not extend to other phonemes affected by the target processes. These investigators defined a correct response as one in which the target process was suppressed. In other words, production of any fricative was considered a correct response to the goal of suppressing stopping of fricatives (Ingram, 1976; Monahan, 1986; Weiner, 1981). These decisions were made on the assumption that the children would become aware of the need for the contrast and produce it. In this study, the children were unable to produce the target sound and were confused by the reinforcement of any fricative, i.e., [f] for /s/. It is not known how children who have some productive knowledge of the target sound would have responded to the same treatment, but reinforcement of any sound that results in a process change, rather than a correctly produced target, has not proven to be an effective strategy.

Since these early studies that investigated the application of phonological processes to treatment, experiments have shown that complexity is likely the most robust predictor of phonological change as a result of treatment, i.e. treatment of more complex targets such as typologically marked properties, non-stimulable sounds, sounds excluded from the phonetic inventory and sounds in words from low-density neighborhoods (cf. Gierut, 1998, 2001). These and other complexity factors may not always be apparent from phonological process analysis.

Regardless of the theoretical basis of an analysis used to describe a phonological system, treatments may not differ greatly. This is not usually the fault of the theory, but rather lies in the clinical application of bits and pieces without an understanding of the larger picture. As described above, current phonological process approaches do not usually distinguish between processes used by typically developing children and those that may be described as deviant or atypical. Furthermore, diverse labeling procedures lead to the lack of a clear understanding of a child's system. As a result, crucial information for designing efficacious treatments may be ignored.

25.6 Contributions of Phonological Process Analysis to Phonological Disorders

Effective clinical assessment requires knowledge of typical phonological development. The attention paid to describing the many processes that occur across children and across languages has advanced our understanding of typical acquisition. Although the physiological underpinnings of phonological processes are often ignored, natural phonology has led to positive changes in how clinicians look at children's phonological systems by calling attention to patterns. Clinicians learned how sounds fall into natural classes and that phonological problems may relate to entire sound classes or levels above the segment. Despite the criticisms of process analysis or its clinical implementation, it has led to the recognition of multiple levels of the phonological hierarchy and the subsequent application of principles from a number of phonological theories to clinical issues (Ball & Kent, 1997).

Nonlinear theories now influence both assessment and treatment (see Bernhardt & Stemberger, chapter 26 in this volume, and Dinnsen & Gierut, chapter 27). Some of these approaches are nonlinear extensions of generative linguistics, but they are also heavily influenced by natural phonology and its ability to describe patterns above the level of the segment. As more attention is turned to current theories, it is important to remember that some of the recent developments are linked to previous work in natural phonology and phonological processes.

REFERENCES

Ball, M. J. and Kent, R. D. (eds.) (1997). *The New Phonologies: Developments in Clinical Linguistics*. San Diego: Singular Publishing.

Bortolini, U. and Leonard, L. B. (1991). The speech of phonologically disordered children acquiring Italian. *Clinical Linguistics and Phonetics*, 8, 283–93.

Chomsky, N. and Halle, M. (1968). *The Sound Pattern of English*. New York: Harper & Row.

Dean, E. C., Howell, J., Hill, A., and Waters, D. (1990). *Metaphon Resource Pack*. Windsor, Berks: NFER-Nelson.

Dinnsen, D. A. (1984). Methods and empirical issues in analyzing functional misarticulation. In M. Elbert, D. A. Dinnsen, and G. Weismer (eds.), *Phonological Theory and the Misarticulating Child*, ASHA Monographs, 22 (pp. 5–17). Rockville, MD: ASHA.

Donegan, P. J. and Stampe, D. (1979). The study of natural phonology. In D. A. Dinnsen (ed.), *Current Approaches to Phonological Theory* (pp. 126–73). Bloomington: Indiana University Press.

Edwards, M. L. (1992). In support of phonological processes. *Language, Speech and Hearing in Schools*, 23, 233–40.

Edwards, M. L. (1997). Historical overview of clinical phonology. In B. W. Hodson and M. L. Edwards (eds.), *Perspectives in Applied Phonology* (pp. 1–18). Gaithersburg, MD: Aspen.

Elbert, M. and McReynolds, L. (1985). The generalization hypothesis: Final consonant deletion. *Language and Speech*, 28, 281–94.

Gierut, J. A. (1998). Treatment efficacy: Functional phonological disorders in children. *Journal of Speech, Language and Hearing Research*, 41, S85–S100.

Gierut, J. A. (2001). Complexity in phonological treatment: Clinical factors. *Language, Speech, and Hearing Services in Schools*, 32, 229–41.

Grunwell, P. (1982). *Clinical Phonology*. Rockville, MD: Aspen.

Grunwell, P. (1985). *Phonological Assessment of Child Speech (PACS)*. Windsor, Berks: NFER-Nelson.

Hodson, B. W. (1980). *The Assessment of Phonological Processes*. Danville, IL: Interstate.

Hodson, B. (1983). A facilitative approach for remediation of a child's profoundly unintelligible phonological system. *Topics in Language Disorders*, 3, 24–34.

Hodson, B. W. (1997). Disordered phonologies: What have we learned about assessment and treatment? In B. W. Hodson and M. L. Edwards (eds.), *Perspectives in Applied Phonology* (pp. 197–224). Gaithersburg, MD: Aspen.

Ingram, D. (1976). *Phonological Disability in Children*. New York: Elsevier.

Ingram, D. (1981). *Procedures for the Phonological Analysis of Children's Language*. Baltimore, MD: University Park Press.

Ingram, D. (1997). The categorization of phonological impairment. In B. W. Hodson and M. L. Edwards (eds.), *Perspectives in Applied Phonology* (pp. 19–42). Gaithersburg, MD: Aspen.

Kenstowicz, M. (1994). *Phonology in Generative Grammar*. Cambridge, MA: Blackwell.

McReynolds, L. and Elbert, M. (1981). Criteria for phonological process analysis. *Journal of Speech and Hearing Disorders*, 46, 197–204.

Miccio, A. W. (1995). Metaphon: factors contributing to treatment outcomes. *Clinical Linguistics and Phonetics*, 9, 28–36.

Monahan, D. (1986). Remediation of common phonological processes: Four case studies. *Language, Speech and Hearing Services in Schools*, 17, 199–206.

Pye, C., Ingram, D., and List, H. (1987). A comparison of initial consonant acquisition in English and Quiché. In K. Nelson and A. van Kleeck (eds.), *Children's Language*, vol. 6 (pp. 175–90). Hillsdale, NJ: Erlbaum.

Saben, C. and Costello Ingham, J. (1991). The effects of minimal pairs treatment on the speech-sound production of two children with phonologic disorders. *Journal of Speech and Hearing Research*, 34, 1023–40.

Shriberg, L. D. and Kwiatkowski, J. (1980). *Natural Process Analysis*. New York: John Wiley.

So, L. K. H. and Dodd, B. (1994). Phonologically disordered Cantonese-speaking children. *Clinical Linguistics and Phonetics*, 8, 235–55.

Stampe, D. (1979). *A Dissertation on Natural Phonology*. New York: Garland.

Stoel-Gammon, C. and Dunn, C. (1985). *Normal and Disordered Phonology in Children*. Austin, TX: Pro-Ed.

Velleman, S. L. (1998). *Making Phonology Functional: What do I Do First?* Boston: Butterworth-Heinemann.

Vihman, M. M. (2004). Later phonological development. In J. Bernthal and N. Bankson (eds.), *Articulation and Phonological Disorders*, 5th ed. (pp. 105–38). Boston: Allyn and Bacon.

Vihman, M. M. and Velleman, S. L. (2000). Phonetics and the origins of phonology. In N. Burton-Roberts, P. Carr, and G. Docherty (eds.), *Phonological Knowledge: Its Nature and Status* (pp. 305–39). Oxford: Oxford University Press.

Weiner, F. (1979). *Phonological Process Analysis*. Baltimore, MD: University Park Press.

Weiner, F. (1981). Treatment of phonological disability using the method of meaningful minimal contrast: Two case studies. *Journal of Speech and Hearing Disorders*, 46, 97–103.

Yavas, M. and Lamprecht, R. (1988). Processes and intelligibility in disordered phonology. *Clinical Linguistics and Linguistics*, 2, 329–45.

26 Constraints-Based Nonlinear Phonological Theories: Application and Implications

BARBARA M. H. BERNHARDT AND
JOSEPH P. STEMBERGER

26.1 Introduction

The current chapter describes the clinical application of constraints-based nonlinear phonological theories. The first part of the chapter presents an overview of the theories, focusing on those constructs that have been applied clinically concerning phonological hierarchies, the autonomy and interaction of phonological elements, feature status, and syllable structure. The second part of the chapter discusses clinical applications.

26.2 Phonological Theories over Time

Speech-language pathology has tracked changes in phonological theory for the past 60 years. Structuralist theories of linguistics (e.g. Hockett, 1955) treated phonological representations as a string of segments (phonemes) with phonological properties such as voicing and frication; consequently, 'articulation' therapy focused on the 'sounds' (Van Riper & Irwin, 1959). Generative phonological theories (e.g. Chomsky & Halle, 1968) expanded the focus on features, viewed as defining natural classes of segments that patterned in similar ways. Phonological phenomena came to be described in terms of rules or processes that altered phonological representations by changing features, or by inserting or deleting whole segments. Child pronunciations were considered a result of such rules or processes. Some argued that children's processes were universal (e.g. Stampe, 1972), while others assumed that rules or processes could vary across children (e.g. Smith, 1973). Clinical applications followed these theoretical changes, with approaches using distinctive features, phonological rules (Blache, 1978; Dinnsen & Elbert, 1984; McReynolds & Engmann, 1975), and phonological processes (e.g. Edwards & Bernhardt, 1973; Grunwell, 1985; Hodson, 1986; Ingram, 1976, Shriberg & Kwiatkowski, 1980; Weiner, 1979). Key to many theoretical views of phonology before the mid-1970s was that phonological phenomena could be described in terms of (linear) sequential CV strings. Chomsky and Halle (1968) claimed that there was no need to group segments into larger units such as syllables in phonological representations.

A shift in phonological theory occurred in the 1970s, in which phonology came to be viewed as hierarchically organized (nonlinear). Phonologists such as Fudge (1969), Hooper (1976) and Kahn (1976) asserted that syllable structure is needed in phonological representations, thus harking back to concepts of some earlier accounts of phonology (including Hockett, 1955). Features also came to be viewed differently. Goldsmith (1976) demonstrated that features often acted autonomously (i.e., not as inherent properties of segments) in deletion, addition or assimilation patterns. The work of Goldsmith (1976) and Kahn (1976) led to a major shift in phonological theory. Phonological representations were described not as a single string of *segments*, but as 'nonlinear', i.e. made up of many different lines ('tiers' or 'levels'), each containing different information and extending over different periods of time. For example, features could be as short as half a segment or extend across (be linked to) many segments; similarly, segments could extend across more than one syllable position ('ambisyllabic'). Segments were considered only one level of representation; they were dominated by and incorporated into increasingly larger units, i.e., syllables, feet (two or more syllables) and phonological words (one or more feet). (See figures 26.1 and 26.2.) Below the level of the segment, features were also seen as hierarchically organized (e.g. Clements, 1985; Sagey, 1986; McCarthy, 1988). Manner, place and laryngeal features were grouped together separately from each other, but linked together by major organizing 'cover' features (or 'nodes') of Place, Laryngeal and Root (Manner) (see figure 26.2). Although each feature was still considered autonomous (Goldsmith, 1976), groupings of features reflected patterns observed in phonological phenomena.

The feature, rather than the segment, thus became a major element of focus for describing many phonological phenomena. Beyond the concepts of hierarchical structure and relative autonomy, feature theory developed further in terms of the status of feature values. From early accounts of features (Chomsky & Halle, 1968; Jakobson, 1968), it had been posited that, given two values for a feature (plus and minus), one was more 'marked' (less common, more complex) than the other. In the 1980s, the term 'default' came to be used to describe the least marked feature value from a set of competing feature values, whether binary (two-valued) features such as [continuant] or monovalent (single-valued) features such as [Coronal]. High-frequency (unmarked) default features were posited to have special properties, including (1) a tendency to be acquired early and to substitute for lower-frequency (marked) 'non-default' features, and (2) a tendency to be replaced by low-frequency non-default

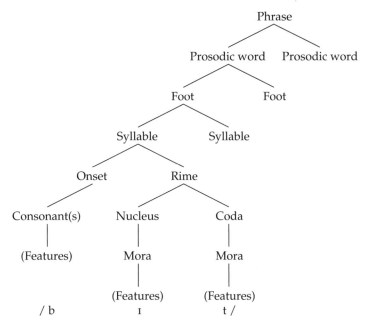

Figure 26.1   The phonological hierarchy from the level of the prosodic phrase to the moras (weight or timing units).

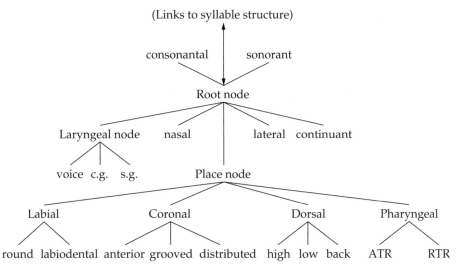

Figure 26.2   The feature hierarchy, showing Root (manner) features, Laryngeal features, and Place features. Note: s.g. = spread glottis, c.g. = constricted glottis; ATR = advanced tongue root, RTR = retracted tongue root. The Root node links upward to the prosodic tiers and downward to manner features and the Laryngeal and Place nodes.

features under some conditions. For example, default [Coronal] ('alveolar') initially substitutes for non-default [Dorsal] ('velar') (e.g., *cow* [tʰaʊ]), but later tends to be replaced by [Dorsal] in consonant harmony (e.g. *duck* [gak]). Both patterns can be accounted for if [Coronal] is left unspecified (as a default) in lexical representations. Thus, *unless* place of articulation is supplied in some other way, such as [Dorsal] spreading in from another segment via the process of assimilation, the default [Coronal] will be supplied automatically by the phonological system. Accounts of child phonology have often included mention of "systematic sound preferences" in a child's speech (Edwards & Shriberg, 1983). The concept of default is consistent with the phenomenon of systematic sound preferences, which implies widespread overgeneralization of high-frequency default features (Bernhardt & Stemberger, 1998). (Note that child defaults do not necessarily match those of adult systems.) In essence, treating each feature as an independent autonomous element allows surface phonological representations to be constructed from incomplete lexical representations, with certain consequences for development, such as use of 'systematic sound preferences', high frequency of defaults in substitutions, elimination of defaults in assimilation patterns and constraints on combinations of more complex, non-default features (Bernhardt & Stemberger, 1998).

The description of phonological tiers above the segment (syllable, foot, prosodic word) also evolved. For example, phonological phenomena such as compensatory lengthening, where vowel lengthening compensated for missing syllable-final consonants (codas), suggested that durational information was also part of phonological representation. This led to the positing of a 'timing' tier between the features and the syllable. The ultimate syllable theory posited 'moras' ('weight' or timing units), which could appear only in the rime of the syllable (see e.g., Kenstowicz, 1994). It had often been observed that 'light' syllables (with a short vowel and no coda) patterned differently than 'heavy' syllables (which have a long vowel, a diphthong, and/or a coda), and that this had consequences for stress and vowel length among other patterns. It was suggested that short vowels have one mora (and a coda may also have one in some languages, including English), but a long vowel or a diphthong has two (e.g., Hayes, 1989, 1995; Kenstowicz, 1994) (see figure 26.1.) Moras divide syllables into an onset, which has no weight, and a rime, which may have one or two weight units; there is a sense in which the words *kitty* (with one mora on /ɪ/ and one on /i/) and *sit* (with one mora on /ɪ/ and one on /t/) have parallel rhythmical patterns (see figure 26.1).

Introduction of multiple tiers and hierarchical structure had other effects on the description of phonological phenomena. For example, the notion of adjacency (which elements are 'next to' each other) changed. Adjacency was considered a critical factor for triggering of phonological alternations, but in earlier approaches to phonology, two elements were considered adjacent only if they were in immediately neighboring segments. Phonological rules thus had difficulty explaining how two segments that were not immediately next to one another could interact, as in, for example, vowel harmony 'across' consonants or consonant harmony 'across' vowels, e.g. [gɪg] for /dɪg/. Nonlinear descriptions solved this theoretical puzzle by showing how elements could be adjacent on one tier even if non-adjacent on some other tier. Figure 26.3 shows adjacency of the feature [Labial] in the word *plum*. Since the /l/ and the vowel in the word *plum* are not labial, the [Labial] feature of the /p/ is adjacent to the [Labial] feature of the /m/. However, the place features of the /p/ and the /l/ are also adjacent, because they have adjacent Place nodes.

Vowel harmony across intervening consonants was possible because the vowels were adjacent on a vowel 'tier' (e.g. Kenstowicz, 1994), and, similarly, consonant harmony was possible (e.g. [pɑp] for *top*) because consonants were adjacent on a consonant tier (e.g. Stemberger, 1988; Stemberger & Stoel-Gammon, 1991).

A key theoretical development throughout this period concerned the role of constraints. While elements of the phonological hierarchy were considered autonomous, it was also argued (e.g., Goldsmith, 1976) that representations and phonological patterns were subject to ('well-formedness') constraints. For example, segments could only rarely be specified for two competing features (e.g. with a change from [+nasal] to [−nasal] in the middle of a single segment). In addition, a constraint on repetition was posited: two identical elements should not occur next to other on a given tier (the 'Obligatory Contour Principle', or 'OCP').

Paradis (1988), for example, proposed that all processes were driven by constraints on outputs. If a language had a constraint that codas were impossible, and there were consonants that would have been expected to wind up in codas, then a process was needed to 'repair' the phonological representation so that the constraint was not 'violated': the consonant could be deleted, or made syllabic, or made the onset of a syllable. For a given constraint, only a very small number of processes could repair a violation (deriving a predicted cross-linguistic typology of repairs for a given constraint). Constraints and processes remained two separate theoretical mechanisms, however. Prince and Smolensky (1993) and McCarthy and Prince (1993) introduced Optimality

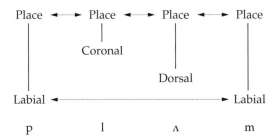

Figure 26.3 Feature adjacency. Note: Segments can be adjacent (next to each other) at the level of general Place of articulation (e.g., *p* and *l*). The /p/ and /m/ are also adjacent because they share [Labial].

Theory (OT), taking their inspiration from the theory of constraints and repairs, but generalizing constraints in a way that even eliminated the need for processes (see Dinnsen and Gierut, chapter 27 in this volume, for more details on OT). Constraints were viewed as relative to one another (some high-ranked or more powerful than others which are low-ranked). In its ranking of constraints, OT is another instantiation of hierarchy in phonological theory.

Constraints lead to a different way of viewing phonological patterns, especially concerning phonological development. Processes seem like entirely arbitrary mechanisms that add complexity to human language for no obvious purpose. For example, child language processes reflect a situation where the child's phonology is like the adult's phonology, but with many extra processes (e.g. Stampe, 1972), contradicting our general impression that child language is simplified and reduced relative to adult language. Constraints take the point of view that there are limitations on phonology (as on all human behavior), and that there are far more limitations on what children are capable of producing than on what adults are capable of producing; phonological reductions in child phonology are more easily explained from the perspective of constraints than from the perspective of processes and rules (see Bernhardt & Stemberger, 1998; Stemberger & Bernhardt, 1997, for in-depth discussions of OT from a developmental psycholinguistic perspective). While the focus of research in OT has been on the constraints, nonlinear representations were incorporated into the constraint-based accounts, and are taken for granted in almost all of the current work in phonological theory (see Bernhardt & Stemberger, 1998; Dinnsen & Gierut, chapter 27 in this volume; Stemberger & Bernhardt, 1997). The following section outlines clinical applications of the nonlinear theories in the last two decades.

26.3　Clinical Application of Constraints-Based Nonlinear Phonological Theories

Clinical applications of nonlinear phonology began in the 1980s. Spencer (1984) convincingly applied nonlinear concepts concerning the syllable and the autonomy of phonological elements to explain unusual patterns of reduplication in a 6-year-old with a phonological impairment. At the end of the paper, he suggested that the "repercussions for diagnosis and treatment of phonological disability . . . [were] self-evident" (p. 347), a challenge which resulted in a dissertation and several subsequent studies applying nonlinear phonological theory to intervention (e.g. Bernhardt, 1990; Bernhardt, 1992a, 1992b; Bernhardt, 1994b; Bernhardt, Brooke, & Major, 2003; Bernhardt & Gilbert, 1992; Bernhardt, MacNeill, & Bohlen, 1994; Edwards, 1995; Major & Bernhardt, 1998; Noble-Wiebe, McFarlane, & Bernhardt, 1995; Ullrich & Bernhardt, 2005; Von Bremen, 1990). Most clinical applications have concerned child phonology (e.g. Bernhardt & Stemberger, 2000), with clinical applications for adult neurogenic disorders limited primarily to descriptions concerning effects of syllable structure; for adult disorders, few studies of features have been inspired by a nonlinear approach, particularly for treatment (see section 26.4.5 below).

26.4 Studies of Phonological Intervention for Children Applying Nonlinear Phonological Theory

Clinical studies applying nonlinear frameworks have been conducted over the last two decades with both English- and German-speaking children with moderate to severe phonological (primary) impairments (see references above). The following major concepts of nonlinear phonological theory have been addressed in the various studies: (1) phonological hierarchy, (2) autonomy versus interaction of phonological elements, (3) syllable structure in terms of moras versus the division into onset and rime, and (4) defaults versus non-defaults. Highlights of some of the studies are described below.

26.4.1 *Phonological hierarchy and autonomy of phonological units*

In a series of eight- to 18-week intervention studies conducted in the 1990s, a number of theoretical tenets from nonlinear phonology were examined for English. In order to examine the concepts of phonological hierarchy and autonomy of phonological elements, detailed analyses were first performed for word structure, segments and features. In the intervention studies, separate word-structure and feature/segmental targets were included within each treatment block, with three to four sessions in a row devoted to a particular target. (An exception was Von Bremen, 1990, a study with identical twins, in which one twin had only structural targets and the other had only feature/segmental targets.) For example, in Bernhardt (1992b), the child (age 5;10) had these structural and feature targets in the first six-week treatment block.

1 Word structure: Word-initial clusters with segments already in his phonetic inventory, i.e., stop-/w/ and stop-/j/ clusters.
2 Features:
   [+lateral] (or [+consonantal] and [+sonorant]) for /l/
   Coronal [−anterior] for the palatoalveolars /ʃ/, /tʃ/, /dʒ/, /ʒ/

In addition, in Bernhardt (1990, 1992b) and Bernhardt and Gilbert (1992), (non-default) features at higher and lower positions in the feature hierarchy were contrasted in alternating treatment periods. The features for /l/ were manner features and thus considered 'higher' in the feature hierarchy than the place features for the palatoalveolars (see figure 26.2). In keeping with the notion of autonomy, new features were targeted in available structures and vice versa.

Overall, children showed independent and faster rates of change for word and syllable structure targets than for segmental feature targets in the studies. In Bernhardt's (1990) 18-week study with six children, word-structure targets significantly outstripped segmental targets in the first six-week block of treatment (Wilcoxon's, $p = .015$). For Von Bremen's identical twin participants, the twin assigned to the word-structure condition mastered his targets and the segmental targets of his brother well before the second twin mastered his own or his brother's targets. In a 12-week study (reported in Major and Bernhardt, 1998), word-shape accuracy for 19 children increased by an average of 24%, compared with a 13% gain for segmental accuracy excluding deletions ($t = 2.11038$, $p < .05$). For 12 participants (Bernhardt, Brooke, & Major, 2003), the greatest gain across participants was observed for the CVCV word structure (32.94% gain), with overall structural targets slightly outstripping segmental targets (although not significantly: 21% and 18% gain respectively). Note that the general pattern was not universal in the studies; at least one child showed faster mastery of a feature than of structure (e.g. Bernhardt & Stemberger, 2000; Craig learned [+lateral] for /l/ before mastering CVC and CVCV).

The data suggest that the concepts of autonomy and hierarchy (features versus structures) are relevant in phonological intervention. In the studies conducted in the 1990s, features and structures showed independent developmental trajectories; higher-level structure usually showed earlier gains than lower-level segments and features, with lower-level features occasionally outstripping higher-level structural targets. Including both feature and structural targets in the first block (period) of a treatment program can enhance the child's potential for early change. Note that it is not inefficient to target new segments and features in the first phase of intervention, even if they are not going to be acquired at that time. First of all, different children show different developmental paths as noted above for Craig. Furthermore, if a cyclic approach to intervention (as introduced by Hodson & Paden, 1983) is adopted, the first block of treatment is simply an introduction. In Bernhardt (1992b), the child was not able to articulate palatoalveolars accurately (i.e., was not stimulable) in the first block of treatment, even though he made significant gains in cluster development and some gains for /l/. However, his very first imitation of a palatoalveolar in the second treatment block was accurate in spite of *no* intermediate training on that target. The initial block of treatment had some unobserved impact on his learning of those targets, even though he showed no immediate gains at the end of Block 1. Overall, the independent targeting of features and structures appears to be a reasonable approach to target selection. The exact number, order and type of targets will necessarily reflect the number of structural and feature needs in a child's system, and will also take into account other factors concerning the child (hearing status, oral mechanism constraints, cognitive and general linguistic abilities, attention and focus, and family and clinic/school support, as noted in Bernhardt, Stemberger,

& Major, 2006). Would new features and word structures ever be targeted jointly, e.g., putting fricatives (a new manner category) in codas of CVC, a new structure? If a particular child shows no associated personal or environmental issues (i.e., has excellent perception, attention, oral-motor and cognitive abilities and environmental support), it may be efficient to target new features and word structures jointly, although this has not been studied directly.

Further to the notion of hierarchy, in Bernhardt (1990) and Von Bremen (1990), higher-level features in the hierarchy did show faster gains than lower-level features for seven out of eight participants. Manner (root node) and laryngeal features were learned more quickly than lower-level place features, in accordance with their relative location in the feature hierarchy. Because it is difficult to determine what is 'high' and what is 'low' across phonological systems, however, subsequent studies have contrasted acquisition of new individual (non-default) features with new combinations of non-default features already present.

26.4.2   *Interactions of phonological units*

Two types of phonological targets addressed the interaction of phonological units in the treatment studies. The first concerned the expansion of available segmental/feature content into word positions where that feature/segment did not yet appear, i.e., an interaction between segments and structure. For example, if a child used fricatives only word-finally but had other consonants word-initially, a treatment target might be word-initial fricatives. The second type of interaction addressed within-segment interactions, i.e. combinations of available features into segments that were not yet present. For example, if a pre-treatment inventory included anterior coronal (alveolar) stops, labial stops and labiodental fricatives ([Labial]&[±continuant]&[−sonorant]), a new feature combination would be coronal (alveolar) fricatives ([Coronal, +anterior]&[+continuant]&[−sonorant]) (Mandy, in Bernhardt & Stemberger, 2000, ch. 7).

26.4.3   *Onset–rime versus moras*

Onset–rime syllable divisions versus syllable weight units (moras) have been compared as the focus of treatment for syllable-structure intervention (Bernhardt, 1990, 1994a, 1994b). English content words require a minimum of two moras, and have either at least two syllables, or a single syllable with a long vowel, a diphthong or a coda. A monosyllabic word with a lax vowel and no coda, e.g. */bɪ/, is not possible in English. Thus, lax vowels were used when taking a moraic approach to target CVC, because codas are obligatory in that context. Onset–rime applications involved separate targeting of onsets and rhymes ('*sm*' versus '*all*' for *small*) or moving segments and features to new word positions through 'backwards chaining': ('*ooze-ooze-ooze-oo-zoo*') (Bernhardt, 1990, 1994a; Bernhardt & Stemberger, 2000). Although Bernhardt

(1990) showed no significant difference in acquisition of targets presented with a focus on onsets–rimes versus moras, it is possible that the use of both approaches to presentation of structural stimuli emphasized the various aspects of word structure and syllable timing, facilitating the faster rate of change for syllable and word structure than for segments.

26.4.4   Defaults and non-defaults

Throughout the studies, frequency and substitution patterns were used to determine a child's default values for structures and features. Highly frequent forms were often viewed as defaults, but substitutions or features that were replaced in assimilation (the [Coronal] of the /t/ in *take* as [keɪk]) were also viewed as potential defaults. With the assumption that marked (lower-frequency, non-default) features and structures are more challenging than defaults, treatment typically targeted adult non-defaults. Exceptions occurred when a child had a different default value from that of the adult, e.g., a velar place default, in which case the adult default was the target (here [Coronal] instead of [Dorsal]). Defaults were also exploited in treatment as supports for new phonological elements: default features were often used when targeting new (non-default) syllable structures. Similarly, default structures were often used to target new features and segments. This approach derives assumptions concerning the nature of features versus structures in interactions. In adult phonology, default features are more frequent in marked word positions (e.g. Bernhardt & Stemberger, 1998; Hammond, 1999). The assumption was that it is easier to learn new (non-default) structures when using well-learned (default) features, and vice versa. After a child learned to combine a default and a non-default element, then non-default elements were targeted simultaneously (that is, non-default structure, non-default feature, e.g. with a fricative in a consonant cluster). Again, if a child appears to be an engaged and confident risk-taker during assessment, the double challenge (new non-default feature + new non-default structure) could perhaps be targeted at the outset. The concepts of defaults and non-defaults have proven useful for describing observed phonological patterns and for determining goals for intervention, focusing on the non-defaults (or what needs to be learned, i.e., is not 'given' by the phonological system).

Overall, children made significant gains in the intervention studies conducted, gaining age-appropriate phonology or moving from a severe level of impairment to a mild-moderate level of impairment in an eight- to 18-week period. In a longer-term outcome evaluation (Bernhardt & Major, 2005), all but two of twelve participants (who had moderate to severe phonological impairments pre-treatment) had age-appropriate language and literacy scores, with only five showing any minor articulatory mismatches. These results suggest that a concentrated focus on the various aspects of the phonological system may have long-term benefits for speech and literacy.

26.4.5 *Studies applying nonlinear phonological theory to adults with neurogenic impairments*

A number of studies have addressed the role of syllable structure in neurogenic impairments, but few have addressed notions about features deriving from nonlinear phonology, and application to clinical treatment is almost non-existent.

Nickels and Howard (2004) provide an overview of the literature showing that more marked syllable structures are subject to higher error rates in aphasic disorders. They argue, however, that the effects reported up to that point, and in their own study, could derive just from complexity: words with more phonemes are subject to greater error rates. Romani and Galluzzi (2005) argue that there are indeed effects separate from complexity. They introduce a scale that combines structural and segmental markedness and show that it correlates with error rates, separately from complexity *per se*. Maas, Barlow, Robin, and Shapiro (2002) is one of the few papers attempting clinical applications. On the basis of the treatment of two patients, they argue that treatment with more complex syllables (with three-consonant onsets such as /str/) led to improvement in all onsets regardless of number of consonants, but treatment with simple syllables (with single-consonant onsets) was effective only for treatment of singleton onsets. This could be interpreted as showing that treatment of both structural and segmental targets (e.g., in /str/) leads to improvement in both structure and segments, whereas treatment of only segmental targets leads to improvement only of segments. It should be noted, however, that these authors focus rather on the fact that the more complex treatment targets had more effect overall, and the results are ambiguous between effects of syllables versus effects of the segmental complexity of the treatment syllables.

A few studies have addressed feature issues specifically. For example, Béland, Paradis, and Bois (1993) showed that consonant clusters containing two non-default place features ([Labial], [Dorsal], and [−anterior]) have a higher error rate than clusters involving default [Coronal,+anterior] plus one non-default place feature. We know of no clinical intervention applying nonlinear approaches to feature remediation in adults.

26.5 Talking Back to Theory

The scope and length of this chapter does not allow us to comment on what the clinical data have to say for the theories, but see Bernhardt (1994a), Bernhardt and Stemberger (1998) and Bernhardt and Stemberger (2007) for in-depth discussions of this nature.

26.6   Clinical Application: Present and Future

For clinical purposes, it is important to find efficient and effective methods for assessment and analysis, and to evaluate various intervention methodologies and plans. Some research has been conducted on the outcomes of nonlinear phonological intervention; it is briefly described above.

Concerning assessment, Bernhardt and Holdgrafer (2001a, 2001b) describe procedures for ensuring that all relevant aspects of the phonological hierarchy are probed for speech samples. Qualitative or quantitative analyses can be performed, examining the various levels of the phonological hierarchy (e.g. Bernhardt & Stemberger, 2000; Bernhardt & Stoel-Gammon, 1994). After six to eight data sets of practice, most clinicians can perform a complete scan (non-quantitative) analysis (including intervention planning) for a child with a moderate to severe phonological impairment in less than two hours. With experience, analysis can take less than an hour, depending on the complexity of the sample. Time spent in assessment is time saved during treatment. If quantitative analysis is needed, hand-counting is possible, or a computer program may be utilized, e.g., Long's Computerized Profiling (PROPH; Long, 2006, a free shareware program), or the Computerized Articulation and Phonology Evaluation System (CAPES; Masterson & Bernhardt, 2001). Such methods have primarily been used for child data to date, but there is nothing limiting their use to children's data only. Speech-language pathologists may find the tools helpful also in characterization of adult speech disturbances of a more phonological nature. Extension to languages other than English has begun with German (Ullrich & Bernhardt, 2005), and extensions are planned to Mandarin, Arabic, Slovene, Spanish, Hungarian, Japanese and Zapotec (an indigenous language of Mexico). Although the tools discussed here do not mention OT or constraints, it is assumed throughout that a set of ranked constraints operate to yield a child's pronunciation. Targeting the non-default structures and features promotes faithfulness and helps the child overcome markedness constraints, aligning the child's system with the rankings of the adult system.

It would be a remarkable computer program that could take the raw audio-files of the child, transcribe them reliably, analyze them according to the most elegant phonological theory and present a ranked set of hierarchical targets for implementation and outcomes evaluation. Of course, that computer program would have to be able to take all of a child's other needs into account, including family support, hearing status, physical abilities, personality, motivation and so on. For the foreseeable future, the fuzzy logic of human beings appears to be needed, as flawed as it sometimes can be, and as poor as we may be at predicting outcomes of treatment based on our assessment. As phonological theories develop, the researcher in child phonology may find better ways of interpreting phonological patterns that will lead to more informed choices for analysis and intervention. In the interim, clinicians are encouraged to engage with the constraints-based nonlinear theories of the past 30 years, to see where these concepts and methods may take them and their clients. Further reading can be found in Baker and Bernhardt (2004), Bernhardt (2005), Bernhardt and Stoel-Gammon (1996), Masterson, Bernhardt, and Hofheinz (2005), Stemberger (1991), Stemberger and Bernhardt (1999), Stemberger, Bernhardt, and Johnson (2001), and Stemberger and Middleton (2003).

REFERENCES

Baker, E. and Bernhardt, B. (2004). From hindsight to foresight: Working around barriers to success in phonological intervention. *Child Language Teaching and Therapy*, 20, 287–318.

Béland, R., Paradis, C., and Bois, M. (1993). Constraints and repairs in aphasic speech: A group study. *Canadian Journal of Linguistics*, 38, 279–302.

Bernhardt, B. (1990). Application of nonlinear phonological theory to intervention with six phonologically disordered children. Unpublished PhD dissertation, University of British Columbia.

Bernhardt, B. (1992a). Developmental implications of nonlinear phonological theory. *Clinical Linguistics and Phonetics*, 6, 259–82.

Bernhardt, B. (1992b). The application of nonlinear phonological theory to intervention. *Clinical Linguistics and Phonetics*, 6, 283–316.

Bernhardt, B. (1994a). The prosodic tier and phonological disorders. In M. Yavas (ed.), *First and Second Language Acquisition* (pp. 149–72). San Diego, CA: Singular Press.

Bernhardt, B. (1994b). Phonological intervention techniques for syllable and word structure development. *Clinics in Communication Disorders*, 4(1), 54–65.

Bernhardt, B. (2005). Selection of phonological goals and targets: Not just an exercise in phonological analysis. In A. Kamhi and K. Pollock (eds.), *Phonological Disorders in Children: Clinical Decision-making in Assessment and Intervention* (pp. 109–20). Baltimore, MD: Paul H. Brookes.

Bernhardt, B., Brooke, M., and Major, E. (2003). Acquisition of structure versus features in nonlinear phonological intervention. Poster presented at the Child Phonology Conference, July, University of British Columbia, Vancouver.

Bernhardt, B. and Gilbert, J. (1992). Applying linguistic theory to speech-language pathology: The case for nonlinear phonology. *Clinical Linguistics and Phonetics*, 6, 123–45.

Bernhardt, B. H. and Holdgrafer, G. (2001a). Beyond the Basics I: The need for strategic sampling for in-depth phonological analysis. *Language, Speech, and Hearing Services in Schools*, 32, 18–27.

Bernhardt, B. H. and Holdgrafer, G. (2001b). Beyond the Basics II: Supplemental sampling for in-depth phonological analysis. *Language, Speech, and Hearing Services in Schools*, 32, 28–37.

Bernhardt, B., MacNeill, H., and Bohlen, C. (1994). Nonlinear phonological intervention: Group and individual case study results. Poster presented at the CASPLA Conference, May, 1994, Winnipeg. *Journal of Speech-Language Pathology and Audiology Abstracts*, 17, 45.

Bernhardt, B. and Major, E. (2005). Speech, language and literacy skills three years later: Long-term outcomes of nonlinear phonological intervention. *International Journal of Language and Communication Disorders*, 40, 1–27.

Bernhardt, B. and Stemberger, J. P. (1998). *Handbook of Phonological Development: From a Nonlinear Constraints-based Perspective*. San Diego, CA: Academic Press.

Bernhardt, B. H. and Stemberger, J. P. (2000). *Workbook in Nonlinear Phonology for Clinical Application*. Austin, TX: Pro-Ed.

Bernhardt, B. and Stemberger, J. P. (2007). Phonological impairment. In P. de Lacy (ed.), *Handbook of Phonology* (pp. 575–94). Cambridge: Cambridge University Press.

Bernhardt, B. H., Stemberger, J. P., and Major, E. (2006). General and nonlinear phonological intervention perspectives for a child with a resistant phonological impairment. *Advances in Speech-language Pathology*, 8, 190–206.

Bernhardt, B. and Stoel-Gammon, C. (1994). Nonlinear phonology: Clinical application. *Journal of Speech and Hearing Research*, 37, 123–43.

Bernhardt, B. and Stoel-Gammon, C. (1996). Underspecification and markedness in normal and disordered phonological development. In C. Johnson and J. H. V. Gilbert (eds.), *Children's Language*, vol. 9 (pp. 253–81). Hillsdale, NJ: Lawrence Erlbaum Associates.

Blache, S. E. (1978). *The Acquisition of Distinctive Features*. Baltimore, MD: University Park Press.

Chomsky, N. and Halle, M. (1968). *The Sound Pattern of English*. Cambridge, MA: MIT Press.

Clements, G. N. (1985). The geometry of phonological features. *Phonology Yearbook*, 2, 225–52.

Dinnsen, D. A. and Elbert, M. (1984). On the relationship between phonology and learning. In M. Elbert, D. A. Dinnsen, and G. Weismer (eds.), *Phonological Theory and the Misarticulating Child*, ASHA Monographs, 22 (pp. 59–68). Rockville, MD: American Speech-Language-Hearing Association.

Edwards, M. L. and Bernhardt, B. (1973). Phonological analyses of the speech of four children with language disorders. Unpublished MS. The Scottish Rite Institute for Childhood Aphasia, Stanford University.

Edwards, M. L. and Shriberg, L. (1983). *Phonology: Applications in Communicative Disorders*. San Diego, CA: College-Hill Press.

Edwards, S. M. (1995). Optimal outcomes of nonlinear phonological intervention. Unpublished MA thesis, University of British Columbia.

Fudge, C. C. (1969). Syllables. *Journal of Linguistics*, 5, 193–320.

Goldsmith, J. (1976). *Autosegmental Phonology*. Doctoral dissertation, MIT. Published by Garland Press, New York, 1979.

Grunwell, P. (1985). *Phonological Assessment of Child Speech*. San Diego, CA: College-Hill Press.

Hammond, M. (1999). *The Phonology of English: A Prosodic Optimality-Theoretic Approach*. Oxford: Oxford University Press.

Hayes, B. (1989). Compensatory lengthening in moraic phonology. *Linguistic Inquiry*, 20, 253–306.

Hayes, B. (1995). *Metrical Stress Theory: Principles and Case Studies*. Chicago, IL: University of Chicago Press.

Hockett, C. (1955). *A Manual of Phonology*. Baltimore, MD: Waverly Press.

Hodson, B. (1986). *Assessment of Phonological Processes – Revised*. Danville, IL: Interstate Publishers.

Hodson, B. and Paden, E. (1983). Targeting intelligible speech: A phonological approach to remediation. Austin, TX: Pro-Ed.

Hooper, J. (1976). *Introduction to Natural Generative Phonology*. New York: Academic Press.

Ingram, D. (1976). *Phonological Disabilities in Children*. New York: Elsevier.

Jakobson, R. (1968) (trans. A. R. Keiler). *Child Language, Aphasia, and Phonological Universals*. The Hague: Mouton. Originally published as *Kindersprache, Aphasie, und allgemeine Lautgesetze*. Uppsala: Almqvist and Wiksell, 1941.

Kahn, D. (1976). *Syllable-based Generalizations in English Phonology*. Doctoral dissertation, MIT. Published by Garland Press, New York, 1980.

Kenstowicz, M. (1994). *Phonology in Generative Grammar*. Cambridge, MA: Blackwell.

Long, S. (2006). *Computerized Profiling*. www.computerizedprofiling.org.

Maas, E., Barlow, J., Robin, D., and Shapiro, L. (2002). Treatment of sound errors in aphasia and apraxia of speech: Effects of phonological complexity. *Aphasiology*, 16, 609–22.

Major, E. and Bernhardt, B. (1998). Metaphonological skills of children with phonological disorders before and after phonological and metaphonological intervention. *International Journal of Language and Communication Disorders*, 33, 413–44.

Masterson, J. and Bernhardt, B. (2001). *Computerized Articulation and Phonology Evaluation System (CAPES)*. San Antonio, TX: Psychological Corporation.

Masterson, J., Bernhardt, B., and Hofheinz, M. (2005). A comparison of single words and conversational speech in phonological evaluation. *American Journal of Speech-Language Pathology*, 14, 229–41.

McCarthy, J. J. (1988). Feature geometry and dependency: A review. *Phonetica*, 43, 84–108.

McCarthy, J. J. and Prince, A. S. (1993). *Prosodic Morphology I: Constraint Interaction and Satisfaction*. Rutgers University Center for Cognitive Science Technical Report-3, Piscataway, NJ.

McReynolds, L. V. and Engmann, D. (1975). *Distinctive Feature Analysis of Misarticulations*. Baltimore, MD: University Park Press.

Nickels, L. A. and Howard, D. (2004). Dissociating effects of number of phonemes, number of syllables and syllabic complexity in aphasia: It's the number of phonemes that counts. *Cognitive Neuropsychology*, 21, 57–78.

Noble-Wiebe, S., McFarlane, L., and Bernhardt, B. (1995). Effectiveness of nonlinear theory in phonological intervention. Unpublished paper, University of Alberta.

Paradis, C. (1988). On constraints and repair strategies. *Linguistic Review*, 6, 71–97.

Prince, A. S. and Smolensky, P. (1993). *Optimality Theory: Constraint Interaction in Generative Grammar*. Rutgers University Center for Cognitive Science Technical Report-2, Piscataway, NJ.

Romani, C. and Galluzzi, C. (2005). Effects of syllabic complexity in predicting accuracy of repetition and direction of errors in patients with articulatory and phonological difficulties. *Cognitive Neuropsychology*, 22, 817–50.

Sagey, E. (1986). *The Representation of Features and Relations in Non-linear Phonology*. Doctoral dissertation, MIT. Published by Garland Press, New York, 1991.

Shriberg, L. D. and Kwiatkowski, J. (1980). *Natural Process Analysis*. New York: Academic Press.

Smith, N. (1973). *The Acquisition of Phonology*. Cambridge: Cambridge University Press.

Spencer, A. (1984). A nonlinear analysis of phonological disability. *Journal of Communication Disorders*, 17, 325–84.

Stampe, D. (1972). *How I Spent my Summer Vacation: A Dissertation on Natural Phonology.* PhD dissertation, University of Chicago. Published by Garland Press, New York, 1981.

Stemberger, J. P. (1988). Between-word processes in child phonology. *Journal of Child Language*, 15, 39–61.

Stemberger, J. P. (1991). Apparent anti-frequency effects in language production: The Addition Bias and phonological underspecification. *Journal of Memory and Language*, 30, 161–85.

Stemberger, J. P. and Bernhardt, B. (1997). Optimality theory. In M. Ball and R. Kent (eds.), *The New Phonologies* (pp. 211–45). San Diego, CA: Singular Press.

Stemberger, J. P. and Bernhardt, B. H. (1999). The emergence of faithfulness. In B. MacWhinney (ed.), *The Emergence of Language* (pp. 417–46). Mahwah, NJ: Lawrence Erlbaum.

Stemberger, J. P., Bernhardt, B. H., and Johnson, C. E. (2001). 'Regressions' ('u'-shaped learning) in the acquisition of prosodic structure. *Rutgers Optimality Archive* ROA-471.

Stemberger, J. P. and Middleton, C. M. (2003). Vowel dominance and morphological processing. *Language and Cognitive Processes*, 18, 369–404.

Stemberger, J. P. and Stoel-Gammon C. (1991). The underspecification of coronals: Evidence from language acquisition and performance errors. In C. Paradis and J.-F. Prunet (eds.), *The Special Status of Coronals* (pp. 181–99). San Diego, CA: Academic Press.

Ullrich, A. and Bernhardt, B. (2005). Neue Perspektiven der phonologischen Analyse. Implikationen für die Untersuchung phonologischer Entwicklungsstörungen [New perspectives in phonological analysis: Implications for the investigation of developmental phonological impairments]. *Die Sprachheilarbeit*, 5, 221–33.

Van Riper, C. and Irwin, J. V. (1959). *Voice and Articulation.* London: Pitman Medical Publishing Company.

Von Bremen, V. (1990). A nonlinear phonological approach to intervention with severely phonologically disordered twins. Unpublished MA thesis, University of British Columbia.

Weiner, F. (1979). *Phonological Process Analysis.* Baltimore, MD: University Park Press.

27 Optimality Theory: A Clinical Perspective

DANIEL A. DINNSEN AND JUDITH A. GIERUT

27.1 Introduction

Optimality theory (Prince & Smolensky, 2004) represents a new and revolutionary approach to phonology with several distinct advantages for dealing with some long-standing issues in acquisition and clinical treatment. To illustrate this point, we have selected as our primary focus the problem of children's overgeneralization errors. Overgeneralization errors (recidivism) are typified by a child's accurate production of a set of words at one point in time, followed by the same set of words being produced inaccurately at a subsequent point in time. Moreover, for clinical phonology, overgeneralization errors appear to reflect regressions in a child's knowledge of the target sound system, rather than the anticipated improvements. Overgeneralization errors are a common developmental phenomenon (e.g., Bernhardt & Stemberger, 1998; Gierut, 1998; Leonard & Brown, 1984; Smith, 1973) that has, until now, eluded a satisfactory explanation. Thus, overgeneralization errors have dual relevance to typical and atypical phonological development, and serve especially well to illustrate the workings and insights of optimality theory. In what follows, we first sketch some essentials of optimality theory and then highlight a few of the theory's contributions by considering a representative case study of overgeneralization. We close with a brief mention of some of the theory's other clinical insights. For a more thorough tutorial introduction to optimality theory with special attention to acquisition concerns, see Barlow and Gierut (1999) and Gierut and Morrisette (2005); see also Bernhardt and Stemberger (chapter 26 in this volume).

27.2   Some Essentials of Optimality Theory

Optimality theory differs from earlier approaches to phonology in several significant ways. There are no rules or processes, no serial derivations or rule interactions, and no child-specific restrictions on underlying representations. The central claim of the theory is instead that language is a system of conflicting universal constraints. The constraints evaluate a full set of competing output candidates (potential phonetic representations) for each input representation (underlying representation) and select one as the optimal phonetic output for that input. Constraints are of two fundamental and often antagonistic types, namely markedness constraints and faithfulness constraints. Markedness constraints militate against marked structures and refer exclusively to phonetic output properties without regard to the underlying input representation. For example, one family of markedness constraints expresses a ban on fricatives, which are marked relative to stops. Output candidates with a fricative would violate this constraint, favoring unmarked candidates with a stop. Faithfulness constraints, on the other hand, require that the input and output match, so that properties of the input correspond in identity to those of the output. Output candidates that differ from the input representation violate faithfulness constraints. For example, a change from an input fricative to an output stop would violate a faithfulness constraint that demands identity in terms of manner features. Faithfulness constraints are the antithesis of rules in that they preserve contrasts and disfavor change. The constraints are presumed to be the same across languages and are present in all grammars. The universal character of these constraints helps explain the prevalence and recurrence of phonological phenomena – especially children's error patterns. The conflict between constraints is resolved by rank-ordering the constraints in a language-specific constraint hierarchy. Some constraints will dominate or outrank others. Output candidates that violate highly ranked constraints lose out to candidates that violate lower-ranked constraints. The output candidate that best satisfies the constraint hierarchy is selected as the winning optimal phonetic form and is the one that is actually produced.

One of the other central hypotheses of optimality theory is that markedness constraints outrank faithfulness constraints in the earliest stages of language acquisition. This is intended to explain the preponderance of simplified productions or error patterns in children's early speech. The process of acquisition proceeds by the gradual demotion of the markedness constraints on the basis of positive evidence (e.g., Tesar & Smolensky, 1998). As markedness constraints are demoted in the hierarchy, error patterns are suppressed. For clinical phonology, this implies that the goal of treatment is to demote high-ranked markedness constraints, with the child becoming increasingly faithful to the native language through intervention.

Many of the above points can be exemplified by considering an optimality-theoretic characterization of children's overgeneralization errors. Despite their ubiquity, it has always been unclear how overgeneralization errors arise, or why they occur so often. We will see that optimality theory provides a set of testable hypotheses relating to these questions.

27.3 Overgeneralization Errors

We turn now to a representative case study of overgeneralization for a child with a phonological disorder. Child 78 (age 4;2) produced many sounds in error, scoring at the fifth percentile relative to age-matched peers on the *Goldman–Fristoe Test of Articulation* (Goldman & Fristoe, 1986). She scored within normal limits on all other tests of hearing, oral-motor function and receptive and expressive vocabulary. An extensive speech sample was elicited and revealed that the interdental fricative /θ/ was produced correctly but was also the substitute for all other fricatives.

The data in (1) and (2) from two different points in time illustrate the phenomenon of overgeneralization. More specifically, at the first point in time (age 4;2), the alveolar fricative [s] and the labial fricative [f] did not occur in the child's inventory and were replaced by [θ], as shown in (1a) and (1b), respectively. Target /θ/ was, however, produced correctly, as shown in (1c).

(1) Stage 1 for Child 78 (age 4;2)
    a. Target /s/ replaced by [θ]
        [θoʊp] 'soap'; [maʊθ] 'mouse';
        [θoʊ] 'sew'; [trihaʊθ] 'treehouse'
    b. Target /f/ replaced by [θ]
        [θæt˺] 'fat'; [naɪθ] 'knife';
        [θɪθ] 'fish'; [kɔθ] 'cough'
    c. Target /θ/ realized as [θ]
        [θʌm] 'thumb'; [bæθ] 'bath';
        [θʌndʊː] 'thunder'; [tiθ] 'teeth'

At a second point in time (three months later and after having been taught a word-initial s-cluster), the situation was just the reverse. Note that target /s/ came to be produced correctly, as shown in (2a). In addition, the substitute for target /f/ changed from [θ] at stage 1 to [s] at stage 2 (compare 1b to 2b), suggesting that a new error pattern emerged in the grammar. More importantly, /θ/, which had been produced correctly, was lost from this child's phonetic inventory. At stage 2, /θ/ was now produced in error, being realized as [s], as in (2c). While Child 78 introduced correct realizations of [s] into the inventory, she overgeneralized its use for other target fricatives, creating two new error patterns.

(2)   Stage 2 for Child 78 (age 4;5)
  a.   Target /s/ realized as [s]
      [soʊp] 'soap';   [maʊs]   'mouse';
      [soʊ] 'sew';   [twihaʊs] 'treehouse'
  b.   Target /f/ replaced by [s]
      [sæt] 'fat';   [naɪs]   'knife';
      [sɪs] 'fish';   [kɔs]   'cough'
  c.   Target /θ/ replaced by [s]
      [sʌm]   'thumb';   [bæs] 'bath';
      [sʌndʊ] 'thunder'; [tis] 'teeth'

Prior theories would have attributed overgeneralization errors of this sort to incorrectly internalized underlying representations and rule loss (e.g., Macken, 1980). For example, it would have been claimed that Child 78 at the first stage had incorrectly internalized all fricatives as /s/, and that a rule converted all of those fricatives to [θ]. The loss of the rule at the second stage would reveal those incorrectly internalized underlying representations and result in the observed overgeneralization errors. Such accounts do, however, run counter to the widely held assumption that children's underlying representations are target-appropriate. Optimality theory would seem to be especially challenged to deal with these facts given that the theory claims that children's underlying representations cannot be restricted in the ways allowed by earlier approaches. Additionally, optimality theory has no rules to lose. To see how optimality theory meets these challenges and accounts for the facts, consider first the constraints in (3) which are most relevant to this case.

(3)   Constraints
  Markedness constraints
      *s: Alveolar fricatives are banned
      *θ: Interdental fricatives are banned
      *f: Labial fricatives are banned
  Faithfulness constraints
      IDENT[cont]:   Corresponding input and output segments must be identical in terms of the feature [continuant]
      FAITH: Corresponding input and output segments must be identical

The markedness constraints in (3a) all belong to a family of constraints disfavoring fricatives generally. Each individual constraint militates against a different class of fricatives and each is independently necessary to account for observed individual differences in the occurrence and non-occurrence of particular fricatives across children (Ingram, Christensen, Veach, & Webster, 1980). The fact is that some children exclude all fricatives from their inventories, others exclude only one class or some combination of those classes, and yet others exclude none. While many different fricatives were banned from Child 78's inventory, it is noteworthy that the substitute for all target fricatives was a fricative, specifically an interdental fricative at Stage 1. This is suggestive of a highly ranked faithfulness constraint, IDENT[cont], which demands that the input manner feature [continuant] be preserved in the corresponding output segment. The dominance of this constraint would ensure that a target stop is realized as a stop and a target fricative as a fricative. Furthermore, Child 78's exclusion of labial and alveolar fricatives is indicative of the highly ranked markedness constraints *f and *s. These two markedness constraints are ranked over another generalized family of faithfulness constraints, which we abbreviate as FAITH. FAITH demands that all properties of corresponding input and output segments be the same. By this analysis, it is more important to avoid labial and alveolar fricatives than it is to preserve their various input features. The consequence of these constraints and rankings is that labial and alveolar fricatives would be excluded from the inventory and replaced by the only remaining class of English fricatives, namely interdental fricatives. It is, however, also well known that many children exclude interdental fricatives from their inventories (Smit, 1993), suggesting the need for the additional independent markedness constraint, *θ, which disfavors interdental fricatives. Given that Child 78 produced interdental fricatives target-appropriately at Stage 1 and, in fact, preferred interdentals as the substitute for all other fricatives, *θ must be ranked just low enough that its violation can be tolerated. We will see that *θ must be ranked above FAITH but below the other markedness constraints during the early stage.

The ranking of constraints needed for Stage 1 is schematized in (4). The notation uses solid lines to connect those constraints that are crucially ranked, with the higher-ranked constraints positioned above the lower-ranked constraints. Constraints that cannot be ranked relative to one another are given on the same horizontal plane and are not connected by a line.

(4)   Constraint ranking for Stage 1

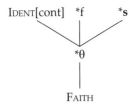

With this ranking of constraints, we can now demonstrate how a particular output candidate is selected as optimal given a specific input representation. It is conventional to use a display known as a tableau for this purpose. Our first tableau is given in (5). In all tableaux, the underlying input representation is given in the upper left corner. Competing output candidates are listed down the left side of the tableau. For expository purposes, we will limit the output candidate set to the most likely competitors. Other competing output candidates that begin with a stop would be eliminated by the highly ranked constraint IDENT[cont], which will not be shown in this or subsequent tableaux. Constraints are listed along the top in accord with their ranking. Crucial rankings are indicated by a solid vertical line between the columns of affected constraints. Constraints whose ranking cannot be determined are separated by a dotted vertical line. A candidate's violation of a constraint is indicated by a '*' in the intersecting cell. A candidate is eliminated from the competition if it incurs a violation of a high-ranked constraint not incurred by some other candidate. The elimination of a candidate from the competition is termed a fatal violation and is indicated by a '!' after the violation mark. The winning or optimal candidate is the one that survives after all competing candidates have been eliminated by violations of higher-ranked constraints. That winning candidate is identified by the manual indicator '☞'.

(5)   Target /s/ realized as [θ] for Stage 1

/soʊp/ 'soap'	*f	*s	*θ	FAITH
a. [foʊp]	*!			*
b. ☞ [θoʊp]			*	*
c. [soʊp]		*!		

To illustrate the evaluation process, the tableau in (5) considers how different output candidates would fare given this ranking of constraints for Child 78. We use as an example an input representation that begins with /s/ as in 'soap'. Candidate (a) with an initial [f] fatally violates the highly ranked markedness constraint *f and is eliminated from the competition. The faithful candidate (c) violates the other highly ranked markedness constraint *s and is also eliminated. Candidate (b) with the interdental is all that remains and is thus selected as optimal in accord with the child's error pattern even though it violates both *θ and FAITH. The lower ranking of those two constraints makes their violations less serious. This illustrates another important point, namely that the constraints can be violated and any winning output candidate will likely violate some constraint.

This same ranking of constraints ensures the target-appropriate realization of /θ/ as shown in the tableau in (6) for an input such as 'thumb'. Candidates (a) and (c) are again eliminated because each violates one of the undominated markedness constraints. The only remaining candidate (b) complies with FAITH and is selected as optimal even though it violates the markedness constraint *θ.

(6) Target /θ/ realized as [θ] for Stage 1

/θʌm/ 'thumb'		*f	*s	*θ	FAITH
a.	[fʌm]	*!			*
b. ☞	[θʌm]			*	
c.	[sʌm]		*!		*

Our ranking of all of the markedness constraints above the generalized faithfulness constraint accords with another fundamental hypothesis of the theory, namely that markedness constraints tend to outrank faithfulness constraints in the early stages of acquisition. In addition, by ranking the markedness constraints relative to one another, specifically both *f and *s above *θ, all but the interdental fricative candidates (5b, 6b) are effectively eliminated. Thus, even though *θ is ranked above FAITH, which would seem to disallow interdentals, interdental fricatives are permitted to survive as optimal. This is because of the greater demand to preserve the manner of the input segment in the corresponding output segment, i.e., as a result of undominated IDENT[cont]. The novel claim of optimality theory is that interdental fricatives are produced not because they are faithful to the input, but because the hierarchy claims that interdentals are better fricatives than [f] or [s]. Thus, interdentals are the last resort in this instance. No matter which fricative the child might have internalized for the underlying representation of a fricative, [θ] would have been the realization. It is also striking that correct realizations of /θ/ resulted from a constraint ranking that does not conform to the target ranking of constraints; in adult English, FAITH dominates *θ. From a clinical perspective, then, a child's correct production cannot necessarily be taken as evidence that the child has arrived at a target-appropriate grammar. This is in keeping with other reports that children may arrive at the 'right' output for the 'wrong' reason (Dinnsen, 1999). Importantly, there was no need to restrict any of this child's underlying representations to incorrectly internalized forms. This accords with a basic tenet of the theory, namely 'richness of the base', which maintains that there can be no language-specific (and by extension, no child-specific) restrictions on input representations.

As a further test of optimality theory, let us now turn to the characterization of Stage 2 and its transition from Stage 1. Given the ranking of constraints for Stage 1 (repeated in (7a)), a coherent account becomes available for the transition to Stage 2 with its target-appropriate realizations of /s/ and the overgeneralization errors associated with the other fricatives. Specifically, the grammar change that took place involves a minimal demotion of *s below *θ, resulting in the new ranking for Stage 2 as shown in (7b). In keeping with clinical interpretations, a possible way that constraint demotion may occur is through treatment on word-initial s-clusters. This reranking is precisely what follows from the constraint demotion algorithm (Tesar & Smolensky, 1998). That is, upon the child's discovery that [s] could occur, she demoted the constraint responsible for the exclusion of [s], namely *s. This is shown in (7b) where *s is demoted just below *θ, which was the highest-ranked constraint that the previous winner violated. This has the effect of bringing *s into the stratum with FAITH. In terms of continuity considerations, the grammars for the two stages otherwise remain the same.

(7)   Constraint demotion for Stage 2

    a.   Stage 1:

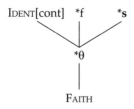

    b.   Stage 2:

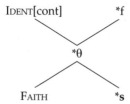

Note that the ranking of *θ over FAITH is retained in the transition from Stage 1 to Stage 2, accounting for the new error pattern where [θ] was no longer in use, with [s] being produced instead. Also common to both stages was the continued dominance of *f, which accounted for the persistent exclusion of labiodental fricatives from the child's inventory.

The effect of the new Stage 2 ranking can be illustrated by considering Child 78's production of target /s/ words. The tableau in (8) provides an example using the word 'soap' to capture the child's accurate productions of /s/ at Stage 2. The faithful candidate (c) only violates the lowest-ranked markedness constraint *s with all of the competitors being eliminated by their violations of the higher-ranked markedness constraints.

(8) Target /s/ realized as [s] for Stage 2

/soʊp/ 'soap'		*f	*θ	FAITH	*s
a.	[foʊp]	*!		*	
b.	[θoʊp]		*!	*	
c. ☞	[soʊp]				*

Recall however that at Stage 2 Child 78 also exhibited overgeneralization errors. Whereas /θ/ had been produced correctly in Stage 1, it now was replaced by [s] in Stage 2. The tableau in (9) shows the overgeneralization effects from the Stage 2 reranking. Given a target word such as 'thumb', candidates (a) and (b) are both eliminated by their fatal violations of the more highly ranked markedness constraints. Candidate (c) with the substitute [s] is selected as optimal in accord with the child's new error pattern even though that candidate violates the two lower-ranked constraints. This also explains why the substitute for /f/ would have changed from [θ] to [s] at the same time. That is, the higher ranking of *f and *θ precludes the occurrence of candidates (a) and (b) independently of the particular fricative that might have been internalized by the child.

(9) Target /θ/ realized as [s] for Stage 2

/θʌm/ 'thumb'		*f	*θ	FAITH	*s
a.	[fʌm]	*!		*	
b.	[θʌm]		*!		
c. ☞	[sʌm]			*	*

The case of Child 78 demonstrates the way in which optimality theory captures overgeneralization errors. The new theory reveals that these errors arise from a characteristic set of grammatical factors and proceed in several crucial incremental steps. The first step in the progression entails an early stage where the error pattern is characterized by several highly ranked and interacting markedness constraints (e.g., *s, *f and *θ). It is equally important for there to be some highly ranked faithfulness constraint (e.g., IDENT[cont]), which favors preservation of a property banned by the highly ranked markedness constraints. The markedness constraints need to be ranked relative to one another, and all need to be ranked above an antagonistic faithfulness constraint (e.g., *s and *f are ranked above *θ, which in turn is ranked above FAITH). The second step in the progression entails the reranking of the markedness constraints so that one is demoted minimally below another (e.g., *s is demoted below *θ). However, because some markedness constraints continue to outrank the general faithfulness constraint (e.g., *θ dominates FAITH), its influence would then become evident with the introduction of a new error pattern. The error pattern induced by the dominance of other markedness constraints during Stage 2 means that yet other changes in the constraint hierarchy must take place before conformity with the target system can be achieved. The clinical implication that derives from this optimality-theoretic analysis is that Child 78 may require successive rounds of treatment. Potential goals of continued treatment would be the labiodental and interdental fricatives. Presumably, this would trigger the demotion of *f and *θ respectively below FAITH. The novel clinical insight is that optimality theory may pinpoint *a priori* when successive rounds of intervention will be needed. Optimality theory also delineates how many rounds of treatment will be required to achieve the necessary constraint demotions for accurate target productions.

Perhaps the most significant distinguishing characteristic of an optimality-theoretic account of overgeneralization is that the substance of a child's underlying representations plays a much smaller role and is less decisive than might have been thought under earlier approaches. We saw, for example, that the underlying specification of target place features did not matter for Child 78, although target manner features did, as captured by the dominance of IDENT[cont]. Importantly, these overgeneralization errors do not require us to abandon the widely held assumption that children's underlying representations are correct relative to the target system. The fact that overgeneralization errors involve correct and incorrect productions during the first two stages of development apparently has less to do with the substance of underlying representations and more to do with the nature of the constraints and the constraint hierarchy. In these circumstances, optimality theory views overgeneralization errors as an expected and unavoidable intermediate step in the right direction, but one that may require multiple rounds of treatment to induce a series of constraint rerankings before conformity with the target language can be achieved. The value of our optimality-theoretic account is supported by its extension to other cases of overgeneralization in both typical and atypical development (e.g., see Dinnsen, 2008, and references therein).

27.4   Conclusion

In summary, our focus on children's overgeneralization errors has allowed us to illustrate some of the workings and insights of optimality theory, leading to a better understanding of a common problem in both typical and atypical phonological development. There are many other developmental phenomena and clinical issues that have also benefited from optimality-theoretic investigations, some of which can only be mentioned in passing. To illustrate, an especially compelling contribution is the theory's explanation of implicational universals (e.g., Jakobson, 1941/1968), including most notably children's feature hierarchies (e.g., Dinnsen, Chin, Elbert, & Powell, 1990). Optimality theory derives implicational universals of this sort from fixed (non-permutable) rankings of constraints (e.g., Dinnsen & O'Connor, 2001; Gierut & Morrisette, 2005). The clinical significance of fixed constraint rankings is that treatment aimed at the demotion of the top-ranked markedness constraint in a fixed hierarchy results in the demotion of the dominated markedness constraints (and hence the suppression of certain other error patterns) without directly treating the sounds associated with those lower-ranked constraints. A second example is optimality theory's characterization of children's error patterns as deriving from an intricate hierarchy of conflicting universal constraints. These hierarchies of conflicting constraints have clinical importance because they bear on both the assessment and treatment of children's phonological errors. From the view of diagnostics, hierarchies of conflicting constraints demonstrate that error patterns, which may at first glance seem 'unusual', are not so very different in substance. This is relevant because 'unusual' errors have been taken as a criterion for differentiating phonological disorder from deviance (Leonard, 1992). Because optimality theory has found that 'unusual' errors fall within the bounds of expected variation in children's grammars, this improves the precision of our diagnostic classification schemes. From the view of treatment, hierarchies of conflicting constraints also reveal why some error patterns are especially resistant to change. That is, some error patterns have been shown to be constituted by multiple independent and highly ranked markedness constraints that need to be demoted in the hierarchy. An in-depth discussion of these and other issues associated with the application of optimality theory to the assessment and treatment of phonological disorders is provided in Dinnsen and Gierut (2008).

The architecture of optimality theory forces us to think about phonology – and especially children's error patterns – in a very different way. The new focus has been shifted to discovering the full set of universal constraints, their ranking and their language-specific versus universal interaction. Clinical assessment and treatment have begun to take advantage of these new insights with promising results, thereby underscoring the mutually beneficial relationship between theory and application. These clinical investigations also serve as a valuable testing ground for the claims of optimality theory.

ACKNOWLEDGMENTS

We are especially grateful to Ashley Farris-Trimble, Michele Morrisette and other members of the Learnability Project at Indiana University for their many contributions to the work described here and elsewhere. This work was supported by a grant from the National Institutes of Health (DC001694).

REFERENCES

Barlow, J. A. and Gierut, J. A. (1999). Optimality theory in phonological acquisition. *Journal of Speech, Language, and Hearing Research*, 42, 1482–98.

Bernhardt, B. H. and Stemberger, J. P. (1998). *Handbook of Phonological Development from the Perspective of Constraint-based Non-linear Phonology*. San Diego, CA: Academic Press.

Dinnsen, D. A. (1999). Some empirical and theoretical issues in disordered child phonology. In W. C. Ritchie and T. K. Bhatia (eds.), *Handbook of Child Language Acquisition* (pp. 647–74). New York: Academic Press.

Dinnsen, D. A. (2008). Recalcitrant error patterns. In D. A. Dinnsen and J. A. Gierut (eds.), *Optimality Theory, Phonological Acquisition and Disorders*, pp. 247–276.

Dinnsen, D. A., Chin, S. B., Elbert, M., and Powell, T. W. (1990). Some constraints on functionally disordered phonologies: Phonetic inventories and phonotactics. *Journal of Speech and Hearing Research*, 33, 28–37.

Dinnsen, D. A. and Gierut, J. A. (2008). *Optimality Theory, Phonological Acquisition and Disorders*. London: Equinox.

Dinnsen, D. A. and O'Connor, K. M. (2001). Implicationally-related error patterns and the selection of treatment targets. *Language, Speech and Hearing Services in Schools*, 32, 257–70.

Gierut, J. A. (1998). Production, conceptualization and change in distinctive featural categories. *Journal of Child Language*, 25, 321–42.

Gierut, J. A. and Morrisette, M. L. (2005). The clinical significance of optimality theory for phonological disorders. *Topics in Language Disorders*, 25, 266–79.

Goldman, R. and Fristoe, M. (1986). *Goldman–Fristoe Test of Articulation*. Circles Pines, MN: American Guidance Service.

Ingram, D., Christensen, L., Veach, S., and Webster, B. (1980). The acquisition of word-initial fricatives and affricates in English by children between 2 and 6 years. In G. H. Yeni-Komshian, J. F. Kavanagh, and C. A. Ferguson (eds.), *Child Phonology. Volume 1: Production* (pp. 169–92). New York: Academic Press.

Jakobson, R. (1941/1968) (trans. A. R. Keiler). *Child Language, Aphasia, and Phonological Universals*. The Hague: Mouton. Originally published as *Kindersprache, Aphasie, und allgemeine Lautgesetze*. Uppsala: Almqvist and Wiksell, 1941.

Leonard, L. B. (1992). Models of phonological development and children with phonological disorders. In C. A. Ferguson, L. Menn, and C. Stoel-Gammon (eds.), *Phonological Development: Models, Research, Implications* (pp. 495–508). Timonium, MD: York Press.

Leonard, L. B. and Brown, B. L. (1984). Nature and boundaries of phonologic categories: A case study of an unusual phonologic pattern in a language-impaired child. *Journal of Speech and Hearing Disorders*, 49, 419–28.

Macken, M. A. (1980). The child's lexical representation: The 'puzzle-puddle-pickle' evidence. *Journal of Linguistics*, 16, 1–17.

Prince, A. and Smolensky, P. (2004). *Optimality Theory: Constraint Interaction in Generative Grammar*. Malden, MA: Blackwell.

Smit, A. B. (1993). Phonologic error distributions in the Iowa–Nebraska Articulation Norms Project: Consonant singletons. *Journal of Speech and Hearing Research*, 36, 533–47.

Smith, N. V. (1973). *The Acquisition of Phonology: A Case Study*. Cambridge: Cambridge University Press.

Tesar, B. and Smolensky, P. (1998). Learnability in optimality theory. *Linguistic Inquiry*, 29, 229–68.

28 Government Phonology and Speech Impairment

MARTIN J. BALL

28.1 Introduction

Government Phonology (Kaye, Lowenstamm, & Vergnaud, 1985, 1990; Harris, 1990, 1994; Harris & Lindsey, 1995) can be seen to some extent as a development of Dependency Phonology (Anderson & Durand, 1986, 1987; Anderson & Ewen, 1987), with the aim of constraining the generative power of this latter approach. Government Phonology (henceforth GovP) is seen by its proponents to be within the generative tradition (and thus part of 'universal grammar'), and it shares with other approaches the insights and developments of feature-geometry, autosegmental, and metrical phonology. In particular we should note that the theory distinguishes a skeletal tier which contains the terminal nodes of syllabic constituents (termed 'constituency') from a segmental one (termed 'melody'), and that the equivalent of features ('elements') are thought to operate on a set of tiers as well. However, despite these similarities, there are major differences – in particular, as the name suggests, the idea of governing or licensing relations between units.

In this chapter, for reasons of space, we will concentrate on pointing out where GovP differs from traditional models of generative phonology, and then turn our attention to how GovP can inform our descriptions of disordered speech.

28.2 Constituency

We noted above that this area of GovP concerns the syllabic tier in traditional parlance. However, we should note that the theory does not, in actual fact, recognize syllables as constituents (although it does as a licensing relation). Harris (1994, p. 45) notes that the notion of the syllable has "no pre-theoretical standing", and Kula (2002, p. 23) states, "there is no notion of *syllable* as understood in the traditional sense; rather, phonological units are regarded as consisting of sequences of Onset–Nuclear (ON) pairs." The concept of the 'phonological word' is used, however, and is deemed to consist of feet, which in turn consist of the units O (onset), N (nucleus) and rime (all of which may potentially be binary-branching, depending on the language concerned). These sequences are located on the tier P^0, which dominates the timing tier (or skeleton) traditionally represented by timing slots x-x-x etc. Kula (2002, p. 23) notes that the skeleton links segmental information to the constituency level, and "the government and licensing relations that hold between them".

While the distinction between rime and nucleus (found in traditional accounts of the syllable) is retained, branching rimes do not contain a traditional coda unit, and in GovP, the coda is not an accepted unit. Syllable-final singleton consonants are always considered to be onsets followed by empty nuclei (see Harris, 1994, for arguments in favor of this viewpoint; theory-independent, empirical reasons for considering final Cs to be onsets are found in Harris & Gussmann, 2002). We can show this in the following examples, where, traditionally, the empty nucleus is normally omitted from the diagram utterance finally:

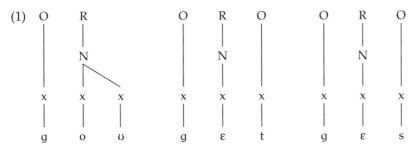

(1)

Branching of the nucleus denotes diphthongs and long vowels, while branching of the onset is used to mark complex onsets. This applies only to non-/s/ -initial two-consonant clusters; with /s/-initial two- or three-consonant clusters the initial /s/ is deemed to be external to the branching onset. Harris (1994) suggests this /s/ may be deemed to be an onset with an empty nucleus. Word-final and word-medial consonant clusters are dealt with by allowing branching rimes. In these cases, the right-hand branch of the rime may contain a consonant, subject to certain restrictions in the case of heavy nuclei (long vowels or diphthongs): consonants can only be fricatives or sonorants, sonorants agree with the place of the following consonant, and the favored such place is coronal (see Harris, 1994, p. 77). These restrictions do not hold on light nuclei. This is illustrated in the following:

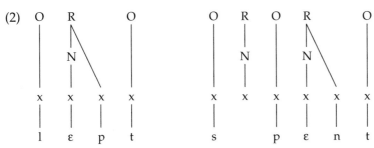

(2)

Clearly, English, for example, allows more complex final consonant clusters, and final two-consonant clusters that do not meet the conditions on branching rimes noted above. In these cases, empty nuclei are posited between the consonants (also we have removed the rime unit from this diagram, as a branching rime plays no part in this example):

(3)

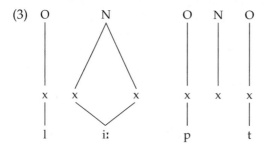

Final three- and four-consonant clusters are accounted for by combinations of branching rimes and empty nuclei, depending on which consonants are involved.

This approach to phonology is termed *government* phonology because its units enter into governing and licensing relations with each other. While this is perhaps most obvious on the melodic tier (see below), there are also relations between the various units we have been considering at the constituency level. We can look at some of the more important of these here. For example the onset, rime and nucleus constituents are subject to the following general principles:

(4)   Every nucleus can and must license a preceding onset.

(5)   Every onset must be licensed by a following nucleus.

Furthermore, it is required that

(6)   Every constituent licenser must dominate a skeletal point.

Given the above, we can derive the following principle:

(7)   Every nucleus must dominate a skeletal point.

Related to these principles is the principle concerning codas, discussed above:

(8)   Coda-licensing principle: Post-nuclear rhymal positions must be licensed by a following onset.

These principles are concerned with the three main units of constituent structure. We may also consider principles concerned with location and direction of government between them. Kula (2002, p. 25) notes that government is subject to the following conditions:

(9) Conditions on government
   a. strict locality: only adjacent positions can constitute a government relation
   b. strict directionality: constituent government goes from left to right and interconstituent government goes from right to left.

Further, she notes a proposal that all governing relations be licensed by a following nucleus. (9) constrains government relations at the constituency tier. So, for example, within a constituent, government is left-headed (so, the first element of an onset cluster is the head of the relation), whereas between constituents, government is left-headed (so, a nucleus governs its preceding onset).

Finally, all governing relations are subject to the projection principle:

(10) Projection principle (Kaye, 1990, p. 321)
   Governing relations are defined at the level of lexical representation and remain constant throughout derivation.

The projection principle implies that "constituent categories may not be altered during the course of derivation; onsets remain onsets, nuclei remain nuclei and the licensing relation between nuclei and onsets remains stable" (Kula, 2002, p. 26).

We have not had the space to examine in detail structures such as the phonological word, and foot, or analyses of prosodic features such as tone. Readers should consult Harris (1994) and Kula (2002) for more information on these areas. We can also note that this summary excludes recent moves towards a more constrained theory, as started in van der Hulst's work on Radical CV Phonology (1989).

28.3 Melody

The main difference at the segmental level between GovP and traditional generative approaches concerns the nature of the smallest phonological unit. The binary feature (that was claimed to be equipollent) was the smallest unit in generative phonology as outlined by Chomsky and Halle (1968) and, until comparatively recently, most theoretical developments within this tradition maintained binary features. In work within feature geometry (Clements, 1985; Halle, 1992; Sagey, 1986; see review in Roca & Johnson, 1999), strict binarity was relaxed to allow nodes with privative, unary features, mixed with binary equipollent ones.

28.3.1 Features

Phonological theories have for a long time posited the need for a phonological unit smaller than the segment. Such units are required if we wish to make statements about classes of sounds (all those that share a particular phonolo-gical aspect), or to describe rules that affect particular sounds or groups of sounds. Since the time of Trubetzkoy (e.g. 1969, originally published 1939), this unit has been the distinctive feature. However, while Trubetzkoy and the Prague School of linguistics considered a range of feature typologies, later work on distinctive features (e.g. Jakobson, Fant, & Halle, 1952; Jakobson & Halle, 1956; Chomksy & Halle, 1968) opted for one particular type: binary, equipollent features. Equipollent features are those where each value (in this case a binary +/− set of values) specifies a particular property. For example, the commonly encountered feature [voice] (as proposed, for example, in Chomsky & Halle, 1968) has a plus value denoting vocal-fold vibration, and a minus value den-oting open vocal folds (i.e. not simply 'not vibrating vocal folds'). Privative features, on the other hand, have a distinction between one value denoting a particular property, and another denoting simply the absence of that property. (In fact, whereas in Chomsky and Halle's 1968 formulation of distinctive fea-tures the authors claim that their features are equipollent, some do not appear to fit within this classification. For example, the feature [high] has a plus value denoting high tongue position, and a minus value denoting not high (mid or low); this would appear to be a privative distinction.)

Feature theory has developed considerably since Chomsky and Halle's groundbreaking work of 1968. We have seen work on the relationship between features (markedness and feature geometry: Clements, 1985; Halle, 1992; Roca & Johnson, 1999; Sagey, 1986), and on economy in segmental feature matrices (underspecification: Archangeli, 1988; Clements, 1988; Steriade, 1987). Some of the work in feature geometry has suggested that some nodes on a feature tree may be best described with privative, unary features rather than with binary equipollent ones (Roca & Johnson, 1999). It is to this notion we turn next.

28.3.2   *Elements*

Dependency phonology (Anderson & Durand, 1986, 1987; Anderson & Ewen, 1987), and related approaches such as Radical CV Phonology (van der Hulst, 1989), and Government Phonology have taken the developments in feature geometry just noted one step farther, and have adopted *elements* rather than features as the basic unit of phonological analysis. These elements are unary (i.e., they are either present or absent in a description, and so also privative), and they are phonetically interpretable in isolation. The main advantage of unary elements is that their use constrains the phonology. Binary features allow a large number of segment classes to be established (those sharing the plus value and those sharing the minus value of a feature); unary elements only allow a class of segments that have that element, not one that does not have it. Harris (1994) also sees unary accounts as a means of reducing the range of phonological processes available to the theory to those that are observed in natural language, thus obviating the need for theoretical add-ons such as markedness conventions.

The advantages claimed for phonetic interpretability of elements include freedom from the need to map non-interpretable distinctive features onto phonetic features late in a derivation, and the fact that we do not need underspecification (or to decide between different models of underspecification). Using phonetically interpretable elements results in all levels of derivation containing segments that are also phonetically interpretable. Harris (1994, p. 96) claims that this approach is arguably more psycholinguistically plausible than traditional ones, and that:

> Since phonological representation uniformly adheres to the principle of full phonetic interpretability, there is no motivation for recognizing an autonomous level of systematic phonetic representation. Any phonological representation at any level of derivation can be directly submitted to articulatory or perceptual interpretation. Derivation is thus not an operation by means of which abstract phonological objects are transformed into increasingly concrete physical objects. Rather it is a strictly generative function which defines the grammaticality of phonological strings.

The appeal to psycholinguistically plausible models of phonology has echoes in recent work within what may be broadly termed cognitive models of linguistics; see, for example, Sosa and Bybee (chapter 30 in this volume). From the point of view of clinical phonology, it might well be more insightful to posit phonetically interpretable phonological elements, rather than uninterpretable binary distinctive features.

28.3.3 Vowel elements

In GovP the phonological primes are termed *elements*, and three elements are proposed for vowels. These, with their pronunciations, are:

(11) **A** [a]
    I [i]
    U [u]

A fourth symbol, @, is also used, but represents a default tongue position, or the carrier signal on which the modulations represented by elements are superimposed (Harris, 2005; Harris & Lindsey, 2002). We noted earlier that, as its name suggests, GovP uses governing relations between its units of description, and this is no less true of the melodic tier than of the constituency one. The combination of elements is regulated by the concept of Licensing Constraints. These constraints provide restrictions on the combinations of elements so that it is possible to derive the set of phonological representations that capture all and only those sound segments relevant to a particular language (Kula, 2002, p. 27).

So, combinations of elements provide a wider vowel set, and in combinations one element is normally considered to be the head (or governor), and others are usually dependent on the head. In GovP formalism, the head element is shown underlined; where no element is underlined then the elements are in a non-governing relationship. English lax vowels illustrate these possibilities:

(12)   [I, @]   /ɪ/
       [A, I, @]   /ɛ/
       [I, A]   /æ/
       [U, A]   /ɒ/
       [U, @]   /ʊ/
       [@]   /ʌ/
       [A, @]   [ɐ]

These combinations illustrate the use of the neutral element [@] as governor of vowels we traditionally term lax. Long vowels, like diphthongs, are deemed to occupy two skeletal slots (as described earlier). Typical examples from English are seen in:

(13)

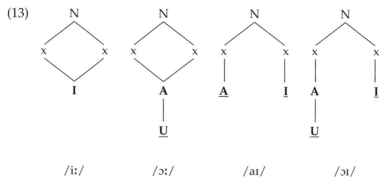

/iː/   /ɔː/   /aɪ/   /ɔɪ/

The layering of the elements in these diagrams reflects the contention that these elements (and the consonant elements of the following subsection) can be thought of as operating on separate tiers.

28.3.4   Consonant elements

The following are the elements most often used to characterize consonants, together with their phonetic exponence and description in more traditional phonological terms. It can be noted that the different exponence of A, I, and U result from their no longer being dominated by a nucleus node in word structure.

(14)   ?   [ʔ]   stop or edge
       h   [h]   noise or aperiodic energy on release
       R   [ɾ]   coronality
       I   [j]   palatality
       U   [w]   labiality
       @   [ɥ]   neutral

    A [ʁ]   present in uvulars and pharyngeals
    N [ŋ]   nasality

There are two further, laryngeal-node, elements used mainly to distinguish voiced from voiceless consonants: **[H]** stiff vocal folds, aspiration, voicelessness, and **[L]** slack vocal folds, voicing. In the following examples we include only voiced sonorants and voiceless obstruents, so have no need of these last two elements.

    Researchers in GovP have sought ways to constrain the theory through the reduction of consonant elements from this original set to seven or five (see Ritter, 1996, as an example). Such reductions have included the removal of the **[N]** element and its replacement by a combination of **[L]** governing **[ʔ]**. For our purposes, we retain a maximal set of elements.

    Illustrations of both place and manner distinctions in consonants can be seen in the following:

(15) **[h, U, ʔ]** [p]
      [h, <u>R</u>, ?] [t]
      [h, @, ?] [k]
      [<u>h</u>, U]   [f]
      [<u>h</u>, R]   [s]
      [h, <u>R</u>]   [θ]
      [<u>h</u>, R, I] [ʃ]
      [h, @]   [x]
      [<u>h</u>, A]   [χ]
      [h, <u>A</u>]   [ħ]
      [N, <u>R</u>, ?] [n]
      [R, ?]   [l]
      [R, @]   [ɹ]

28.3.5　Element geography

We have referred to feature geometry above; those working with GovP have proposed element geometries for similar reasons. As Kula (2002, p. 30) notes,

> Feature geometries have . . . been proposed in order to not only classify natural classes, but also to exclude unnatural ones. . . . The GP view that elements are directly linked to the skeleton implies that they are individually accessible to phonological processing. True as this is, it has also been observed that particular phonological processes do indeed access more than one element at the same time and thus make it necessary for us to conceive of some geometric organisation of elements.

In other words, element geometries allow us to constrain the possible combinations of elements that can be accessed in phonological processes, in a way complementary to that in which licensing constraints restrict the possible combination of elements within the description of a single segment; both are language-specific. While various possible element geometries have been proposed in the literature, we can illustrate the concept with an element tree combined from proposals in Harris (1994) and in Harris and Lindsey (1995):

(16)

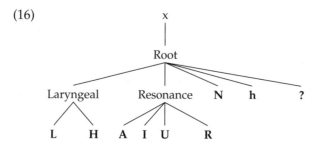

28.4   Government Phonology in Derivation

The mechanisms we have looked at so far are used to describe a range of phonological processes in natural language. We have space here to consider just a couple of examples (both taken from Harris, 1994). First, we can consider vowel syncope. In fast, casual speech, unstressed vowels in certain words are subject to deletion. Examples include *separate* (/'sɛpəɹət/ vs. /'sɛpɹət/); *camera* (/'kæməɹə/ vs. /'kæmɹə/); *opener* (/'oʊpənə/ vs. /'oʊpnə/); and *definite* (/'dɛfɪnət/ vs. /'dɛfnət/). The removal of the unstressed vowel might be thought to result in a resyllabification process. Considering *definite*, we could propose that, in the reduced form, the /f/ could be treated as post-nuclear in a branching rime. However, when we examine the example of *opener*, this solution is not open to us, as /p/ belongs to the class of stops that are not permitted in this position after a heavy nucleus. The solution best fitting the constituent-structure constraints of GovP for *separate* would be to treat *pr* as a complex onset to the second syllable, as follows:

(17)

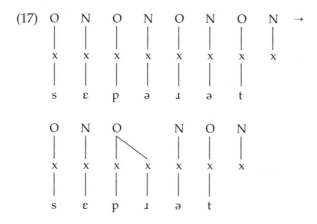

However, in some instances such a strategy will produce onset clusters that are not otherwise found in the language (e.g. /pn/ in /ˈoʊpnə/, /mɹ/ in /ˈkæmɹə/, and /fn/ in /ˈdɛfnət/), or even ones that break the sonority sequencing principle (e.g. /nt/ in /ˈmɒntɹɪŋ/ *mon'toring*). Harris (1994), therefore, argues that a better-motivated solution is to assume that the N slot for the deleted vowel remains in structure at the skeletal tier, but is phonetically empty, i.e. there is no resyllabification, just the phonetic interpretation or non-interpretation of stable syllabic positions. This would give us, for the example *separate*, the following:

(18)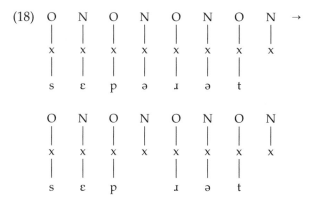

At the melodic level we can consider a commonly occurring example of lenition. In many instances historically original /s/ in a language has weakened to [h] or even been deleted. This is a current change in Cuban Spanish and can also be seen in classical Greek as compared to its reconstructed ancestor language. We also know of many instances of /h/ deletion: in modern English dialects, in fast speech in English with /h/-initial function words, in several Romance languages historically. Lenition of /t/ has also been commonly reported and, although this is more often seen as a change to [θ] (as in Welsh aspirate mutation), a change to [ts] or [s] may also be found (as in Merseyside English, and the German sound shift producing [ts] from earlier [t]). If we put all these lenitions together, we see that GovP provides in its combinations of elements an explanation of these changes through a gradual elimination of melodic material until an empty slot is obtained.

(19) t → s → h → Ø

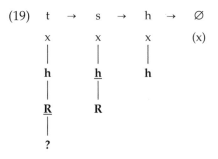

28.5   Government Phonology and Disordered Speech

This model has not been applied often to disordered speech, but note the work of Harris, Watson and Bates (1999), and Ball (2002), and in normal phonological acquisition the work of Ball (1996), and Harrison (1996). Following the example of Ball (1997) regarding Dependency Phonology, we can examine here some of the more commonly reported phonological patterns in disordered speech and see how GovP accounts for them.

We can commence by considering some common patterns in disordered speech at the constituency level. Difficulties with onset clusters are commonly reported in the clinical literature (e.g. Bauman-Waengler, 2003), and indeed, simplifications of these clusters are found in normal phonological development as well. As we have noted earlier, GovP deals with onset clusters in English in two ways: non-/s/-initial clusters are accounted for through binary branching of the onset; /s/-initial clusters, on the other hand, have the /s/ as the onset to an empty nucleus (Harris, 1994, notes that alternative analyses are available, but the /s/ is never part of a branching onset). This distinction does reflect differences in the ways English initial clusters behave in both normal and disordered phonological development (see Gierut, 1999, for evidence of this). Harris (1994) points out that GovP adopts a principles and parameters approach to grammar and so, for the cluster simplification we have been looking at, a change in parameter setting to disallow branching onsets (as is found in many languages, such as Chinese) will account for loss of non-/s/-initial clusters. As the leftmost item in the cluster is the head, this also accounts for the usual pattern in cluster simplification of this type: the retention of the leftmost item, and loss of the right.

To account for simplification in /s/-initial clusters, we have to look beyond the onset to P^0 or even the skeletal tier. We need to ban onsets with empty nuclei to account for these clusters but, all other things being equal, this ban must work only with initial instances. The operation of such a prohibition, then, would remove the /s/ onset and its empty nucleus, leaving (in this case) the rightmost consonant of the (superficial) /s/-initial cluster, as is indeed found in most cases in disordered speech. In normally developing /s/-clusters, and in delayed phonology, an epenthetic vowel may be encountered between the /s/ and the following consonant (e.g. *stop* being realized as [sətɒp]). GovP supplies an elegant account of these forms, whereby we assume the constraint at initial position is not on onsets *and* their following empty nuclei, but just on empty nuclei following initial onsets; the empty nuclei must be phonetically realized, in this case through the addition of the default [@] element.

Another commonly occurring simplification in both developmental and disordered phonology is the deletion of final consonants, whereby *cat* is realized as [kæ], and *dog* as [dɒ]. These, too, can be accounted for by a constraint on onsets and empty nuclei, this time in final position. If final consonant clusters are involved (and if all consonants are deleted), then the parameter setting allowing branching rimes will also need to be turned off. The label 'final consonant deletion' may, however, be overused as, at least on some occasions, final consonants may be replaced by glottal stops. (It is probable that lack of training in detailed phonetic transcription has led to this overuse.) Final glottal replacement involves an interaction between constituency (as this realization is restricted to final position) and melody (in that these consonant slots have had all element material stripped from them except [?]).

Turning now to disordered patterns at the melodic level, we will examine first the commonly reported pattern of velar fronting (we ignore for the purposes of this discussion the debate as to whether this pattern is mainly phonological or articulatory in origin). In traditional binary feature descriptions, a change from target /k/, /g/, /ŋ/ to [t], [d], [n] involves changing the values of the four features [high, back, anterior, coronal]. In GovP we can show that a much simpler account is available where the element [@] is substituted for [R]:

(20) k → t

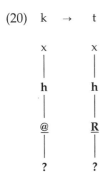

Typical lisp patterns involve the realization of target /s/ and /z/ as dental fricatives or alveolar lateral fricatives. Both of these patterns can be accounted for through simple changes at the melodic level: for the dental fricative a change in head is all that is required, while for the lateral fricative the addition of the [?] element is all that is needed.

(21) s → θ /→ ɬ

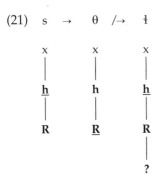

Whereas these lisping patterns (arguably motoric rather than phonological disruption) are relatively straightforward to account for in GovP, more obviously phonological patterns such as fricative simplification are not so easy to deal with. Fricative simplification is a pattern whereby (in English) target dentals are realized as labiodentals, and target postalveolars as alveolars (e.g. /θ, ð/ as [f, v], and /ʃ, ʒ/ as [s, z]). These two patterns can be seen in GovP formalism as follows:

(22)   θ   →   f   ʃ   →   s

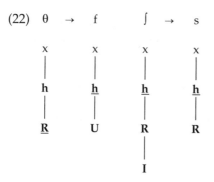

The realization of postalveolars as alveolars is neatly captured through the deletion of the **[I]** element, but the dental to labiodental change requires a switch of elements and a change of head pattern. This last aims to reflect the change from a non-strident to a strident fricative (but, as argued in Ball and Howard, 2004, the classification of labiodentals as strident is not well motivated phonetically or developmentally, and so a simpler change would result if dentals and labiodentals were both classed as non-sibilant fricatives).

Finally, we can briefly consider the work on vowel disorders reported in Ball (1996, 2002) and Harris, Watson, and Bates (1999). Many of the realization patterns described in these publications involved a move to, or towards, the corner vowels [i, a, u]. This can elegantly be captured in GovP by a simplification of vowels to the three elements of **[I, A, U]**.

Other commonly reported patterns in disordered speech (such as context-sensitive voicing, fricative stopping, and liquid gliding) can also, of course, be captured in GovP, but we do not have the space to explore all of these. However, what we do see when we look at accounts of disordered phonology with GovP is the economy of description when we are dealing with unary primes rather than binary features (for example, Grunwell, 1986, argues that a fully specified /r/ to [w] change requires at least six feature changes, whereas in GovP this is accomplished through the removal of two elements and their replacement by one other).

28.6   Conclusion

Government Phonology, and especially the use of phonetically interpretable unary primes, clearly provides more elegant accounts of many aspects of disordered speech than traditional feature-based accounts. However, few studies have yet applied this approach to clinical data, and we await with interest discussion on whether GovP has a role to play in informing intervention as well as analysis.

ACKNOWLEDGMENT

I would like to thank John Harris for his insightful comments on an earlier draft of this chapter. Any remaining faults are solely my own.

REFERENCES

Anderson, J. and Durand, J. (1986). Dependency phonology. In J. Durand (ed.), *Dependency and Non-linear Phonology* (pp. 1–54). London: Croom Helm.

Anderson, J. and Durand, J. (eds.) (1987). *Explorations in Dependency Phonology*. Dordrecht: Foris.

Anderson, J. and Ewen, C. (1987). *Principles of Dependency Phonology*. Cambridge: Cambridge University Press.

Archangeli, D. (1988). Aspects of underspecification theory. *Phonology*, 5, 183–207.

Ball, M. J. (1996). An examination of the nature of the minimal phonological unit in language acquisition. In B. Bernhardt, J. Gilbert, and D. Ingram (eds.), *Proceedings of the UBC International Conference on Phonological Acquisition* (pp. 240–53). Somerville, MA: Cascadilla Press.

Ball, M. J. (1997). Monovalent phonologies. In M. J. Ball and R. D. Kent (eds.), *The New Phonologies* (pp. 127–62). San Diego: Singular.

Ball, M. J. (2002). Clinical phonology of vowel disorders. In M. J. Ball and F. E. Gibbon (eds.), *Vowel Disorders* (pp. 187–216). Boston, MA: Butterworth-Heinemann.

Ball, M. J. and Howard, S. (2004). Is Stridency Deletion really a phonological process? Paper presented at 10th ICPLA Symposium, Lafayette, LA.

Bauman-Waengler, J. (2003). *Articulatory and Phonological Impairments: A Clinical Focus*. 2nd ed. Boston, MA: Allyn and Bacon.

Chomsky, N. and Halle, M. (1968). *The Sound Pattern of English*. Cambridge, MA: MIT Press.

Clements, G. (1985). The geometry of phonological features. *Phonology Yearbook*, 2, 225–52.

Clements, G. (1988). Towards a substantive theory of feature specification. *Proceedings of the North Eastern Linguistic Society*, 18, 79–93.

Gierut, J. A. (1999). Syllable onsets: Clusters and adjuncts in acquisition. *Journal of Speech, Language, and Hearing Research*, 42, 708–46.

Grunwell, P. (1986). *Clinical Phonology*. 2nd ed. London: Croom Helm.

Halle, M. (1992). Phonological features. In W. Bright (ed.), *International Encyclopedia of Linguistics*, vol. 3 (pp. 207–12). Oxford: Oxford University Press.

Harris, J. (1990). Segmental complexity and phonological government. *Phonology*, 7, 255–300.

Harris, J. (1994). *English Sound Structure*. Oxford: Blackwell.

Harris, J. (2005). Vowel reduction as information loss. In P. Carr, J. Durand, and C. Ewen (eds.), *Headhood, Elements, Specification and Contrastivity: Phonological Papers in Honour of John Anderson* (pp. 119–32). Amsterdam: Benjamins.

Harris, J. and Gussmann, E. (2002). Codas, constraints, and coda constraints. *UCL Working Papers in Linguistics*, 14, 1–42.

Harris, J. and Lindsey, G. (1995). The elements of phonological representation. In J. Durand and F. Katamba (eds.), *Frontiers of Phonology* (pp. 34–79). London: Longman.

Harris, J., Watson, J., and Bates, S. (1999). Prosody and melody in vowel disorder. *Journal of Linguistics*, 35, 489–525.

Harrison, P. (1996). The acquisition of melodic primes in infancy. Paper presented at the 4th Phonology Meeting, University of Manchester, May.

Jakobson, R., Fant, G., and Halle, M. (1952). *Preliminaries to Speech Analysis*. Cambridge, MA: MIT Press.

Jakobson, R. and Halle, M. (1956). *Fundamentals of Language*. The Hague: Mouton.

Kaye, J. (1990). Coda-licensing. *Phonology*, 7, 301–30.

Kaye, J., Lowenstamm, J., and Vergnaud, J.-R. (1985). The internal structure of phonological elements: A theory of charm and government. *Phonology Yearbook*, 2, 305–28.

Kaye, J., Lowenstamm, J., and Vergnaud, J.-R. (1990). Constituent structure and government in phonology. *Phonology*, 7, 193–232.

Kula, N. C. (2002). *The Phonology of Verbal Derivation in Bemba*. Utrecht: Netherlands Graduate School of Linguistics.

Ritter, N. (1996). An alternative means of expressing manner. Paper presented at the 4th Phonology Meeting, University of Manchester, May.

Roca, I. and Johnson, W. (1999). *A Course in Phonology*. Oxford: Blackwell.

Sagey, E. (1986). The representation of features and relations in non-linear phonology. PhD dissertation, MIT.

Steriade, D. (1987). Redundant values. *Chicago Linguistic Society*, 23(2), 339–62.

Trubetzkoy, N. (1969). *Principles of Phonology*. Berkeley: University of California Press. (Originally published in 1939.)

van der Hulst, H. (1989). Atoms of segmental structure: Components, gestures and dependency. *Phonology*, 6, 253–84.

29 Articulatory Phonology and Speech Impairment

PASCAL H. H. M. VAN LIESHOUT
AND LOUIS M. GOLDSTEIN

29.1 Introduction

Human beings have a unique ability to interact with each other through the use of a sophisticated symbolic system called language, which allows them to express concepts, feelings and intentions in a way that seems beyond any form of communication used by other animals. The actual expression of these linguistic units requires an effector system that can be controlled in a flexible, fast and accurate manner in order to deal with the high speed and density of information flow in human communication. There are only two motor systems that satisfy these requirements: the vocal tract (and facial structures) and the hands. Apart from the fact that both are used in their own specific way, there is also evidence that they are intrinsically connected in their communicative role (e.g., Treffner & Peter, 2002).

Traditionally, linguistic units are described as discrete mental objects that somehow in their expression through a motor system are transformed or mapped onto dynamic actions, thereby losing part of their identity and distinctiveness. In contrast, the theory that is discussed here, Articulatory Phonology (AP), claims not just that linguistic units are compatible with the output system (vocal tract), but also that their identity is maintained in production and perceived as such by the listener (Goldstein & Fowler, 2003). Section 29.2 describes the origin of AP and its basic principles; section 29.3 is a discussion of its application in the area of speech errors. Building on this information, section 29.4 addresses its usefulness for revealing potential mechanisms that underlie coordination problems in people with speech disorders. In section 29.5, we provide a short outlook on future developments in AP and related areas of research.

29.2   Articulatory Phonology: Origin and Basic Definitions

The origin of AP lies in the late 1970s when researchers at Haskins' Laboratories developed a unique perspective on the representation and nature of action, called Task Dynamics, and applied this to vocal tract actions for speech (Fowler, Rubin, Remez, & Turvey, 1980; Saltzman, 1986). Concepts from dynamical systems were used to develop the idea that the patterns that are observed in motor activities are the result of self-organization in component interactions, constrained by their functional coupling as part of a larger entity, called a synergy or coordinative structure (e.g., Turvey, 1990). When applied to speech, individual articulators form natural functional relationships to perform a common task, for example to create a local vocal tract constriction (e.g., bilabial closure). The advantages of such a system are clear: it provides a low-dimensional, flexible and reliable control system, able to quickly adjust to changes in the positioning of individual articulators, as demonstrated in perturbation studies (e.g., Kelso, Tuller, Vatikiotis-Bateson, & Fowler, 1984).

From here it was a small step to extrapolating the concept of coordinative structures at the level of articulators to the concept of linguistic primitives or gestures as defined in AP (Browman & Goldstein, 1986). Gestures are phonological in the sense that they are discrete and context-free units which can be combined in larger sequences (syllables, words and phrases) to form meaningful language-specific contrasts. For example, the words [bim] and [dim] differ in their initial gesture (bilabial closure vs. tongue tip constriction), similarly to how they would differ in their initial segment according to a more traditional phonology theory. This is not to say that segments and gestures are the same thing; many traditionally defined segments consist of multiple gestures, as in /m/ which requires coordination of velum and bilabial closure gestures.

Gestures are task-specific vocal tract actions, not physical movements of the vocal tract articulators themselves. The latter come into play only during the activation intervals of gestures, when their dynamics guide the articulatory movements in a contextually appropriate manner (see below). With the exception of the velic and glottal gestures, the goals of each gesture are determined by two independent dimensions or tract variables, one specifying constriction location (along a longitudinal dimension) and the other constriction degree (along a vertical dimension) for the particular constricting organ. Different constricting organs (each of which corresponds to a set of articulators) are organized in larger anatomical hierarchies (tongue, oral, vocal tract; Browman & Goldstein, 1990a). Tract variables control the context-free trajectory of motion in their respective dimension according to a second-order dynamical system for a mass-normalized, critically damped harmonic oscillator, which has a single stable solution. The implementation of these control settings is part of the associated Task Dynamic model (Saltzman & Munhall, 1989), which also regulates how discrete tract variable actions are mapped onto the appropriate articulatory subsystems of the vocal tract. The resulting movements of individual articulators lead to changes in vocal tract geometry, with predictable aerodynamic and acoustic consequences.

In the AP model, the production of a given utterance can be described, at one level, as an overlapping sequence of constriction actions of the various articulatory subsystems. This is represented in a gestural score, specifying the temporal intervals during which each constriction task actively controls the vocal tract articulators (Browman & Goldstein, 1992). The fact that discrete gestures overlap in time (and space) provides a natural account of how at one level (phonology) discrete units can be used to build meaningful linguistic contrasts and at the other level (articulation), they combine in a continuous dynamic sequence of individual articulator movements without losing their basic identity (Goldstein & Fowler, 2003).

The gestural score for a particular production of a given word can be estimated from examination of kinematic vocal tract data, finding the points in time at which a constriction begins to be formed, achieves its maximum constriction, and is released. Of course, these particular points in time will vary across exemplars of the same word, as a function of speaking rate, prosodic position, speaker, etc. To capture the lexically significant aspects of coordination that remain constant across exemplars (e.g., the characteristic coordination of gestures in the word 'bad' that distinguish it from 'dab', which is composed of the same gestures), the relationship between individual gestures is specified in terms of phase differences or relative phase (Kelso, Saltzman, & Tuller, 1986). Originally, it was proposed that relative phasing would be more or less fixed for a given gestural combination, regardless of variations in, for example, syllable position and stress (e.g., Kelso & Tuller, 1984). Subsequent experimental studies did not confirm this claim (e.g., Nittrouer, 1991; Shaiman & Porter, 1991), and this has led to a new model for gestural coordination (Goldstein, Byrd, & Saltzman, 2006; Saltzman & Byrd, 2000).

In the new model (figure 29.1), a limit-cycle planning oscillator is associated with each gesture, and the oscillators for a given utterance are coupled to one another in a so-called coupling graph that allows multiple, potentially competing coupling specifications (Browman & Goldstein, 2000; Goldstein, Byrd, & Saltzman, 2006; Nam & Saltzman, 2003; Saltzman, Nam, Goldstein, & Byrd, 2006). The coupling graph provides a gestural alternative to the segment-based mental lexicons assumed in the linguistic literature (e.g., Levelt, Roelofs, & Meyer, 1999). During the 'planning' process, the system of oscillators settles into a stable pattern of relative phases, and these phases are used to trigger the activation of the gestures. The coupling specifications take advantage of intrinsically stable modes of coordination – in-phase and anti-phase (Haken, Kelso, & Bunz, 1985). For example, the consonant and vowel gestures of a CV syllable are coupled in-phase. A syllable-final consonant is coupled anti-phase with respect to the vowel. The topology of specifications in the coupling graph has been shown to account not only for the phasing of gestures in different syllable positions (Browman & Goldstein, 2000), but also for the relative amount of

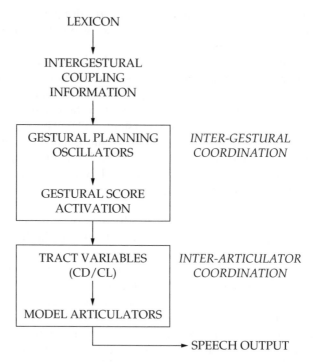

Figure 29.1   A schematic and simplified representation of the revised AP model, based on coupled nonlinear oscillators (from Goldstein, Byrd, & Saltzman, 2006; Nam & Saltzman, 2003; Saltzman & Byrd, 2000). The intergestural coupling information refers to the coupling graph. Note: CD = constriction degree; CL = constriction location (see text for more details).

phase variability in different positions (Nam & Saltzman, 2003; Saltzman, Nam, Goldstein, & Byrd, 2006). Variability is a function of coupling strength (in-phase is strongest) and the number of paths that link a pair of gestures. Coupling strength is a function of the complexity of the coupling and the speed at which the coupling needs to be maintained (Goldstein & Fowler, 2003; Saltzman, Nam, Goldstein, & Byrd, 2006; van Lieshout, Hulstijn, Alfonso, & Peters, 1997). The complexity of the coupling can be determined by the ratio of movement frequencies for the coupled structures. This is why the new model incorporates multi-frequency couplings, that is, when one articulator moves at a different frequency than the one to which it is coupled (Saltzman & Byrd, 2000). Complex couplings underlie the rhythmic organization of speech in the way faster-moving smaller units are coupled to slower-moving larger units; for example, syllable (vowel) oscillators couple to foot oscillators, which in turn couple to phrase level oscillators (Cummins & Port, 1998).

AP also claims that the gesture is the common code shared by communicators for production and perception (Goldstein & Fowler, 2003). The specific aspects of speech perception as related to gestures are formalized in the theory of Direct Perception (Fowler, 1996). Recent studies have provided data in support of the potential role of gestures in (multimodal) speech perception (e.g., Fowler, Brown, Sabadini, & Weihing, 2003; Kerzel & Bekkering, 2000; Watkins, Strafella, & Paus, 2003).

Finally, AP attributes a crucial role to non-verbal phylogenetically older oral motor behaviors in the origin and development of speech. Space limitations do not allow us to elaborate, but review papers provide a detailed account of this topic (Goldstein, Byrd, & Saltzman, 2006; Studdert-Kennedy & Goldstein, 2003).

29.3   Articulatory Phonology: Gestural Overlap and Speech Errors

As mentioned in section 29.2, gestures have an inherent temporal structure, which allows them to overlap during speech production. The amount of overlap is assumed to be a function of various factors, including speech rate, style (casual vs. formal speech), the organs used for making the constrictions, and linguistic constraints (Goldstein & Fowler, 2003). Studies have shown how gestural overlap in casual speech can be used to explain events like segment assimilation, deletion and insertion, which in traditional accounts are associated with language-specific phonological rules (e.g., Browman & Goldstein, 1990b). The concept of gestural overlap and its perceptual consequences have also been used to explain systematic patterns of change in language-specific phonological inventories (Browman & Goldstein, 1991).

More recently, the application of gestures and their ability to overlap in time has been broadened to include an account of speech errors in normal speech production (Goldstein, Pouplier, Chen, Saltzman, & Byrd, 2007) and their perception (Pouplier & Goldstein, 2005). Traditionally, phonologically based speech errors are described in terms of whole-segment operations (e.g., Dell, 1984) as in the substitution between /k/ and /p/ in 'poffee cot' instead of 'coffee pot'. These interpretations are based on phonetic transcriptions (Meyer, 1992). However, perception can be quite deceptive when it comes to detecting changes in speech output (Kent, 1996). This issue was first addressed in a kinematic study by Boucher (1994), showing that segments that were perceived as being substituted were still present in the actual articulation of the word. Mowrey and MacKay's study (1990) pushed this issue further in demonstrating that many of the speech errors they elicited in their speakers, and which were either interpreted as phonemic errors or missed all together, showed a variety of (subtle and non-phonemic) variations in muscle output. Since individual muscles may not signal what is actually going on in terms of gestural activity, Goldstein and colleagues (Goldstein, Pouplier, Chen, Saltzman, & Byrd, 2007) used kinematic data to study the nature of speech errors as elicited by the repetition of bisyllabic sequences with alternating syllable-onset consonants (e.g., 'cop top' and 'tip kip'). Their results showed that errors can be described and explained more adequately as a dynamic process operating on controlled constricting actions than as substitutions of abstract phonemic segments. Typically, error patterns consisted of gestural intrusion errors, in which the intended gesture was co-produced with a gesture for the conflicting consonant. In the majority of cases, extra gestures were not at the expense of the earlier intended gesture, so true substitutions were rare. This is clearly in contrast to the observations based on segmental transcriptions. The phonotactically illegal co-production of these gestures also contradicts the often reported principle that units containing speech errors remain well-formed phonological sequences (e.g., Dell, Reed, Adams, & Meyer, 2000). In addition, the intrusion gesture varied in degree of constriction, which influenced how they were perceived (Pouplier & Goldstein, 2005; see also Mowrey & MacKay, 1990). In terms of rate, it was found that faster speech rates led to an increase in gestural intrusion errors. Goldstein and colleagues (Goldstein, Pouplier, Chen, Saltzman, & Byrd, 2007) explained their findings by means of the notion of frequency locking. Tongue tip and tongue dorsum gestures both showed a multi-frequency coupling relationship (2:1) with the lip gesture at the end of the word ('cop' 'top'), which is intrinsically less stable (Nam & Saltzman, 2003), especially under fast rate conditions. The gestural intrusion corrects this situation, yielding a more stable harmonic relationship among tongue tip, dorsum, and lip gestures (see also Saltzman & Byrd, 2000; van Lieshout, Hijl, & Hulstijn, 1999).

29.4   Articulatory Phonology: Speech Impairments

In the previous sections we have outlined the basic principles of AP for speech production and perception, including its view on the nature and occurrence of speech errors. Research on speech disorders using concepts of AP is still limited (van Lieshout, 2004). Due to space limitations, we can only present a selection of studies on coordination issues in people with speech disorders. For ease of exposition, their findings are organized along the types of coordination that can be distinguished in AP: coordination between individual articulators (intra-gestural coupling), coordination between individual gestures (intergestural coupling), and gestural intrusion. This does not mean that problems at one level cannot extend to other levels; in fact most likely they do (Saltzman, Löfqvist, Kay, Kinsella-Shaw, & Rubin, 1998).

29.4.1   Gestural overlap

In the area of stuttering, Ward (1997) reported on higher variability in the phase coupling between lips and jaw in the fluent production of bilabial closure gestures in people who stutter (PWS), especially at faster speech rates and in conditions where stress alterations were required. Since the study by Ward used adult stuttering subjects, it remains unclear if the findings are causally related to stuttering or rather an adaptation or symptom of the disorder itself. Therefore, it is interesting to look at data from children who stutter, as their motor behaviors may more directly reflect the underlying mechanisms involved in stuttering.

Chang and colleagues (Chang, Ohde, & Conture, 2002) used F2 information in CV syllables as an acoustic measure of gestural overlap of C and V productions. While they could not find a systematic difference between children who stutter (CWS) and age-matched controls in the amount of gestural overlap in CV onsets, they did find a trend for less differentiation between bilabial and alveolar places of articulation in their youngest stuttering subjects. It is possible that this lack of differentiation is due to a problem in intra-gestural coordination. The jaw is an articulator that forms part of the functional synergy for both tongue tip and lip gestures, in addition to the unshared articulators specific to the two gestures (tongue and lips, respectively). If intra-gestural coordination is problematic (as suggested above for adult PWS), so that too much of the task-directed motion is contributed by the jaw, then large, passive decreases in the size of lip opening (due to jaw-raising) will occur during tongue tip stops, and conversely, decreases in the distance of the tongue tip from the palate during bilabial stops. These will have the consequences that the coronals and labials will be more acoustically similar than they would be for controls. If this can be confirmed in future studies, the tendency to increase jaw movements would fit assumptions about a more general preference in PWS to increase movement range in order to maintain coupling stability (van Lieshout, Hulstijn, & Peters, 2004). For children, the jaw is a likely candidate to implement such a strategy as they show more stable control of this structure compared to the lips (e.g., Green, Moore, Higashikawa, & Steeve, 2000).

29.4.2 *Intergestural coupling and coordination*

A different line of research with patients with speech problems has focused on gestural overlap. According to AP (Browman & Goldstein, 1990b), the nature of overlap differs between gestures that share the same constricting organ and tract variables (homorganic) and gestures that do not (heterorganic). Whereas the former will lead to gestural blending (interaction), the latter form of co-production preserves the identity of the individual gestures. Depending on the amount of overlap, gestures may lack acoustic consequences and may be perceptually 'hidden' (Surprenant & Goldstein, 1998). Taking these notions as a basis, Huinck and colleagues (Huinck, Peters, van Lieshout, & Hulstijn, 2004) investigated the effects of gestural overlap using acoustic measures of reaction time and word duration in homorganic and heterorganic clusters within and across syllable boundaries in PWS and matched controls. They found that both groups were virtually identical in their responses, except for a three-way interaction found for reaction times: PWS showed longer reaction times for homorganic clusters, but only across syllable boundaries. According to AP, bonding strength (cohesiveness of gestural constellations) is particularly strong for gestures forming syllable onsets because the gestures are coupled in-phase with the syllable's vowel gesture (Goldstein, Byrd, & Saltzman, 2006; see also section 29.2 above). In contrast, consonant clusters across syllable boundaries may not be directly coupled to one another at all, which results in much greater phase variability. Nam (forthcoming) has shown in a reaction-time study that structures that are more loosely coupled take longer to plan. This would apply even more to gestures which share the same constricting organ and have to blend. Limitations in speech motor skill in PWS (van Lieshout, Hulstijn, & Peters, 2004) may include difficulties in gestural planning, which could provide an explanation for the findings reported by Huinck, Peters, van Lieshout, & Hulstijn (2004).

Other studies have focused on formant measures as an estimate for gestural overlap. For example, Tjaden (2000) studied F2 and center of gravity values of consonant noise spectra in CV syllables in patients with Parkinson's disease (PD) and matched controls. In general, the PD subjects were found to show more coarticulatory overlap between consonant and vowel productions. In the new AP model, the C and V gestures are hypothesized to be coupled in-phase in terms of generalized relative phase, but the C oscillator has a higher frequency than the V oscillator, as consistent with the slower movement and longer duration for vowels. As a result of this coupling structure, C and V gestures begin synchronously, but the V gesture takes longer to get to its target, and it is active for a longer period of time. The behavior of PD subjects reported in Tjaden could result from a preference for C and V gestures to exhibit 1:1 frequency mode locking, the simplest (and most stable) kind of coupling. If the gestures have the same frequencies, the V gesture will be fully formed at the same time as the C gesture, leading to the reported increase in measured coarticulation during the consonant production.

Hertrich and Ackermann (1999) investigated coarticulation in patients with ataxic dysarthria using an acoustic variable based on spectral dissimilarity. Their findings suggested a specific decrease in (anticipatory) CV coarticulation and a tendency towards a stronger influence of vowel articulation on the following segments. Whereas they interpreted the first phenomenon as being related to articulatory imprecision, they related their second finding to the typical slower speech rate of these patients. In terms of AP, both findings can be related to the effect of speech rate on gestural overlap, if we assume that V gestures are proportionally more affected by speech rate than are C gestures (Klatt, 1976). If C and V gestures are synchronized at their onset, as discussed above, and if V gestures are slowed proportionally more than C gestures, then at the moment the C gesture reaches its target, the V gesture will be further from its target at a slow rate than at a fast rate, resulting in a reduced CV co-articulation measurement. By the same logic, a C that begins when the V reaches its target (a coda C or the initial C of the following syllable) will be more overlapped by that V at a slow rate than a fast rate, because at the slow rate, the V will move away from its target toward the next V at a slower rate.

Potential problems in gestural coordination are also reported for patients with apraxia of speech (e.g., van Lieshout, Bose, Square, & Steele, 2007; Ziegler & von Cramon, 1986). The latter study also indicates that variation in movement amplitude could be related to changes in the stability of coordination (see also section 29.5).

29.4.3 *Gestural intrusion*

In a review, Pouplier & Hardcastle (2005) compared several articulatory studies on patients with aphasia and apraxia, concluding that the (partial) co-production of segments/gestures in speech errors in these populations seems a rather common mechanism, even if the error is perceived as being a whole segment substitution. Thus, there is a striking similarity to the mechanisms reported in section 29.3 for speech errors in normal speakers.

Gestural intrusion may also be partly the source of decreased distinctiveness in the VOT distribution and/or increase in VOT variability found for different patient populations, when compared to control speakers (see Auzou, Ozsancak, Morris, et al., 2000, for a review of this literature). One way to have less distinctiveness is to produce voiced stops by adding a glottal abduction gesture that is not normally present, thus making them sound more like voiceless stops.

This selective review of the literature on differences in coordination in patients with speech problems provides a small window on the potential of AP to provide a systematic and principled account of the source of speech errors and coordination instability. There is obviously still a lot of work to be done in this area and some of the directions this research might take are addressed in the next section.

29.5 Articulatory Phonology: Future Developments

Gestural accounts of speech production (and perception) will need to demonstrate that their models provide an economical and efficient way to explain known phenomena in normal and disordered speech, both in adults and during development. This will include studies in the area of multimodal perception in adults and young infants to access their ability to use this information to identify and control gestures (Goldstein & Fowler, 2003). Future studies will also have to explore more systematically the role of specific movement variables on the nature and stability of coupling relationships in speech (Saltzman & Byrd, 2000; van Lieshout, 2004). Recent work has suggested that nonlinear variations in speech movement amplitude (and/or peak velocity) may influence coordination stability in normal speakers (van Lieshout, 2001) and in patient populations with structural (van Lieshout, Rutjens, & Spauwen, 2002) or neurological problems, as in apraxia of speech (van Lieshout, Bose, Square, & Steele, 2007).

Other issues that need to be explored in greater detail include the relationship between the concept of gestures and other (more traditional) linguistic units (segments, syllables, words, phrases). Finally, future studies will have to deal with methodological issues in relating behavioral aspects of intra- and intergestural coordination to corresponding dynamics in brain activity (cf., Kelso, Fuchs, Lancaster, et al., 1998). More generally, AP model abstractions will have to be related to neural control networks in the central and peripheral nervous system in order to predict the potential effects of lesions in patient populations. Work along the lines described above will determine the future success of the theory in both basic and applied research.

ACKNOWLEDGMENTS

This work was undertaken, in part, thanks to funding from the Canada Research Chairs Program, the Canadian Institutes of Health Research (CIHR), the Natural Sciences and Engineering Research Council of Canada (NSERC), the Canada Foundation for Innovation (CFI) and the Ontario Innovation Trust (OIT).

REFERENCES

Auzou, P., Ozsancak, C., Morris, R. J., Jan, M., Eustache, F., and Hannequin, D. (2000). Voice onset time in aphasia, apraxia of speech and dysarthria: A review. *Clinical Linguistics and Phonetics*, 14, 131–50.

Boucher, V. J. (1994). Alphabet-related biases in psycholinguistic inquiries: Considerations for direct theories of speech production and perception. *Journal of Phonetics*, 22, 1–18.

Browman, C. P. and Goldstein, L. (1986). Towards an articulatory phonology. *Phonology Yearbook*, 3, 219–52.

Browman, C. P. and Goldstein, L. (1990a). Tiers in articulatory phonology, with some implications for casual speech. In J. Kingston and M. E. Beckman (eds.), *Papers in Laboratory Phonology. Volume I: Between the Grammar and Physics of Speech* (pp. 341–76). Cambridge: Cambridge University Press.

Browman, C. P. and Goldstein, L. (1990b). Gestural specification using dynamically-defined articulatory structures. *Journal of Phonetics*, 18, 299–320.

Browman, C. P. and Goldstein, L. (1991). Gestural structures: Distinctiveness, phonological processes, and historical change. In I. G. Mattingly and M. Studdert-Kennedy (eds.), *Modularity and the Motor Theory of Speech Perception* (pp. 313–38). Hillsdale, NJ: Lawrence Erlbaum Associates.

Browman, C. P. and Goldstein, L. (1992). Articulatory phonology: An overview. *Phonetica*, 49, 155–80.

Browman, C. P. and Goldstein, L. (2000). Competing constraints on intergestural coordination and self-organization of phonological structures. *Les Cahiers de l'ICP, Bulletin de la Communication Parlée*, 5, 25–34.

Chang, S. E., Ohde, R. N., and Conture, E. G. (2002). Coarticulation and formant transition rate in young children who stutter. *Journal of Speech, Language, and Hearing Research*, 45, 676–88.

Cummins, F. and Port, R. F. (1998). Rhythmic constraints on stress timing in English. *Journal of Phonetics*, 26, 145–71.

Dell, G. S. (1984). Representation of serial order in speech: Evidence from the repeated phoneme effect in speech errors. *Journal of Experimental Psychology: Learning, Memory and Cognition*, 10, 222–33.

Dell, G. S., Reed, K. D., Adams, D. R., and Meyer, A. S. (2000). Speech errors, phonotactic constraints, and implicit learning: A study of the role of experience in language production. *Journal of Experimental Psychology: Learning, Memory and Cognition*, 26, 1355–67.

Fowler, C. A. (1996). Listeners do hear sounds, not tongues. *Journal of the Acoustical Society of America*, 99, 1730–41.

Fowler, C. A., Brown, J. M., Sabadini, L., and Weihing, J. (2003). Rapid access to speech gestures in perception: Evidence from choice and simple response time tasks. *Journal of Memory and Language*, 49, 396–413.

Fowler, C. A., Rubin, P., Remez, R., and Turvey, M. T. (1980). Implications for speech production of a general theory of action. In B. Butterworth (ed.), *Language Production. Volume 1: Speech and Talk* (pp. 373–420). London: Academic Press.

Goldstein, L. M., Byrd, D., and Saltzman, E. (2006). The role of vocal tract gestural action units in understanding the evolution of phonology. In M. A. Arbib (ed.), *From Action to Language: The Mirror Neuron System* (pp. 215–49). Cambridge: Cambridge University Press.

Goldstein, L. M. and Fowler, C. (2003). Articulatory phonology: A phonology for public language use. In A. S. Meyer and N. O. Schiller (eds.), *Phonetics and Phonology in Language Comprehension and Production: Differences and Similarities* (pp. 159–207). Berlin: Mouton de Gruyter.

Goldstein, L., Pouplier, M., Chen, L., Saltzman, E., and Byrd, D. (2007). Dynamic action units slip in speech production errors. *Cognition*, 103, 386–412.

Green, J. R., Moore, C. A., Higashikawa, M., and Steeve, R. W. (2000). The physiologic development of speech motor control: Lip and jaw coordination. *Journal of Speech, Language, and Hearing Research*, 43, 239–55.

Haken, H., Kelso, J. A., and Bunz, H. (1985). A theoretical model of phase transitions in human hand movements. *Biological Cybernetics*, 51, 347–56.

Hertrich, I. and Ackermann, H. (1999). Temporal and spectral aspects of coarticulation in ataxic dysarthria: An acoustic analysis. *Journal of Speech, Language, and Hearing Research*, 42, 367–81.

Huinck, W. J., Peters, H. F. M., van Lieshout, P. H. H. M., and Hulstijn, W. (2004). Gestural overlap in consonant clusters: Effects on the fluent speech of stuttering and non-stuttering subjects. *Journal of Fluency Disorders*, 29, 3–25.

Kelso, J. A., Fuchs, A., Lancaster, R., Holroyd, T., Cheyne, D., and Weinberg, H. (1998). Dynamic cortical activity in the human brain reveals motor equivalence. *Nature*, 392, 814–18.

Kelso, J. A. S., Saltzman, E., and Tuller, B. (1986). The dynamical theory in speech production: Data and theory. *Journal of Phonetics*, 14, 29–60.

Kelso, J. A. and Tuller, B. (1984). Converging evidence in support of common dynamical principles for speech and movement coordination. *American Journal of Physiology*, 246, R928–R935.

Kelso, J. A., Tuller, B., Vatikiotis-Bateson, E., and Fowler, C. A. (1984). Functionally specific articulatory cooperation following jaw perturbations during speech: Evidence for coordinative structures. *Journal of Experimental Psychology: Human Perception and Performance*, 10, 812–32.

Kent, R. D. (1996). Hearing and believing: Some limits to the auditory-perceptual assessment of speech and voice disorders. *American Journal of Speech-Language Pathology*, 5, 7–23.

Kerzel, D. and Bekkering, H. (2000). Motor activation from visible speech: Evidence from stimulus response compatibility. *Journal of Experimental Psychology: Human Perception and Performance*, 26, 634–47.

Klatt, D. H. (1976). Linguistic uses of segmental duration in English: Acoustic and perceptual evidence. *Journal of the Acoustical Society of America*, 59, 1208–21.

Levelt, W. J., Roelofs, A., and Meyer, A. S. (1999). A theory of lexical access in speech production. *Behavioral and Brain Sciences*, 22, 1–38.

Meyer, A. S. (1992). Investigation of phonological encoding through speech error analyses: Achievements, limitations, and alternatives. *Cognition*, 42, 181–211.

Mowrey, R. A. and MacKay, I. R. (1990). Phonological primitives: Electromyographic speech error evidence. *Journal of the Acoustical Society of America*, 88, 1299–1312.

Nam, H. (forthcoming). A competitive, coupled oscillator model of moraic structure: Split-gesture dynamics focusing on positional asymmetry. In J. Cole and J. Hualde (eds.), *Papers in Laboratory Phonology 9*. Berlin: Mouton de Gruyter.

Nam, H. and Saltzman, E. (2003). A competitive, coupled oscillator of syllable structure. In M. J. Solé, D. Recasens, and J. Romero (eds.), *Proceedings of the XIIth International Congress of Phonetic Sciences, Barcelona* (pp. 2253–6). Rundle Mall, Adelaide: Causal Productions.

Nittrouer, S. (1991). Phase relations of jaw and tongue tip movements in the production of VCV utterances. *Journal of the Acoustical Society of America*, 90, 1806–15.

Pouplier, M. and Goldstein, L. (2005). Asymmetries in the perception of speech production errors. *Journal of Phonetics*, 33, 47–75.

Pouplier, M. and Hardcastle, W. (2005). A re-evaluation of the nature of speech errors in normal and disordered speakers. *Phonetica*, 62, 227–43.

Saltzman, E. (1986). Task dynamic coordination of the speech articulators: A preliminary model. *Experimental Brain Research*, Suppl. 15, 129–44.

Saltzman, E. and Byrd, D. (2000). Task-dynamics of gestural timing: Phase windows and multifrequency rhythms. *Human Movement Science*, 19, 499–526.

Saltzman, E., Löfqvist, A., Kay, B., Kinsella-Shaw, J., and Rubin, P. (1998). Dynamics of intergestural timing: A perturbation study of lip–larynx coordination. *Experimental Brain Research*, 123, 412–24.

Saltzman, E. L. and Munhall, K. (1989). A dynamical approach to gestural patterning in speech production. *Ecological Psychology*, 1, 333–82.

Saltzman, E., Nam, H., Goldstein, L., and Byrd, D. (2006). The distinctions between state, parameter and graph dynamics in sensorimotor control and coordination. In A. G. Feldman (ed.), *Progress in Motor Control: Motor Control and Learning over the Lifespan* (pp. 63–73). New York: Springer.

Shaiman, S. and Porter, R. J. (1991). Different phase-stable relationships of the upper lip and jaw for production of vowels and diphthongs. *Journal of the Acoustical Society of America*, 90, 3000–7.

Studdert-Kennedy, M. and Goldstein, L. (2003). Launching language: The gestural origin of discrete infinity. In M. H. Christiansen and S. Kirby (eds.), *Language Evolution* (pp. 235–54). Oxford: Oxford University Press.

Surprenant, A. M. and Goldstein, L. (1998). The perception of speech gestures. *Journal of the Acoustical Society of America*, 104, 518–29.

Tjaden, K. (2000). An acoustic study of coarticulation in dysarthric speakers with Parkinson disease. *Journal of Speech, Language, and Hearing Research*, 43, 1466–80.

Treffner, P. J. and Peter, M. (2002). Dynamics of speech-hand gestures. *Human Movement Science*, 21, 641–97.

Turvey, M. T. (1990). Coordination. *American Psychologist*, 45, 938–53.

van Lieshout, P. H. H. M. (2001). Coupling dynamics of motion primitives in speech movements and its potential relevance for fluency. *Society for Chaos Theory in Psychology and Life Sciences Newsletter*, 8(4), 18.

van Lieshout, P. H. H. M. (2004). Dynamical systems theory and its application in speech. In B. Maassen, R. Kent, H. Peters, P. van Lieshout, and W. Hulstijn (eds.), *Speech Motor Control in Normal and Disordered Speech* (pp. 51–82). Oxford: Oxford University Press.

van Lieshout, P. H. H. M., Bose, A., Square, P. A., and Steele, C. A. (2007). Speech motor control in fluent and dysfluent speech production of an individual with apraxia of speech and Broca's aphasia. *Clinical Linguistics and Phonetics*, 21 (3), 159–88.

van Lieshout, P. H. H. M., Hijl, M., and Hulstijn, W. (1999). Flexibility and stability in bilabial gestures. 2: Evidence from continuous syllable production. In J. J. Ohala, J. J. Hasegawa, M. Ohala, D. Granville, and A. C. Bailey (eds.), *Proceedings XIVth International Congress of Phonetic Sciences* (pp. 45–8). San Francisco: American Institute of Physics.

van Lieshout, P., Hulstijn, W., Alfonso, P. J., and Peters, H. F. (1997). Higher and lower order influences on the stability of the dynamic coupling between articulators. In W. Hulstijn, H. F. Peters, and P. van Lieshout (eds.), *Speech Production: Motor Control, Brain Research and Fluency Disorders* (pp. 161–70). Amsterdam: Elsevier.

van Lieshout, P. H. H. M., Hulstijn, W., and Peters, H. F. M. (2004). Searching for the weak link in the speech production chain of people who stutter: A motor skill approach. In B. Maassen, R. Kent, H. Peters, P. van Lieshout, and W. Hulstijn (eds.), *Speech Motor Control in Normal and Disordered Speech* (pp. 313–56). Oxford: Oxford University Press.

van Lieshout, P. H. H. M., Rutjens, C. A. W., and Spauwen, P. H. M. (2002). The dynamics of interlip coupling in speakers with a repaired unilateral cleft-lip history. *Journal of Speech, Language, and Hearing Research*, 45, 5–19.

Ward, D. (1997). Intrinsic and extrinsic timing in stutterers' speech: Data and implications. *Language and Speech*, 40, 289–310.

Watkins, K. E., Strafella, A. P., and Paus, T. (2003). Seeing and hearing speech excites the motor system involved in speech production. *Neuropsychologia*, 41(8), 989–94.

Ziegler, W. and von Cramon, D. (1986). Timing deficits in apraxia of speech. *European Archives of Psychiatry and Neurological Sciences*, 236, 44–9.

30 A Cognitive Approach to Clinical Phonology

ANNA VOGEL SOSA AND JOAN L. BYBEE

30.1 Introduction

The task of the clinical phonologist is to evaluate the speech production abilities of children and adults with speech difficulties, aiding the speech-language pathologist in assessing the need for treatment, and helping monitor progress during and after treatment. This task has remained and probably will remain fairly constant over the years; the tools that are used to perform it, however, have changed and will continue to change over time. Not surprisingly, the practice of clinical phonology is greatly influenced by current trends in general phonological theory, which in turn alter according to which linguistic theory is presently popular.

30.1.1 Linguistic theory in developmental phonology

The history of the field of developmental phonology provides an excellent example of how general linguistic theory is extended to work in related disciplines. Roman Jakobson, in his seminal paper on phonological acquisition and phonological disorder associated with aphasia (Jakobson, 1968), applied principles of early structural linguistics, which was popular at the time, to arrive at his conclusions regarding the universal order of acquisition of phonemic contrasts. Later, with the rise of generative approaches to phonology after the publication of Chomsky and Halle's *Sound Pattern of English* (1968), scholars of child language began to describe phonological acquisition in terms of abstract underlying representations and obligatory realization rules. Stampe's *natural phonology* (Stampe, 1969; see also Miccio and Scarpino, chapter 25 in this volume) led to the discussion of innate phonological processes in children's speech, while the advent of optimality theory (Prince & Smolensky, 1993; see also Dinnsen & Gierut, chapter 27 in this volume) has generated an extensive literature about the ranking and reranking of constraints during the developmental process. Many of these individual approaches to the study of phonology have left permanent traces in the clinical world. For example, children are often diagnosed as disordered on the basis of Jakobson-like ideas of a universal order and a universal timetable of acquisition of individual speech sounds. Meanwhile, the most enduring influence of Stampe's natural phonology is probably the role that phonological processes continue to play in the description of the systematic errors that occur both in typical development and in children with phonological disorders.

This chapter will introduce a relatively new approach to phonology, *cognitive phonology*, and will discuss how this theory may prove useful for the work and thinking of clinical phonologists. Although the innovative ideas of cognitive phonology are certainly relevant to all clinical populations, discussion in this chapter regarding clinical applications will focus primarily on developmental phonology and the remediation of phonological disorders in young children.

30.1.2   The terms: Cognitive vs. usage-based

The term *cognitive phonology* should be taken as a general descriptor for the phonological theory that will be described here rather than as a hard and fast label. In fact, the same general approach has probably gone by a variety of different names in the existing literature and the term 'cognitive phonology' has certainly been used for a variety of different approaches that may have important differences. Our preferred terminology is *usage-based phonology*; this is the term used by Bybee in her 2001 book *Phonology and Language Use*, which provides an in-depth discussion of her theory. The theory discussed in this chapter is grounded in Bybee's concept of usage-based phonology.

30.2   Usage-Based Linguistics

The term 'usage-based' was first introduced in 1987 by Ronald Langacker in his book *Foundations of Cognitive Grammar*. In this book he described a usage-based model of language as one in which "Substantial importance is given to the actual use of the linguistic system and a speaker's knowledge of the full range of linguistic conventions" (Langacker, 1987, p. 494). This approach stands in stark contrast to the generative position which distinguishes competence from performance and takes competence to be representative of the true nature of the linguistic system. Most notably, a usage-based framework for linguistic study assumes an intimate relationship between language use and language structure, with structure seen as both a generator and a product of language use. With specific reference to phonology, a usage-based account will emphasize the role that language use plays in shaping a linguistic sound system (Bybee, 2001), while a usage-based approach to phonological acquisition will highlight the important role of input and use in the instantiation and ongoing modification of the child's phonological system.

Several key characteristics of a usage-based approach to linguistics in general, and phonology in particular, are outlined below (see also Kemmer & Barlow, 2000). For readers familiar with more traditional phonological theory, the notable differences between usage-based phonology and other rule- or constraint-based theories will be evident. For readers with a background in clinical phonology, the fundamentals of usage-based phonology may seem quite obvious and very compatible with their clinical experiences.

30.2.1   Language use creates structure

As the term implies, a usage-based approach to linguistics assumes a *close relationship between linguistic structure and instances of language use*. Specifically, the linguistic system itself is a product of a speaker's experience with specific instances of language production and comprehension. This approach de-emphasizes the abstract/concrete dichotomy that is such an important feature of generative accounts of phonology. While generative theory assumes stripped-down, abstract phonological representations, a usage-based approach denies the existence of abstract structure in the absence of a direct link to a specific instance of use; linguistic structure itself is dynamic, and is constantly being changed by use. This emphasis on individual instances of language use allows word-specific phonetic detail to be part of our linguistic system. This view-point is compatible with an exemplar model of lexical storage. In general terms, exemplar theory holds that all instances of a particular token (a word, for example) are stored whole and relationships develop among the different tokens according to phonetic similarities and patterns of use (Johnson, 1997; Pierrehumbert, 2001). Certain categories may emerge from these relationships, centering on the best or most frequent exemplars, but these categories are flexible and are subject to modification depending on the nature of the input. Exemplar models allow for associations at numerous levels of representation, from the phrase to the phoneme (or its equivalent) and even the feature. While exemplar theory itself is not intrinsic to usage-based approaches to linguistics, the emphasis on experience, on use creating structure, and on structure as a dynamic property influenced by instances of production and comprehension is certainly consistent with usage-based linguistics.

30.2.2   Frequency

A second, and extremely important, aspect of usage-based theories is the *emphasis on the role of frequency in the shaping of linguistic structure*. The role of frequency in language processing is a well-established phenomenon. In perception, for example, more frequent forms are accessed more quickly and more accurately. In production, a number of different effects have been noted. For example, Bybee (2000) describes a significant effect of token frequency on the deletion of final /t/ and /d/ in American English. Two thousand tokens of words with final t/d targets were analyzed. The results of the transcription-based analysis indicate that word frequency is a significant factor affecting the deletion of final t/d; final /t/ and /d/ were deleted significantly more often in the high-frequency forms (see also Gregory, Raymond, Bell, Fosler-Lussier, & Jurafsky, 1999). The explanation for this effect is that sound changes affect words 'opportunistically' each time they are produced. Therefore, frequent words are exposed to the sound change more often, and the lexical representation adjusts so that the changed form becomes a more central member of the category.

30.2.2.1   Token frequency

The frequency effect discussed in the above section represents the influence of token frequency. As defined by Bybee, token frequency is "the frequency of occurrence of a unit, usually a word, in running text" (2001, p. 10). Token frequency can be counted for a theoretically infinite number of linguistic structures, including phrases, words, syllables, phoneme combinations, and individual phonemes. The first phonological effect of token frequency is illustrated in the above description of t/d deletion. Words and constructions that are more frequent are more likely to undergo processes of phonetic reduction; therefore, sound change that is motivated by articulatory forces will affect high-frequency forms first. Another effect of token frequency is that it renders high-frequency forms less susceptible to change associated with grammatically based analogical forces. This phenomenon is best explained with reference to the notion of lexical strength, as a product of frequency. A stored item accrues lexical strength by repeated use: each instance of use has the effect of strengthening the representation of an item, making it more accessible (Bybee, 1985). If a form is readily accessible, it is less likely to undergo change influenced by similarities to other recurring patterns. For example, there are relatively few irregular past-tense verbs in English. Many of those individual forms, however, are highly frequent. Because the high-frequency past tense *went* is easily accessed, it is unlikely to become regularized to *goed*. On the other hand, less frequent irregular past-tense forms such as *wept* or *crept* are much more likely to undergo the process of regularization, becoming *weeped* or *creeped*.

30.2.2.2   Type frequency

Token frequency represents only one way to count frequency. The other way to count yields type frequency, which plays a major role in the determination of productivity of patterns of linguistic use. Type frequency describes the relative frequency of a pattern or schema. That is, the greater the number of items that a specific pattern applies to, the higher its type frequency. To return to the English past-tense example, the regular past-tense morpheme has a very high type frequency since most verbs are regular and therefore fit the pattern of the English regular past tense. Therefore, when a new verb or a nonce form is presented, it is this most frequent inflectional pattern that will usually apply in the formation of the past tense of the novel form. In phonology, type frequency may be defined in a number of different ways. For example, all words that share a common onset may be thought of as conforming to a specific schema. In developmental phonology, children in early stages of word learning often seem to come upon a preferred production pattern that is then extended to other words that share some acoustic or articulatory property with the pattern (Stoel-Gammon & Cooper, 1984; Vihman, 1992). Vihman called these preferred production patterns *vocal motor schemes*; these vocal motor schemes allow children to make rapid progress in the development of a productive lexicon, creating many near-homophones in the early vocabulary. These words would all conform to the same basic phonological pattern, which would be considered to have a high type frequency.

30.2.3   Emergence

Another important feature of most usage-based accounts is the notion that *linguistic representation is emergent*, not stored as a fixed entity. This approach rejects the rule/list dichotomy advocated by Pinker (1991, 1999), among others, that the language system consists of a static list of lexical forms and a separate store of rules that operate on those lexical forms. Instead, linguistic units are seen as cognitive routines that emerge by generalizing over existing forms and extracting patterns of similarity, or 'schemas', to use Langacker's term, of different levels of generality (Langacker, 2000). Since the patterns that emerge are entirely dependent on instances of language use, there are no *a priori* limitations on the levels of representation that may exist; schemas may describe grammatical constructions, words, syllables, phonemes, features, or gestures. In the process of phonological acquisition, this notion of emergence would not assume the existence of phoneme-like categories. Instead, phonological knowledge is a gradient property that is extracted from similarity relationships between individual items in the lexicon.

The basic idea behind emergence, as described by Bybee (2001), is that complex structure can be created through the repeated application of simple properties; something much more complex than the sum of the individual instances can emerge. An important implication of this is that complex linguistic structure can be created; it need not be the product of innate mental programs.

In a usage-based model, linguistic categories emerge from the organized lexical storage in which associations form between phonetically and semantically related items. Some associations are stronger than others, depending on the degree of similarity, how often the items are accessed together, and the lexical strength of individual items. Both token and type frequency will influence the relative strength of individual representations as well as the strength of the associations between lexical items. In Bybee's (2001) view, storage is redundant in that multimorphemic words, including regularly inflected words, may be stored holistically, and even multiple representations of the same word may exist. The similarity associations between forms give rise to the generalizations or schemas, allowing morphological and phonological structure to emerge.

30.2.4   Use of data

Another characteristic of a usage-based theory of language, which distinguishes it from more traditional approaches, is the *importance of using data in theory construction*. As opposed to the acceptability judgments that constituted the majority of the evidence for generative accounts, usage-based theorists assume that the object of study is the language that people actually produce and understand. Thus, theory based on the study of large spoken and written corpora, as well as some experimental work, is making its way into general linguistic theory. This change in approach to theory building parallels the change that occurred in the study of developmental phonology, when researchers began to look closely at the speech of more and more children and discovered that the theories based on a few limited observations or anecdotal reports were not adequate. Furthermore, within a usage-based framework, attention should be paid not only to those forms that are consistent with the general patterns, but also to exceptions and marginal cases. From a clinical perspective, this is an extremely important aspect of usage-based phonology; the variability that is often observed in certain clinical populations may prove to be a valuable source of information about the nature of phonological representations and associations between those forms.

30.2.5   Language as a general cognitive function

Usage-based accounts relate language learning to other types of learning that exploit the same necessary mental capacities such as memory, motor control, categorization, and inference making, to name a few (Bybee, 2001). This is the basis of Langacker's use of the term 'cognitive grammar'; grammar is derived from general cognitive capacities, thereby minimizing the role of innate structures (Langacker, 2000). Bybee (2001) adds to this the notion of grammar as procedural knowledge; through practice and repetition, aspects of language become quite automatic and are executed in much the same way as other types of highly practiced motor routines. Phonology, as a highly redundant system of repetition of a limited number of patterns, is part of the articulatory and perceptual procedure for producing and understanding language.

30.2.6   Importance of context

Finally, usage-based models of linguistics emphasize the *importance of context in the acquisition and operation of the linguistic system*. Instances of language use include specifics about the context of the usage event, including non-linguistic and social factors. Context-dependent use of language in the early stages of acquisition is a well-known phenomenon, the ability to de-contextualize language in both comprehension and production involves a process of generalizing over multiple instances of use of similar patterns, thereby extracting schemas that can be used in novel situations. Linguistic structure, however, is never entirely de-contextualized, even in fully mature systems; abstractions are always linked to individual instances of use.

The preceding discussion of the aspects of a usage-based model of linguistics may be succinctly summarized using Langacker's three descriptive terms for cognitive linguistics: maximalist, non-reductive, and bottom-up (Langacker, 2000). In other words, storage and representation is thought to be highly redundant, concrete as opposed to abstract, and phonological generalizations arise out of specific instances of use.

30.3   Clinical Applications of Cognitive Phonology

Thinking about language use and the importance of context is certainly not a strange concept for most practicing clinicians. When the language system is impaired, the role of context and functional use is almost always considered in planning intervention. For example, augmentative devices are often arranged so that the most frequently used words and phrases are most easily accessed. Similarly, treatment may include specific work on words, phrases, and even entire dialogues that are most useful in the daily communicative interactions of the individual client. This focus on context and patterns of use, however, is usually not extended to the treatment of children or adults with phonological disorders. Thus, a usage-based approach to clinical phonology will differ considerably from a more traditional approach in that great importance will be placed on the role of individual patterns of use in both the evaluation and treatment of phonological disorders.

30.3.1   *The object of study*

Perhaps the biggest difference in terms of clinical thinking, however, will stem from the idea that phonological competence in a usage-based approach is not described merely in terms of the mastery of individual features, contrasts, or sounds, as is typical of most clinical practice. From a usage-based perspective, phonology does not exist in isolation, but only in relation to stored lexical items. Furthermore, the underlying representations for these items are thought to be concrete, as opposed to abstract, and productions would not be described in terms of rules or processes that change a correct underlying form into the erred production. Thus, analysis would consist of looking at existing networks of lexical items that are either sufficient or insufficient for the emergence of individual phonological patterns and units. Therefore, clinical phonological analysis will go well beyond the phonemic inventory and the description of existing phonological processes, and will include analysis of the individual lexical items that are present in the child's vocabulary and the specific patterns of use of those items.

30.3.2 Phonology and the lexicon

The idea of an important link between phonology and the lexicon is certainly not a new one in the field of clinical phonology and phonological development. In the 1970s, child phonologists began to acknowledge an important relationship between phonological and lexical development. Ferguson and Farwell (1975), for example, highlighted the importance of the 'lexical parameter' in phonological acquisition. In this view, phonological development is not just a matter of change in the system (rules), but may take place on a word-by-word basis, reflecting the individual experiences and preferences of the child. This position was extremely influential in the field of developmental phonology for many years. However, recent attempts to integrate developmental phonology with mainstream phonological theory, most notably Optimality Theory, have again minimized the role of lexical-phonological interactions in development. Usage-based phonology, with its emphasis on language use and emergence of phonological structure, may provide an opportunity to merge developmental phonology with mainstream phonology without minimizing the importance of the relationship between phonology and the lexicon (Pierrehumbert, 2003).

30.3.3 Predictions of usage-based phonology

Usage-based phonology makes testable predictions regarding patterns of phonological development that one would expect to see. Specifically, the role of frequency (both token and type frequency) would be predicted to have an observable influence in typical development, and may be exploited in planning treatment for individuals with delayed or disordered development.

Unfortunately, the data regarding the role of frequency in the diffusion of developmental sound change in typical development are limited. A few studies, however, suggest that accurate productions may emerge first in high-frequency words (Leonard & Ritterman, 1971; Tyler & Edwards, 1993; but see Velten, 1943) and in high-frequency/-probability sound sequences (Beckman & Edwards, 2000; Zamuner, Gerken, & Hammond, 2004). Other predictions include differential roles for production vs. perception frequency; for example, a word that is heard infrequently, but produced often, may be less accurate than words that are heard more frequently. Usage-based phonology also makes specific predictions regarding the role of frequency in the process of sound change. For example, high-frequency words are more susceptible to change caused by articulatory forces (as seen in the example of final t/d deletion discussed above). Low-frequency words, however, are more susceptible to change by analogy; that is, low-frequency items are more likely to conform to a high type frequency pattern. The goal of the clinical phonologist is to cause change in the disordered sound system of an individual; thus, understanding and employing these principles of usage-based phonology may prove very beneficial in promoting sound change. While a more complete understanding of the role of token frequency and type frequency in typical development is necessary, some attempts have been made to use frequency as a parameter in the selection of treatment targets for children with phonological delay.

30.3.4   *Word frequency and neighborhood density in phonological treatment*

The majority of the work in this area comes from Gierut and colleagues in their investigations of the role of lexical factors such as word frequency and phonological neighborhood density on patterns of change in the productive phonology of children with functional phonological delay (Gierut & Storkel, 2002; Gierut, Morrisette, & Champion, 1999; Morrisette, 1999). Phonological neighborhood density refers to similarity relationships among words in an individual's lexicon; the lexicon is thought to be organized around groups of words that share similar phonological properties. Most often, phonological neighbors are defined as words that differ from each other by only one phoneme substitution, deletion, or addition in any position (Luce & Pisoni, 1998). Thus, the words *hat*, *cap*, and *cast* would all be neighbors of the word *cat*. Words that have many neighbors are said to reside in high-density neighborhoods, while words that have few or no neighbors are said to reside in low-density or sparse neighborhoods. Phonological neighborhood density may be compared to the usage-based concept of type frequency; phoneme sequences that occur in many words would have high type frequency and would create high-density phonological neighborhoods. The studies of Gierut and colleagues provide some evidence that the use of high-frequency and low-density words as treatment targets significantly facilitates generalization of the treated sounds to untreated words (Gierut, Morrisette, & Champion, 1999). In almost all cases, treatment using high-frequency words promoted generalization when compared to all other conditions, and treatment using high-density words inhibited generalization.

In one of the few articles to consider clinical applications of a usage-based phonology, Ball (2003) notes that this approach suggests that stressing contrast is less important in disordered phonology than the reinforcement of networks containing sounds and sequences of sounds that are problematic for the client.

30.4   Conclusion

A usage-based framework may offer an excellent opportunity for the integration of developmental and clinical phonology with general linguistic theory. Specifically, the emphasis placed on the intimate relationship between the lexicon and other aspects of the grammar, including phonology, may help us better understand phonological phenomena observed in children with both typical and disordered phonology. Furthermore, this new way of thinking about phonology may lead to important changes in treatment for phonological disorders. Many clinicians have probably selected treatment words for individual children simply because it's a word that the child says a lot; further research evaluating treatment techniques grounded in usage-based phonology may show that those clinical intuitions were right on the mark.

REFERENCES

Ball, M. J. (2003). Clinical applications of a cognitive phonology. *Phoniatrics, Logopedics, Vocology*, 28, 63–9.

Beckman, M. E. and Edwards, J. (2000). Lexical frequency effects on young children's imitative productions. In M. B. Broe and J. B. Pierrehumbert (eds.), *Acquisition and the Lexicon*, Papers in Laboratory Phonology, V (pp. 208–18). Cambridge: Cambridge University Press.

Bybee, J. (1985). *Morphology: A Study of the Relation between Meaning and Form*. Amsterdam: John Benjamins.

Bybee, J. (2000). The phonology of the lexicon: Evidence from lexical diffusion. In M. Barlow and S. Kemmer (eds.), *Usage-based Models of Language* (pp. 65–85). Stanford, CA: CSLI Publications.

Bybee, J. (2001). *Phonology and Language Use*. Cambridge: Cambridge University Press.

Chomsky, N. and Halle, M. (1968). *The Sound Pattern of English*. New York: Harper & Row.

Ferguson, C. A. and Farwell, C. B. (1975). Words and sounds in early language acquisition. *Language*, 51, 419–39.

Gierut, J., Morrisette, M., and Champion, A. (1999). Lexical constraints in phonological acquisition. *Journal of Child Language*, 26, 261–94.

Gierut, J. and Storkel, H. (2002). Markedness and the grammar in lexical diffusion of fricatives. *Clinical Linguistics and Phonetics*, 16, 115–34.

Gregory, M., Raymond, W., Bell, A., Fosler-Lussier, E., and Jurafsky, D. (1999). The effect of collocational strength and contextual predictability in lexical production. *Chicago Linguistic Society*, 35, 151–66.

Jakobson, R. (1968) (trans. A. R. Keiler). *Child Language, Aphasia, and Phonological Universals*. The Hague: Mouton. Originally published as *Kindersprache, Aphasie, und allgemeine Lautgesetze*. Uppsala: Almqvist and Wiksell, 1941.

Johnson, K. (1997). Speech perception without speaker normalization. In K. Johnson and W. Mullennix (eds.), *Talker Variability in Speech Processing* (pp. 145–65). San Diego, CA: Academic Press.

Kemmer, S. and Barlow, M. (2000). Introduction: A usage-based conception of language. In M. Barlow and S. Kemmer (eds.), *Usage-based Models of Language* (pp. vii–xxviii). Stanford, CA: CSLI Publications.

Langacker, R. (1987). *Foundations of Cognitive Grammar. Volume 1: Theoretical Prerequisiites*. Stanford, CA: Stanford University Press.

Langacker, R. (2000). A dynamic usage-based model. In M. Barlow and S. Kemmer (eds.), *Usage-based Models of Language* (pp.1–63). Stanford, CA: CSLI Publications.

Leonard, L. and Ritterman, S. (1971). Articulation of /s/ as a function of cluster and word frequency of occurrence. *Journal of Speech and Hearing Research*, 14, 476–85.

Luce, P. A. and Pisoni, D. B. (1998). Recognizing spoken words: The neighborhood activation model. *Ear and Hearing*, 19(1), 1–36.

Morrisette, M. (1999). Lexical characteristics of sound change. *Clinical Linguistics and Phonetics*, 13, 219–38.

Pierrehumbert, J. (2001). Exemplar dynamics: Word frequency, lenition and contrast. In J. Bybee and P. Hopper (eds.), *Frequency and the Emergence of Linguistic Structure* (pp. 137–57). Amsterdam: John Benjamins.

Pierrehumbert, J. (2003). Phonetic diversity, statistical learning, and acquisiiton of phonology. *Language and Speech*, 46, 115–54.

Pinker, S. (1991). Rules of language. *Science*, 253, 530–5.

Pinker, S. (1999). *Words and Rules: The Ingredients of Language*. New York: Basic Books.

Prince, A. and Smolensky, P. (1993). *Optimality Theory: Constraint Interaction in Generative Grammar*. Malden, MA: Blackwell.

Stampe, D. (1969). The acquisition of phonetic representation. Papers from the Fifth Regional Meeting of the Chicago Linguistic Society, 443–54.

Stoel-Gammon, C. and Cooper, J. (1984). Patterns of early lexical and phonological development. *Journal of Child Language*, 11, 247–71.

Tyler, A. and Edwards, J. (1993). Lexical acquisition and acquisition of initial voiceless stops. *Journal of Child Language*, 20, 253–73.

Velten, H. V. (1943). The growth of phonemic and lexical patterns in infant language. *Language*, 19, 231–92.

Vihman, M. M. (1992). The construction of a phonological system. In B. de Boysson-Bardies, S. de Schonen, P. Jusczyk, P. MacNeilage, and J. Morton (eds.), *Developmental Neurocognition: Speech and Face Processing in the First Year of Life*. Dordrecht: Kluwer Academic Publisher.

Zamuner, T. S., Gerken, L., and Hammond, M. (2004). Phonotactic probabilities in young children's speech production. *Journal of Child Language*, 31, 515–36.

31 Neurophonetics

WOLFRAM ZIEGLER

31.1 The Scope of Neurophonetics

Neurophonetics deals with neurogenic impairments of the motor act of speaking and of the perceptual processes of spoken language understanding, with the aim of unraveling the neural organization of speech motor control and speech perception. To the extent that phonetics is a subdiscipline of linguistics, neurophonetics can be viewed as a subdiscipline of *neurolinguistics*. In this view, the field focuses on the 'front-ends' of the neural apparatus devoted to spoken language processing, neglecting the more central issues of lexical, syntactic, semantic, or pragmatic processing. The notoriously difficult problem of drawing a clear taxonomic line between phonetics and phonology also extends to neurophonetics. It will be shown later in this chapter that the distinction between phonological encoding, phonetic encoding, and speech motor execution is among the most controversial issues in the understanding of neurogenic speech disorders.

Neurophonetic research is in large part based on classical phonetic methodologies, such as instrumental assessment of the dynamics and kinematics of impaired speech movements, measurement of the aerodynamic and the acoustic events resulting from such movements, auditory analyses of the utterances of impaired speakers, or perceptual experiments taxing the auditory speech processing capabilities of patients with brain lesions (see chapters 19–24 in this volume). More recently, the development of functional brain imaging and electrophysiological techniques has opened new windows onto the neural machinery controlling the motor act of speaking and the perceptual act of deciphering the acoustic speech code. These approaches demarcate a boundary between *cognitive neuroscience* and *neurophonetics*.

Since it is not possible to give a full account of all relevant syndromes, this overview is rather selective and reflects my individual perspective and my personal focus on adult disorders. The chapter contains two major sections, devoted to motor and perceptual aspects. Within the speech production section

I further distinguish between acquired neurogenic impairments in adults and developmental impairments in children, whereas the section on perceptual neurophonetics will be confined to adult disorders. In a final section I cover a few issues concerning the impact of neurophonetics on mainstream linguistic accounts of spoken language processing.

31.2   Disorders of Speech Production

31.2.1   *Acquired disorders in adults*

Acquired neurogenic disorders of speech production are conventionally classified into three categories: dysarthria, apraxia of speech, and aphasic phonological impairment. These categories correspond with three different levels distinguished in most theories of spoken language generation, namely speech motor execution, phonetic encoding, and phonological encoding (figure 31.1).

31.2.1.1   *Dysarthria*

The dysarthrias are acquired neurogenic disorders of the speech motor execution apparatus. They comprise several syndromes which have in common that they correspond to the motor impairments known from neurologic disorders of the limb motor system, such as paresis, ataxia, akinesia, rigidity, different types of dyskinesias and dystonias, and tremor. It is important to mention that

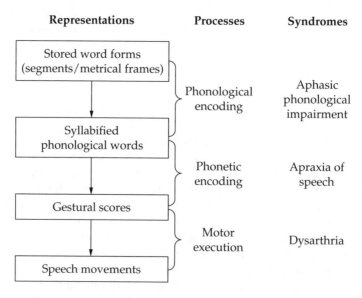

Figure 31.1   From stored lexical forms to speech movements (adapted from Levelt, Roelofs, & Meyer, 1999). The three major classes of neurogenic speech impairment can be allocated to three consecutive components of the speech production process.

the clinical and physiological criteria by which these pathomechanisms can be verified are typically defined for the upper and lower limb motor systems and cannot easily be transferred to the speech musculature. Clinical assessment of limb paresis or rigidity is, for instance, based on examinations of muscular resistance to passive stretching, but these examinations can certainly not be applied to the soft palate or the vocal folds. Application of the neuromotor taxonomy to the speech motor apparatus is therefore predominantly based on analogies rather than on neurophysiologic data.

Paretic dysarthria of the *flaccid* type, to begin with, is usually caused by lesions to the final neuromotor pathway, i.e., the lower motor neurone or the neuromuscular junction. Lesions to these structures prevent the afflicted muscles from receiving sufficient innervation. This results in significant muscular weakness and a flaccid appearance of the muscles. Depending on which subsystem is affected, problems of respiration, phonation, resonance, and/or articulation arise. In patients with progressive disorders afflicting the motor nuclei in the brainstem, a generalized flaccid syndrome is observed, with slowed speech, hypernasal resonance, imprecise articulation, weak and breathy voice, and increased inspiration rate. Since the lesion affects the *peripheral* nervous system, muscular contraction is impeded for all movement conditions, i.e., reflexive, involuntary, or volitional.

Paretic dysarthria of the *spastic* type results from lesions to the inferior part of the rolandic motor cortical region, or to the fiber tracts descending from there to the brainstem motor nuclei (*upper motor neurone*). Since most of the speech muscle pairs receive input from both hemispheres, the sequelae of uni-lateral lesions can usually be compensated for within several days or weeks, and severe persisting impairments are confined to patients with bilateral lesions (Urban, Wicht, Vukurevic, et al., 2001). The presence of spasticity, as defined in the limb motor system (i.e., acceleration-dependent increase of the resistance to passive movement), cannot be verified in most speech muscles, but the spastic dysarthria syndrome differs from its flaccid counterpart by the appearance of an *increased* muscular tension. Since functional weakness may result from spastic co-contractions of agonist and antagonist muscles, many features of spastic dysarthria (e.g., slow rate, hypernasality, imprecise consonants) resemble those of the flaccid type, with the exception of a strained-strangled voice quality resulting from hyper-adduction of the vocal folds in spastic dysarthria. In patients with lesions to the upper motor neurone or the rolandic motor cortex the brainstem motor nuclei may still receive input from other motor cortical areas, such as mesial premotor cortex or anterior cingulate cortex. Hence, emotional vocal or facial expression (e.g. voiced laughing or crying) can be preserved even in patients with severely impaired speech.

Ataxic dysarthria is a syndrome resulting from cerebellar disease or from lesions to the afferent or efferent pathways of the cerebellum. The pathomechanism of ataxia interferes with movement coordination and with the temporal and spatial precision of motor execution. Dyscoordination may be seen, for instance, in the thoracic-abdominal speech breathing pattern or in the interplay between laryngeal and articulatory gestures, dysmetria and impaired timing may result in a variable articulatory accuracy or in intermittent disturbances of the nasal-oral distinction. Cerebellar tremor of 2–3 Hz may be present in the laryngeal or the supralaryngeal system. As in limb ataxia, patients with ataxic speech may tend to compensate for their problems by increasing their muscular tension, e.g., in order to suppress tremor or dysmetic aberrations. This may, for instance, lead to a tense voice quality.

Akinesia and *rigidity* are two mutually independent pathomechanisms which may typically co-occur in patients with basal ganglia disorders, e.g., Parkinsonism. Akinesia denotes a condition characterized by impoverished motor activity, with impaired movement initiation, reduced movement amplitudes (*hypokinesia*) and slowed movements (*bradykinesia*). Rigidity describes an increased stiffness of the musculature, i.e., increased resistance to passive movement, which is caused by an increase of agonist and antagonist muscular tone. In patients with Parkinson's disease dysarthria occurs with an incidence of between 60 and 80 percent. In these patients, speech movements are considered to be impaired by hypokinesia and rigidity, while the presence of bradykinesia is controversial. Their voice is soft and breathy, their intonation is flat, and their articulation is undershooting. Unlike those with most other syndromes, patients with a hypokinetic-rigid dysarthria may often speak at a normal rate or even sound hasty. Akinesia may also occur in patients with lesions to mesial-frontal cortex, especially anterior cingular cortex and supplementary motor area. Since these cortical sites are part of a motor loop which also includes basal ganglia structures, akinetic speech can be considered as a symptom of the fronto-striatal motor system, resulting from an interruption of motivational input from mesio-frontal cortex to the speech motor system. After bilateral mesial-frontal lesions, enduring mutism may occur as part of a syndrome of generalized immobility (*akinetic mutism*). After (left) unilateral lesions mutism is usually transient and recovery is characterized by a hypophonic and breathy voice and a monotonous intonation (Mega & Cohenour, 1997).

Dyskinesia and *dystonia* are collective terms denoting conditions of involuntary muscle contractions leading to uncontrolled movements (hyperkinesias, tics) or abnormal postures (*dystonia*). Hyperkinetic movements are for instance present in Huntington's chorea, where they may interfere with the control of speech movements. Focal dystonia may occur in the laryngeal muscles, causing strained-strangled and rough voice quality and voice tremor (*spasmodic dysphonia*), or in the oromandibular system, where alterations of muscle tone may interfere with articulation (*oromandibular dystonia*).

For comprehensive clinical descriptions of these syndromes, readers are referred to Duffy (2005).

31.2.1.2   Acquired apraxia of speech

Apraxia of speech is a speech motor impairment which is clinically distinguishable from the dysarthrias. A definition relating this syndrome to psycholinguistic models of spoken language production postulates that it is an impairment of the *phonetic encoding* of words and sentences. According to this view, apraxic speakers have (1) a preserved knowledge of the phonological form of the words they intend to produce (which is considered to distinguish them from patients with aphasic-phonological impairment; see below), and (2) no significant paresis, ataxia, akinesia, or other motor execution problem which would prevent them from performing the required speech movements (which distinguishes them from dysarthric patients). Instead, their problem is in transforming the more abstract representations of word forms into the motor commands guiding the articulators (Code, 1998).

This definition suffers from the weakness that it relies on model-based terms, such as *phonetic encoding*, whose semantics is not sufficiently clear to make the concept clinically useful. A clinical definition of the disorder would therefore focus on the most salient symptoms of apraxia of speech, i.e. dysfluent, groping, and effortful speech with phonetic distortions and phonemic paraphasias, and a frequent occurrence of false starts and restarts (table 31.1).

Effortful and phonetically distorted speech are suggestive of the motor nature of the disorder, the presence of groping movements and of self-initiated corrections indicates that the patient struggles for the realization of some internalized, stable phonological target, and the fact that the symptoms are variable and inconsistent is taken as evidence against more elementary, dysarthric pathomechanisms. A point of debate concerns the nature of the phonemic

Table 31.1   The symptoms of apraxia of speech (adapted from Ziegler, 2007)

Segmental impairment

Phonetic distortions	Phonemic paraphasias
gradual aberrations from target phonemes	*categorical* aberrations from target phonemes
phonemes sound phonetically *ill-formed*	phonemes sound *well-articulated*

Error variability

Errors are *inconsistent*: a patient may produce a phoneme accurately or inaccurately, and multiple inaccurate productions may have different phonetic qualities.
Islands of unimpaired speech: Even severely impaired speakers may at times produce entirely accurate words or phrases.

Prosodic impairment

Speech is hesitant and halting, with pauses between syllables or words, with false starts, repairs, and repetitive attempts at initiating speech. Pauses are often accompanied by prolonged articulatory groping. Dysfluent articulation corrupts the regular rhythm and melody of speech.

paraphasias observed in apraxia of speech, since this symptom may also occur in aphasic phonological impairment (see below), where it is generally interpreted as a mis-selection of abstract phonological units rather than as a motor problem. However, discrete, categorical (i.e. phonemic) errors can easily be explained as a surface phenomenon resulting from gradual, phonetic aberrations, if one considers that discontinuity may arise (1) in the motor system itself (as a consequence of the 'quantal nature of speech' or of phase-coupling principles governing the organization of articulatory gestures (Goldstein, Pouplier, Chen, Saltzman, & Byrd, forthcoming), (2) in the movement-to-aerodynamics or the aerodynamics-to-acoustics mapping, or (3) in the ear of the examiner (categorical perception, phoneme restoration).

Unlike the dysarthrias, apraxia of speech is a syndrome of the language-dominant cerebral hemisphere, occurring almost exclusively after lesions to the anterior language zone. Broca's area, left anterior insular cortex, and the anterior portion of left inferior motor cortex are considered most relevant in the genesis of the impairment, and lesions to the white matter underlying these cortical regions may contribute to its persistence and severity. The French neurologist Paul Broca, who was the first to explicitly describe this syndrome, characterized it as a loss of the "faculty of articulate language", not caring much about a conceptual distinction between the motor and the linguistic aspects of spoken language production. In later theories, a strict dualism between linguistic and motor processes was postulated which left no room for a clinical condition situated between disorders of elementary motor execution (dysarthria) on the one hand and disorders of the generation of an abstract, amodal, phonological code (aphasia), on the other (Ziegler, 2007). At that time, the debate about apraxia of speech was dominated by the question of whether it is aphasic or dysarthric. In modern psycholinguistic theories of speech production and in theories of general action control, however, the existence of a separate phonetic encoding or a motor programming level is undisputed, and apraxia of speech has been broadly acknowledged as an impairment located to this level.

The new model-based account of the disorder has stimulated discussions about the structure of phonetic representations, especially about the role of the syllable in the generation of speech motor plans. The observation that the apraxic speech error mechanism is sensitive to syllable frequency and syllable structure has been interpreted as evidence that syllabicity is an important structural property of the phonetic code (Aichert & Ziegler, 2004). More recent research has shown that the structure of phonetic plans is probably still more complex, since an influence of the frequency of syllable onsets on apraxic speech errors can also be demonstrated. Furthermore, the results of a nonlinear predictive modeling of word accuracy in apraxic speech (Ziegler, 2005) suggested that the phonetic code obviously inherits the metrical tree structure of the phonological make-up of words, and that within this structure the substructures that are linked on different layers have different strengths of connectivity. More specifically, the binding of a syllable nucleus with one or more coda consonants within a syllabic rhyme turned out to be significantly more stable than the attachment of one or more onset consonants to a rhyme, which is compatible with phonetic data demonstrating an asymmetric shape of syllable-internal articulations (Krakow, 1999). Another particularly stable junction in the metrical tree structure of phonetic plans, as revealed by apraxic speech error patterns, was at the level where two syllables are attached to form a trochaic foot (Ziegler, 2005). This result is compatible with phonological evidence concerning the unmarkedness of the trochaic stress pattern in German lexical phonology and suggests that such phonological regularities are handed down to the level of phonetic encoding or speech motor programming. On the whole, this work opens up a discussion on how the nature of phonetic processes and the make-up of phonetic representations should be conceived of.

31.2.1.3 *Aphasic phonological impairment*

The occurrence of phonemic errors in speech production is an ubiquitous aphasic symptom. The term 'phonemic error' comprises phoneme substitutions (*gat for cat), omissions (*bue for blue), additions (*grose for rose), or complex combinations of these types (*det for nest). These errors sometimes appear to be triggered by immediate phonological context, as in anticipatory (*bobacco for tobacco), perseveratory (*fif for fish) or metathetic errors (*motato for tomato). Phonemic paraphasia occurs in almost all aphasic syndromes. In a subtype of Wernicke's aphasia, i.e., phonemic jargon, the phonological forms of words can be corrupted to an extent that the target word is no longer recognizable ('abstruse neologisms'). The syndrome which is mentioned most often in the context of phonemic paraphasia is *conduction aphasia*, where the occurrence of paraphasic errors is not substantially contaminated by lexical, semantic, or comprehension problems.

An important criterion to distinguish patients with aphasic phonological impairment from those with apraxia of speech is that their entire speech output is well articulated and fluent. The fact that phonetic distortions do not occur in these patients is considered an indication of the non-motor nature of the underlying pathomechanism. Explanations of phonemic paraphasias as a surface phenomenon of an underlying motor impairment, as in apraxia of speech (see above), is usually considered inappropriate in these patients since such an impairment would probably also entail a significant number of phonetic errors.

Some neurolinguistic theories assume that phonemic paraphasias may arise at at least two sites: first, the entries in the word form lexicon (a long-term memory system containing the phonological information for each word of our language) can be corrupted, or, second, errors may occur during one of the postlexical phonological processing steps, or in a short-term store where phonological information is buffered before it is fed into lower processing stages of the motor system. In Levelt's word production model (Levelt, Roelofs, & Meyer, 1999), postlexical errors of a phonemic type may occur during the reading out of the segmental constituents of a lexical unit, during syllabification, or during access to the syllabic units stored in the syllable lexicon. The finding of a syllable frequency effect in patients with aphasic phonological impairment suggests that phonemic errors arise at a point where the mental syllabary is addressed (Laganaro, 2005).

Other models dispense with such serial processing assumptions, postulating a spreading of activation between the layers of a connectionist network (Dell, Schwartz, Martin, Saffran, & Gagnon, 1997). In the connectionist approach, no distinction is made between lexical and postlexical stages of phonological encoding, and phonemic errors are modeled by varying the strengths of connections or the rate of activation decay in the network. One of the constraints of existing connectionist models of word production is that they end at the phonemic level. From there on, information flow is only top-down. Hence, these models cannot be used to discuss the phonetic-phonemic dichotomy of speech error types and the distinction between phonological impairment and apraxia of speech.

31.2.2   Developmental apraxia of speech (DAS)

Developmental apraxia of speech (DAS) is a syndrome which occurs during speech development in early childhood. It resembles acquired apraxia of speech in adults in that it is characterized by a corruption of the sound structure of spoken words, with distorted articulation, phonemic errors, and severe dysfluency (Shriberg, Aram, & Kwiatkowski., 1997). Comparisons of adult apraxia of speech with DAS are hampered by the problem that DAS interferes with the early motor learning stage of speech acquisition, with the consequence that a normal development of speech perception and of phonological, lexical, or syntactic aspects of language is prevented. While in the adult speech production system a tripartite organization can be postulated, with separate phonological and phonetic encoding components and a distinct motor execution stage (cf. figure 30.1), this organization must be considered to be still nascent and not fully developed in young children developing DAS. Hence, a conceptual separation between impairments of phonological or phonetic encoding, or of motor execution, is even more intricate in developmental speech disorders than it is in adults.

Retrospective analyses of speech acquisition in children with DAS often reveal that the children had delayed or reduced babbling and reduced oral motor capabilities during infancy. Hence, the relative contributions of early auditory-perceptual, oral motor, and speech-specific factors to the genesis of the disorder cannot easily be disentangled (Groenen, Maassen, Crul, & Thoonen, 1996). Although a neurogenic basis of the disorder appears certain, there are no consistent findings regarding the localization of a potentially underlying structural lesion, and in many cases neuroanatomical findings were unremarkable. Today, a genetic origin of DAS is hypothesized, on the basis of the discovery of a mutation of the *FOXP2*-gene in the DAS-afflicted members of the 'KE-family' which, over three generations, has shown a high incidence of the disorder (Vargha-Khadem et al., 2005). Variants of this mutation have now also been discovered in DAS-patients from other families (Shriberg, Ballard, Tomblin, et al., 2006).

Data from patients with genetically based developmental apraxia of speech suggest that mutation of the *FOXP2* gene results in an abnormal development of volitional oral motor control more generally (Alcock et al., 2000) and that, probably on the basis of this, the development of normal speech motor control is prevented.

31.2.3 *Methodologies*

The *methods* used in neurophonetic investigations of dysarthric, apraxic, or phonologically impaired speech cover virtually the whole range of phonetic methodologies, extending from the deep level of muscle action potentials in the speech motor system to the surface level of the audible features of disordered speech. Here is a collection of examples.

(1) Several influential studies of the speech motor impairment of Parkinson's disease have used surface EMG of the lips to verify the presence of rigidity in the perioral muscles or of Parkinsonian tremor (Hunker & Abbs, 1990). Clinically, EMG of the tongue muscles plays an important role in the differential diagnosis of motor neurone disease.

(2) Measurement of muscular forces in the oral motor system is confined to *isometric* forces, hence to nonspeech oral motor activities. Two major applications were (a) maximum force measurements, with the aim of quantifying the degree of weakness in the articulatory muscles, e.g. in *amyotrophic lateral sclerosis* (DePaul & Abbs, 1987), and (b) visuo-motor tracking of constant or varying target force levels, with the aim of examining fine motor adaptation skills or the acquisition of motor routines by feedback-based learning (McNeil, Weismer, Adams, & Mulligan, 1990).

(3) Articulator movement kinematics have been investigated in many syndromes and with many different techniques, aiming to uncover the details of articulatory impairment in dysarthric and apraxic speech (Bose, van Lieshout, & Square, 2003).

(4) Aerodynamic measures like airflow rate have been applied as a control signal in visuo-motor tracking tasks, e.g., to study respiratory control and motor learning in cerebellar ataxic patients (Deger, Ziegler, & Wessel; 1999).

(5) Acoustic analyses of the speech signal have a long-standing tradition in neurophonetics. Most of them are focused on the speech wave correlates of certain pathologic conditions, such as ataxic, hypokinetic, or apraxic speech (Kent, Weismer, Kent, Vorperian, & Duffy, 1999; Kent & Kim, chapter 22 in this volume).

(6) Despite the increasing role of instrumental assessment techniques, perceptual analyses still constitute the gold standard of clinical neurophonetics. The comprehensive catalogue of auditory features of dysarthria established by Darley, Aronson, and Brown (1975) continues to provide a

basis for clinical assessment, although modifications have been proposed. Auditory analyses are also used as a research tool, e.g. in studies of apraxia of speech and aphasic phonological impairment.

31.3   Disorders of Speech Perception in Adults

Brain lesions may at different levels of the central nervous system interfere with auditory processing, especially with the processing of the speech signal. A long-standing debate in phonetics concerns the question whether the auditory processing of speech sounds is performed by a specialized auditory-phonetic module, or whether it is merely one of many equivalent tasks performed by a multi-purpose auditory-perceptual system (Liberman & Whalen, 2000). This issue has also been debated in clinical investigations of patients with neurogenic auditory and speech processing impairments.

A very basic impairment of auditory perception may occur after bilateral lesions to the ascending auditory tracts, from the cochlear nuclei in the brainstem via pontine and midbrain nuclei and the dorsal thalamus to the primary auditory cortices in the superior temporal gyri. Because of the bilateral, redundant organization of the system, unilateral lesions do not cause clinically or behaviorally significant impairment. Bilateral involvement of the auditory afferent projections causes 'central auditory impairment' affecting perception of all kinds of auditory stimuli, i.e., ambient noise, music, and speech. In the most severe cases (which are very rare), total deafness results (Egan, Davies, & Halmagyi, 1996).

Beyond these rare cases of complete neurogenic deafness, researchers have been attracted by syndromes characterized by selective impairments of the processing of distinct classes of auditory events, such as environmental sounds, music, or speech. These syndromes are termed *auditory agnosias*. A small number of patients have, for instance, been reported who, mostly after bilateral temporal lesions, are 'word-deaf', i.e., unable to understand speech, although they have normal hearing (as revealed by audiometry) and are relatively unimpaired in the processing of music or environmental sounds (Praamstra, Hagoort, Maassen, & Crul, 1991). In other cases, auditory processing of speech may be preserved, but music processing is significantly impaired (Satoh, Takeda, Murakami, et al., 2005). Only a few well-documented case reports have described agnosias for environmental sounds, with preserved processing of speech and sometimes also music (Fujii, Fukatsu, Watabe, et al., 1990). Finally, a syndrome called *phonagnosia* has been described which is characterized by an inability to recognize the identity of a speaker, although the processing of the phonological patterns of words and phrases is unimpaired (Van Lancker, Kreiman, & Cummings, 1989).

Pure word-deafness occurs mostly after bilateral and rarely after left-unilateral temporal lesions, but never after unilateral lesions to the non-dominant hemisphere, suggesting that auditory processing of speech patterns is left-dominant. On the contrary, impaired processing of music, of environmental sounds, and of speaker characteristics appears to be lateralized predominantly to the right hemisphere (cf. Scott & Wise, 2004).

The auditory agnosias are conventionally seen as disorders affecting higher processing levels of sound recognition rather than the more elementary processes by which the acoustic features of an auditory event are analyzed. Consistently with this view, the lateralization of specialized sound processing abilities to either the left or the right hemisphere is ascribed to the cross-talk of auditory processing areas proper with the more abstract representations of the different categories of auditory events, i.e., language, music, etc. From this perspective, the primary stages of auditory processing are genuinely bilateral and not specific to any particular domain (e.g. Price, Thierry, & Griffiths, 2005). Contrasting with this view, Zatorre, Belin, and Penhune (2002) claim that the two hemispheres have complementary skills as far as the temporal and spectral resolution of acoustic patterns is concerned, with the right hemisphere acting as a spectral analyzer with a broader time-window, hence a poor time resolution and a good frequency resolution, and the left hemisphere having poor spectral resolution skills, to the benefit of time resolution. In their interpretation, functional specializations of the two hemispheres, as they become apparent in the auditory agnosia syndromes, can be explained by specific auditory-perceptual mechanisms of the left and the right temporal cortex.

31.4   What may Neurophonetics Tell Us about Phonetic Theories?

The major objective of neurophonetic research is to understand the mechanisms underlying the different neurogenic impairments of producing or of perceiving spoken language. Therefore, neurophonetic evidence may influence mainstream phonetic theories at many levels. In this chapter, two particularly controversial issues may deserve specific consideration: (1) the question whether speech is special, and (2) the question of how perception and action interact in speech.

31.4.1   Is speech special?

This question was originally raised for the issue of speech perception (Liberman, 1982), asking if auditory processing of spoken language is achieved by a specialized neural machinery, or if it constitutes one out of many domains of a multi-purpose perceptual system. A similar question may also be formulated for speech production, asking if the motor processes implied in speaking are *a priori* phonetic, or if oral motor control is universal for all kinds of motor activities, like emotional expression, chewing, swallowing, or mouth movement imitation (Liberman & Whalen, 2000).

Some of the clinical data from disorders of auditory processing might, on a first view, be interpreted to substantiate the claim that speech perception is highly specific, since observations of dissociations between word-deafness, sound agnosia, and amusia suggest the existence of modular perceptual systems. However, there are two major problems with this interpretation: first, the specific nature of the processing of speech may not arise at a genuinely perceptual stage, but may rather be attributable to the point where auditory perception interfaces with higher linguistic or cognitive processes, and, second, the dissociation between impairments of auditory speech vs. nonspeech perception may simply result from the fact that the auditory events from different domains (speech, music, environment) differ in their complexity and their spectral-temporal properties. Functional imaging research is currently being undertaken to resolve these issues (e.g. Price, Thierry, & Griffiths, 2005).

The situation is similar for the motor domain: clinical data strongly suggest that impairments of speech motor control can be dissociated from impairments of vegetative, emotional, or voluntary nonspeech motor activities of the muscles implied in speaking (Bonilha, Moser, Rorden, Baylis, & Fridriksson, 2006; Ziegler, 2006). Does this necessarily imply that our brain disposes of motor mechanisms which are specific to the production of spoken language? There is one strong, although indirect, argument in favor of this conclusion: during the first decade of our life and even beyond, the oral motor system is extensively trained for the particular motor activity of producing acoustic communicative signals. From what we know about the plasticity of the nervous system in response to motor learning, it is very plausible that a motor circuitry develops over time which is specifically geared to serve this behavioral purpose. If it is true that life experience and learning mold the motor system for linguistic purposes, an analogous case can be made for the auditory-perceptual system. Taken together this would imply that speech is special not from birth, but rather as a result of extensive motor and perceptual learning. What distinguishes humans from non-human primates, on this issue, is (1) our anatomical and neuronal endowments for fine motor adaptations of the upper and lower vocal tract, and (2) our outstanding vocal imitation and vocal learning capacities.

31.4.2   *Action and perception*

Human vocal imitation and learning is based on our ability to acquire and flexibly adapt movement patterns appropriate for the voluntary generation of distinct acoustic events, i.e. speech sounds. This capability presumably depends on the existence of a massive fiber-connection between auditory and motor cortical areas of the human brain, the *arcuate fascicle*, which guarantees a fast and accurate cross-talk between the perceptual and the motor representations involved in spoken language processing. However, auditory-motor interactions are not confined to the situation where new speech motor patterns are acquired: it is for instance known that the left superior temporal gyrus, a structure involved in auditory functions, is also activated in speech *production*. Likewise, perceptual tasks operating on the segmental aspects of spoken words typically involve activation of anterior language areas implied in higher speech motor functions (Hickok & Poeppel, 2004).

The hypothesis that we perceive speech by mapping the incoming auditory patterns onto the motor representations associated with these patterns has been a central and much debated issue of the motor theory of speech perception (Liberman, Cooper, Shankweiler, & Studdert-Kennedy, 1967). The importance of perception–action interactions is no longer a controversial issue, and since the discovery of mirror neurones in monkeys (Rizzolatti & Arbib, 1998) a proliferation of mirror systems has been postulated to accommodate action with movement perception in our brain. Pulvermüller, Huss, Kherif, et al. (2006) have verified a rather specific prediction of the motor theory of speech perception, i.e., that auditory perception of labial and lingual consonants is associated with activations of motor cortical sites linked with the motor production of these consonants. However, the functional role of this motor coactivation is still unresolved. More specifically, it is questionable if such auditory-motor interactions are relevant in speech understanding, i.e., in listening for meaning. For instance, it appears that the integrity of motor representations for speech in patients with left cortical lesions is not a necessary requirement for them to understand spoken language, since patients with severe apraxia of speech may nonetheless have normal auditory comprehension. Furthermore, focal brain lesions may selectively impair a patient's ability to analyze the phonological make-up of a spoken word, but leave her spoken language comprehension intact. This finding may indicate that only the explicit processing and segmentation of spoken words is interlinked with the speech motor system, while listening for meaning is not.

REFERENCES

Aichert, I. and Ziegler, W. (2004). Syllable frequency and syllable structure in apraxia of speech. *Brain and Language*, 88, 148–59.

Alcock, K. J., Passingham, R. E., Watkins, K. E. and Vargha-Khadem, F. (2000). Oral dyspraxia in inherited speech and language impairment and acquired dysphasia. *Brain and Language*, 75, 17–33.

Bonilha, L., Moser, D., Rorden, C., Baylis, G. C., and Fridriksson, J. (2006). Speech apraxia without oral apraxia: Can normal brain function explain the physiopathology? *NeuroReport*, 17, 1027–31.

Bose, A., van Lieshout, P., and Square, P. A. (2003). Speech coordination in individuals with aphasia and normal speakers. *Brain and Language*, 87, 158–9.

Code, C. (1998). Models, theories and heuristics in apraxia of speech. *Clinical Linguistics and Phonetics*, 12, 47–65.

Darley, F. L., Aronson, A. E., and Brown, J. R. (1975). *Motor Speech Disorders*. Philadelphia, PA: W. B. Saunders.

Deger, K., Ziegler, W., and Wessel, K. (1999). Airflow tracking in patients with ataxic disorders. *Clinical Linguistics and Phonetics*, 13, 433–47.

Dell, G. S., Schwartz, M. F., Martin, N., Saffran, E. M., and Gagnon, D. A. (1997). Lexical access in aphasic and nonaphasic speakers. *Psychological Review*, 104, 801–38.

DePaul, R. and Abbs, J. H. (1987). Manifestation of ALS in the cranial motor nerves: Dynamometric, neuropathologic, and speech motor data. *Neurologic Clinics*, 5, 231–50.

Duffy, J. R. (2005), *Motor Speech Disorders: Substrates, Differential Diagnosis, and Management*. St. Louis, MO: Elsevier Mosby.

Egan, C. A., Davies, L., and Halmagyi, G. M. (1996). Bilateral total deafness due to pontine hematoma. *Journal of Neurology, Neurosurgery, and Psychiatry*, 61, 628–31.

Fujii, T., Fukatsu, R., Watabe, S., Ohnuma, A., Teramura, K., Kimura, I., Saso, S., and Kogure, K. (1990). Auditory sound agnosia without aphasia following a right temporal lobe lesion. *Cortex*, 26, 263–8.

Goldstein, L., Pouplier, M., Chen, L., Saltzman, E., and Byrd, D. (forthcoming). Dynamic action units slip in speech production errors. *Cognition*.

Groenen, P., Maassen, B., Crul, T. and Thoonen, G. (1996). The specific relation between perception and production errors for place of articulation in developmental apraxia of speech. *Journal of Speech and Hearing Research*, 39, 468–82.

Hickok, G. and Poeppel, D. (2004). Dorsal and ventral streams: A framework for understanding aspects of the functional anatomy of language. *Cognition*, 92, 67–99.

Hunker, C. J. and Abbs, J. H. (1990). Uniform frequency of Parkinsonian resting tremor in the lips, jaw, tongue, and index finger. *Movement Disorders*, 71, 71–7.

Kent, R. D., Weismer, G., Kent, J. F., Vorperian, H. K., and Duffy, J. R. (1999). Acoustic studies of dysarthric speech: Methods, progress, and potential. *Journal of Communication Disorders*, 32, 141–86.

Krakow, R. A. (1999). Physiological organization of syllables: A review. *Journal of Phonetics*, 27, 33–54.

Laganaro, M. (2005). Syllable frequency effect in speech production: Evidence from aphasia. *Journal of Neurolinguistics*, 18, 221–35.

Levelt, W. J. M., Roelofs, A., and Meyer, A. S. (1999). A theory of lexical access in speech production. *Behavioral and Brain Sciences*, 22, 1–38.

Liberman, A. M. (1982). On finding that speech is special. *American Psychologist*, 37, 148–67.

Liberman, A. M., Cooper, F. S., Shankweiler, D. P., and Studdert-Kennedy, M. (1967). Perception of the speech code. *Psychological Review*, 74, 431–61.

Liberman, A. M. and Whalen, D. H. (2000). On the relation of speech to language. *Trends in Cognitive Sciences*, 4, 187–96.

McNeil, M. R., Weismer, G., Adams, S., and Mulligan, M. (1990). Oral structure nonspeech motor control in normal, dysarthric, aphasic and apraxic speakers: Isometric force and static position control. *Journal of Speech and Hearing Research*, 33, 255–68.

Mega, M. S. and Cohenour, R. C. (1997). Akinetic mutism: Disconnection of frontal-subcortical circuits. *Neuropsychiatry, Neuropsychology, and Behavioral Neurology*, 10, 254–9.

Praamstra, P., Hagoort, P., Maassen, B., and Crul, T. (1991). Word deafness and auditory cortical function: A case history and hypothesis. *Brain*, 114, 1197–1225.

Price, C., Thierry, G., and Griffiths, T. (2005). Speech-specific auditory processing: Where is it? *Trends in Cognitive Sciences*, 9, 271–6.

Pulvermüller, F., Huss, M., Kherif, F., del Prado Martin, F. M., Hauk, O., and Shtyrov, Y. (2006). Motor cortex maps articulatory features of speech sounds. *Proceedings of the National Academy of Sciences of the USA*, 103, 7865–70.

Rizzolatti, G. and Arbib, M. A. (1998). Language within our grasp. *Trends in Neurosciences*, 21, 188–94.

Satoh, M., Takeda, K., Murakami, Y., Onouchi, K., Inoue, K., and Kuzuhara, S. (2005). A case of amusia caused by the infarction of anterior portion of bilateral temporal lobes. *Cortex*, 41, 77–83.

Scott, S. K. and Wise, R. J. (2004). The functional neuroanatomy of prelexical processing in speech perception. *Cognition*, 92, 13–45.

Shriberg, L. D., Aram, D. M., and Kwiatkowski, J. (1997). Developmental apraxia of speech: I. Descriptive and theoretical perspectives. *Journal of Speech and Hearing Research*, 40, 273–85.

Shriberg, L. D., Ballard, K. J., Tomblin, J. B., Duffy, J. R., Odell, K. H., and Williams, C. A. (2006). Speech, prosody, and voice characteristics of a mother and daughter with a 7;13 translocation affecting *FOXP2*. *Journal of Speech, Language, and Hearing Research*, 49, 500–25.

Urban, P. P., Wicht, S., Vukurevic, G., Fitzek, C., Fitzek, S., Stoeter, P., Massinger, C., and Hopf, H. C. (2001). Dysarthria in acute ischemic stroke: Lesion topography, clinicoradiologic correlation, and etiology. *Neurology*, 56, 1021–7.

Van Lancker, D. R., Kreiman, J., and Cummings, J. (1989). Voice perception deficits: Neuroanatomical correlates of phonagnosia. *Journal of Clinical and Experimental Neuropsychology*, 11, 665–74.

Vargha-Khadem, F., Gadian, D. G., Copp, A., and Mishkin, M. (2005). FOXP2 and the neuroanatomy of speech and language. *Nature Reviews Neuroscience*, 6, 131–8.

Zatorre, R. J., Belin, P., and Penhune, V. B. (2002). Structure and function of auditory cortex: music and speech. *Trends in Cognitive Sciences*, 6, 37–46.

Ziegler, W. (2005). A nonlinear model of word length effects in apraxia of speech. *Cognitive Neuropsychology*, 22, 603–23.

Ziegler, W. (2006). Distinctions between speech and nonspeech motor control: A neurophonetic view. In M. Tabain and J. Harrington (eds.), *Speech Production* (pp. 41–54). Oxford: Psychology Press.

Ziegler, W. (2007). Apraxia of speech. In G. Goldenberg and B. Miller (eds.), *Handbook of Clinical Neurology*, vol. 88 (3rd series), pp. 269–85. London: Elsevier.

32 Coarticulation and Speech Impairment

BILL HARDCASTLE AND
KRIS TJADEN

32.1 Coarticulation: The Concept

Coarticulation is a term used to describe the ubiquitous overlapping of articulatory movements associated with separate sound segments. The phenomenon can best be seen in instrumental records, which track the movements of speech organs during continuous speech. For example, in a word like 'stew', the lip rounding associated with the vowel [u] begins at the same time (i.e. 'coarticulates') with tongue tip raising for the [s]. This is an example of labial coarticulation with the lips moving forward during the [s] in anticipation of the rounded vowel. The [s] produced in this environment would thus be quite different acoustically from the [s] in a word like 'stair', where no such lip rounding occurs. One of the consequences of coarticulation is therefore that speech sounds vary (both acoustically and physiologically) according to the context in which they are produced and the nature of sounds which precede or follow them.

This is the sense in which the term coarticulation is often used nowadays, referring to the variation in speech sound production according to context. In this broader usage the term is frequently used interchangeably with 'assimilation', which also refers to the influence of context on speech sounds. Terms like 'place' assimilation are used to describe the 'instability' of alveolar stops in the environment of a following velar or bilabial (e.g. in sequences like 'red car' where the [d] may assimilate into the following [k], or 'voice' assimilation in a phrase like 'I have to' in which the voiced [v] assimilates into the voiceless [t] to become the perceived voiceless [f]; see also Howard, Wells, & Local, chapter 36 in this volume). Some investigators, including the originator of the term 'coarticulation', Paul Menzerath (Menzerath & Lacerda, 1933), restrict 'coarticulation' to the physiological mechanisms underlying the coordination of the organs of speech production and reserve 'assimilation' for audible change to specific sounds often resulting in the perception of a different phoneme (/k/ or /g/ for /d/, /f/ for /v/ in the above examples).

Coarticulation effects are often described in terms of the direction of influence and extent of influence. Right-to-left or anticipatory coarticulation such as the labial coarticulation illustrated above in the word 'stew' occurs when a speech sound (e.g. [s]) is influenced by a following sound (e.g. [u]). If a sound shows influence of a preceding sound this is carry-over or perseverative (left-to-right) coarticulation.

The temporal domain of influence may also be relevant in a description of coarticulatory effects. In the 'stew' example above, the lip rounding influence spreads at least two segments in advance of the vowel. Earlier studies (e.g. Benguerel & Cowan, 1974) found lip rounding influence extending up to six segments in advance. The notion of coarticulatory influence spreading across many segments was conceptualized in the computer model proposed by Henke (1966), which came to be characterized by a 'feature-spreading' model. These early models proposed that a coarticulatory effect begins as early as possible in a string of segments as long as there are no adverse perceptual consequences of such spreading.

An alternative view is that coarticulatory influences are time-locked and that the component gestures of a segment begin a fixed interval of time before the phonetic target is achieved (see e.g. Bell-Berti & Harris, 1982). The time-locking approach is closely allied to an action-theory view of speech production using the notion of coordinative structures. In this approach, the underlying units of speech production are not segments but gestures, which can be defined as speech-relevant goals containing spatio-temporal information about speech articulation (see van Lieshout and Goldstein, chapter 29 in this volume). An example of an articulatory gesture in this framework would be a bilabial closing gesture, which consists of a unique combination of upper lip, jaw and lower lip movements irrespective of context. Contextual effects arise from overlapping (co-production) with other gestures. In this coordinative structure framework, coarticulation is seen as the automatic consequence of the inherent kinematic properties of the speech production mechanism.

Explanations for coarticulation tend to vary depending on whether it is of the carry-over or of the anticipatory type. Carry-over effects are often attributed to inherent kinematic characteristics of the speech organs, for example a relatively slow velum-raising movement during the vowel in a sequence such as /mi/ after maximum lowering during the /m/. Anticipatory coarticulatory effects are more difficult to explain and are generally regarded to be a characteristic of all skilled motor behavior. At a cognitive level, anticipatory movements are evidence of a universal tendency for the brain to 'scan ahead of time' (cf. Lashley, 1951) and it is suggested that such anticipation may be disrupted in many types of speech disorders affecting normal speech motor control (see below). In addition, it has been suggested that anticipatory coarticulation may aid perceptual processes. For example, the prior acoustic knowledge of an upcoming segment provided by anticipatory coarticulation may facilitate a more accurate perception of a segment than would be the case if all acoustic cues were confined within the temporal boundaries of that segment (Kühnert & Nolan, 1999).

Coarticulatory effects are subject to a variety of constraints. These may be related to physiological features of the articulators (cf. the notion of 'coarticulatory resistance', Bladon & Al-Bamerni, 1976; Fowler & Brancazio, 2000; Recasens, 1985) and to a variety of suprasegmental features such as stress patterns, prosodic and syntactic boundaries, syntactic structure, rate of articulation, clarity, and speech style (see, e.g., Engstrand, 1988; Lindblom, 1963; Hardcastle, 1985; Matthies, Perrier, Perkell, & Zandipour, 2001). The phonological structure of a particular language also may constrain the type and extent of coarticulatory influences (see e.g., Clumeck, 1976; Manual, 1999).

32.2   Measurement of Coarticulation

Coarticulatory processes may be measured directly with instrumental techniques that can accurately track the movements of individual speech organs in time. Such techniques include electromagnetic articulography (EMA), X-ray (including the X-ray microbeam system), real-time magnetic resonance imaging (MRI) and optoelectronic techniques such as VICON and SELSPOT (for visible organs such as the lips and jaw). Electropalatography (EPG) can be used but it records spatio-temporal details of tongue contacts with the palate, so will give only indirect information on actual lingual movement trajectories. (These techniques and their use in recording and analyzing coarticulatory events are described in detail in Hardcastle & Hewlett, 1999; see also Gibbon, chapter 19 in this volume.)

For measuring coarticulation in people with speech disorders, most researchers have used relatively more indirect techniques such as acoustic analysis, mainly because of the practical difficulties associated with the types of physiological techniques mentioned above. Acoustic analysis by itself cannot provide precise quantitative information about the onset, amplitude and velocity of movements of specific organs such as the tongue. However, acoustic analysis is valuable for recording general contextual effects that occur as a result of coarticulatory processes – for example, the effect of V2 on both V1 or C in a VCV sequence – and in fact is widely used. This pertains to the broader use of the term 'coarticulation' alluded to above in section 32.1.

The following is a brief overview of some of the techniques and measurements that have been used to record and analyze coarticulation in people with speech impairment.

32.2.1   *Kinematic techniques*

Direct measurement techniques have been used to record different articulatory movements in speakers with a variety of speech disorders. For example: Itoh, Sasanuma, and Ushijima (1979) and Itoh, Sasanuma, Hirose, Yoshida, and Ushijima (1980) used the X-ray microbeam system to record velum lowering in a speaker with apraxia of speech; Bartle, Goozée, Scott, Murdoch, and Kuruvilla (2006) and Jaeger, Hertrich, Stattrop, Schönle, and Ackermann (2000) used EMA to record lip, jaw and tongue movement in speakers with traumatic brain injury; Katz, Machetanz, Orth and Schönle (1990) used EMA to record the kinematics of articulatory movement in anterior aphasics; and Weismer, Yunusova and Westbury (2003) used the X-ray microbeam system and acoustic reference points to measure coordination in speakers with motor speech disorders associated with amyotrophic lateral sclerosis (ALS) and Parkinson's disease (PD). These techniques offer direct and quantifiable means of measuring the temporal coordination between different speech organs as well as offering the possibility of measuring the dynamics of the articulatory movements such as velocity and acceleration. They can show accurately, for example, the onset of lip movement in a word such as 'stew' (mentioned in section 32.1), in relation to other articulatory events such as the closure for the /t/ measured by, for example, the drop in tongue velocity. Kinematic measures can also usefully be combined with acoustic measures, as described in Weismer, Yunusova, and Westbury (2003). Here the F2 low point during the vowel in 'suit' was compared to local maxima and minima in the traces of the tongue dorsum and lip movement, as measured by the X-ray microbeam system.

32.2.2 *Acoustic techniques*

32.2.2.1 *F2 ratios*

F2 ratios usually involve tracking frequency influences on preceding C or V using minimal pairs. A typical paradigm involves measuring F2 ratios using pairs such as ə'bi versus ə'ba. If there is no change in /ə/ midpoint there is minimal coarticulation. The higher the F2 in ə'bi and the lower the F2 at the same point in ə'ba, the greater the degree of anticipation of the upcoming V (see, for example, Nittrouer, Studdert-Kennedy, & McGowan, 1989; Nijland, Maassen, van der Meulen, et al., 2002). The paradigm used by Ziegler and von Cramon (1985, 1986) involved a test sequence (gətVtə, where V = /i, y, u, a/) spoken in a carrier phrase to avoid the problems of a possibly highly variable speech-ready gesture if the test items are spoken in isolation. Using a similar VCV sequence, it is possible to measure the effects of V2 on the C by using acoustic measures such as first-moment coefficients (see, for example, Nittrouer, Studdert-Kennedy, & McGowan, 1989; Tjaden & Wilding, 2005).

32.2.2.2 *F2 locus equations*

Many researchers have used F2 locus equations as a metric for C–V coarticulation (e.g. Chang, Ohde, & Conture, 2002; Krull, 1987; Lindblom, 1963; Sussman, McCaffrey, & Matthews, 1991). The locus equation plots F2 at vowel onset against the target frequency of the same vowel at a so-called steady-state location. The plots are compiled mainly for voiced stops and fricatives across different vowels (e.g. /i, a, u/) and the slope is said to be linked to the degree of coarticulation (Krull, 1987). Minimum coarticulation is where the locus equation has a relatively fixed F2 onset frequency across vowel contexts and maximum coarticulation is where the F2 onset frequency varies systematically with F2 vowel target frequency. Steep functions for labials and velars compared to alveolars are said to indicate places of articulation where following vowels greatly influence preceding consonants. (But see Löfqvist, 1999, p. 2022, who concluded that no measures based on EMA data showed support for the assumption that the slope serves as an index of the degree of coarticulation between C and V.)

32.2.2.3   Centroid frequency

Centroid frequency is a weighted average of spectral peak frequencies. The measure is often used for fricatives and stop releases in showing evidence of labial and lingual anticipation of an upcoming rounded V (e.g., Baum, 1998).

32.2.2.4   Auditory-perceptual measures

Ziegler and von Cramon (1985, 1986) used a gating technique where the gated speech segments contained coarticulatory information relating to different vowels presented to listeners for a V identification task. The conclusion from one of these studies (Ziegler & von Cramon, 1985) was that individuals with apraxia of speech begin the V gesture in CV syllables later than their normal controls (see also Tuller & Seider-Story, 1987).

32.3   Coarticulation in Clinical Populations: General Issues

Clinical populations of interest in studies of coarticulation generally fall into one of three categories, namely (1) hearing-impaired or deaf speech, (2) aphasia, and (3) speech motor control disorders. For the purpose of the current chapter, this latter category includes stuttering, dysarthria, acquired apraxia of speech (AOS) and the developmental form of apraxia, hereafter referred to as childhood apraxia of speech (CAS). Before we summarize research findings for each of these populations, it is useful to consider the rationale for studying coarticulation in persons with speech impairment and what might be gained from these kinds of studies.

32.3.1   Rationale for studying coarticulation in clinical populations

Studies investigating coarticulation in clinical populations have been undertaken for a variety of reasons; accordingly, the nature of the information gained from these studies varies. Some studies seek to enhance understanding of normal sensorimotor speech processes or to evaluate predictions suggested by theories and models of normal speech production. The notion that studies of clinical populations have the potential to provide insight into normal speech processes or can be used as a test case for evaluating predictions suggested by normal speech production theory may seem contradictory. This idea makes sense, however, insofar as clinical populations may be viewed as a variation from the normal mechanism rather than as a transformation of the normal mechanism to a completely different one (Bernstein & Weismer, 2000). For example, a gesture-based account of speech suggests specific predictions concerning the overlapping and sliding of speech events and their acoustic consequences (Browman & Goldstein, 1997; Fowler & Saltzman, 1993; van Lieshout & Goldstein, chapter 29 in this volume). Predictions concerning the co-production of speech events have been tested in a variety of speech motor control disorders, with the bulk of studies providing only modest support for a gesture-based account of speech (e.g., Huinck, van Lieshout, Peters, & Hulstijn, 2004; Tjaden, 1999; Weismer, Tjaden, & Kent, 1995). Relatedly, research investigating coarticulation in cochlear implant users who are postlingually deafened has helped clarify the role of audition in the mature sensorimotor speech mechanism (Lane, Matthies, Perkell, Vick, & Zandipour, 2001). That is, postlingually deafened speakers acquire speech and language while they can still hear themselves and others, and thus have normal auditory models for speech-language acquisition. Studies investigating changes in speech for postlingually deafened speakers pre- versus post-implant – after which hearing is at least partially restored – therefore shed light on the role of audition in the speech mechanism of persons who have acquired their native language under normal auditory conditions. Similarly, because AOS and CAS are widely considered to be disorders of speech motor programming, studies comparing coarticulatory patterns in speakers with apraxia and normal controls provide insight regarding the role of motor programming in coarticulation. Studies of clinical populations with identifiable focal lesions of the nervous system further allow testing of hypotheses concerning the neural representation of normal speech processes. For example, on the basis of a review of studies investigating coarticulation in AOS and cerebellar ataxia, Katz (2000) concluded that anticipatory coarticulation has a multifocal representation in the nervous system and that perseveratory coarticulation is regulated, at least in part, by the cerebellum.

Studies investigating coarticulation in speakers with impaired speech production also have obvious importance for advancing understanding of the disorders themselves, which ultimately has implications for diagnosis and treatment of speech impairment. Stuttering, for example, has been hypothesized to stem from a breakdown in coarticulation or difficulty transitioning between sounds (van Riper, 1982; Wingate, 1969). Studies reporting coarticulatory deviancies in persons who stutter not only would support this suggestion, but also might indicate that therapeutic efforts should focus on facilitating more normal coarticulatory patterns. As discussed below in section 32.4, however, findings from studies investigating coarticulation in persons who stutter are equivocal. Relatedly, studies of dysarthria, apraxia, and hearing-impaired speech have been undertaken to determine whether coarticulatory abnormalities might help to explain deviant perceptual characteristics, such as reduced intelligibility or scanning speech – a perceptual label referring to slow speech rate, reduced segment duration contrasts, prolonged transitions, and segregated syllables. Most of these studies have focused on characterizing coarticulatory patterns for persons with speech impairment, however, and comparatively few studies have systematically examined the perceptual consequences of coarticulation in clinical populations, perhaps with the exception of AOS (e.g., Baum, 1998; Southwood, Dagenais, Sutphin, & Garcia, 1997; Tjaden & Sussman, 2006; Ziegler & von Cramon, 1985). Some studies also have explored how therapeutic strategies used in the treatment of dysarthria or AOS impact coarticulation (e.g., Southwood, Dagenais, Sutphin, & Garcia, 1997; Tjaden, 2000; Tjaden & Wilding, 2005).

32.3.2   *Methodological challenges in studying coarticulation in clinical populations*

It is worth noting that the literature investigating coarticulation in clinical populations is relatively modest in size compared to the literature investigating coarticulation in typically developing children and normal adults. On the one hand, this should not come as a surprise given the long-standing prominence of coarticulation in theories and models of normal speech production. It stands to reason that constructs of theoretical importance would be a major focus of research, and a good understanding of normal coarticulatory patterns is obviously necessary for identifying and interpreting coarticulatory deviancies in clinical populations. Nonetheless, methodological factors associated with studying clinical populations probably help to explain why few studies have investigated coarticulation in clinical populations.

Compared to normal speakers, clinical populations are arguably more challenging to identify and recruit for study. Finding adequate numbers of clinical-research participants is especially challenging in studies employing a between-groups design because this type of design requires a group of homogeneous clinical participants. For example, if findings for a group of speakers with hearing impairment are to be compared to a group of normally hearing speakers, it is important that the former group have a similar degree of hearing impairment. This is necessary because degree of hearing impairment covaries with severity of speech production impairment, so that speakers with more severe hearing impairment tend to have more severely affected speech (see review in Pratt & Tye-Murray, 1997). Thus, speech severity will be a confounding variable in studies employing a between-groups design if degree of hearing impairment is substantially different among speakers. Similar statements apply to the timing of hearing loss, as speech is more severely impaired in prelingually than in postlingually deafened persons. Some studies have addressed the severity issue by treating individual speakers as separate experiments and also by supplementing group findings with individual speaker data (Lane, Matthies, Perkell, Vick, & Zandipour, 2001; Okalidou & Harris, 1999).

Difficulties in identifying homogeneous groups in populations with impaired speech are not unique to studies of hearing impairment. Studies to date investigating coarticulation in dysarthria secondary to Parkinson's disease (PD) have thus far excluded persons who have received neurosurgical treatment for PD as well as individuals who have received certain forms of speech therapy (e.g., Tjaden, 2003; Tjaden & Wilding, 2005; Weismer, Yunusova, & Westbury, 2003). These kinds of inclusionary criteria help to ensure a relatively homogeneous group of speakers, but also limit the pool of potential participants. Difficulty in identifying adequate numbers of clinical speakers for research is further exacerbated by the fact that certain types of communication disorders are rare in their 'pure' form. AOS is a good example. Cerebrovascular accident or stroke is a common cause of AOS, but rarely does a stroke produce an AOS without an accompanying dysarthria or aphasia (McNeil, Robin, & Schmidt, 1997). Yet, if a study seeks to determine whether impaired speech motor programming in AOS affects coarticulation, it is important that findings cannot be attributed to a coexisting impairment.

In addition to the difficulties of identifying and recruiting clinical populations, individuals with impaired speech present challenges to measurement. One issue that arises in studies of apraxia is whether to restrict analyses to error-free or 'on target' productions or whether to extend analyses to 'off-target' productions, defined as utterances containing perceptually identifiable phoneme substitutions or distortions. Restricting the data set to on-target productions facilitates quantitative, parametric analysis of the data, but excludes potentially interesting and revealing information (Liss & Weismer, 1992; Sussman, Marquardt, MacNeilage, & Hutchinson, 1988). A related issue in the stuttering literature is whether to study speech tokens that are perceptually fluent or dysfluent (Armson & Kalinowski, 1994). In addition, many studies of coarticulation have used acoustic analyses to quantify coarticulation, although EPG and techniques that measure articulatory kinematics have been used a fair amount to study coarticulation or coordination in AOS. There are a variety of advantages to acoustic analyses, such as the noninvasive nature and portability of the instrumentation and the fact that there is a large comparison literature describing acoustic characteristics of normal speech, including studies of coarticulation. Alterations in voice quality and resonance in populations such as dysarthria and hearing impairment contribute to poor resolution of formant structure, however, thereby increasing the difficulty in identifying segmental acoustic landmarks that often are necessary for acoustic measures of coarticulation. This is not to say that acoustic measures of coarticulation in clinical populations cannot be reliably obtained. Rather, compared to normal populations, acoustic analyses in clinical populations are more time-intensive and require significant investigator expertise.

Hertrich and Ackermann (1999) attempted to address the issue of formant resolution in clinical populations by developing acoustic measures of coarticulation that do not rely on identification of formant structure. These measures present their own challenges, however, because the link to the underlying speech events is not particularly obvious; nor can findings be easily compared to studies utilizing more 'traditional' acoustic measures of coarticulation, such as the acoustic ratios developed by Nittrouer and her colleagues (Nittrouer, 1993; Nittrouer, Studdert-Kennedy, & Neely, 1996). Of course, instrumental techniques like EPG do not pose the same types of measurement problems in clinical populations (see Wood & Hardcastle, 2000).

Finally, abnormalities in articulatory rate and scaling that are common in clinical populations like apraxia, hearing impairment, and dysarthria can complicate interpretation of coarticulatory effects, and thus need to be considered in the experimental design. At least some studies suggest that strength or amount of coarticulation is affected by articulatory rate, so that relatively slower rates are associated with reduced coarticulation. Thus, a slower-than-normal articulatory rate in clinical speakers can contribute to the appearance of reduced coarticulation, if articulatory rate is not appropriately controlled in the data analyses or is not considered in the experimental design. Relatedly, it is not uncommon for persons with hearing impairment, dysarthria or apraxia to produce speech movements that are reduced in size or amplitude. Reduced articulatory scaling in clinical populations, as indexed by an acoustic measure like vowel space area, also can contribute to the appearance of reduced coarticulation and thus needs to be appropriately controlled in the design and data analysis.

32.4   Coarticulation in Specific Clinical Populations

The remainder of the chapter is devoted to summaries of studies investigating coarticulation in hearing impairment, aphasia, and speech motor control disorders. The review is necessarily selective, as the intent is to provide a broad overview of the literature. Readers are encouraged to consult Katz (2000) for a comprehensive treatment of studies investigating anticipatory coarticulation in AOS or Broca's aphasia, as well as Wood and Hardcastle (2000) for a summary of relevant EPG studies. Relatedly, Pratt and Tye-Murray (1997) review most of the literature focusing on coarticulation in hearing impairment, and Tjaden (2006) summarizes studies investigating coarticulation in dysarthria. Finally, it should be noted that the studies reviewed in this section have used a variety of terms to refer to the construct of coarticulation, including gestural overlap, coordination, interarticulator timing, context effects, and sound-transitional effects, among others.

32.4.1   *Hearing impairment*

Most of what is known about coarticulation in persons with hearing impairment comes from studies investigating speakers with prelingual deafness or hearing impairment. By and large, these studies indicate reduced context effects for children and adults with prelingual hearing impairment or deafness (e.g., Baum & Waldstein, 1991; Monsen, 1976; Okalidou & Harris, 1999; Rothman, 1976; Tye-Murray, 1987; Tye-Murray, Zimmerman, & Folkins, 1987; Waldstein & Baum, 1991, 1994). For example, Okalidou and Harris (1999) used vowel F2 measures to quantify coarticulation in three prelingually deafened adults and three normally hearing adults for 'schwa plus CVC' utterances like /əbib/ and /əbub/. Deaf speakers demonstrated reduced anticipatory vowel-to-vowel coarticulation in utterances containing bilabial, but not alveolar consonants. Deaf speakers also showed reduced anticipatory consonant effects during the preceding schwa, as well as reduced perseveratory or carry-over consonant effects on the upcoming corner vowel. The authors concluded that the speech of deaf and normally hearing adults is guided by different gestural organization – a conclusion more or less consistent with the notion that hearing facilitates coarticulation, at least in persons who are prelingually deafened (Lane, Matthies, Perkell, Vick, & Zandipour, 2001).

To further evaluate the role of hearing in coarticulation, Lane and colleagues investigated anticipatory coarticulation in seven postlingually deafened adults who had received prosthetic hearing in the form of a cochlear implant. Deaf speakers were audio-recorded multiple times both pre- and post-implant, and two normally hearing adults were studied for comparison purposes. A variety of acoustic measures were used to quantify anticipatory vowel coarticulation in CV syllables, including locus equations and vowel F2 ratios. Results indicated that hearing status had little effect on the acoustic measures of coarticulation. The implication is that hearing does not have a direct role in regulating anticipatory coarticulation in adult speakers. Finally, Waldstein and Baum (1994) conducted one of the few studies formally investigating perception of vowel coarticulatory information in hearing-impaired speech. Previous production studies indicated less robust anticipatory and perseveratory vowel coarticulation in syllables produced by children with profound prelingual hearing loss, as compared to normally hearing children (Baum & Waldstein, 1991; Waldstein & Baum, 1991). Listeners in the perceptual study were presented with the aperiodic portion of consonants extracted from syllables like /si/ and /is/, and were asked to identify the vowel. In general, listeners were able to identify the absent vowel from presentation of the neighboring consonant at better than chance levels, but identification accuracy was better for tokens produced by normally hearing children. These perceptual findings support the production studies reporting reduced coarticulation in speech of prelingually deafened children. Although it has been hypothesized that reduced context effects reported in these and other studies of hearing-impaired speech might help to explain reductions in speech intelligibility, studies formally evaluating this suggestion are needed.

32.4.2 *Aphasia*

Following Katz (2000), the articulatory impairment in AOS and Broca's aphasia are considered to be equivalent for the purposes of the current chapter. Studies investigating coarticulation in patients with Broca's or nonfluent aphasia therefore are discussed under the topic heading of apraxia. Persons with other types of aphasia, such as Wernicke's aphasia and anomic aphasia, produce speech that is more fluent and better articulated than that of persons with nonfluent or Broca's aphasia. Persons with Wernicke's aphasia and even anomic aphasia may demonstrate articulatory deficits that are not perceptually obvious, however. Thus, several studies have examined articulatory coordination or coarticulation in aphasias characterized by relatively fluent speech production. Results of acoustic-perceptual studies suggest normal or preserved patterns of anticipatory coarticulation in Wernicke's aphasia (e.g., Baum, 1998; Katz, 1988; Tuller & Seider-Story, 1987). The implication is that any subtle articulatory deficit associated with Wernicke's aphasia does not compromise sound-transitional aspects of speech. However, EPG data for a speaker with anomic aphasia suggests intrusive articulatory movements for perceptually accurate productions (Hardcastle, Ellis, Wood, & Gibbon, 2001). Thus, at least some individuals with 'fluent' forms of aphasia seem to exhibit deficits of articulatory coordination.

32.4.3   Speech motor control disorders

32.4.3.1   Stuttering

Studies investigating coarticulation in persons who stutter (PWS) vary in terms of the age group of interest, the methodology or measures used to infer coarticulation, and the speech sample – which in the case of stuttering means whether perceptually fluent or dysfluent tokens were of interest. It probably is not surprising then that a consistent picture has yet to emerge as to whether coarticulation is deviant for PWS. Descriptive and quantitative measures of F2 vowel transitions have been used in many studies to infer coarticulation, although at least one study has used locus equations to index coarticulation (Chang, Ohde, & Conture, 2002) and another recent study used word-duration and reaction-time measures to infer variation in gestural overlap (Huinck, van Lieshout, Peters, & Hulstijn, 2004). The bulk of studies focusing on dysfluent utterances of PWS suggest atypical or absent F2 transitions (Harrington, 1987; Howell & Vause, 1986; Yaruss & Conture, 1993). Thus, coarticulation in dysfluencies of PWS appears to differ from normally fluent speech, at least as inferred from F2 transition characteristics. On the other hand, studies investigating coarticulation in perceptually fluent tokens of PWS report mixed findings, with some studies suggesting essentially normal F2 transition characteristics in fluent speech of PWS and other studies reporting differences in F2 transition characteristics for fluent speech of PWS and persons who do not stutter (e.g., Howell & Vause, 1986; Robb & Blomgren, 1997; Zebrowski, Conture, & Cudahy, 1985; Zimmerman, 1980). Moreover, the nature of the differences in F2 transition characteristics for PWS and persons who do not stutter vary in these studies of perceptually fluent speech. Some studies report steeper F2 transitions in PWS, while other studies report shallower or absent F2 transitions in PWS.

In contrast to studies inferring coarticulation from F2 transitions, Chang, Ohde and Conture (2002) used locus equations to infer coarticulation in perceptually fluent tokens of children who stutter (CWS) and children who do not stutter. F2 transition-rate measures were used to infer rate of vocal tract shape change. Findings revealed similar locus equation slopes and y-intercepts for the CWS and control children, indicating developmentally appropriate or intact patterns of coarticulation in CWS. Results further indicated that CWS do not distinguish F2 transition rates as a function of place of articulation as much as children who do not stutter. This latter finding was interpreted to suggest that the organization of formant transition rate is not as refined in CWS owing to difficulty in the speed of speech-language production, which in turn may contribute to disrupted speech fluency.

32.4.3.2 Dysarthria

With a few exceptions, studies investigating coarticulation or coordination in dysarthria have been conducted during the last decade. For example, earlier kinematic studies by Kent and colleagues indicated no major disruption in the temporal sequencing of supraglottal articulatory motions for phonetic events in dysarthria secondary to a variety of neurological impairments (Kent, Netsell, & Bauer, 1975; Netsell & Kent, 1976). Similar results concerning regularity in the timing of supraglottal articulatory gestures have been reported by Weismer, Yunusova, and Westbury (2003) for dysarthria secondary to ALS or PD, although results suggested a trend toward subtle coordination deficits in dysarthria, especially in ALS. Bartle, Goozée, Scott, Murdoch, and Kuruvilla (2006) also failed to find robust group differences in tongue–jaw timing or spatial coordination for speech produced by healthy talkers and a group of talkers with dysarthria secondary to traumatic brain injury. Consistently with the findings of Weismer, Yunusova, and Westbury (2003) for ALS, however, Bartle and colleagues identified a subgroup of individuals with TBI who showed evidence of articulatory incoordination. In contrast to these studies indicating largely normal coordination of supraglottal articulatory gestures, laryngeal-supralaryngeal incoordination in dysarthria is suggested by studies showing that speakers with dysarthria have difficulty stopping vocal-fold vibration at the interface of a vowel and a voiceless obstruent, as for the word 'it' (e.g., Tjaden & Watling, 2003; Weismer, 1984).

Acoustic studies investigating coarticulation in dysarthria report mixed findings. Some studies suggest increased or reduced coarticulation for speakers with dysarthria compared to healthy controls, although the differences were quite subtle (Hertrich & Ackermann, 1999; Tjaden, 1999, 2000). Yet, other studies suggest essentially normal patterns of coarticulation in dysarthria (Tjaden, 2003; Tjaden & Wilding, 2005). Given that the bulk of studies indicate only the most subtle of deficits in coordination or coarticulation in dysarthria, the contribution to perceived articulatory imprecision, irregular articulatory breakdown or reduced intelligibility is unclear. Further, even when normal talkers and speakers with dysarthria produce similar amounts of coarticulatory information, listeners may not be sensitive to these cues in the acoustic signal of dysarthria. To elaborate, a recent study showed that listeners had difficulty identifying the vowel /i/ in 'seed' produced by speakers with PD when presented with only the prevocalic /s/, although the strength of anticipatory vowel coarticulation was the same for normal and PD stimuli (Tjaden & Sussman, 2006). Further, difficulty in perceiving anticipatory vowel information in the prevocalic consonant of PD stimuli had no effect on word-level intelligibility. One implication is that information that is meaningful in a simple vowel identification task may not be indicative of the importance of that information for recovering the speaker's intended message. That being said, methodological limitations of at least some studies to date suggest additional studies are warranted. In addition, studies to date have mostly focused on speakers with relatively mild dysarthria, and coordination or coarticulatory deficits may only be evident for persons with more severe dysarthria.

32.4.3.3   Apraxia of speech

Far more studies have investigated coarticulation or coordination in apraxia of speech (AOS) as compared to other clinical populations, likely because incoordination is thought to play such a prominent role in the articulatory impairment in AOS. Several sources provide a more comprehensive treatment of the literature than we are able to within the constraints of the current chapter. For example, Katz (2000) summarizes findings from 15 studies investigating intrasyllabic anticipatory coarticulation in AOS, while Wood and Hardcastle (2000) review a variety of EPG studies suggestive of difficulties in articulatory coordination or timing in AOS.

Voice onset time (VOT) studies are one category of research that has provided insight concerning coordination or interarticulator timing in AOS. These studies indicate overlap of VOT values for voiced and voiceless consonants in AOS, even for consonants that listeners perceive as accurate (Blumstein, Cooper, Goodglass, Statlender, & Gottlieb, 1980; Blumstein, Cooper, Zurif, & Caramazza, 1977; see also Hardcastle, Morgan Barry, & Clark, 1985, for EPG data). Speakers with AOS also show large variability in VOT values for the same consonant. The overlap of VOT values for voiced and voiceless stops coupled with observations of greater variability have been interpreted as evidence that the timing of laryngeal and supralaryngeal events in AOS is poorly coordinated. Because VOT abnormalities are so pervasive in AOS, it seems AOS may be especially vulnerable to disruptions in timing or coordination between articulators.

A kinematic study by Itoh and Sasanuma (1984) further illustrates how deficits in articulatory timing or coordination contribute to impaired speech sound production in AOS. Velar movement for a patient with AOS as well as for a normal control was observed using fiberoscopy and the X-ray microbeam system. For a syllable sequence such as /dini/, the speaker with AOS showed substantial variability in the amount and duration of velar displacement, and this was accompanied by a perceived phonemic change from /n/ to /d/. This type of careful analysis of both instrumental and perceptual data – even for a single speaker – has been important for revealing underlying timing or coordination deficits in AOS as well as for showing how those deficits might contribute to perceived speech sound errors (for similar examples using EPG see Hardcastle & Edwards, 1992). Variability in timing in AOS is also suggested in many of the studies of anticipatory coarticulation reviewed by Katz (2000). That is, about half of the 15 studies reviewed support the conclusion that coarticulation is variable in AOS, but the overall pattern is largely normal (e.g., Baum, 1998; Katz, 1988; Sussman, Marquardt, MacNeilage, & Hutchinson, 1988). Other studies reviewed by Katz (2000) support the conclusion that coarticulation is delayed in AOS (e.g., Liss & Weismer, 1992; Ziegler & von Cramon, 1985). Given such mixed findings, it is difficult to draw any strong conclusions concerning anticipatory coarticulation in AOS. This is not to say that AOS is not characterized by some form of incoordination, but rather that studies of anticipatory coarticulation may not be particularly sensitive to the nature of the incoordination in AOS.

Similarly, a clear picture concerning coarticulation or coordination in CAS has yet to emerge. Some studies report that anticipatory vowel effects during a preceding consonant occur earlier and are stronger in children with CAS than in age- and sex-matched typically developing children (Maassen, Nijland, & van der Meulen, 2001; Nijland, Maassen, van der Meulen, et al., 2003). Other studies have found reduced anticipatory coarticulation in CAS, however (Nijland, Maassen, & van der Meulen, 2003). Still other studies report more variable and idiosyncratic patterns of coarticulation or coordination in children with CAS compared to typically developing children (Nijland, Maassen, Hulstijn, & Peters, 2004; Nijland, Maassen, van der Meulen, et al., 2002). Finally, a study employing locus equations to infer anticipatory vowel coarticulation in children with CAS concluded that these children do not differentiate coarticulatory extent across stop place of articulation to the same extent as normally developing children (Sussman, Marquardt, & Doyle, 2000). This was interpreted to mean that children with CAS are unable to refine coarticulation levels to maximally distinguish and acoustically contrast stop place categories. Sussman and colleagues further hypothesized that the lack of contrastiveness in coarticulatory extent across stop place of articulation contributes to reduced intelligibility in CAS.

32.5 Conclusion

As is clear from the above review, research into coarticulatory patterns in different types of speech impairment has produced somewhat equivocal results. This is perhaps not surprising given the often subtle nature of coarticulatory effects, the difficulties associated with undertaking research on clinical populations, and the inherently limited nature of many of the methodologies and measures used to analyze coordination between speech organs. More refined analysis techniques are warranted, ideally involving the simultaneous recording of both acoustic and kinematic aspects of speech production processes. We should then be able to specify more confidently the nature of the subtle abnormalities in coordination between speech organs that may signal the underlying nature of the disorder and thus have clinical significance in providing more refined assessment and diagnosis.

ACKNOWLEDGMENT

The writing of this chapter was supported by NIH R01DC004689 and MRC G0401388.

REFERENCES

Armson, J. and Kalinowski, J. (1994). Interpreting results of the fluent speech paradigm: Difficulties in separating cause from effect. *Journal of Speech and Hearing Research*, 37, 69–82.

Bartle, C. J., Goozée, J., Scott, D., Murdoch, B. E., and Kuruvilla, M. (2006). EMA assessment of tongue–jaw co-ordination during speech in dysarthria following traumatic brain injury. *Brain Injury*, 20, 529–45.

Baum, S. R. (1998). Anticipatory coarticulation in aphasia: Effects of utterance complexity. *Brain and Language*, 63, 357–80.

Baum, S. R. and Waldstein, R. S. (1991). Perseveratory coarticulation in the speech of profoundly hearing-impaired and normally hearing children. *Journal of Speech and Hearing Research*, 34, 1286–92.

Bell-Berti, F. and Harris, K. S. (1982). Temporal patterns of coarticulation: Lip rounding. *Journal of the Acoustical Society of America*, 71, 449–54.

Benguerel, A. P. and Cowan, H. (1974). Coarticulation of upper lip protrusion in French. *Phonetica*, 30, 41–55.

Bernstein, L. E. and Weismer, G. (2000). Basic science at the intersection of speech science and communication disorders. *Journal of Phonetics*, 28, 225–32.

Bladon, R. A. W. and Al-Bamerni, A. (1976). Coarticulation resistance in English /l/. *Journal of Phonetics*, 4, 137–50.

Blumstein, S. E., Cooper, W. E., Goodglass, H., Statlender, S., and Gottlieb, J. (1980). Production deficits in aphasia: A voice-onset time analysis. *Brain and Language*, 9, 153–70.

Blumstein, S., Cooper, W. E., Zurif, E., and Caramazza, A. (1977). The perception and production of voice-onset time in aphasia. *Neuropsychologia*, 155, 371–83.

Browman, C. P. and Goldstein, L. (1997). The gestural phonology model. In W. Hulstijn, H. F. M. Peters, and P. H. H. M. van Lieshout (eds.), *Speech Production: Motor Control, Brain Research and Fluency Disorders* (pp. 57–71). Amsterdam: Elsevier.

Chang, S., Ohde, R. N., and Conture, E. G. (2002). Coarticulation and formant transition rate in young children who stutter. *Journal of Speech, Language, and Hearing Research*, 45, 676–88.

Clumeck, H. (1976). Patterns of soft palate movement in six languages. *Journal of Phonetics*, 4, 337–51.

Engstrand, O. (1988). Articulatory correlates of stress and speaking rate in Swedish VCV utterances. *Journal of the Acoustical Society of America*, 83, 1863–75.

Fowler, C. A. and Brancazio, L. (2000). Coarticulatory resistance of American English consonants and its effects on transconsonantal vowel-to-vowel coarticulation. *Language and Speech*, 43, 1–41.

Fowler, C. A. and Saltzman, E. (1993). Coordination and coarticulation in speech production. *Language and Speech*, 36, 171–95.

Hardcastle, W. J. (1985). Some phonetics and syntactic constraints on lingual coarticulation during /kl/ sequences. *Speech Communication*, 4, 247–63.

Hardcastle, W. J. and Edwards, S. (1992). EPG-based description of apraxic speech errors. In R. D. Kent (ed.), *Intelligibility in Speech Disorders: Theory, Measurement and Management* (pp. 287–328). Amsterdam: John Benjamins.

Hardcastle, W. J., Ellis, L., Wood, W. E., and Gibbon, F. E. (2001). EPG/EMA studies of speech motor co-ordination. In B. Maassen, W. Hulstijn, R. Kent, H. F. M. Peters, and P. H. M. M. van Lieshout (eds.), *Speech Motor Control in Normal and Disordered Speech* (pp. 16–19). Nijmegen: Uitgeverij Vantilt.

Hardcastle, W. J. and Hewlett, N. (1999). *Coarticulation: Theory, Data and Techniques*. Cambridge: Cambridge University Press.

Hardcastle, W. J., Morgan Barry, R. A., and Clark, C. J. (1985). Articulatory and voicing characteristics of adult dysarthric and verbal dyspraxic speakers: An instrumental study. *British Journal of Disorders of Communication*, 20, 249–70.

Harrington, J. (1987). Coarticulation and stuttering: An acoustic and electropalatographic study. In H. F. M. Peters and W. Hulstijn (eds.), *Speech Motor Dynamics in Stuttering* (pp. 381–92). New York: Springer-Verlag.

Henke, W. L. (1966). *Dynamic Articulatory Model of Speech Production Using Computer Simulation*. PhD dissertation, Massachusetts Institute of Technology.

Hertrich, I. and Ackermann, H. (1999). Temporal and spectral aspects of coarticulation in ataxic dysarthria: An acoustic analysis. *Journal of Speech, Language, and Hearing Research*, 42, 367–81.

Howell, P. and Vause, L. (1986). Acoustic analysis and perception of vowels in stuttered speech. *Journal of the Acoustical Society of America*, 79, 1571–9.

Huinck, W. J., van Lieshout, P. H. H. M., Peters, H., and Hulstijn, W. (2004). Gestural overlap in consonant clusters: Effects on the fluent speech of stuttering and non-stuttering subjects. *Journal of Fluency Disorders*, 29, 3–25.

Itoh, M. and Sasanuma, S. (1984). Articulatory movements in apraxia of speech. In J. C. Rosenbek, M. R. McNeil, and A. E. Aronson (eds.), *Apraxia of Speech: Physiology, Acoustics, Linguistics, Management*. San Diego, CA: College-Hill Press.

Itoh, M., Sasanuma, S., Hirose, H., Yoshida, H., and Ushijima, T. (1980). Abnormal articulatory dynamics in a patient with apraxia of speech: X-ray microbeam observations. *Brain and Language*, 11, 66–75.

Itoh, M., Sasanuma, S., and Ushijima, T. (1979). Velar movements during speech in a patient with apraxia of speech. *Brain and Language*, 7, 227–39.

Jaeger, M., Hertrich, I., Stattrop, U., Schönle, P., and Ackermann, H. (2000). Speech disorders following severe traumatic brain injury: Kinematic analysis of syllable repetitions using electromagnetic articulography. *Folia Phoniatrica et Logopaedica*, 52, 178–86.

Katz, W. F. (1988). Anticipatory coarticulation in aphasia: Acoustic and perceptual data. *Brain and Language*, 35, 340–68.

Katz, W. F. (2000). Anticipatory coarticulation and aphasia: Implications for phonetic theories. *Journal of Phonetics*, 28, 313–34.

Katz, W. F., Machetanz, J., Orth, U., and Schönle, P. (1990). A kinematic analysis of anticipatory coarticulation in the speech of anterior aphasic subjects using electromagnetic articulography. *Brain and Language*, 38, 555–75.

Kent, R. D., Netsell, R., and Bauer, L. L. (1975). Cineradiographic assessment of articulatory mobility in the dysarthrias. *Journal of Speech and Hearing Disorders*, 40, 467–80.

Krull, D. (1987). Second formant locus patterns as a measure of consonant–vowel coarticulation. *Phonetic Experimental Research at the Institute of Linguistics, PERILUS*, 5, 43–61.

Kühnert, B. and Nolan, F. (1999). The origin of coarticulation. In W. J. Hardcastle and N. Hewlett (eds.), *Coarticulation: Theory, Data and Techniques* (pp. 7–30). Cambridge: Cambridge University Press.

Lane, H., Matthies, M., Perkell, J., Vick, J., and Zandipour, M. (2001). The effects of changes in hearing status in cochlear implant users on the acoustic vowel space and CV coarticulation. *Journal of Speech, Language, and Hearing Research*, 44, 552–63.

Lashley, K. S. (1951). The problem of serial order in behavior. In L. A. Jeffress (ed.), *Cerebral Mechanisms in Behavior* (pp. 112–36). New York: Wiley.

Lindblom, B. (1963). Spectographic study of vowel reduction. *Journal of the Acoustical Society of America*, 35, 1773–81.

Liss, J. M. and Weismer, G. (1992). Qualitative acoustic analysis in the study of motor speech disorders. *Journal of the Acoustical Society of America*, 92, 2984–7.

Löfqvist, A. (1999). Interarticulator phasing, locus equations, and degree of coarticulation. *Journal of the Acoustical Society of America*, 106(4), 2022–30.

Maassen, B., Nijland, L., and van der Meulen, S. (2001). Coarticulation within and between syllables by children with developmental apraxia of speech. *Clinical Linguistics and Phonetics*, 15, 145–50.

Manual, S. (1999). Cross-language studies: Relating language-particular coarticulation patterns to other language-particular facts. In W. J. Hardcastle and N. Hewlett (eds.), *Coarticulation: Theory, Data and Techniques* (pp. 179–98). Cambridge: Cambridge University Press.

Matthies, M., Perrier, P., Perkell, L. S., and Zandipour, M. (2001). Variation in anticipatory coarticulation with changes in clarity and rate. *Journal of Speech, Language and Hearing Research*, 44(2), 340–53.

McNeil, M. R., Robin, D. A., and Schmidt, R. A. (1997). Apraxia of speech: Definition, differentiation and treatment. In M. R. McNeil (ed.), *Clinical Management of Sensorimotor Speech Disorders* (pp. 311–44). New York: Thieme.

Menzerath, P. and Lacerda, A. (1933). *Koartikulation, Steuerung und Lautabgrenzung*. Berlin: Fred. Dummlers.

Monsen, R. B. (1976). Second formant transitions of selected consonant–vowel combinations in the speech of deaf and normal-hearing children. *Journal of Speech and Hearing Research*, 19, 279–89.

Netsell, R. and Kent, R. D. (1976). Paroxysmal ataxic dysarthria. *Journal of Speech and Hearing Disorders*, 41, 93–109.

Nijland, L., Maassen, B., Hulstijn, W., and Peters, H. (2004). Speech motor coordination in Dutch-speaking children with DAS studied with EMMA. *Journal of Multilingual Communication Disorders*, 2, 50–60.

Nijland, L., Maassen, B., and van der Meulen, S. (2003). Evidence of motor programming deficits in children diagnosed with DAS. *Journal of Speech, Language and Hearing Research*, 46, 437–50.

Nijland, L., Maassen, B., van der Meulen, S., Gabreels, F., Kraaimaat, F. W., and Schreuder, R. (2002). Coarticulation patterns in children with apraxia of speech. *Clinical Linguistics and Phonetics*, 16, 461–83.

Nijland, L., Maassen, B., van der Meulen, S., Gabreels, F., Kraaimaat, F. W., and Schreuder, R. (2003). Planning of syllables in children with developmental apraxia of speech. *Clinical Linguistics and Phonetics*, 17, 1–24.

Nittrouer, S. (1993). The emergence of mature gestural patterns is not uniform: Evidence from an acoustic study. *Journal of Speech and Hearing Research*, 36, 959–72.

Nittrouer, S., Studdert-Kennedy, M., and McGowan, R. S. (1989). The emergence of phonetic segments: Evidence from the spectral structure of fricative–vowel syllables spoken by children and adults. *Journal of Speech and Hearing Research*, 32, 120–32.

Nittrouer, S., Studdert-Kennedy, M., and Neely, S. T. (1996). How children learn to organize their speech gestures: Further evidence from fricative–vowel syllables. *Journal of Speech and Hearing Research*, 39, 379–89.

Okalidou, A. and Harris, K. S. (1999). A comparison of intergestural patterns in deaf and hearing adult speakers: Implications from an acoustic analysis of disyllables. *Journal of the Acoustical Society of America*, 106, 394–410.

Pratt, S. R. and Tye-Murray, N. (1997). Speech impairment secondary to hearing loss. In M. R. McNeil (ed.), *Clinical Management of Sensorimotor Speech Disorders* (pp. 345–87). New York: Thieme.

Recasens, D. (1985). Coarticulatory patterns and degrees of coarticulatory resistance in Catalan CV sequences. *Language and Speech*, 28, 97–114.

Robb, M. and Blomgren, M. (1997). Analysis of F2 transition in the speech of stutterers and nonstutterers. *Journal of Fluency Disorders*, 22, 1–16.

Rothman, H. (1976). A spectrographic investigation of consonant–vowel transitions in speech of deaf adults. *Journal of Phonetics*, 4, 129–36.

Southwood, H., Dagenais, P. A., Sutphin, S. M., and Garcia, J. M. (1997). Coarticulation in apraxia of speech: A perceptual, acoustic, and electropalatographic study. *Clinical Linguistics and Phonetics*, 11, 179–203.

Sussman, H. M., Marquardt, T. P., and Doyle, J. (2000). An acoustic analysis of phonemic integrity and contrastiveness in developmental apraxia of speech. *Journal of Medical Speech-Language Pathology*, 8, 301–13.

Sussman, H., Marquardt, T., MacNeilage, P. F., and Hutchinson, J. A. (1988). Anticipatory coarticulation in aphasia: Some methodological considerations. *Brain and Language*, 35, 369–79.

Sussman, H., McCaffrey, H., and Matthews, S. (1991). An investigation of locus equations as a source of relational invariance for stop place categorization. *Journal of the Acoustical Society of America*, 90, 1309–25.

Tjaden, K. (1999). Can a model of overlapping gestures account for scanning speech patterns? *Journal of Speech, Language, and Hearing Research*, 42, 604–17.

Tjaden, K. (2000). An acoustic study of coarticulation in dysarthric speakers with Parkinson's disease. *Journal of Speech, Language, and Hearing Research*, 43, 1466–80.

Tjaden, K. (2003). Anticipatory coarticulation in Multiple Sclerosis and Parkinson's disease. *Journal of Speech, Language, and Hearing Research*, 46, 990–1008.

Tjaden, K. (2006). Segmental articulation in motor speech disorders. In G. Weismer (ed.), *Motor Speech Disorders* (pp. 151–86). San Diego, CA: Plural Publishing.

Tjaden, K. and Sussman, J. (2006). Perception of coarticulatory information in normal speech and dysarthria. *Journal of Speech, Language, and Hearing Research*, 49, 888–902.

Tjaden, K. and Watling, E. (2003). Characteristics of diadochokinesis in multiple sclerosis and Parkinson's disease. *Folia Phoniatrica Logopaedica*, 55, 241–59.

Tjaden, K. and Wilding, G. E. (2005). Effects of rate reduction and increased loudness on acoustic measures of anticipatory coarticulation in Multiple Sclerosis and Parkinson's disease. *Journal of Speech, Language, and Hearing Research*, 48, 1–17.

Tuller, B. and Seider-Story, R. (1987). Anticipatory coarticulation in aphasia. In J. Ryalls (ed.), *Phonetic Approaches to Speech Production in Aphasia* (pp. 243–60). San Diego, CA: College-Hill Press.

Tye-Murray, N. (1987). Effects of vowel context on the articulatory closure postures of deaf speakers. *Journal of Speech and Hearing Research*, 30, 90–104.

Tye-Murray, N., Zimmerman, G., and Folkins, J. (1987). Movement timing in deaf and hearing speakers: Comparison of phonetically heterogeneous syllable strings. *Journal of Speech and Hearing Research*, 30, 411–17.

Van Riper, C. (1982). *The Nature of Stuttering*. 2nd ed. Englewood Cliffs, NJ: Prentice-Hall.

Waldstein, R. S. and Baum, S. R. (1991). Anticipatory coarticulation in the speech of profoundly hearing-impaired and normally hearing children. *Journal of Speech and Hearing Research*, 34, 1276–85.

Waldstein, R. S. and Baum, S. R. (1994). Perception of coarticulatory cues in the speech of children with profound hearing loss and children with normal hearing. *Journal of Speech and Hearing Research*, 37, 952–9.

Weismer, G. (1984). Articulatory characteristics of Parkinsonian dysarthria: Segmental and phrase-level timing, spirantization and glottal-supraglottal coordination. In M. R. McNeil, J. C. Rosenbek, and A. E. Aronson (eds.), *The Dysarthrias: Physiology, Acoustics, Perception, and Management* (pp. 101–30). San Diego, CA: College-Hill Press.

Weismer, G., Tjaden, K., and Kent, R. D. (1995). Can articulatory behaviour in motor speech disorders be accounted for by theories of normal speech production? *Journal of Phonetics*, 23, 149–64.

Weismer, G., Yunusova, Y., and Westbury, J. R. (2003). Interarticulator coordination in dysarthria: An X-ray microbeam study. *Journal of Speech, Language, and Hearing Research*, 46, 1247–61.

Wingate, M. (1969). Stuttering as a phonetic transition defect. *Journal of Speech and Hearing Disorders*, 34, 107–8.

Wood, S. and Hardcastle, W. J. (2000). Instrumentation in the assessment and therapy of motor speech disorders: A survey of techniques and case studies with EPG. In I. Papathanasiou (ed.), *Acquired Neurogenic Communication Disorders: A Clinical Perspective* (pp. 203–48). London: Whurr Publishers.

Yaruss, J. and Conture, E. (1993). F2 transitions during sounds/syllable repetitions of children who stutter and predictions of stuttering chronicity. *Journal of Speech and Hearing Research*, 36, 883–96.

Zebrowski, P., Conture, E., and Cudahy, E. (1985). Acoustic analysis of young stutterers' fluency: Preliminary observations. *Journal of Fluency Disorders*, 10, 173–92.

Ziegler, W. and von Cramon, D. R. (1985). Anticipatory coarticulation in a patient with apraxia of speech. *Brain and Language*, 26, 117–30.

Ziegler, W. and von Cramon, D. R. (1986). Disturbed coarticulation in apraxia of speech. *Brain and Language*, 29, 34–47.

Zimmerman, G. (1980). Articulatory dynamics of fluent utterances of stutterers and non-stutterers. *Journal of Speech and Hearing Research*, 23, 95–107.

33 Vowel Development and Disorders

CAROL STOEL-GAMMON AND KAREN POLLOCK

33.1 Introduction

This chapter provides an overview of vowel development and vowel disorders in children. The focus is primarily on investigations of English-speaking children although studies of other languages are included where appropriate. The body of work on the acquisition of vowels is very small compared with research on consonants. Most studies are based on phonetic transcription and focus on patterns of accuracy in word productions and types of errors that occur. Hence, these are the studies that will be reviewed in the next sections. The chapter begins with a feature description of the vowel system of American English; this description will serve as a framework for the discussion of vowel acquisition and vowel disorders that follows.

In terms of physiology, vowels are characterized as having no obstruction in the vocal tract. In terms of articulation, there is a fundamental difference between 'place of articulation' for vowels and consonants: consonant place distinctions are discrete – a consonant stop is labial or coronal but not somewhere in between, whereas 'place' features for vowels are continuous, varying in small steps from high to low, or front to back. In terms of phonology, vowels differ from consonants regarding their role within a word, phrase, or sentence: they are the elements that carry stress, pitch and basic aspects of rhythm. They are also the elements that tend to differ most across dialects.

Regardless of the language, articulatory descriptions of vowels include a basic set of features: (1) vowel height, based on tongue and jaw position; (2) front–back, based on the position of the tongue, and (3) rounding (or not), based on the lips. The acoustic realization of tongue height is the first formant (F1), which is inversely related to tongue height (i.e., high vowels have low F1 values and low vowels have high F1 values), while the acoustic realization of tongue advancement is directly related to the second formant, or F2 (front vowels have high F2 values and back vowels have low F2 values). Tongue height appears to be more important to vowel identity than tongue advancement and some languages, e.g., Kabardian, have vowel systems that differ only along the height dimension. For many vowel systems, additional features are used to distinguish phonemic contrasts; common secondary features include phonemic distinctions based on vowel length, nasalization, rounding, or vocal quality, i.e., creaky vs. normal phonation. Many languages also have complex vowels, such as diphthongs and triphthongs. Diphthongs have two different targets within the same nucleus, one of which is more prominent. Similarly, triphthongs have three different targets. In English, the first target of a diphthong is always prominent; this type of diphthong is called a 'falling' diphthong. However, other languages have 'rising' diphthongs, in which the second element is more prominent.

Languages vary in the number of vowels in their phonological system, from as few as two phonologically contrastive vowels (e.g., Margi) to 16 or more (e.g., Swedish, Urdu). The number of diphthongs and triphthongs also varies considerably, with some languages (e.g., Spanish) having none, and others having more than 10 (e.g., Cantonese). However, the number of diphthongs reported is related to the phonological description of the language in question. Phonetically similar complex vowels may be described in one language as diphthongs and in another as a sequence of vowel+glide or glide+vowel. For example, in English, the pronunciation of the word 'why' is generally interpreted as glide + diphthong ([waɪ]), but a phonetically similar sound might be interpreted as a triphthong ([u͡aɪ]) in Cantonese. Diphthongs occur in approximately one third of the world's languages, but triphthongs are relatively rare. A majority of languages have between three and nine vowel phonemes (Maddiesson, 1984), with the most common vowel system being the triangular five-vowel system: /i, e, a, o, u/.

33.2   The Vowel System of American English

Figure 33.1 shows the articulatory features associated with the vowels of American English. This dialect of English is typically described as having five front

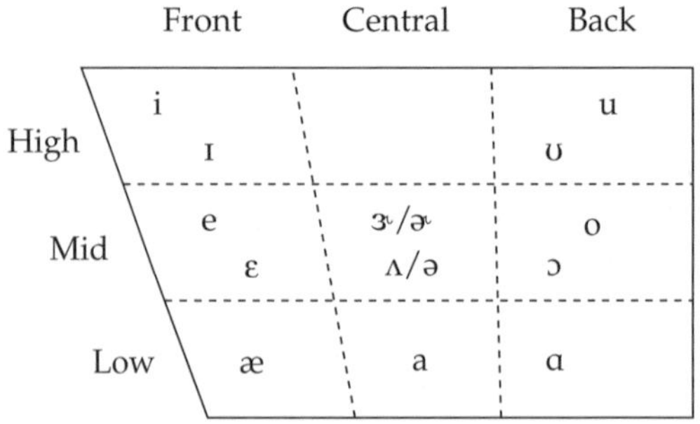

Figure 33.1   Monophthongs of American English plotted on a vowel quadrilateral.

vowel phonemes: [i, ɪ, e, ɛ, æ], and five back vowel phonemes: [u, ʊ, o, ɔ, ɑ]. There is some disagreement on the number and type of central vowels: some descriptions include two mid-central non-rhotic (i.e., not r-colored) vowels, [ə] and [ʌ], with the first vowel (schwa) occurring in unstressed syllables and the second in stressed syllables. In like fashion, there is a lack of agreement regarding mid-central rhotic vowels: unstressed [ɚ] and [ɝ]. In addition, the inclusion of a low central vowel [a] is not uniform. In most of the studies discussed in the sections that follow, the vowels [ɪ, ɛ, æ, ʌ, ʊ, ɔ] are classified as 'lax', a feature that we will also use.

English has three non-rhotic phonemic diphthongs: /âɪ/, /âʊ/, and /ôɪ/. The most commonly occurring of these diphthongs is /âɪ/, followed by /âʊ/ and then /ôɪ/; /ôɪ/ is the least common of all the vowel sounds in English. The vowels /e/ and /o/ are also typically diphthongized in English (e.g., [êɪ] and [ôʊ]), but the diphthongization is not phonemic. In addition, some phoneticians consider postvocalic /r/ to be part of a rhotic diphthong, with a rhotic vowel [ɚ] as the second vowel target (e.g., /îɚ/ /âɚ/).

33.3   Development of Vowels in Infancy

33.3.1   *Perception*

Since the work of Eimas, Siqueland, Jusczyk, and Vigorito was published in 1971, research on infant speech perception has shown that, months before they begin to babble and a year before they begin to produce words, babies are capable of distinguishing fine phonetic contrasts including those that do not occur in their language environment. Although the bulk of studies have focused on consonants, investigations of vowels (e.g., Swoboda, Morse, & Leavitt, 1976; Trehub, 1976) indicate that infants as young as two months can distinguish between phonetically similar vowels. Studies with older infants suggest that between six and 12 months, there is a shift from 'universal' perception, whereby babies can distinguish phonetic contrasts from many (perhaps all) of the world's languages, to 'language-specific phonetic perception', whereby speech perception becomes attuned to the ambient language and certain abilities decline (Werker, 1992).

33.3.2   *Production*

In the first six months of life babies produce a variety of sounds, some more speech-like than others (Vihman, 1996). In terms of speech-like productions, central, low vowels predominate. In the first few months, these vowel-like sounds (sometimes called 'vocants' or 'vocoids') are perceived as being very nasal. With changes in the infant vocal structures that occur in the first months, the separation between the velum and the epiglottis grows and vowels become less nasal.

Around 6–7 months, babies begin to produce consonant–vowel (CV) syllables such as [mɑ] or [dæ] which exhibit adult-like timing and often resemble real words. The great majority of vowels produced in CV syllables are perceived as being front or central, and mid or low (Bond, Petrosino, & Dean, 1982; Buhr, 1980; Lieberman, 1980). According to Kent and Bauer (1985) the most frequent vowel types produced by one-year-old infants were mid central [ʌ, ə]; other vowels occurring frequently in the speech samples they analyzed were [ɛ, æ, ʊ]. MacNeilage and Davis propose that the basic CV syllable type developed from the closing (for consonant production) and opening (for vowels) mandibular movements associated with chewing and sucking. These movements constitute the 'frame' of a syllable and the particular consonants and vowels within the frame form the 'content', hence the term 'Frame/Content theory' of the evolution of speech (MacNeilage, 1998; MacNeilage & Davis, 2000, 2001). According to MacNeilage (1998), the content that occurs within the syllable frame is influenced by movements of the jaw with no independent movements of the tongue, resulting in the likelihood of more frequent occurrences of particular consonant–vowel (CV) sequences. Specifically, it is argued that (1) consonants produced with a constriction in the front of the mouth are more likely to precede front vowels (e.g., [dɪ], (2) consonants produced with the lips (i.e., with no tongue involvement) will be strongly associated with central vowels (e.g., [bɑ]), and (3) consonants produced with a constriction in the back of the mouth will be associated with back vowels (e.g., [ku]).

Changes in vowel productions in the first year are usually attributed to maturational changes of the oral-motor structures and neurophysiological system (Kent, 1992; Kent & Murray, 1982). In addition, hearing status plays a role in the emergence of vowels. In a study of a boy with profound hearing loss, Kent, Osberger, Netsell, and Hustedde (1987) analyzed vowels acoustically and reported that, from eight to 15 months of age, the boy's F1–F2 vowel space became more restricted while the vowel space of his twin brother with normal hearing increased and became more like that of adult speakers in the environment.

33.3.3   *Production: From babble to speech*

It is well documented that the set of consonants occurring frequently in babble, namely stops, nasals and glides, are (1) the same consonants that appear frequently in a child's early word productions and (2) the consonants that tend to be produced accurately. The same pattern does not hold for vowels. Front and central lax vowels predominate in prespeech utterances (Kent & Bauer, 1985), yet analyses of accuracy of production indicate that it is precisely these vowels that are often in error in meaningful speech. Furthermore, the set of vowels that is frequent in babble is not the same set that is frequent in early words (Davis & MacNeilage, 1991).

Jakobson (1968) proposed that children would follow a universal pattern of acquisition of consonants and vowels in their early word productions, beginning with the greatest differentiation between segments (e.g., labial stop and open vowel yielding /pa/) and proceeding to finer and finer distinctions. For vowels, Jakobson claimed that children begin with a three vowel system, usually the 'fundamental' vowel triangle /i/ – /a/ – /u/, and then acquire vowels that fall between the extreme points of the triangle. The minimal three-vowel system that serves as the starting point is, Jakobson notes, the same minimal system found in many of the languages of the world.

33.4   Vowel Acquisition in Meaningful Speech

Vowels in the speech of children between 12 and 24 months have been examined using *independent* and *relational* analyses. An independent analysis is based on the children's productions regardless of accuracy; this type of analysis can include glossable forms, i.e., those for which a target word can be identified, and non-glossable forms, i.e., babble or unintelligible speech. A relational analysis is based on a comparison of a child's productions with the target form and provides information on accuracy of production and on error patterns (Stoel-Gammon & Dunn, 1985). Independent analyses are used to determine a child's 'phonetic inventory' – the phones that occur in his or her speech. In a longitudinal study of vowel inventories based on analyses of conversational interactions, Selby, Robb, and Gilbert (2000) described the inventories of four children aged 15–36 months; a vowel was considered to be part of the group inventory at a particular age if it occurred in the sample of three of the four children. At 15 months the group inventory was limited to four vowels [ɑ, ɪ, ʊ, ʌ] Notably lacking are the high tense 'corner' vowels [i] and [u]. By 18 months, the group inventory had expanded to include these corner vowels, and the inventories at 21 and 24 months, taken together, include all target vowels of American English except the rhotic vowels. Thus the size of vowel inventories across the four children increased rapidly between 15 and 24 months.

33.4.1   Accuracy of production

Although the study by Selby, Robb, and Gilbert (2000) indicates that the full range of vowels are produced by 21–24 months, relational analyses indicate that accuracy is not uniform across vowel targets (e.g., Hare, 1983; Olmsted, 1971; Paschall, 1983; Templin, 1957; Wellman, Case, Mengert, & Bradbury, 1931). Reports of vowel accuracy vary somewhat from one study to another in part because some investigations (e.g., Otomo & Stoel-Gammon, 1992; Pollock & Berni, 2003; Templin, 1957) were based on analysis of elicited single-word targets while others (e.g., Hare, 1983; Olmsted, 1971; Paschall, 1983) analyzed vowels in spontaneous utterances. Pollock (2002) presents findings from three types of data: a single-word elicitation task, a story-retelling task, and a controlled imitation task. Taken together, the research indicates that accurate vowel production of nearly all vowel targets is achieved by the age of 36 months.

In terms of individual vowel phonemes, Paschall (1983) found that, at 16–18 months of age, the 20 American children in her study produced the targets /i, ɪ, ʊ, ʌ, ɑ/ with accuracy rates of 73–81% in conversational speech. Only the rhotic vowels and /e/ and /ɛ/, both non-rhotic, mid-front vowels, exhibited accuracy rates that were lower than 50%. Using the same methodology as Paschall, Hare (1983) examined vowel accuracy in productions of children of 21–24 months. The findings indicate a substantial increase in accuracy of production: the vowels /i, æ, u, ʊ, o, ɔ, ɑ, ʌ/ were correct in over 91% of target words; accuracy rates for /e, ɛ, ə, ɪ/ were also high, ranging from 84 to 89%. In this age range, only the r-colored vowels were produced with less than 50% accuracy.

Findings from studies of vowels in single-word productions also indicate that, except for the r-colored vowels, production accuracy is quite high. Templin (1957) analyzed word productions of 480 children aged 3–8 years and reported that, across all vowels, accuracy was 93% in the group of three-year-old children and did not change between ages three and eight years. In an earlier cross-sectional study of single-word productions, Wellman, Case, Mengert and Bradbury (1931) investigated speech development in 204 children aged 2–6 years. Using correct production by 75% of children in a particular age group as the criterion for 'mastery' of a vowel phoneme, Wellman showed that the vowels /i, ɑ, u, ʊ, o, ʌ, ə/ were mastered by age 2;0; mastery of /e, ɔ/ occurred at age 3;0, and /ɪ, ɛ, æ, ʊ/ were mastered at 4;0. More recently, in a study of 162 children aged 18–83 months, Pollock (2003) reported mean vowel accuracies for non-rhotic vowels exceeding 92% by 24 months. By 36 months, mean accuracy levels exceeded 97%. The notable exception is the r-colored vowels which are mastered later, typically after four years (Pollock & Berni, 2003).

Overall, the acquisition of vowels of English can be described by the following general patterns: (1) corner vowels (except /æ/) are acquired before non-corner vowels, (2) tense vowels are acquired before their lax counterparts, and (3) rhotic vowels are acquired later than non-rhotic vowels.

33.4.2   *Suprasegmental aspects of vowel acquisition*

Descriptions of vowel acquisition should include studies focusing not only on vowel quality, but also on the suprasegmental features of vowels associated with stress, rhythm and timing. In English, these features interact in predictable ways: vowels in stressed syllables tend to be longer, louder and higher-pitched than vowels in unstressed syllables. As a result, the 'rhythm' of English is described as 'stress-timed' (i.e., having approximately equal intervals between stressed syllables in a word or phrase). Although it has been shown that the intervals are not exactly equal, the rhythmic pattern of stress-timed languages such as English and Dutch is notably different from the pattern of 'syllable-timed' languages such as Spanish and Hindi in which the timing of each syllable is said to be approximately the same regardless of stress placement (see Ramus, Nespor, & Mehler, 1999, for a discussion of the rhythmic properties of languages traditionally classified as syllable-timed or stress-timed).

In terms of suprasegmental properties, productions of young children acquiring English are clearly affected by the stress patterns of words and phrases. In American English, syllables that receive primary stress are longer, louder, and higher-pitched than unstressed syllables, as noted above. In addition, these syllables tend to have 'clearer' vowel articulations than the vowels of unstressed syllables. In general, segmental accuracy, including vowel accuracy, is greater in stressed than in unstressed syllables. In the early stages of word production, unstressed syllables, particularly those in word-initial position, may be omitted, leading to the production of [nænə] for *banana* and [ɛfɪnt] for *elephant*. Unstressed syllables at the ends of words are omitted much less frequently. Acoustic analyses of American children's disyllabic word productions indicate that stressed syllables in the adult form are characterized by greater duration, greater amplitude, and longer duration – the three features associated with stress in English (Kehoe, Stoel-Gammon, & Buder, 1995; Pollock, Brammer, & Hageman, 1989). Researchers have noted, however, that young children appear to have difficulty with the timing pattern of unstressed syllables. Allen and Hawkins (1980) reported that American children have problems reducing the vowel of unstressed syllables, thereby diminishing the durational differences between stressed and unstressed vowel. This finding was further explored by Kehoe, Stoel-Gammon, and Buder (1995) who compared the syllable durations of phonetically controlled word pairs such as *key–monkey* where the syllable [ki] was produced as a stressed monosyllable in the first word and as an unstressed syllable in the disyllabic form. The researchers found that the ratio of the duration of the unstressed to the stressed syllable was .51 in adult productions (i.e., the unstressed syllable was half as long as the stressed syllable) and was .75 for children aged 18–30 months; thus the children distinguished between stressed and unstressed syllables, but the length distinction was less marked in the children than in adults.

33.4.3   Vowel errors in the speech of children with typical development

Analysis of errors in consonant productions tends to be fairly straightforward as it is easy to identify changes on the basis of place or manner classes. Thus, in the speech of young children, velar consonants are often produced as alveolars, and liquids as glides. Descriptions of vowel errors are somewhat messier; in some cases a target vowel is raised (i.e., /ɪ/ is produced as [i]); in other cases the same vowel may be lowered (/ɪ/ produced as [ɛ]) or centralized (i.e., /ɪ/ produced as [ʌ]). Pollock (1991) identified a wide range of possible error patterns for vowels, including feature changes (e.g., backing and fronting, raising and lowering, tensing and laxing, rounding and unrounding), complexity changes (e.g., diphthong reduction and diphthongization), and harmony (i.e., assimilation) patterns. Some error patterns apply to a limited set of target vowels (e.g., unrounding can only apply to round vowels), and some patterns are affected by word stress and complexity of the vowel target (e.g., monophthongal vs. diphthongal vowels).

Donegan (2002), using a slightly different framework for identifying vowel errors, distinguishes between context-sensitive and context-free error patterns. An example of the former is the raising and diphthongization of /æ/ or /ɛ/ to [êɪ] in words like *bag, thank,* and *leg,* i.e., when /æ/ or /ɛ/ precedes a velar consonant. Other context-sensitive errors are likely to occur when a vowel precedes liquid /l/ as in *milk* produced as [mʊk]. Context-free errors, in contrast, are not affected by phonetic environment.

Bleile (1989) presented analyses of vowel errors in two young children aged 22 to 26 months. Patterns he noted were (1) substitution of the diphthong [âɪ] for the front vowels [æ] and [êɪ], (2) lowering of /i/ to [ɛ], and (3) 're-syllabification', in which a syllable was epenthesized to monosyllabic words ending in /âʊ/ or /ɔ̂ɪ/. Bleile reported that some of these error patterns were similar to those reported in diary studies of children in the same age range.

As with consonants, vowel errors may change with development. In a longitudinal study focusing on front vowels in a controlled set of words, Otomo and Stoel-Gammon (1992) noted that, at 22 months, children often produced /ɪ/ as [i], accounting for 30% of the incorrect productions, an error which could be classified as 'raising' and 'tensing' of /ɪ/. At 30 months, the most common error for /ɪ/ was that it was 'lowered' to [ɛ]; at this age, the use of [i] as a substitute had declined to 3%. Otomo and Stoel-Gammon also reported that productions of /ɛ/ were often inaccurate at 22 and 26 months, but there was no obvious developmental pattern and no single substitution that was most common. The most frequent substitutions for /ɛ/ at these ages were [e], [æ] and [ʌ]. At 30 months, the most frequent substitutions were [e] (raising and tensing of the target) and [æ] (lowering of the target). At 30 months, the accuracy levels for the lax targets /ɪ/ and /ɛ/ were the lowest of the phonemes studied, at 40% and 49% respectively.

33.4.4   *Vowel acquisition in other languages*

Relatively few studies of vowel acquisition in other languages are available. Reports of Dutch and Cantonese vowel acquisition (Beers, 1995; Tse, 1991) suggest that corner vowels emerge first, followed by a tense–lax distinction, with the rounding contrast emerging later. These findings are consistent with Jakobson's predictions of unmarked segments developing first. However, [u] was late to develop in Cantonese, and is also the least frequent vowel in Cantonese, suggesting that ambient frequency also plays a role in the order of acquisition.

Stokes and Wong (2002) investigated the vowel and diphthong development of 40 Cantonese-speaking children ranging from 10 to 27 months of age. Cantonese has eight contrastive vowels that can be classified on the four dimensions of height, anteriority, tenseness, and roundness, and 10 contrastive diphthongs. They found that feature complexity and ambient frequency affected the accuracy of vowels production. Their data also suggested that feature complexity is more important initially (15–18 months) but is superseded by ambient language influences by 24 months.

Zajdó (Zajdó, 2002; Zajdó & Stoel-Gammon, 2003) carried out a large study on the acquisition of Hungarian vowels by 80 children aged two to four years. Hungarian has a relatively large vowel inventory, with 14 monophthong vowels that vary along four dimensions: front–back, high–mid–low, round–unround (of both front and back vowels), and long–short. Cross-sectional data revealed that, by 2;6, accuracy levels of simple CVCV forms exceeded 90 percent for most vowels. Rounded vowels were acquired later than unrounded vowels; in particular, the mid front rounded pair /ø/ and /ø:/ and the high front rounded pair /y/ and /y:/ exhibited low levels of accuracy until 3;6–4;0.

33.5 Vowel Production in Children with Phonological Disorder

33.5.1 Incidence of vowel errors

Vowel errors are less common than consonant errors in children with phonological disorders and thus have received less attention in the literature and in clinical practice. Pollock and Berni (2003) investigated the incidence of non-rhotic vowel errors in 149 children (30 to 81 months of age) with delayed/disordered phonology, and found that the incidence of vowel errors ranged from 11 to 32 percent, depending on the criteria used, i.e. whether the percentage of vowels correct (PVC) was set at < 85, < 90, or < 95. Furthermore, the incidence of vowel errors appeared to be related to the severity of consonant errors. Children exhibiting severe consonant errors (percentage of consonants correct (PCC) < 50) were three to four times more likely to also have vowel errors than children who had mild (PCC > 85) or mild-to-moderate (PCC = 66–84) consonant errors. However, it was also noted that not all children with severe consonant errors had vowel errors. Thus far, no studies have compared the types of consonant errors produced by children with and without vowel errors.

The incidence of vowel errors also varies from language to language and appears to be related to the complexity of the language's vowel system. For example, vowel errors are relatively infrequent in phonologically disordered children learning Spanish, which has a simple five-vowel system (e.g., Goldstein & Pollock, 2000; Meza, 1983), and more common in children learning languages with more complex vowel systems such as Swedish or Cantonese (e.g., Nettelbladt, 1983; So & Dodd, 1994).

33.5.2 Vowel error patterns in children with phonological disorder

There appears to be considerable variation in the types of vowel errors produced by children with phonological disorder, based on a review of individual case studies (Gibbon, Shockey, & Reid, 1992; Hargrove, 1982; Harris, Watson, & Bates, 1999; Khan, 1988; Penny, Fee, & Dowdle, 1994; Pollock, 1991, 1994; Pollock & Swanson, 1986) and small-group studies (Pollock & Keiser, 1990; Reynolds,

1990, 2002; Stoel-Gammon & Herrington, 1990; Watson, Bates, Sinclair, & Hewlett, 1994). However, some general trends are apparent. For example, the corner vowels (/i, u, ɑ/) and the mid back vowel (/o/) were rarely in error. Rhotic vowels and diphthongs were most often incorrect. Among the non-rhotic vowels, mid and low front vowels (/e, ɛ, æ/), high lax vowels (/ɪ, ʊ/), and diphthongs (/aɪ, aʊ, ɔɪ/) were most frequently in error.

Backing, lowering, and diphthong reduction were the most common error patterns observed for non-rhotic vowels in studies of American English-speaking children. Backing most often affected the low front vowel (e.g., /æ/ produced as [a] or [ɑ]), and lowering occurred most frequently with the mid front vowels (/e, ɛ/ produced as [æ] or [a]). Diphthong reduction resulted in the loss of the offglide, sometimes (but not always) accompanied by a length-ening of the vowel remaining (e.g., /aʊ/ produced as [a] or [a:]). Loss of con-trast between tense/lax vowel pairs was also common, with individual children exhibiting either tensing or laxing patterns. Mid vowels also appear to be highly susceptible to error.

Interestingly, an asymmetry has been observed in errors on mid vowels, with mid front vowels /e, ɛ/ often produced incorrectly and mid back vowels /o, ɔ/ generally produced correctly (e.g., Pollock, 2002; Stoel-Gammon & Herrington, 1990). However, this may be specific to American English speakers, as the same asymmetry has not been noted in speakers of other varieties of English (e.g., Reynolds, 1990; Watson, Bates, Sinclair, & Hewlett, 1994) or in Spanish (e.g., Goldstein & Pollock, 2000). Other differences across varieties of English have also been observed. Children learning West Yorkshire English (Reynolds, 1990, 2002) did not use backing, as /æ/ is not part of the target vowel system. However, fronting of the very low back /ɒ/ to [a] was com-monly observed. It appears then, that the American English backing of /æ/ and the West Yorkshire English fronting of /ɒ/ may both serve to reduce the front–back distinction among the low vowels. Another common error observed in children speaking West Yorkshire English was an avoidance of central vowels, by either fronting or lowering, possibly reflecting a preference for a more peripheral vowel quality (Reynolds, 2002). The finding of different patterns in different varieties of English highlights the need to consider both cross-dialectal and cross-linguistic perspectives in the study of vowel errors.

Pollock, Meeks, Stepherson, and Berni (2004) investigated the types of vowel errors produced by a group of 47 children with phonological disorder, ranging in age from 30 to 81 months, and a comparison group of 40 younger typically developing children, 18–49 months of age, all speaking some variety of southern American English (e.g., Southern White Vernacular English, African American Vernacular English). These children were selected from the larger group of children in Pollock and Berni's (2003) study because they produced at least 5 percent of their vowels incorrectly. Dialectally appropriate productions, such as monophthongization of /aɪ/ or merger of /ɪ/ and /ɛ/ before nasals, were accepted as correct. For both groups, the vowels most often in error were diphthongs, mid front vowels, and lax vowels. There was no significant group difference in the frequency of different vowel error types; that is, the children with phonological disorder appeared to use the same types of errors as younger typically developing children. However, there was considerable variability among children in terms of the error types produced, with several of the children with phonological disorder exhibiting highly persistent and/or idiosyncratic error patterns. To illustrate this, the vowel errors of one child from each group (matched on PCC and PVC) were compared. Both had a high use of diphthong reduction (29–36%). They also showed many of the same vowel error patterns (fronting, backing, raising, lowering, centralization), but the frequency of usage differed across the two children. The typically developing child (18 months of age) showed relatively modest usage (3–11%) of six different error types, but the child with phonological disorder (43 months of age) had a much higher usage of backing (34%) and lowering (23%) and only minimal usage (2–3%) of the other error patterns. Pollock and colleagues concluded that further exploration of other individual children's vowel error patterns was needed to determine whether or not this type of difference was characteristic of the two groups.

Although the majority of vowel errors produced by children with phonological disorder may follow the common trends noted above, there is ample evidence across many studies that considerable individual variation exists. Stoel-Gammon and Herrington (1990) hypothesized two subgroups of children with vowel errors, based on a review of studies at that time. Children in the first subgroup have large vowel repertoires but produce many errors, most often on mid vowels, high lax vowels, and rhotic vowels. Children in the second group have restricted vowel inventories consisting of two to three lax vowels; their systems resemble those of infants in the prelinguistic period, with tense vowels missing from the inventory. Beyond differences in which error types are produced and the relative frequency of occurrence of error types, Reynolds (2002) points out the use of idiosyncratic vowel error patterns in a number of children with phonological disorder in his sample. For example, one child simplified diphthong productions by introducing a schwa offglide, in essence changing the original offglide to a glide and adding another syllable (e.g., down produced as [daʊ̯ən]). Another produced the high back vowels (/u, ʊ/) as unrounded back vowels ([ɯ]) or as front rounded vowels ([y]). Pollock (1994) also reported an idiosyncratic vowel error pattern in a 3-year-old girl. She substituted [eɪ] for lax non-rhotic vowels (e.g., /ɪ, ɛ, æ, ʊ/), rhotic vowels (/ɝ/), and rhotic diphthongs with front vowels (e.g., /ɪɚ/, /ɛɚ/).

33.5.3 Vowel errors in children with phonological disorder learning other languages

A small number of studies have looked at vowel error patterns in languages other than English. For example, Nettelbladt (1983) identified three vowel error patterns in a sample of four to seven-year-old Swedish-speaking children with phonological disorders. Swedish has a relatively complex vowel system, with a length distinction and rounded front vowels. Interestingly, the two most commonly observed vowel errors involved laxing, or loss of the length contrast, and unrounding, suggesting that the more 'marked' features of the Swedish vowel system were most susceptible to error. So and Dodd (1994) described vowel error patterns in two of the 17 children in their study of 3- to 6-year-old Cantonese-speaking children with phonological disorders. Cantonese also has a complex vowel system, including front rounded vowels and a large number of diphthongs. Examples of errors produced included backing in the context of a following velar nasal, confusion of /ɛ/ and /ɐ/, and substitution of [a] for /ɐ/. Stokes, Lau, and Ciocca (2002) provided a detailed investigation of diphthong errors in Cantonese-speaking children. They constructed a metric of diphthong complexity based on the number of features differences between component monophthongs. For example, the vowels comprising /ei̯/ have a difference of only one feature, height, whereas the component vowels in /au̯/ differ on roundness, height, and anteriority. Results indicated that feature complexity and ambient frequency together predicted a ranking of diphthong production accuracy. When diphthongs were incorrect, over 80 percent of the time they were reduced to monophthongs.

33.5.4   *Vowel errors and intelligibility*

Errors on vowels can have a significant effect on intelligibility, as noted in studies of hearing-impaired and dysarthric speakers (e.g., Ansell, 1987; Metz, Schiavetti, Samar, & Sitler, 1990; Monsen, 1978). In an experimental study of the relative effects of different consonant and vowel error patterns on intelligibility, Vaughn and Pollock (1997) found that vowel and consonant errors had similar effects on listeners' ability to identify words when other factors were controlled. However, for both consonants and vowels, the type of error played a significant role. For example, substitutions of tense vowels for lax vowels resulted in a 12% decrease in intelligibility, but the opposite pattern where lax vowels replaced tense vowels resulted in a 40% decrease. Errors involving more distant substitutions (e.g., backing and lowering) resulted in even larger reductions (up to 71%). In addition, the combined effects of both consonant and vowel errors in the same utterance, which is the more common situation encountered clinically, resulted in a 79% reduction in intelligibility, compared to an average reduction of 47% for either consonant or vowel errors alone.

33.6   Vowel Errors as a Marker of Childhood Apraxia of Speech (CAS)

33.6.1   *Vowel accuracy and error patterns in CAS*

Vowel errors are an oft-cited characteristic of childhood apraxia of speech (CAS), and many consider vowel errors to be a marker useful in the differential diagnosis of CAS (Davis, 2003; Hall, Jordan, & Robin, 1993; Rosenbek & Wertz, 1972). Although vowel errors are frequently cited as occurring in the speech of children with CAS, very few studies have provided detailed descriptions of the vowel errors produced by children with CAS. Pollock and Hall (1991) analyzed the vowel errors produced by five children, with severe CAS (8;2 to 10;9 years at time of testing). They found that all of the children had difficulty with rhotic vowels and diphthongs, but there was a wide range of non-rhotic vowel accuracy scores (56–96% correct). However, all of the children had been receiving speech-language intervention services through the public schools since five years of age, and vowels had been previous remediation targets for three of the children, including those with the highest non-rhotic vowel accuracy scores (90% and 96% correct). Thus, all of the children had experienced difficulties with the production of vowels at some point in time. Four of the five children produced each non-rhotic vowel/diphthong correctly at least once, but the fifth child (who also had the lowest overall accuracy rate, 56%) appeared to have phonetic inventory constraints, with four phonemes (/êɪ/, /aɪ/, /aʊ/, and /ɔɪ/) never produced in the sample. The most frequent errors on non-rhotic vowels included diphthong reduction, laxing, backing, tensing, and lowering, patterns also commonly seen in children with phonological disorders. The three children with vowel accuracy rates < 90% were reassessed one year later. Two showed modest improvement in their vowel production accuracy (from 80 to 90% and 71 to 87%), but the child with the lowest accuracy and inventory constraints showed no change.

Children with CAS are often reported to have an increase in errors with increased utterance length or complexity. Pollock and Hall (1991) compared accuracy rates in monosyllabic and multisyllabic words for their five participants. For four children, accuracy was slightly (4 to 14%) higher in monosyllabic words. The fifth and most severely involved child showed the opposite pattern (52% accuracy in monosyllabic words, 59% accuracy in multisyllabic words). They also looked at the effects of stress on vowel production in multisyllabic words, and found no difference in accuracy for vowels in stressed and unstressed syllables.

In another study of vowels in children with CAS, Davis, Jacks, and Marquardt (2005) investigated the vowel inventories and accuracy patterns of three children (P1, P2 and P3: 4;6, 5;6, and 5;10 at first testing) over a three-year period during which they were receiving intervention services. At each test period, all three children showed relatively complete vowel inventories, with the exception of rhotic vowels. However, accuracy of vowel production was low, ranging from 61 to 85% correct overall. Non-rhotic vowel accuracy was slightly higher (68 to 92% correct), while rhotic vowel accuracy was quite low (0 to 48% correct). In contrast to Pollock and Hall's (1991) findings, the children in this study did not show high rates of diphthong reduction, with diphthong accuracy ranging from 63 to 100% correct. No consistent vowel error patterns were observed, although tongue advancement errors were slightly more common than height errors, and errors involving small changes (e.g., tensing/laxing) were slightly more frequent than other errors. Vowel accuracy was not related to utterance length and only slightly reduced with increased syllable or word complexity. Two of the three children showed consistent improvement in vowel accuracy over the three-year time period (from 61 to 85% correct for P1 and from 65 to 86% correct for P3), but the third showed a less predictable pattern, with vowels rising from 74% correct at Time 1 to 85% at Time 2, but then dropping to 71% correct at Time 3. Despite intervention, all three children showed persistent vowel errors over time, with overall vowel accuracy rates remaining below 85% at the third test time (6;5 to 7;7).

33.6.2   *Disordered prosody and timing as a marker of CAS*

The suprasegmental features of timing and prosody are also mentioned as a characteristic of CAS, with the speech patterns described as 'robotic' or 'monopitch' (e.g., Davis, Jakielski, & Marquardt, 1998; Shriberg, Aram, & Kwiatkowski, 1997a, 1997b). In a study of lexical stress in bisyllabic words, Shriberg, Campbell, Karlsson, Brown, McSweeny, and Nadler (2003) examined correlates of stress (frequency, intensity, and duration) in terms of a stressed/unstressed ratio. Findings indicated that those participants who met the authors' criteria for CAS produced the majority of the highest and lowest lexical stress ratios, compared to the control participants, who had other diagnoses of speech disorders of unknown origin (see also work on lexical stress by Munson, Bjorum, & Windsor, 2003).

Peter and Stoel-Gammon (2005, 2006) hypothesized that the control of movement timing rather than vocal characteristics such as intensity and pitch may contribute most substantially to the perceivable deficits in lexical stress production in children with CAS. They examined the productions of two children whose speech was consistent with a diagnosis of CAS and those of two age-matched controls during a variety of tasks including sentence imitation, non-word imitation, singing a familiar song, clapped rhythm imitation, and paced repetitive tapping. The timing accuracy in the productions of the controls was found to be higher in all tasks, compared to the participants with the speech disorder.

Although more research with larger numbers of children is needed, these studies suggest that children with CAS exhibit prosody and timing patterns that differ from those of children with typical development and children with other types of phonological disorders. Thus, this area of speech production may ultimately be useful in the diagnosis of CAS.

33.7   Clinical Assessment of Vowel Errors

As noted earlier, the bulk of research in phonological development and disorders has focused on consonants. In this regard, Davis and MacNeilage (1990) stated: "until the neglect of vowels is rectified, it is doubtful that any major issue in child phonology can be satisfactorily addressed." The lack of attention to vowels is evident in the clinical tests that are used to assess children with suspected articulatory and phonological disorders. Pollock (1991) suggested that an adequate sample for vowel assessment ought to provide multiple opportunities to produce each vowel and diphthong, ideally in a variety of different contexts (e.g., monosyllabic and multisyllabic words, stressed and unstressed syllables, and in a variety of phonetic contexts). A review of the target items from five commonly used articulation/phonology tests found considerable variability in the number and type of stimuli but, in general, they were not adequate for vowel assessment (Pollock, 1991). In fact, three of the five did not include any words with the high, back lax vowel /ʊ/ and three did not include the diphthong /ɔ̃ɪ/. Across the five tests, /æ/ occurred in 49 words, /i/ occurred in 24 words, while /ɑ/ occurred in only 11 words. Another shortcoming with most tests is that they lack stimuli that can provide opportunities to assess the vowels in both stressed and unstressed syllables.

Pollock and colleagues (Pollock, 1994, 2002; Pollock & Keiser, 1990) developed a set of stimuli designed specifically for the analysis of vowel productions of children with phonological disorders. In the most recent version of the stimulus list, described in Pollock (2002), each vowel (including diphthongs) was targeted in 6–9 words; at least three of these words were monosyllablic and at least two were multisyllabic. If possible, the position of the vowel in the target word was also varied so that vowels were assessed in both open and closed syllables and in syllables receiving primary and non-primary stress. For example, the diphthong /aʊ/ was assessed in the words: *cow* (open monosyllable), *couch* and *mouth* (closed monosyllable), *cowboy* and *flowers* (primary stress; multisyllable word), and *outside* (secondary stress; multisyllable word). Words with postvocalic /l/ were avoided, as vowels are frequently altered in this context (Pollock & Keiser, 1990; Reynolds, 1990).

In the clinical assessment of a child's phonological system it is important to distinguish between segmental errors (incorrect productions) and dialect differences. Within the United States, vowels are more affected by regional differences than consonants. For example, speakers on the west coast do not differentiate between *cot* and *caught* or *don* and *dawn*. All four words are produced with a low back unrounded vowel. In other parts of the country, these word pairs contain two different vowels. It would, then, be inappropriate for a speech language pathologist working with children in the west to identify lack of /ɔ/ as a vowel error. Other dialectal differences include lack of rhotic vowels in some northeastern dialects (the unstressed syllable of *father* or *Harvard* is produced with a schwa rather than a rhotic vowel), while in many southern dialects [ɛ] and [ɪ] are merged before nasals (e.g., *pen* and *pin* are both pronounced [pɪn]). Many dialect features are inherently variable; that is, they occur in some contexts but not others. For example, although monophthongization (e.g., *pie* produced as [paː] is a common feature of southern American English dialects, it occurs most frequently in /aɪ/, rarely in /aʊ/, and generally only before /l/ in /ɔɪ/. Furthermore, in African American Vernacular English, monophthongization of /aɪ/ does not occur before voiceless consonants. Therefore, across-the-board patterns of diphthong reduction in children with phonological disorder cannot be attributed to dialect (Pollock, 2002). A thorough knowledge of the local dialect and associated vowel patterns is thus essential to accurate identification of vowel errors in children. A summary of vowel variation in major dialects of American English was provided by Pollock and Berni (2001).

As with younger typically developing children, analyses of vowel errors in children with phonological disorders also include both independent and relational analyses (Pollock, 1994, 2002). An inventory of the vowels produced, regardless of whether they are produced correctly or not, provides an overview of the range of vowels produced and points out any gaps in the child's use of the vowel space. The vowel inventory may also have prognostic significance, as vowels missing from the inventory are less likely to be acquired without direct intervention (Pollock, 1994). Relational analyses typically include vowel accuracy measures, such as the percentage of vowels correct (PVC) and descriptions of the types of errors that occur. Pollock (2002) recommends the use of a vowel correspondence chart, which identifies correct vowel productions as well as vowel substitution errors, and an analysis of the frequency and distribution of vowel error patterns, such as lowering, fronting, backing, and so forth. The combined results from these analyses can provide a basis for determining the selection of appropriate vowel targets for intervention, if needed.

33.8   Treatment of Vowels

Very little information is available on the selection or sequencing of vowel targets in therapy or on specific procedures and techniques for treating vowel errors in children with phonological disorders or childhood apraxia of speech. Most children with vowel errors also have difficulty with consonant production, often leading to an unstated assumption that if the consonants are treated first the vowels may improve without direct intervention (Stoel-Gammon, 1990). Although this observation appears to hold true for some children (e.g., the child studied by Robb, Bleile, & Yee, 1999, and one of the children with CAS followed by Pollock & Hall, 1991), there are other reports of children for whom vowel errors did not spontaneously improve following intervention for consonants (e.g., Pollock, 1994; Pollock & Hall, 1991; Pollock & Swanson, 1986). Gibbon and Beck (2002) suggest that vowels be targeted as part of a treatment program because their improved accuracy is likely to lead to improved speech intelligibility and acceptability. In addition, they argue that because the vowel system is typically mastered earlier than the consonant system, vowel errors should be targeted before consonant errors in order to restore a normal developmental pattern.

In the few case study reports of direct intervention for vowel errors in children with phonological disorders, the techniques utilized were similar to those commonly used with consonants, but represented a wide range of therapy approaches and targeted vowel error patterns. Several studies reported the use of minimal pair activities in which the contrast included the target vowel and the child's error production. For example, Khan (1988) used primarily minimal pair activities with a child who centralized most vowel targets. Pollock and Swanson (1986) and Pollock (1994) also used minimal pair activities with their clients (both 4-year-old boys with diphthong reduction and lowering/backing of mid front vowels), but only after they were able to establish correct production of the target vowel(s) through imitation, successive approximation, and drill activities. Finally, in a therapy program for a 4-year-old boy who reduced diphthongs, described by Gibbon, Shockey, and Reid (1992), the first step was establishing a suitable vocabulary for discussing the distinguishing features of monophthongs and diphthongs, in this case a sliding analogy to represent the articulatory movement between the two components of the diphthong. Minimal pair word pictures were then used to encourage the production of a monophthong/diphthong contrast.

Other studies reported the use of more traditional articulation approaches to intervention. Hargrove, Dauer, and Montelibano (1989) described a program for remediating a pattern of vowel prolongation in 4-year-old twins, which involved targeting vowels in increasingly demanding contexts (i.e., starting with imitation of vowel targets in isolation and ending with correct spontaneous productions in connected speech). Strategies included the use of contingent reinforcement, verbal feedback, auditory/visual cues, imitation, and modeling. Penney, Fee, and Dowdle (1994) used a similar progression from isolation to spontaneous speech in intervention for /u/ and /æ/ targets for a 4-year-old girl with a reduced vowel inventory and low overall vowel accuracy, but included perceptual strategies (e.g., auditory detection, auditory bombardment, vowel discrimination) as well as production strategies (e.g., phonetic placement).

In all of the cases reported, direct intervention resulted in improvement in vowel accuracy, although the extent of improvement and degree of carryover was variable. In at least some of the studies (e.g., Pollock, 1994; Pollock & Swanson, 1986), baseline measures and monitoring of untreated control sounds provided evidence that the direct vowel treatment, and not maturation, was responsible for the improvement. However, more research is clearly needed to establish the efficacy of vowel treatment and to compare different approaches to vowel treatment.

Gibbon and Beck (2002) provided an overview of general principles for vowel therapy and a description of treatment approaches developed for consonants that might be adapted for use with vowels. The principles include the need for clinicians to have good perceptual skills for analyzing vowels, knowledge of the sociolinguistic variations expected in the child's community, and production skills adequate for modeling target vowel qualities. Another principle is the need to select appropriate targets and treatment approaches based on a detailed assessment including phonetic and phonological analyses and an assessment of speech and language processing in order to determine whether the deficits are auditory/perceptual, cognitive-linguistic, or motor/articulatory. The treatment approaches reviewed included those that focus on the development of auditory/perceptual skills (e.g., auditory input therapy, auditory bombardment), linguistic/phonological abilities (e.g., minimal pairs contrasts, Metaphon), and motor/articulatory skills (e.g., phonetic placement, contextual facilitation).

Gibbon and Beck (2002) also provided an overview of a variety of treatment approaches that utilize computer technology to provide visual feedback for vowel production. This feedback is based on either acoustic or physiological information. Such feedback may be particularly useful for the establishment of new vowels in the phonetic inventory, as articulatory placement awareness for vowels (with the exception of high vowels such as /i/ and /ɪ/) is difficult to teach due to the lack of tactile feedback. For example, a number of acoustic feedback programs have been designed for teaching vowels to children with hearing impairment, and these may be useful for children with phonological disorder or CAS. Important considerations in selecting such a program are the timing of the feedback (e.g., it must be quick enough to allow children to associate tactile and kinesthetic cues with the acoustic feedback, but not so transitory as real-time displays which do not give sufficient time for children to interpret the feedback) and the type of visual display (e.g., whether the visual display is a representation of articulatory information or an abstract display unrelated to speech production that serves to maintain attention and reward success). Acoustic feedback systems are most useful in differentiating gross vowel categories, but may be less accurate in detecting subtle vowel differences. In addition, the utility of such feedback needs to be interpreted cautiously given the signal-processing difficulties often associated with the high F0, low intensity, and nasality of children's speech.

Physiological feedback systems, such as glossometry, electropalatography, and ultrasound, may also be useful in providing direct articulatory information such as tongue height and advancement. These systems have an advantage over acoustic feedback systems in that the articulatory feedback can be directly related to instructional cues for correcting vowel errors. Although many of these technologies have been shown to be effective in improving vowel production in children with hearing impairment, their use in treating vowel errors in children with phonological impairment or CAS has been largely untested. Furthermore, despite the exciting opportunities offered by these new technologies, Gibbon and Beck (2002) caution that their widespread clinical use is unlikely in the near future given the financial costs involved and the limited availability of such equipment in pediatric speech-language clinics and schools. In addition, the procedural demands of techniques such as glossometry and electropalatography may be too difficult for young children such as those most often seen for phonological intervention.

33.9   Summary and Conclusion

This chapter has provided an overview of vowel development and disorders in children, including clinical assessment and treatment. It is clear that, compared with consonants, our understanding of acquisition in children with typical development and in children with speech disorders is limited. Many of the investigations cited are case studies or studies of relatively few children; several of the larger studies provided little detail on vowels, focusing only on accuracy, with little information on error types and even less on suprasegmental aspects of vowel productions. The picture of vowel development and disorders is further complicated by lack of agreement on a feature system to describe accurate productions and errors.

Based on the American English data of children with typical and atypical phonological development, the generalizations listed below appear to be valid. In many cases, the same tendencies have been reported for children acquiring languages other than English.

- Corner vowels tend to be acquired (i.e., produced correctly) before non-corner vowels.
- Monophthongs tend to be acquired before diphthongs.
- Non-rhotic vowels tend to be acquired before rhotic vowels.
- Vowels in stressed syllables tend be more accurate than vowels in unstressed syllables.
- Adultlike timing of stressed vs. unstressed syllables is achieved later than adultlike accuracy of segments.

Although the patterns of accuracy and errors are similar across children with typical and atypical phonological development, some possible differences have emerged. First, it appears as though vowel errors in children with atypical development often affect a larger number of vowel types. Second, children with atypical development, especially those with childhood apraxia of peech (CAS), may exhibit greater variability in their vowel errors. Lastly, a subset of children with phonological disorders exhibit prosodic patterns not seen in children with typical development; these differences are particularly apparent in the features of stress and timing.

As noted above, literature on treatment of vowels is very sparse. Traditionally, clinicians have been inclined to treat consonants before attempting to treat vowels and many children may never receive intervention on vowels in spite of obvious errors. Unlike assessment and treatment for consonants, there are no accepted guidelines for intervention with vowels and little material available for use in a pediatric clinical setting. It is clear that this is an area that deserves more attention.

REFERENCES

Allen, G. and Hawkins, S. (1980). Phonological rhythm: Definition and development. In G. Yeni-Komshian, J. Kavanagh, and C. Ferguson (eds.), *Child Phonology. Volume 1: Production* (pp. 227–56). New York: Academic Press.

Ansell, B. (1987). *Acoustic Predictors of Speech Intelligibility in Cerebral Palsied–Dysarthric Adults*. Blooomington: Indiana University Linguistics Club.

Beers, M. (1995). *The Phonology of Normally Developing and Language-Impaired Children*. Dordrecht: Institute for Functional Research into Language and Language Use.

Bleile, K. (1989). A note on vowel patterns in two normally developing children. *Clinical Linguistics and Phonetics*, 3, 201–12.

Bond, Z. S., Petrosino, L., and Dean, C. R. (1982). The emergence of vowels: 17 to 26 months. *Journal of Phonetics*, 10, 417–22.

Buhr, R. (1980). The emergence of vowels in an infant. *Journal of Speech and Hearing Research*, 23, 73–94.

Davis, B. (2003). Developmental apraxia of speech. In R. Kent (ed.), *Encyclopedia of Communication Sciences and Disorders*. Boston, MA: MIT Press.

Davis, B., Jacks, A., and Marquardt, T. (2005). Vowel patterns in developmental apraxia of speech: Three longitudinal case studies. *Clinical Linguistics and Phonetics*, 19, 249–74.

Davis, B., Jakielski, K., and Marquardt, T. (1998). Developmental apraxia of speech: determiners of differential diagnosis. *Clinical Linguistics and Phonetics*, 12, 25–45.

Davis, B. and MacNeilage, P. (1990). Acquisition of correct vowel production: A quantitative case study. *Journal of Speech and Hearing Research*, 33, 16–27.

Davis, B. and MacNeilage, P. (1991). The articulatory basis of babbling. *Journal of Speech and Hearing Research*, 38, 1199–1211.

Donegan, P. (2002). Normal vowel development. In M. Ball and F. Gibbon (eds.), *Vowel Disorders* (pp. 1–35). Boston, MA: Butterworth-Heinemann.

Eimas, P. D., Siqueland, E. R., Jusczyk, P., and Vigorito, J. (1971). Speech perception in infants. *Science*, 171, 303–6.

Gibbon, F. E. and Beck, J. M. (2002). Therapy for abnormal vowels in children with phonological impairment. In M. Ball and F. Gibbon (eds.), *Vowel Disorders* (pp. 217–48). Boston, MA: Butterworth-Heinemann.

Gibbon, F., Shockey, L., and Reid, J. (1992). Description and treatment of abnormal vowels in a phonologically disordered child. *Child Language Teaching and Therapy*, 8, 30–59.

Goldstein, B. and Pollock, K. (2000). Vowel errors in Spanish-speaking children with phonological disorders. *Clinical Linguistics and Phonetics*, 14, 217–34.

Hall, P. K., Jordan, L. S., and Robin, D. A. (1993). *Developmental Apraxia of Speech: Theory and Clinical Practice*. Austin, TX: Pro-Ed.

Hare, G. (1983). Development at 2 years. In J. V. Irwin and S. P. Wong (eds.), *Phonological Development in Children: 18 to 72 Months* (pp. 55–88). Carbondale: Southern Illinois University Press.

Hargrove, P. (1982). Misarticulated vowels: A case study. *Language, Speech, and Hearing Services in Schools*, 13, 86–95.

Hargrove, P., Dauer, K., and Montelibano, M. (1989). Reducing vowel and final consonant prolongations in twin brothers. *Child Language Teaching and Therapy*, 5, 49–63.

Harris, J., Watson, J., and Bates, S. (1999). Prosody and melody in vowel disorder. *Journal of Linguistics*, 35, 489–525.

Jakobson, R. (1968) (trans. A. R. Keiler). *Child Language, Aphasia, and Phonological Universals*. The Hague: Mouton. Originally published as *Kindersprache, Aphasie, und allgemeine Lautgesetze*. Uppsala: Almqvist and Wiksell, 1941.

Kehoe, M., Stoel-Gammon, C., and Buder, E. H. (1995) Acoustic correlates of stress in young children's speech. *Journal of Speech and Hearing Research*, 38, 338–50.

Kent, R. (1992). The biology of phonological development. In C. Ferguson, L. Menn, and C. Stoel-Gammon (eds.), *Phonological Development: Models, Research, Implications* (pp. 65–90). Timonium, MD: York Press.

Kent, R. D. and Bauer, H. R. (1985). Vocalizations of one year olds. *Journal of Child Language*, 12, 491–526.

Kent, R. D. and Murray, A. (1982). Acoustic features of infant vocalic utterances at 3, 6, and 9 months. *Journal of the Acoustical Society of America*, 72, 353–65.

Kent, R. D., Osberger, M. J., Netsell, R., and Hustedde, C. (1987). Phonetic development in identical twins differing in auditory function. *Journal of Speech and Hearing Disorders*, 52, 64–75.

Khan, L. (1988). Vowel remediation: A case study. Paper presented at the annual convention of the American Speech-Language-Hearing Association, Boston, November.

Lieberman, P. (1980). On the development of vowel production in young children. In G. H. Yeni-Komshian, J. F. Kavanagh, and C. A. Ferguson (eds.), *Child Phonology. Volume 1: Production* (pp. 113–42). New York: Academic Press.

MacNeilage, P. F. (1998). The frame/content theory of evolution of speech production. *Behavioral and Brain Sciences*, 21, 499–546.

MacNeilage, P. F. and Davis, B. L. (2000). Origin of the internal structure of words. *Science*, 288, 527–31.

MacNeilage, P. F., and Davis, B. L. (2001). Motor mechanisms in speech ontogeny: Phylogenetic and neurobiological and linguistic implications. *Current Opinion in Neurobiology*, 11, 696–700.

Maddiesson, I. (1984). *Patterns of Sounds*. New York: Cambridge University Press.

Metz, D., Schiavetti, N., Samar, V., and Sitler, R. (1990). Acoustic dimensions of hearing-impaired speakers' intelligibility: Segmental and suprasegmental characteristics. *Journal of Speech and Hearing Research*, 33, 476–87.

Meza, P. (1983). Phonological analysis of Spanish utterances of highly unintelligible Mexican-American children. Unpublished master's thesis, San Diego State University, San Diego, CA.

Monsen, R. (1978). Toward measuring how well hearing-impaired children speak. *Journal of Speech and Hearing Research*, 21, 197–219.

Munson, B., Bjorum, E. M., and Windsor, J. (2003). Acoustic and perceptual correlates of stress in nonwords produced by children with suspected developmental apraxia of speech and children with phonological disorder. *Journal of Speech, Language, and Hearing Research*, 46, 189–202.

Nettelbladt, U. (1983). *Developmental Studies of Dysphonology in Children*. Lund: CWK Gleerup.

Olmsted, D. (1971). *Out of the Mouth of Babes*. The Hague: Mouton.

Otomo, K. and Stoel-Gammon, C. (1992). The acquisition of unrounded vowels in English. *Journal of Speech and Hearing Research*, 35, 604–16.

Paschall, L. (1983). Development at 18 months. In J. V. Irwin and S. P. Wong (eds.), *Phonological Development in Children: 18 to 72 Months* (pp. 27–54). Carbondale: Southern Illinois University Press.

Penny, G., Fee, E. J., and Dowdle, C. (1994). Vowel assessment and remediation: A case study. *Child Language Teaching and Therapy*, 10, 47–66.

Peter, B. and Stoel-Gammon, C. (2005). Timing errors in children with suspected childhood apraxia of speech (sCAS) during speech and music-related tasks. *Clinical Linguistics and Phonetics*, 19, 67–87.

Peter, B. and Stoel-Gammon, C. (2006). Typology of primary speech disorder based on multivariate classification. Seminar presented at the Annual Convention of the American Speech-Language-Hearing Association, Miami, November 16–18.

Pollock, K. E. (1991). The identification of vowel errors using traditional articulation or phonological process test stimuli. *Language, Speech, and Hearing Services in Schools*, 22, 39–50.

Pollock, K. E. (1994). Assessment and remediation of vowel misarticulations. *Clinics in Communication Disorders*, 4, 23–37.

Pollock, K. E. (2002). Identification of vowel errors: Methodological issues and preliminary data from the Memphis Vowel Project. In M. Ball and F. Gibbon (eds.), *Vowel Disorders* (pp. 83–113). Boston: Butterworth-Heinemann.

Pollock, K. E. and Berni, M. C. (2001). Transcription of vowels. *Topics in Language Disorders*, 21, 22–40.

Pollock, K. E. and Berni, M. C. (2003). Incidence of non-rhotic vowel errors in children: Data from the Memphis Vowel Project. *Clinical Linguistics and Phonetics*, 17, 1–9.

Pollock, K. E., Brammer, D. M., and Hageman, C. F. (1989). An acoustic analysis of young children's productions of word stress. In *Papers and Reports on Child Language Development*, 28, 140–7 (*Proceedings of the Annual Meeting of the Child Language Research Forum*, Stanford, CA, April 7–9, 1989).

Pollock, K. E. and Hall, P. (1991). An analysis of the vowel misarticulations of five children with developmental apraxia of speech. *Clinical Linguistics and Phonetics*, 5, 207–24.

Pollock, K. E. and Keiser, N. (1990). An examination of vowel errors in phonologically disordered children. *Clinical Linguistics and Phonetics*, 4, 161–78.

Pollock, K. E., Meeks, M., Stepherson, E., and Berni, M. C. (2004). Types of vowel errors in children: More data from the Memphis Vowel Project. Paper presented at the annual Child Phonology Conference, Tempe, AZ, May.

Pollock, K. E. and Swanson, L. (1986). Analysis of vowel errors in a disordered child during training. Paper presented at the annual convention of the American Speech-Language-Hearing Association, Detroit, MI, November.

Ramus, F., Nespor, M., and Mehler, J. (1999). Correlates of linguistic rhythm in the speech signal. *Cognition*, 73, 265–92.

Reynolds, J. (1990). Abnormal vowel patterns in phonological disorder: Some data and a hypothesis. *British Journal of Disorders of Communication*, 25, 115–48.

Reynolds, J. (2002). Recurring patterns and idiosyncratic systems in some English children with vowel disorders. In M. J. Ball and F. E. Gibbon (eds.), *Vowel Disorders*. Boston: Butterworth-Heinemann, pp. 115–43.

Robb, M., Bleile, K., and Yee, S. (1999). A phonetic analysis of vowel errors during the course of treatment. *Clinical Linguistics and Phonetics*, 13, 309–21.

Rosenbek, J. and Wertz, R. (1972). A review of fifty cases of developmental apraxia of speech. *Language, Speech, and Hearing Services in Schools*, 3, 23–33.

Selby, J., Robb, M., and Gilbert, H. (2000). Normal vowel articulations between 15 and 36 months of age. *Clinical Linguistics and Phonetics*, 14, 255–65.

Shriberg, L. D., Aram, D. M., and Kwiatkowski, J. K. (1997a). Developmental apraxia of speech: II. Toward a diagnostic marker. *Journal of Speech, Language, and Hearing Research*, 40, 286–312.

Shriberg, L. D., Aram, D. M., and Kwiatkowski, J. K. (1997b). Developmental apraxia of speech: III. A subtype marked by inappropriate stress. *Journal of Speech, Language, and Hearing Research*, 40, 313–37.

Shriberg, L. D., Campbell, T. F., Karlsson, H. B., Brown, R. L., McSweeny, J. L., and Nadler, C. J. (2003). A diagnostic marker for childhood apraxia of speech: The lexical stress ratio. *Clinical Linguistics and Phonetics*, 17, 549–74.

So, L. and Dodd, B. (1994). Phonologically disordered Cantonese-speaking children. *Clinical Linguistics and Phonetics*, 8, 235–55.

Stoel-Gammon, C. (1990). Issues in phonological development and disorders. In J. Miller (ed.), *Progress in Research on Child Language Disorders*. Austin, TX: Pro-Ed.

Stoel-Gammon, C. and Dunn, C. (1985). *Normal and Disordered Phonology in Children*. Austin, TX: Pro-Ed.

Stoel-Gammon, C. and Herrington, P. (1990). Vowel systems of normally-developing and phonologically-disordered children. *Clinical Linguistics and Phonetics*, 4, 145–60.

Stokes, S. F., Lau, J., and Ciocca, V. (2002). The interaction of ambient frequency and feature complexity in the diphthong errors of children with phonological disorders. *Journal of Speech, Language, and Hearing Research*, 45, 1188–1201.

Stokes, S. F. and Wong, I. M. (2002). Vowel and diphthong development in Cantonese-speaking children. *Clinical Linguistics and Phonetics*, 16, 597–617.

Swoboda, P. J., Morse, P. A., and Leavitt, L. A. (1976). Continuous vowel discrimination in normal and at-risk infants. *Child Development*, 47, 459–65.

Templin, M. (1957). Certain language skills in children: Their development and inter-relationships. *Institute of Child Welfare Monographs*, 26. Minneapolis: University of Minnesota Press.

Trehub, S. E. (1976). Infants' sensitivity to vowel and tonal contrasts. *Developmental Psychology*, 9, 466–72.

Tse, A. C. Y. (1991). The acquisition process of Cantonese phonology: A case study. Unpublished doctoral dissertation, University of Hong Kong.

Vaughn, A. and Pollock, K. E. (1997). The relative contribution of vowel and consonant errors to intelligibility. Poster presentation at the annual convention of the American Speech-Language-Hearing Association, Boston, November.

Vihman, M. (1996). *Phonological Development: The Origins of Language in the Child*. Cambridge, MA: Blackwell.

Watson, J., Bates, S., Sinclair, A., and Hewlett, N. (1994). Unusual vowel systems in some Edinburgh children with phonological disorder. Poster presented at the annual convention of the American Speech-Language-Hearing Association, New Orleans, LA, November.

Wellman, B., Case, I., Mengert, I., and Bradbury, D. (1931). Speech sounds of young children. *University of Iowa Studies in Child Welfare*, 5(2), 7–82.

Zajdó, K. (2002). Vowel acquisition in Hungarian: A first look at the data. In J. Larson and M. Paster (eds.), *Proceedings of the Twenty-Eighth Annual Meeting of the Berkeley Linguistics Society*, pp. 363–74. Berkeley, CA: Berkeley Linguistics Society.

Zajdó, K. and Stoel-Gammon, C. (2003). The acquisition of vowels in Hungarian: Developmental data. In M. J. Solé, D. Rescasens, and J. Romero (eds.), *Proceedings of the 15th International Congress of Phonetic Sciences, Barcelona, 3–9 August, 2003*, vol. 3, pp. 2229–32. Barcelona: Universitat Autónoma de Barcelona.

34 Prosodic Impairments

BILL WELLS AND
SANDRA WHITESIDE

34.1 What is a Prosodic Impairment?

Every time we speak, we have to do something with the pitch, loudness and duration of the utterance. Linguists sometimes refer to these features as 'suprasegmental', suggesting that they are somehow above a string of consonants and vowels. This connotation is misleading: rather, in speech the string of consonants and vowels is overlaid onto a base of phonation (voicing) generated by an airstream from the lungs passing through the larynx, which results in fluctuations in pitch (height and movement) and loudness distributed over phonatory chunks of varying durations. The term 'prosody', and the related adjective 'prosodic', are commonly used to refer to features of pitch, loudness and duration in speech, in a broad sense, encompassing their use on individual words (e.g. in lexical stress, duration of the syllable or part of syllable, and lexical tones), as well as the use of these features over longer stretches of speech (phrases, complete utterances, and conversational turns), the latter being the focus of the present chapter.

There are at least two good reasons why clinical linguists and speech and language pathology professionals should study prosody. First, there are some clients who present with unusual prosodic patterns, and it is important to investigate why this might be. Second, if prosody is a relative strength for many people with speech and language difficulties, how might it be used to support or compensate for other aspects of language? In the case of prosody, the basis for postulating an impairment is likely to be the auditory impression of listeners that the speaker's use of prosodic features is in some way atypical for that speech community, but that its atypicality cannot be attributed to other causes, such as being a non-native speaker whose prosody in the second language is influenced by the mother tongue. Beyond that, identification, description and explanation of the impairment are theory-dependent. The investigator can adopt one or more relatively distinct though complementary approaches.

34.2   Phonetic Approach

Atypical prosody can arise in both developmental disorders of speech (e.g. developmental apraxia of speech (DAS), stuttering, Williams syndrome, autism and Asperger's syndrome) and acquired ones (e.g. acquired apraxia of speech (AOS), foreign accent syndrome (FAS), and the acquired dysarthrias (e.g. hypokinetic and hyperkinetic)). It can be explored using a range of methodologies which are based on auditory-perceptual, acoustic-phonetic and experimental methodologies (e.g. Odell & Shriberg, 2001). Although this discussion will focus on the latter set of approaches, the combination of acoustic and perceptual methods is both strongly advocated (Kent & Kim, 2003), and employed in the profiling of prosody (Bunton, Kent, Kent, & Rosenbek, 2000).

Prosody is related to a number of perceptual dimensions, and includes, though not exhaustively, features of pitch, loudness and duration. All of these features can be explored instrumentally using a range of techniques which include acoustically based methods (Kent & Kim, 2003), and other techniques like laryngography (see Fourcin, 1986, for a description of the methodology). Quantitative information on fundamental frequency (F0), intensity and duration can be employed independently to profile prosody. However, a multidimensional approach which combines aspects of F0, intensity and duration allows a more comprehensive assessment and characterization of atypical prosody.

The perception of pitch is partly determined by F0, which therefore forms an important part in the investigation and profiling of atypical prosody. Various F0-related parameters can be explored instrumentally and quantified for any isolated word or any type of connected speech utterance with this aim in mind. These parameters could include mean F0, the standard deviation of F0, F0 range, and the shape of fundamental frequency contours. Information gleaned from parameters such as a limited F0 range can provide quantifiable acoustic information on an adult with dysarthria, or a child with autism who may, for example, present with monotonous-sounding speech.

The perception of loudness is partly determined by intensity, which can be quantified in a number of ways, and could include information on mean intensity, the standard deviation of intensity, intensity range, the shape of the intensity envelope, and intensity decay. For example, patterns of diminishing intensity (or intensity decay) have been observed in the speech of individuals with Parkinsonian dysarthria (Ho, Iansek, & Bradshaw, 2001). However, there is also evidence to suggest that intensity decay is not consistent across different individuals with Parkinson's disease, and that patterns of intensity decay may also vary across different speech tasks (Rosen, Kent, & Duffy, 2005). This highlights the role of individual variability, and the effect of different speech tasks in the assessment of prosody (Lowit-Leuschel & Docherty, 2001). In contrast to Parkinsonian dysarthria, speakers with AOS who are perceived as having abnormal stress patterns may display a limited variation in the intensity of syllables across an utterance.

The aspect of prosody which relates to the durational dimension of speech includes parameters such as utterance duration, articulation rate, mean pause duration, the incidence of pauses, the ratio between articulation time and pause time and mean stressed vowel duration. As an illustration, speakers with moderate to severe AOS may show evidence of a high number of pauses in relation to articulation time, which, when combined with the excessively long syllables, goes some way toward explaining their atypical prosody patterns (Whiteside & Varley, 1998).

Most studies of atypical prosody focus on the acoustic parameters related to the primary features of pitch (via fundamental frequency), loudness (via amplitude) and duration. However, other acoustic cues related to various dimensions of voice quality at both the laryngeal and supralaryngeal levels have been identified in the perception and production of emotion and affect in healthy individuals (Banse & Scherer, 1996). This therefore deserves further investigation in studies of individuals who may display impairment in the production and perception of affective prosody. A more comprehensive set of acoustic parameters may also prove useful in furthering our understanding of the perception and production of atypical linguistic prosody.

34.3   Linguistic Approach

Prosodic features serve to realize linguistic systems such as tone (in tone languages), stress and intonation. From this perspective a prosodic impairment impacts on the linguistic system in question, with the result that the meaning (in its broadest sense) of the speaker's utterance may be obscured. Identification of a linguistic impairment of intonation, for example, is therefore dependent on the analyst having a description of the intonation system of the language. Such descriptions are available for a growing number of languages; in this chapter examples are taken from English to illustrate general principles.

Various approaches to the systematic description of intonation have been adopted over the last 100 years or so. The Tones and Break Indices (ToBI) notational system, derived from autosegmental-metrical theory (Ladd, 1996), is currently the most widely adopted within phonetic and speech technology research (e.g. speech synthesis). However, it has so far been applied little to clinical analysis or to studies of children's intonation development, where versions of analyses that follow a tradition established by David Crystal (e.g. 1987) have tended to be used.

In what follows, we briefly outline how a linguistic description of English prosody can be used to draw attention to atypical prosodic patterns. This is illustrated in the following transcript of an interaction between John (J), a 23-year-old man with acquired aphasia, and a speech and language therapist (T):

1 T: ‖ 'what 'sort of 'things `do you 'watch ‖
2 J: ‖ 'it's er (1.0) `first of all it's (.) er (0.5) ‖ `not er 'good (0.5) ‖ er (.) `watching

3   (.) the 'box hh and er (.) like (1.5) ‖ `mystery (.) er (1.5) ‖
4   or s er (0.5) 'de`tective er hh ‖ `but ‖
5 T: ‖ you 'don't like 'Starsky and `Hutch then ‖
6 J: *(laughs)* ‖ `yeah ‖ I `watch it (.) ‖ `yeah (.) hh (0.5) ‖ 'you 'watch it ‖
7 T: ‖ `no ‖ 'actually I `don't ‖ but I 'watch `Kojak ‖

It is likely that all languages have an equivalent of the English systems of Tonality and Tone, i.e. a way of chunking the utterance prosodically in different ways, and a choice of pitch direction (Halliday, 1967). English intonation makes use of a third major system that is more restricted in its distribution across languages. This is Tonicity, the location of the tonic syllable, which serves to highlight important information in the utterance and to background less important information. For example the location of the tonic on 'do' in line 1 may carry an implication that the co-participants have already been talking about TV programs that John doesn't watch.

Each of these systems may be impaired, and John's contribution in the extract above illustrates some ways in which this happens. His extended turn (lines 2–4) is delivered at a slow rate, and is characterized by a number of prominent syllables, each marked by a falling pitch movement, notated [`], from relatively high in the speaker's pitch range, accompanied by relative loudness. Between them occur non-prominent syllables, some of which are audible hesitation tokens (transcribed 'er') and also silences of up to 1.5 seconds. One analytic strategy is to transcribe such data using the conventions of English intonation, as has been done above. This can serve to highlight the impact on meaning caused by prosodic patterns such as John's. Following this approach, the prominent syllables are transcribed as tonic syllables. In some cases, this conforms to the typical English use of tonic prominence to highlight informationally important elements, e.g. 'mystery', 'detective'. Elsewhere, tonic prominence is not aligned with information focus: in J's production of 'watching the box', the location of the accent on 'watching' is hard to make sense of, given that watching TV is already well established as the topic of the interchange.

The occurrence of a tonic syllable entails the occurrence of a tone unit, and thus raises the issue of where to locate tone unit boundaries, notated ‖. This is not straightforward even when transcribing typical English speakers. According to Cruttenden (1997), the principal cues are potential for pause and change in pitch direction. These criteria coincide for the first three boundaries in the turn; however, following 'watching the box' there is a step up in pitch to 'and', with no pause, followed by a long pause before 'mystery'. This gives the effect of a word-search pause, as opposed to a tone unit boundary pause, as the pause is located within what appears to be the intonational head of the tone unit, preceding an important and accented lexical item, 'mystery'. The upshot is a series of short tone units, each with its tonic syllable. Grammatically these mainly map onto short phrases or single words, rather than clauses.

Turning to the system of Tone, in John's speech there is an overwhelming preponderance of falls, which suggests that this may be a default tone for him. This is reinforced by the occurrence of a fall on 'but' in line 4: as a connective, this word rarely constitutes a tonic syllable, and where that does happen in John's accent of English it is more likely to be with a level or fall–rise, projecting further talk from the speaker. If there were no evidence of other tones, we could reasonably infer that John has lost the ability to use the tonal system. However, in line 6 John uses a rise on 'you watch it'. This reinforces the questioning function of the turn (in the absence of syntactic inversion), thereby suggesting that John does retain some kind of Tone system.

This linguistic approach to prosodic assessment is associated particularly with Crystal, who formalized it into a profile (Crystal, 1992). An example of a fully worked-through study using this approach, of a client with dysarthria, is presented in Vance (1994). Because of the detailed and time-consuming nature of linguistic analysis, the case study is the preferred method, although linguistically based test batteries may also be used (e.g. Samuelsson & Nettelbladt, 2004). The particular value of the linguistic approach is to tell us what is going wrong linguistically with a speaker's output, and to suggest how it might affect meaning and intelligibility. It also indicates rather directly what would need to be changed in order to improve intelligibility. Moreover, while a linguistic description does not itself indicate directly what the underlying causes of the client's prosodic problems might be, it provides a systematic basis for generating hypotheses about causation.

34.4   Interactional Approach

The interactional approach resembles the linguistic approach in that it involves the analysis of spontaneous speech data, on the basis of careful transcription, including phonetic notation. Studies of prosody in conversational interaction have revealed the complex and subtle ways in which speakers deploy prosodic features in order to negotiate everyday talk (Couper-Kuhlen & Selting, 1996). This approach tends to take as its starting point basic interactional phenomena, frequently turn organization, though it could also be repair organization, or topic management, for example. In clinical analysis, the focus is on how the client manages (or doesn't manage) the business of maintaining the social interaction, in the face of prosodic or other limitations.

A case study by Wells and Local (1993) of a boy with speech and language difficulties illustrates the approach. At the age of 5;4, David invariably located the main pitch movement on the final syllable of his turn at talk, and it was invariably a rising pitch. Words preceding this final syllable were produced with level pitch around the middle of the pitch range. The direction of final pitch movement was more or less appropriate for the variety of English which David was exposed to (West Midlands of England), but, from a linguistic perspective, the *invariable* location of the main pitch movement on the final syllable of the utterance was not, since in English the location of the tonic or nuclear tone varies in position according to considerations of context and information focus. David was receiving speech and language therapy, but this was not targeted at prosodic features. Recordings made one year later showed that this pattern had been superseded by the more usual one for his variety of British English, whereby position of nuclear tone is determined by considerations of information focus as well as turn completion. Partly as a consequence, David displayed much greater variety in pitch height and movement. This was accompanied by a marked improvement in his overall intelligibility. Wells and Local argued that at 5;4, David's idiosyncratic prosodic pattern served to mark the end of his turns at talk in a clear, consistent and unambiguous way, which was useful for him and his co-participants given the unintelligibility of his speech. By clearly signaling the end of his turn at talk, David managed to maintain interactions with others without an unusual amount of overlap or interruption by co-participants.

34.5   Psycholinguistic Approach

With prosody as with other levels of linguistic analysis, the structures posited by linguists can be taken as a testable hypothesis as to how linguistic knowledge is represented in adult speakers' minds. It can thus be hypothesized that the English speaker has to learn to draw on representational distinctions, of the type encoded in the three systems of intonation (Tonality, Tonicity, Tone) described above, both in comprehension and in production (cf. Levelt, 1989, ch 10). For example, if, in comprehension, a client interprets /CHOCOLATE AND HONEY/ as having its main focus on CHOCOLATE rather than on HONEY, one possibility is that he or she has not learned the systemic significance of Tonicity. Such an immature or inaccurate prosodic representation may have consequences for the speaker's own production. If the distinction between non-final and final tonic placement (Tonicity) is lacking at the representational level, we might anticipate that the speaker will mix up the form in his or her own production, i.e., may on occasion use a final tonic in a context which requires non-final focus, and vice versa. Thus inaccurate uses of intonation, in terms of both comprehension and production, may be attributed to imprecise representations, i.e. to 'high-level' factors.

However, low-level influences may also be involved. On the input side, the client may have deficits in hearing or in auditory processing that block access to prosodic details of the incoming signal (Barry, Blamey, Martin, et al., 2002). Such deficits are likely to give rise to imperfect processing and comprehension of the heard utterance, and in the longer term the construction of inaccurate prosodic representations. On the output side, a speaker with a prosodic impairment may have accurate representations but be unable to realize them accurately, due to limitations on his or her ability to execute complex prosodic patterns/contours, arising, for example, from laryngeal anomalies or respiratory difficulties (Heselwood, Bray, & Crookston, 1995).

Within this psycholinguistic framework, in the case of a person with impaired prosodic output we can ask the question: What is the level of breakdown? Is it in input, representations, or output, or a mix of these? In order to address such questions systematically, it is usual to use a battery of tasks that tap different levels of processing.

PEPS-C represents an attempt to devise a systematic and comprehensive prosodic test battery (Wells & Peppé, 2003). It incorporates the following dimensions: *Input* (perception/comprehension) vs. *Output* (generation/production); and *Form* (referring to lower-level phonetic processing, where meaning is not involved) vs. *Function* (involving higher-level processing, drawing on stored knowledge, relating phonetic form to meaning). PEPS-C covers four *communicative areas* where intonation is generally agreed to have an important role:

1   Chunking: prosodic delimitation of the utterance into units for grammatical, semantic or pragmatic purposes, e.g. /COFFEE-CAKE/AND HONEY/ vs. /COFFEE/ CAKE/AND HONEY/.
2   Affect: expressing strong liking as opposed to reservation with the syllable 'M', by using rise–fall vs. fall–rise pitch movement.
3   Interaction: PEPS-C used the prosodic opposition between a low fall meaning 'yes I understand'; as opposed to a high rise meaning 'no I didn't understand, please repeat'.
4   Focus: the speaker's use of phonetic prominence (tonicity) to indicate which item is most important in an utterance, e.g. /CHOCOLATE AND HONEY/ vs. /CHOCOLATE AND HONEY/.

Each of the four communicative areas is tested for both Input and Output, with different assessments for Form and Function, giving a total of sixteen tasks. The battery has been employed in order to characterize clinical groups, e.g. developmental speech and language impairment, with respect to prosody, compared to typical populations (Wells & Peppé, 2003). It can also be used to profile the prosodic abilities of individual clients, thus providing a basis for individually tailored intervention. Wells and Peppé (2001) profile two contrasting eight-year-old boys diagnosed as having a specific language impairment, and compare their pattern of performance on various prosodic tasks against data from a normative study of prosodic development (Wells, Peppé, & Goulandris, 2004). Jonathan and Robin had each been identified as having language difficulties serious enough to warrant special educational provision.

The following observations were made of Jonathan's prosody in spontaneous speech, compared to normally developing children of a similar age: (1) many syllables are unusually loud; (2) his speech is slow overall; (3) at the end of utterances, Jonathan often has level pitch or moves rapidly from one level to another; (4) he lengthens vowels very noticeably in the final syllables of his utterances. Jonathan's speech has a 'sing-song' character, deriving from his pervasive use of level pitch, as well as sustained vowels in some positions (as opposed to dynamic falls and rises). This intonation was regarded as unusual by his parents, as well as by professionals and others outside the family. They noted that this feature started some time after his seventh birthday, and had become increasingly evident.

Pervasively poor performance on the PEPS-C Output tasks suggests that Jonathan may have problems with output representation for some items in the intonation lexicon. He may also have low-level motor execution deficits. This ties in with the observations of his conversational speech. However, on the Affect Output Function task his performance was flawless, suggesting that Jonathan is not incapable of using prosody deliberately to express his meaning; moreover it was for Affect that he made his highest score on an Input Function task (15/16). On other Input Function tasks he scored less well, suggesting that his representation of some intonational meanings may be imprecise. This may in turn contribute to inaccurate output.

In Robin's spontaneous speech, by contrast, there are few strikingly unusual prosodic features. It is therefore quite surprising to discover that on the PEPS-C he had difficulties with both Input and Output. On Input Function, he scored below normal limits on all communicative areas except Chunking; in fact, he performed worse than Jonathan. Robin's difficulties with Input Function suggest that he has problems interpreting pragmatic aspects of prosody. This is likely to be one of the factors responsible for his difficulties with social interaction, and may therefore be a suitable area for intervention. Robin was successful on three of the four Output Function tasks. This is somewhat paradoxical, given his failure on two of these (Affect, Focus) on Input Function. It suggests that a child may sound quite typical in terms of his own prosody, yet still have problems making sense of intonation. This can be described as a covert prosodic deficit.

The contrasting profiles of Jonathan and Robin indicate the value of psycholinguistic profiling in the area of prosody, potentially as a basis for targeted intervention. The method enables the identification of areas of prosodic strength and prosodic weakness, neither of which may be evident from the study of spontaneous output alone. That said, psycholinguistic testing of intonation presents considerable challenges. For example, production on output tasks is subject to contextual effects: the test situation is a social interaction of a kind, and intonation is very susceptible to interactional factors. The test demands of a battery like PEPS-C are such as to preclude its use with preschool children, and with older clients who are not at a sufficient cognitive level. Furthermore, while the interpretation of scores depends on comparison with matched typical children or adults, there is a lot of variability in the adult population (Peppé, Maxim, & Wells, 2000) and among children of different age ranges (Dankovičová, Pigott, Peppé, & Wells, 2004; Wells, Peppé, & Goulandris, 2004), which means that considerable caution must be exercised when diagnosing a prosodic impairment on the basis of such test results.

34.6   Prosodic Impairments in Developmental Disorders

Prosody in people with autistic spectrum disorders (ASD) has been the subject of a growing number of studies reviewed by McCann & Peppé (2003) (see also Paul, Augustyn, Klin, & Volkmar, 2005; Peppé, McCann, Gibbon, O'Hare, & Rutherford, 2006, 2007, for recent group studies of prosody in high level ASD). Single case studies of children with severe autism (Local & Wootton, 1995; Tarplee & Barrow, 1999), focusing on immediate and delayed echoes, have illustrated the value of the interactional approach in cases where testing is impossible and linguistic comparison with the adult system would be unrevealing: the child's echoes are well-formed phonetically, in terms of typical English prosody; it is their frequency and precise distribution, in relation to the interaction in progress, that is anomalous.

Some other developmental disorders have been the subject of the occasional study. Catterall, Howard, Szczerbinski, Stojanovik, and Wells (2006) used the PEPS-C battery to profile two adolescents with Williams syndrome. Different profiles of strengths and weaknesses were revealed for the two subjects. The results support the growing view that people with Williams syndrome are a heterogeneous population in terms of linguistic abilities. Other clinical groups of children who do not have a primary language impairment have been shown to have poor comprehension of affective prosody, including boys suffering from depression (Emerson, Harrison, & Everhart, 1999) and girls with Ullrich–Turner syndrome (Ross, Stefanatos, Roeltgen, Kushner, & Cutler, 1995). More sustained investigation of prosody in specific speech and language impairments is reviewed in the following sections.

34.6.1   *Specific language impairments (SLI)*

As a clinical entity SLI is notoriously difficult to define (Bishop, 1997), and the studies of prosody in SLI use a wide range of inclusion/exclusion criteria, with a wide age range. Perhaps in part as a consequence, the findings are rather mixed, and hard to interpret.

Snow (1998) examined two specific prosodic features associated with sentence-final position: final pitch movement and final lengthening. Ten children with SLI and ten children with normally developing language between the ages of 4;0 and 4;11 were age-matched within three months of each other. Children took part in play sessions centered on a baby doll, and the sessions were recorded. Specific spontaneous utterances were then measured for mean length of utterance (MLU), duration and F0 contour. Analysis of variance was used to evaluate the mean final–nonfinal differences between language groups, alongside a minimum perceptual criterion known as 'just noticeable difference' (JND). Snow found that both groups used final-syllable lengthening to some degree, and all children had control of the final pitch fall.

Snow had hypothesized that the phrase-final features of greater tone contour and syllable lengthening might not be found to the same degree in the SLI group, since their grammatical abilities were less than those of the normally developing children. In the event, both groups showed similar use of these parameters. This suggests that the prosodic features studied by Snow are not associated directly with syntax, i.e., they are not serving as exponents of syntactic boundaries in his data. Snow's results support the view that these children are not impaired in this area of prosodic output. He suggests that this relatively intact prosodic ability could be used as a strength, for therapy.

In a subsequent study, Snow (2001) investigated SLI children's prosodic production abilities by using an imitation task. He focused specifically on rising and falling intonational contours, which the children were encouraged to imitate in an appropriate pragmatic and linguistic context, at the end of a play session. The subjects were 11 four-year-olds with SLI, and a group of 11 chronological-age-matched controls. Acoustic measures of the falls and rises used by the children revealed no differences between the two groups.

Weinert (1996) gave a sentence imitation task to 24 children with SLI (mean age 6;5), matched for memory span to younger normal-language children. The sentences were presented under two prosodic conditions: normal prosody or monotone. There was no difference between groups in the monotone condition, but on the normal prosody condition, the SLI group had a poorer performance. Weinert interpreted this as evidence for a specific deficit in prosodic processing in the children with SLI. Weinert and Mueller (1996) tested 11 children with SLI in a similar way, but this time using three prosodic conditions: monotone, normal, and exaggerated sentence prosody, the latter resembling 'motherese' in its prosodic features. Exaggerated prosody performance did not improve performance for the group as a whole; however, some of the older SLI children, who had better language abilities, did improve their sentence reproductions under the exaggerated condition. This suggests that for these children prosodic processing ability may be relatively preserved.

Van der Meulen, Janssen, and Den Os (1997) studied prosodic production in groups of four-, five- and 6-year-old Dutch children, diagnosed as having a severe language delay. The children had to imitate ten sentences, each of which embodied a particular emotional or linguistic use of prosody. The children's responses were judged for accuracy of imitation. The children with language impairment performed consistently more poorly on this task than normally developing children matched for chronological age, though performance of both language-impaired and normal groups improved significantly with age. The authors point out that the discrepancy between language-impaired and normal groups does not necessarily mean that the language-impaired children have a primary deficit in prosodic production. Their poor performance may be the consequence of other speech and/or language difficulties.

Wells and Peppé (2003) studied a group of 18 eight-year-old children with speech and/or language impairments (LI), using the PEPS-C battery described above. Scores were compared to those from a chronological-age-matched (CA) group and a language-age group matched individually on grammatical comprehension (LA). The LI group performed below the LA group on just two out of 16 tasks. On seven out of 16 tasks, the LI group did not differ significantly from the CA group. There were few significant correlations between the prosodic measures and measures of grammatical comprehension, expressive language and articulation. The results support the view that in general intonation is relatively discrete from other levels of speech and language.

A basic dichotomy in the PEPS-C procedure is between Form and Function. The generally good scores on Function tasks suggest that for children with speech and language impairment, intonation may be an island of relative strength in their communicative repertoire, enabling them to convey linguistically important areas of meaning without having recourse solely to grammatical and lexical means. Nevertheless, some specific problems were indicated. For the group as a whole, the pattern of results on the Input Form tasks suggested that the children with language impairments may find it difficult to store and process long prosodic strings. This points to an auditory memory deficit that may be responsible for their difficulties with language development. The other area of difficulty for the group was in using prosody for pragmatic/interactional purposes. However, there was a lot of variation across individuals, in the profile of scores on the PEPS-C battery. This points to the importance of individual profiling as a basis for clinical intervention; Robin and Jonathan, described earlier in the chapter, were participants in this study.

It could be predicted that expressive prosodic difficulties may give rise to *pragmatic* difficulties in conversation and other forms of spoken interaction, given that the functions of prosody, particularly intonation, include the conveying of interactional and affective meaning. Having found that LI children with morphosyntactic difficulties have normal prosody, Snow (1998) leaves open that other groups of LI children, such as pragmatic language-impaired children, may have prosodic output deficits. This idea has been around among clinicians for a long time. Nevertheless, there is a lack of studies investigating prosodic processing in children diagnosed as having pragmatic language impairments. Wells and Peppé (2003) included a subgroup of SLI children with pragmatic language difficulties. Interestingly, their performance on the more pragmatically oriented of the PEPS-C tasks was at least as good as that of children with SLI who were not thought to have pragmatic difficulties.

In sum, research suggests that while many children diagnosed as SLI do not appear to have overt prosodic difficulties in their speech output (at least by the time they are diagnosed), they may still have subtle hidden problems with processing prosody, which might affect either their language production, or their comprehension, or both. This possibility cannot be discounted on the basis of analysis of their speech output alone.

34.6.2 Specific speech impairments

Shriberg, Aram, and Kwiatkowski (1997) investigated the possibility that there is a particular subgroup of speech-impaired children for whom the diagnostic marker is prosodic, a deficit in lexical and phrasal stress production. They compared the spontaneous spoken output of children who met clinical criteria for developmental apraxia of speech (DAS) (n = 53) with that of children diagnosed as having speech delay (SD) (n = 73). In an attempt to determine whether there was a single diagnostic criterion that would distinguish children with suspected DAS from others with speech delay, a very comprehensive range of segmental and prosodic features were examined. The only one that appeared to distinguish a sizable subgroup of the children with suspected DAS from the other speech-delayed/disordered group was the feature 'inappropriate stress'. They found that just over half the DAS group had inappropriate (excessive, equal or misplaced) stress, compared to 10 percent of the SD group. The authors suggest that the children in the DAS group who had inappropriate stress may represent a specific subtype of severe speech disorder.

Shriberg and colleagues argue that inappropriate stress is likely to result from a deficit in the linguistic representation of stress, rather than in motor planning or execution. They speculate that this may link to deficits in stress comprehension or perception, but their study did not look at the children's input processing. They go so far as to suggest that the segmental difficulties that these children have may arise from the prosodic deficit. Further, they argue that the stress deficit they discovered is independent of segmental phonological difficulties, on the grounds that some of the older children with inappropriate stress had only mild segmental difficulties. This parallels one conclusion of Snow's (1998) study of SLI children, where he also argued for a dissociation between segmental phonology and prosody, on the grounds of poor correlation between scores of consonantal accuracy and prosodic performance.

A subgroup of the children studied by Wells and Peppé (2003) had speech difficulties at the segmental level. These were more likely to have a low score on the PEPS-C Output Form tasks, which involved imitation of a short phrase, including its prosodic pattern. This result suggests a relationship between the ability to pronounce segments accurately and prosodic contours. It seems plausible that difficulty with segmental articulation might disrupt the planning and execution of prosodic structures and systems, but the opposite relation cannot be discounted: problems with prosodic organization may affect the production of segments (see also Howard, Wells, & Local, chapter 36 in this volume).

34.7 Prosodic Impairments in Acquired Disorders

The first part of this section provides a brief review of the prosodic patterns of two types of acquired speech impairment: acquired apraxia of speech (AOS) and foreign accent syndrome (FAS). The second part focuses on prosodic processing in individuals with left-hemisphere (LH) and right-hemisphere (RH) brain damage impairments.

34.7.1   *Prosody in acquired apraxia of speech (AOS)*

Acquired apraxia of speech (AOS) is a motor deficit typically associated with left-hemisphere (LH) damage; it interferes with the programming and sequencing of movements in the volitional articulation of speech (Varley & Whiteside, 2001). Studies on AOS have reported a wide range of speech characteristics that typify this motor speech disorder. In addition to groping behaviors commonly observed in speakers with AOS, at the segmental level their speech characteristics include inconsistent and variable articulatory movements, increased word and vowel duration patterns, voicing errors, segmental errors, and reduced coarticulation patterns (see Whiteside & Varley, 1998, for a review). In addition, effortful speech which is produced in a word-by-word, phrase-by-phrase fashion, and a generally slowed rate of speaking with prolongations of transitions, segments and intersyllabic pauses have been observed. These features, together with a limited variation in peak intensity across syllables, result in the perception of abnormal stress and rhythm patterns, a general impression of atypical prosody in AOS (Kent & Rosenbek, 1983).

Because speech production in AOS is impaired phonetically at both the segmental and suprasegmental levels, it is likely that suprasegmental characteristics in emotional or affective prosody may also be affected. On this basis, Van Putten and Walker (2003) investigated the ability of one healthy speaker, one speaker with moderate AOS, and another with mild AOS to produce emotional prosody using sentences. The emotions investigated were happy, sad and neutral. Both repetition and reading tasks were employed in the study. Ten sets of phonetically balanced and semantically neutral sentences were produced with a happy, sad or neutral voice. The sentences produced by all subjects were analyzed using a range of acoustic parameters. Results indicated that the speakers with AOS were not able to produce significant differences in F0, duration and amplitude to signal the three different emotions, as a consequence of their groping, intersyllabic pauses and word initiation difficulties. The severity of AOS did not appear to be a factor; both subjects had an impaired capacity to signal emotional prosody. In addition, although naive listeners were able to identify the emotional intent of the control subject's productions, this was not the case for the AOS samples. These results suggest that in addition to linguistic prosody, the production of affective prosody is impaired in speakers with AOS.

34.7.2   *Prosody in foreign accent syndrome (FAS)*

There is a group of speakers with brain damage who display speech characteristics which are suggestive of a failure to produce smooth and fully integrated speech movements. They are described as having 'foreign accent syndrome' (FAS), a rare neurogenic speech disorder in which an individual produces altered speech which is perceived as sounding like that of a non-native speaker of the language in question. The disorder may occur in relative isolation or be accompanied by aphasia, AOS, or dysarthria (Varley, Whiteside, Hammill, & Cooper, 2006). In common with other acquired neurogenic speech and language disorders, there is considerable variability in the phonetic behaviors demonstrated across individual patients with FAS. The changes in speech production patterns are generally within the boundaries of permissible phonological and phonetic variants of a language and, as a result, the intelligibility of speech remains high and the speaker is perceived as 'foreign' rather than 'disordered'. For example, segmental changes in vowel realizations, increased diphthongization (Dankovičová, Gurd, Marshall, et al., 2001; Fridriksson, Ryalls, Rorden, et al., 2005), consonant cluster reduction, consonant substitution and vowel epenthesis (Varley, Whiteside, Hammill, & Cooper, 2006) have all been observed. In addition, prosodic changes are documented for some cases of FAS (Monrad-Krohn, 1947; Varley, Whiteside, Hammill, & Cooper, 2006), and for some cases, segmental alterations such as vowel epenthesis can contribute to altered speech rhythm and prosodic changes (e.g. Varley, Whiteside, Hammill, & Cooper, 2006). Although prosodic changes are widely reported in FAS, these altered patterns vary from case to case. For example, the FAS subject reported by Monrad-Krohn (1947) displayed lexical overemphasis and the use of raised pitch (rather than an expected pattern of lowered pitch) for words in phrase-final position. However, Dankovičová, Gurd, Marshall, et al. (2001) report less significant prosodic changes in a patient with FAS, which highlights the variable constellation of segmental and suprasegmental characteristics which are present in FAS speech.

34.7.3   Processing prosody in individuals with left-hemisphere and right-hemisphere lesions

Because prosody signals both linguistic and emotional information, it provides a useful basis for exploring the traditional view of left-hemisphere dominance for linguistic processing vs. right-hemisphere dominance for the processing of emotion and affect. Several theories have been proposed on the roles of the left and right hemispheres in the processing of prosody. One hypothesis relates to functional lateralization (FLH for our purposes here); here, the left and right hemispheres are viewed as being primarily responsible for linguistic prosody and emotional prosody respectively. Another view is that the processing of prosody is stimulus driven ('cue lateralization hypothesis'; CLH for our purposes here), and that it relates to the lateralization of different acoustic cues; here individual acoustic cues to prosody are lateralized to different hemispheres so that frequency-determined acoustic cues such as fundamental frequency (F0) are processed by the right hemisphere (RH), whereas those that have a temporal component are processed by the left hemisphere (LH) (e.g. Van Lancker

& Sidtis, 1992). There is some direct evidence for CLH from neuroscientific studies which have investigated the processing of acoustic cues. For example, in a study by Zatorre and Belin, (2001) when participants were asked to make phonetic judgments of CVC syllables, which contain temporal and frequency changes, Broca's area was activated. However, when participants were required to make pitch judgments of the same CVC syllables, the right prefrontal area became activated, suggesting that hemispheric specialization for the perception of prosody may be stimulus-driven. This view is supported by behavioral (Brancucci, Babiloni, Rossini, & Romani, 2005) and imaging evidence (e.g. Liebenthal, Binder, Spitzer, Possing, & Medler, 2005).

However, the evidence on the organization and the processing of prosodic information in individuals with acquired brain damage presents a complex picture. Although there is evidence to support the FLH and CLH positions in studies of both RHD and LHD patients and the processing of linguistic and emotional prosody (Perkins Walker, Daigle, & Buzzard, 2002), there are individual differences in the nature, location and extent of brain lesions. This, coupled with the multidimensional nature of acoustic parameters which function in the processing of both linguistic and affective prosody, suggests that further research is required to develop and refine the FLH and CLH (see Baum & Pell, 1999, for a review). In addition, a substantial number of instrumental studies of prosodic processing have focused on the primary features of pitch (via fundamental frequency) and duration (e.g. Baum, 1998; Pell, 1998). Given the wide range of acoustic cues which have been identified in the processing of emotion and affect in healthy individuals (Banse & Scherer, 1996), this deserves further consideration in experimental studies of individuals who display impairments in the processing of affective and linguistic prosody.

34.8 Future Directions

Developmental and acquired disorders of spoken communication make up the bulk of the caseload of speech and language pathologists and are an important focus for research. A reliable picture of typical prosodic systems and their development is therefore very important. However, it is not at all easy to attain. Prosody is resistant to testing, and the measures used throw up large individual differences (cf. Peppé, Maxim, & Wells, 2000). While significant headway has been made on early prosodic development (e.g. Snow, 2006), much research remains to be done.

While the phonetic, linguistic, interactional and psycholinguistic approaches to prosodic impairment have been differentiated, it will be clear that they are interlocking. Phonetic observation and description of prosodic patterns remain the indispensable foundations on which a linguistic account, relating prosodic form to meaning, can be erected. Psycholinguistic investigations are themselves dependent on linguistic and phonetic expertise, notably in the construction of test stimuli, if they are to produce valid and reliable results.

Interactional analysis is an extension of the linguistic approach that takes account systematically of the place of utterances, and their prosodic components, within sequences of talk.

Group studies are important in establishing the prosodic components in particular clinical entities. However, case studies have a key role in the research endeavor, in generating hypotheses to be tested experimentally. Clinically, case studies can provide concrete suggestions as to how to identify and describe the prosodic difficulties of individual clients – an essential prerequisite for intervention.

REFERENCES

Banse, R. and Scherer, K. R. (1996). Acoustic profiles in vocal emotion expression. *Journal of Personality and Social Psychology*, 70(3), 614–36.

Barry, J. G., Blamey, P., Martin, L., Lee, K., Tang, T., Ming, Y. Y., and van Hasselt, C. (2002). Tone discrimination in Cantonese-speaking children using a cochlear implant. *Clinical Linguistics and Phonetics*, 16(2), 79–99.

Baum, S. R. (1998). The role of fundamental frequency and duration in the perception of linguistic stress by individuals with brain damage. *Journal of Speech, Language, and Hearing Research*, 41, 31–40.

Baum, S. R. and Pell, M. D. (1999). The neural bases of prosody: Insights from lesion studies and neuroimaging. *Aphasiology*, 13, 581–608.

Bishop, D. (1997). *Uncommon Understanding: Development and Disorders of Language Comprehension in Children*. Hove, Sussex: Psychology Press.

Brancucci, A., Babiloni, C., Rossini, P. M., and Romani, G. L. (2005). Right hemisphere specialization for intensity discrimination of musical and speech sounds. *Neuropsychologia*, 43, 1916–23.

Bunton, K., Kent, R. D., Kent, J. F., and Rosenbek, J. C. (2000). Perceptuo-acoustic assessment of prosodic impairment in dysarthria. *Clinical Linguistics and Phonetics*, 14, 13–24.

Catterall, C., Howard, S., Szczerbinski, M., Stojanovik, V., and Wells, B. (2006). Investigating prosody in Williams Syndrome. *Clinical Linguistics and Phonetics*, 20(7–8), 531–8.

Couper-Kuhlen, E. and Selting, M. (1996). *Prosody in Conversation: Interactional Studies*. Cambridge: Cambridge University Press.

Cruttenden, A. (1997). *Intonation*. 2nd ed. Cambridge: Cambridge University Press.

Crystal, D. (1987). *Clinical Linguistics*. 2nd ed. London: Edward Arnold.

Crystal, D. (1992). *Profiling Linguistic Disability*. 2nd ed. London: Whurr.

Dankovičová, J., Gurd, J. M., Marshall, J. C., MacMahon, M. K. C., Stuart-Smith, J., Coleman, J. S., and Slater, A. (2001). Aspects of non-native pronunciation in a case of altered accent following stroke (foreign accent syndrome). *Clinical Linguistics and Phonetics*, 15, 195–218.

Dankovičová, J., Pigott, K., Peppé, S., and Wells, B. (2004). Temporal markers of prosodic boundaries in children's speech production. *Journal of the International Phonetic Association*, 34, 17–36.

Emerson, C. S., Harrison, D. W., and Everhart, D. E. (1999). Investigation of receptive affective prosodic ability in school-aged boys with and without depression. *Neuropsychiatry, Neuropsychology, and Behavioral Neurology*, 12(2), 102–9.

Fourcin, A. (1986). Electrolaryngographic assessment of vocal fold function. *Journal of Phonetics*, 14, 435–42.

Fridriksson, J., Ryalls, J., Rorden, C., Morgan, P. S., George, M. S., and Baylis, G. C. (2005). Brain damage and cortical compensation in foreign accent syndrome. *Neurocase*, 11, 319–24.

Halliday, M. A. K. (1967). *Intonation and Grammar in British English*. The Hague: Mouton.

Heselwood, B., Bray, M., and Crookston, I. (1995). Juncture, rhythm and planning in the speech of an adult with Down's syndrome. *Clinical Linguistics and Phonetics*, 9(2), 121–37.

Ho, A. K., Iansek, R., and Bradshaw, J. L. (2001). Motor instability in Parkinsonian speech intensity. *Neuropsychiatry, Neuropsychology, and Behavioral Neurology*, 14, 109–16.

Kent, R. D. and Kim, Y.-J. (2003). Toward an acoustic typology of motor speech disorders. *Clinical Linguistics and Phonetics*, 17(6), 427–45.

Kent, R. D. and Rosenbek, J. C. (1983). Acoustic patterns of apraxia of speech. *Journal of Speech and Hearing Research*, 26, 231–49.

Ladd, D. R. (1996). *Intonational Phonology*. Cambridge: Cambridge University Press.

Levelt, W. (1989). *Speaking: From Intention to Articulation*. Cambridge, MA: MIT Press.

Liebenthal, E., Binder, J. R., Spitzer, S. M., Possing, E. T., and Medler, D. A. (2005). Neural substrates of phoneme perception. *Cerebral Cortex*, 15, 1621–31.

Local, J. and Wootton, T. (1995). Interactional and phonetic aspects of immediate echolalia in autism: A case study. *Clinical Linguistics and Phonetics*, 9, 155–84.

Lowit-Leuschel, A. and Docherty, G. J. (2001). Prosodic variation across sampling tasks in normal and dysarthric speakers. *Logopaedics, Phoniatrics and Vocology*, 26, 151–64.

McCann, J. and Peppé, S. (2003). Prosody in autism spectrum disorders: A critical review. *International Journal of Language and Communication Disorders*, 38, 325–50.

Monrad-Krohn, G. H. (1947). Dysprosody or altered 'melody of language'. *Brain*, 70, 405–15.

Odell, K. H. and Shriberg, L. D. (2001). Prosody-voice characteristics of children and adults with apraxia of speech. *Clinical Linguistics and Phonetics*, 15, 275–307.

Paul, R., Augustyn, A., Klin, A., and Volkmar, F. R. (2005). Perception and production of prosody by speakers with autism spectrum disorders. *Journal of Autism and Developmental Disorders*, 35, 205–20.

Pell, M. D. (1998). Recognition of prosody following unilateral brain lesion: Influence of functional and structural attributes of prosodic contours. *Neuropsychologia*, 36, 701–15.

Peppé, S., Maxim, J., and Wells, B. (2000). Prosodic variation in Southern British English. *Language and Speech*, 43(3), 309–34.

Peppé, S., McCann, J., Gibbon, F., O'Hare, A., and Rutherford, M. (2006). Assessing prosodic and pragmatic ability in children with high-functioning autism. *Journal of Pragmatics*, 38, 1776–91.

Peppé, S., McCann, J., Gibbon, F., O'Hare, A., and Rutherford, M. (2007). Receptive and expressive prosody in children with high-functioning autism. *Journal of Speech, Language, and Hearing Research*, 50, 1015–28.

Perkins Walker, J., Daigle, T., and Buzzard, M. (2002). Hemispheric specialisation in processing prosodic structures: Revisited. *Aphasiology*, 16, 1155–72.

Rosen, K. M., Kent, R. D., and Duffy, J. R. (2005). Task-based profile of vocal intensity decline in Parkinson's disease. *Folia Phoniatrica et Logopaedica*, 57, 28–37.

Ross, J. L., Stefanatos, G., Roeltgen, D., Kushner, H., and Cutler, G. B. (1995). Ullrich–Turner syndrome: Neurodevelopmental changes from childhood through adolescence. *American Journal of Medical Genetics*, 58(1), 74–82.

Samuelsson, C. and Nettelbladt, U. (2004). Prosodic problems in Swedish children with language impairment: towards a classification of subgroups. *International Journal of Language and Communication Disorders*, 39(3), 325–44.

Shriberg, L., Aram, D., and Kwiatkowski, J. (1997). Developmental apraxia of speech: III. A subtype marked by inappropriate stress. *Journal of Speech, Language, and Hearing Research*, 40, 313–37.

Snow, D. (1998). Prosodic markers of syntactic boundaries in the speech of four-year-old children with normal and disordered language development. *Journal of Speech, Language, and Hearing Research*, 41, 1158–70.

Snow, D. (2001). Imitations of intonation contours by children with normal and disordered language development. *Clinical Linguistics and Phonetics*, 15(7), 567–84.

Snow, D. (2006). Regression and reorganization of intonation between 6 and 23 months. *Child Development*, 77(2), 281–96.

Tarplee, C. and Barrow, E. (1999). Delayed echoing as an interactional resource: A case study of a 3-year-old child on the autistic spectrum. *Clinical Linguistics and Phonetics* 13(6), 449–82.

Vance, J. (1994). Prosodic deviation in dysarthria: A case study. *European Journal of Disorders of Communication*, 29, 61–76.

Van der Meulen, S., Janssen, P., and Den Os, E. (1997). Prosodic abilities in children with specific language impairment. *Journal of Communication Disorders*, 30, 155–70.

Van Lancker, D. and Sidtis, J. (1992). The identification of affective-prosodic stimuli by left- and right-hemisphere-damaged subjects: All errors are not created equal. *Journal of Speech and Hearing Research*, 35, 963–70.

Van Putten, S. M. and Walker, J. P. (2003). The production of emotional prosody in varying degrees of severity of apraxia of speech. *Journal of Communication Disorders*, 36, 77–95.

Varley, R. A. and Whiteside, S. P. (2001). What is the underlying impairment in acquired apraxia of speech? *Aphasiology*, 15, 39–49.

Varley, R., Whiteside, S., Hammill, C., and Cooper, K. (2006). Phases in speech encoding and foreign accent syndrome. *Journal of Neurolinguistics*, 19, 356–69.

Weinert, S. (1996). Prosodie–Gedächtnis–Geschwindigkeit: Eine vergleichende Studie zu Sprachverarbeitungsdefiziten dysphasisch-sprachgestörter Kinder. *Sprache and Kognition*, 15(1–2), 46–69.

Weinert, S. and Mueller, C. (1996). Erleichtert eine akzentuierte Sprachmelodie die Sprachverarbeitung? Eine Untersuchung zur Verarbeitung rhythmisch-prosodischer Informationen bei dysphasisch-sprachgestörten Kindern. *Zeitschrift für Entwicklungspsychologie und Pädagogische Psychologie*, 28(3), 228–56.

Wells, B. and Local, J. (1993). The sense of an ending: A case of prosodic delay. *Clinical Linguistics and Phonetics*, 7(1), 59–73.

Wells, B. and Peppé, S. (2001). Intonation within a psycholinguistic framework. In J. Stackhouse and B. Wells (eds.), *Children's Speech and Literacy Difficulties. 2: Identification and Intervention*. London: Whurr Publishers.

Wells, B. and Peppé, S. (2003). Intonation abilities of children with speech and language impairments. *Journal of Speech, Language, and Hearing Research*, 46, 5–20.

Wells, B., Peppé, S., and Goulandris, A. (2004). Intonation development from five to thirteen. *Journal of Child Language*, 31, 749–78.

Whiteside, S. P. and Varley, R. A. (1998). A reconceptualisation of apraxia of speech. *Cortex*, 34, 221–31.

Zatorre, R. J. and Belin, P. (2001). Spectral and temporal processing in human auditory cortex. *Cerebral Cortex*, 11, 946–53.

35   Speech Intelligibility

GARY WEISMER

35.1   Introduction: What is Speech Intelligibility?

The concept of speech intelligibility has for many years been central to studies of speech communication in both normal speakers and speakers with various types of speech disorders. Speech intelligibility measures, originally developed in the 1920s to assess the quality of telephone transmission systems, consisted of syllable, word, or sentence tests in which the proportion of correctly identified items was taken as an estimate of 'true' speech intelligibility. This basic line of reasoning is still in practice today, not only in evaluation of speech transmission systems but, as the topic of this chapter suggests, in the evaluation of a speaker's ability to communicate when he or she has some type of speech disorder.

When the original speech intelligibility tests were being refined at Bell Laboratories and Harvard University between the 1920s and the 1940s (see Egan, 1948; and review in French & Steinberg, 1947), a major concern was to limit potential influences on intelligibility measures to those associated with the speech acoustic signal. Factors including linguistic cues, gesture, and visual information associated with movements of the speech mechanism were known to have an impact on speech intelligibility, but the desired estimate was a purified one in which the clarities of consonants and vowels were the only contributing variables. The *articulation index*, a statistical model of the predictability of speech intelligibility scores from speech acoustic characteristics (see French & Steinberg, 1947), emphasized this 'pure' view of the process and has influenced contemporary models of speech intelligibility in speech disorders, as reviewed below. This index, generated from the spectral characteristics of isolated syllables (e.g., of CV form) and from certain other factors such as overall signal level and degree of distortion in the transmission medium, typically varies between 0.0 and 1.0, where zero equals complete unintelligibility and unity equals perfect intelligibility.

As a baseline for understanding the effectiveness of communication, an articulation index approach to speech intelligibility is a good starting point. As pointed out by French and Steinberg (1947), however, such an evaluation is not particularly useful unless it can be applied to real-world situations. There is some limited evidence for normal speakers that the quality of their acoustic-phonetic signals distinguishes their marginally different speech intelligibilities (Bradlow, Torretta, & Pisoni, 1996), but in the case of speakers with disorders the situation is decidedly more complicated.

Thus a straightforward answer to the question 'What is speech intelligibility?' is not immediately apparent. As summarized by Licklider and Miller (1951) long before such measures were used as an index or explanation of speech disorders, speech intelligibility depends minimally on speaker characteristics, speech material, specifics of the listening medium, and listener characteristics. In the history of work on speech intelligibility in persons with speech disorders, speaker characteristics have been studied most often, but some attention has been paid to speech materials (see the empirical work of Monsen, 1983; and reviews in Sell, 2005; Whitehill, 2002) and more recently to the listener's contribution to intelligibility deficits (e.g., Klasner & Yorkston, 2005; Liss, Spitzer, Caviness, & Adler, 2002; Liss, Spitzer, Caviness, Adler, & Edwards, 2000; Monsen, 1983).

For now, we will offer a tentative answer to the question 'What is speech intelligibility?' by distilling comments of Monsen (1983) that he based on his study of speech intelligibility in persons with hearing impairment. Speech intelligibility is a *relative* measure of the degree to which a speaker's speech signal is understood, the relativity depending at a minimum on the identities of speaker and listener, what is spoken and where it is spoken. Thus a particular degree of speech intelligibility – for example, a speaker who is said to be 75 percent intelligible – is not interpretable unless a good deal of additional information is available. In the present chapter, we will turn a necessarily selective focus on different measures of speech intelligibility and their interpretation. Most specifically, our interest is in the use of speech intelligibility measures to understand the underlying communication disorder, rather than as a simple index of the magnitude of the disorder. Citations of several review papers are made throughout this brief essay, many of which provide information on other topics relevant to speech intelligibility among persons with speech disorders.

35.2 Measures of Speech Intelligibility

Measures of intelligibility for speech disorders can be divided into four broad classes. The first of these involves a forced-choice format, much like the diagnostic rhyme tests used in standard assessments of intelligibility (e.g., House, Williams, Hecker, & Kryter, 1965); we refer to these as 'feature-analytic' measures because they are presumed to allow specification of the underlying reasons, in terms of reduced, distorted, or lost articulatory contrasts, for an intelligibility deficit. A second class includes transcription measures, which can take the form of orthographic renderings of single word and/or sentence utterances (Yorkston & Beukelman, 1981), or phonetic transcriptions of target segments or syllables (Sell, Grunwell, Mildenhall, et al., 2001). A third class of measures requires the assignment of a numerical scale value to an utterance, whether it is single words, phrases, or even extended passages spanning several phrases (Schiavetti, 1992). The fourth and final class of measures is the rarest, and involves an inference of speech intelligibility from a related measure such as a listener's accuracy in answering questions based on a speaker's utterances, or some other measure of speech involvement (such as severity) assumed to reflect a speaker's 'true' intelligibility (see Beukelman & Yorkston, 1979; Klasner & Yorkston, 2005). The remainder of this essay will be devoted primarily to feature-analytic and transcription measures of intelligibility, because these are the ones most often associated with explanation of intelligibility deficits.

35.2.1   Feature-analytic measures

Speech intelligibility for speakers with disorders has often been evaluated using single-word materials. Single-word tests, such as those described by Kent, Weismer, Kent, and Rosenbek (1989), Yorkston and Beukelman (1978), Liu, Tsao, and Kuhl (2005), Hazan and Markham (2004), Whitehill and Chau (2004), and Monsen (1981), are typically developed for a particular population or application. For example, Kent, Weismer, Kent, and Rosenbek (1989) developed a single-word, forced-choice test designed to probe phonetic contrasts known or strongly suspected to be vulnerable to the effects of neuromotor diseases. Each of 19 phonetic contrasts was represented by at least one target word and three foils, each of which differed from the target by a single feature. Each of the 19 contrasts was also supported by an acoustic measurement, well attested in the literature on normal speech production and presumed to apply more or less in the same way among speakers with dysarthria. For example, the phonetic contrast of word-initial voicing for stops was represented by a target such as *bad* and a foil *pad*, and supported acoustically by voice onset time (VOT) measures. In a sense the contrast-based test construction represented a hypothesis, that speakers with roughly the same intelligibility deficit expressed as a percentage of correctly heard words might nevertheless have very different reasons for their scores. More specifically, a *phonetic contrast error profile* could be derived from this test, for each speaker, and those contrasts most frequently in error would best 'explain' the intelligibility deficit (Weismer & Martin, 1992; see Boothroyd, 1985, and Whitehill, 2002, for similar approaches for speakers with hearing impairment and cleft palate respectively). A clinician could take these contrasts and target them in therapy, as their remediation would be expected to have a high-yield effect on overall intelligibility. Moreover, the frequently occurring contrast errors may differ for different types of disorders (e.g., types of dysarthria, cleft, or hearing loss, and even different speakers within a disorder type).

Other single-word intelligibility tests constructed on the same or similar principles include one described by Liu, Tsao, and Kuhl (2005), who were interested in the relationship between the size of the acoustic vowel space (see Turner, Tjaden, & Weismer, 1995) and vowel and word intelligibility among Mandarin-speaking persons with cerebral palsy. Liu and colleagues developed a word test incorporating the vowels of interest /i/, /a/, /u/ and correlated the acoustic spaces derived from the first two formants of these vowels with intelligibility scores. This vowel-specific word test allowed the investigators to calculate both segment-level (that is, vowel) and word-level intelligibility scores. Other selected examples of combined segment and word intelligibility tests specially constructed for specific populations have been published by Jeng, Weismer, and Kent (2006) for Mandarin speakers with dysarthria, Whitehill and Chau (2004) for Cantonese speakers with cleft palate, and Rogers and Dalby (2005) for native Mandarin speakers producing English as a second language.

In the original incarnation of speech intelligibility tests, in which attributes of the signal (spectrum and overall loudness) and the transmission channel (noisiness and distortion) could be linked directly to variation in the percentage of words heard correctly, the magnitude of an intelligibility score had a straightforward meaning. In early versions of intelligibility testing in persons with speech disorders (e.g., Tikofsky & Tikofsky, 1964; see reviews in Kent, Miolo, & Bloedel, 1994, and Weismer & Martin, 1992), the score was viewed as an objective index of speech involvement, preferable to a qualitative judgment or coarse-grained measurement such as 'highly intelligible' vs. 'somewhat intelligible', and so forth. Monsen's (1983) careful analysis of the relative nature of speech intelligibility scores in persons with hearing impairment pointed to one significant weakness of these simple indices of severity, and prompted investigators to design the kinds of tests described above to produce data more relevant to the specifics of intelligibility deficits. The construction of each of these tests was therefore motivated by an expectation of enhancing the interpretation of intelligibility scores. The desired enhancement was to generate from the test explanatory observations concerning an intelligibility deficit.

Single-word intelligibility tests constructed in a rhyme-test format, as well as segment-specific intelligibility tests, can be criticized for a number of reasons, some logical and others empirical. For example, Ziegler and Hartmann (1996) noted that single-word, multiple-choice tests may not reveal real differences among speakers who have the ability to produce fairly intelligible, isolated word forms even if they are substantially more unintelligible in connected speech. If the typical perception of connected speech is largely geared toward rapid and efficient lexical access based on word-boundary identification (e.g., Luce & McLennan, 2005; Stevens, 2002), a single-word test may tap a listening strategy very different from that used in typical communication (see Liss, Spitzer, Caviness, Adler, & Edwards, 1998, 2000; Liss, Spitzer, Caviness, & Adler, 2002). A second problem concerns the test materials, and specifically the way in which contrasts are represented by target–foil pairs. Weismer and Martin (1992) were the first to suggest possible biases in these kinds of tests, as a result of either uneven representation of phonetic contrasts across the word list or lack of symmetry in the assessment of a given contrast. Whereas some authors (e.g., Whitehill & Chau, 2004, p. 345) have argued that a differential representation of contrast examples within a test should not affect the contrast error results, an empirical evaluation of this issue is not available in the literature. The symmetry issue is (according to current opinion) a more serious concern. When a contrast such as 'initial stop voicing' is included in these tests, directionality is not specified and the unstated assumption is that there will be as many errors in one direction (e.g., voiced for voiceless) as the other (voiceless for voiced). Phonemic errors derived from perceptual analyses, however, are known to be asymmetrical for many contrasts (e.g., see confusion matrices in Miller & Nicely, 1955), and the few relevant analyses for errors produced by persons with speech disorders suggest the same phenomenon (see Niemi, Koivuselkä-Sallinen, & Hänninen, 1985; Platt, Andrews, & Howie, 1980). This problem is compounded in tests such as Kent, Weismer, Kent, and Rosenbek (1989) and Whitehill and Chau (2004), where the test items and their foils do not allow equal opportunities for errors in either direction. In simple terms, the structure of the tests may create biases in the types and frequencies of observed contrast errors. The evidence and nature of such biases is currently unknown.

An indirect manifestation of these biases may be found in work reported by Bunton and Weismer (2001, 2002). Errors from the high–low vowel, stop voicing, and glottal–null word-onset contrasts produced by speakers with dysarthria were evaluated for correspondence with the speech acoustic signal. For example, a high-for-low vowel error (*bit* chosen instead of target *bat*) would be predicted to result from a first formant frequency lower than expected for a low-front vowel; similarly, a null-for-/h/ error (as in *at* chosen for target *hat*) would be expected to have minimal or absent /h/ noise preceding the vowel. Surprisingly, Bunton and Weismer (2001, 2002) failed to find systematic correspondences between the well-attested acoustic manifestations of these contrasts and the phonetic contrast errors derived from the multiple-choice intelligibility test of Kent, Weismer, Kent, and Rosenbek (1989). This counterintuitive finding did not seem to be the result of poorly or incompletely measured speech signals; rather, it seemed the availability of a choice close to the target may have biased listeners to select it when the actual production was a 'noisy', but not incorrect, version of the target segment. Consider the following scenario from the Kent, Weismer, Kent, and Rosenbek (1989) test: The target word *geese* has the foils *goose*, *guess*, and *gas*, the second and third of which are probes for the high–low vowel contrast. A speaker produces *geese* with a poor version of /i/, but not a version that would be transcribed as /ɛ/ or /æ/ by an expert phonetician. The question is: Will a listener be more likely to select *guess* or *gas* in response to a poor /i/ in *geese* simply because they are options? Would the response patterns change if the foils were different – the most extreme case being if there were no high–low vowel contrast options? Bunton and Weismer (2001) reported a small-scale experiment that seemed to support the idea of the test foils distorting the real perceptual phenomena. Words in which high–low vowel errors were made in the multiple choice test were transcribed phonetically, with no choices available to the listener other than the symbols known to be used in the International Phonetic Alphabet (International Phonetic Association, 1999). The transcription exercise revealed vowel segments different from the ones selected in the multiple-choice format. This finding – and it is a tentative one – suggests caution in interpreting the phonetic basis of an intelligibility deficit when it is derived from the kind of multiple-choice tests under discussion.

35.2.2   *Transcription measures*

Intelligibility estimates can be derived from orthographic or phonetic transcriptions. Orthographic transcription of either word or sentence material is the basis for one well-known intelligibility test (Yorkston & Beukelman, 1981). Relatively infrequent use has been made of phonetic transcription to generate or understand intelligibility scores, but examples can be found in the literature on developmental speech delay (e.g., Shriberg, Flipsen, Kwiatkowski, & McSweeny, 2003; Yavas & Lamprecht, 1988), motor speech disorders in adults (Platt, Andrews, Young, & Quinn, 1980), and cleft palate (Sell, Grunwell, Mildenhall, et al., 2001).

Orthographic transcription measures have been used to generate intelligibility indices of severity, especially in sentence intelligibility tests that express transcribed word accuracy as a percentage of the total number of words in the sentence material (e.g., Yorkston & Beukelman, 1981). The purpose of such a measure is to have a metric of speech involvement, presumably reflecting the magnitude of a patient's functional impairment. Sentence measures obtained in this way from speakers with dysarthria have been shown to correspond fairly well with single-word intelligibility scores and various psychophysical estimates of intelligibility across speakers with varying levels of speech involvement (Hustad, 2006; Platt, Andrews, Young, & Quinn, 1980; Yorkston & Beukelman, 1978). As pointed out by Yunusova, Weismer, Kent, and Rusche (2005), however, such correlations between different kinds of speech material or different measurement scales are not surprising, as any and all measures of speech intelligibility are likely to be correlated with overall severity of involvement, and thus with each other. Such correlations are likely to be high especially when speakers are chosen to span a wide range of speech intelligibilities as in Yorkston and Beukelman (1978). In her extensive review of intelligibility studies in persons with cleft palate, Whitehill (2002) does not mention studies comparing transcriptional measures of word and sentence intelligibility across speakers, or between scaled and transcribed intelligibility, but if such studies used speakers with widely ranging intelligibilities, high correlations between measures using different speech materials or measurement approaches would be expected.

35.3   Predicting Speech Intelligibility

35.3.1   *Segmental articulation and intelligibility*

A number of investigators have been interested in the predictability of speech intelligibility from error analyses derived from phonetic transcription. The more specific question seems to be: To what extent do the number and/or type of errors predict a speaker's intelligibility? An early, indirect answer to this question for speakers with dysarthria associated with cerebral palsy was reported by Platt, Andrews, Young, and Quinn (1980) who noted that even with an average single-word speech intelligibility of only 50 percent, 78 percent of consonants and vowels within intelligibility test words were transcribed as 'correct'. This curious finding may reflect, in part, a difference between the expertise of the phonetic transcriptionist and the naive listeners who responded to the single-word test. Whitehill (2002, pp. 50–1), however, in her review of work on correspondences between articulatory errors and speech intelligibility among speakers with cleft palate, notes some studies showing a close relation between the two measures but others showing somewhat surprising and contradictory dissociations. For example, Subtelny, van Hattum and Myers (1972) found that among a group of speakers with velopharyngeal incompetence (VPI) and phonetic errors judged as 'severe', only a few were judged to have unintelligible speech. This is reminiscent of the findings of Platt, Andrews, Young, and Quinn (1980), but reversed: the speakers with dysarthria in that study had better phoneme scores than intelligibility scores! Earlier work by Subtelny (Subtelny, Koepp-Baker, & Subtelny, 1961; Subtelny & Subtelny, 1959) had shown strong correlations between stop but not fricative errors and speech intelligibility in speakers with VPI associated with cleft palate. Hardin, Lachenbruch, and Morris (1986), however, found the proportion of correctly produced fricatives to be the *best* predictor of scaled speech proficiency for a group of females with VPI.

  The relationship of segmental integrity to speech intelligibility has also been investigated in developmental phonological disorders. Weston and Shriberg (1992) summarized the evidence on correlational relations between speech intelligibility and the number of correctly articulated segments, and concluded that the shared variance was typically no more than 20 percent. A similar indeterminate relationship seems to emerge from the literature on type and frequency of phonological processes and speech intelligibility among children with either typical or atypical developmental speech errors. Even when there is evidence of a strong relationship between number of segmental errors and speech intelligibility, as in Smith's (1975) well-known study of speech intelligibility of hearing-impaired children, individual children show dissociations between number of segmental errors and speech intelligibility.

If we reflect on the original goal of speech intelligibility tests, the dissociation between segmental errors and speech intelligibility may, at first glance, seem confusing. After all, speech intelligibility tests were meant to reflect *only* segmental integrity, as influenced by characteristics of the transmission channel. Clearly, speakers with disorders have segmental articulation problems as a prominent if not dominant feature of their communication deficit, so why do their segmental measures correlate only weakly with speech intelligibility? One explanation is that the highly controlled transmission-channel characteristics – presentation level, distortion, and frequency response – of the original speech intelligibility tests are augmented or replaced in speech disorders by other factors not under experimental control and, in some cases, lacking measurement specificity. A whole host of phonetic and linguistic variables, including at a minimum position-induced allophonic variation, context, voice quality, prosody, *speaker* voice level, and speaking rate, cannot be controlled when a speaker with a disorder produces single words, sentences, or a connected discourse. Moreover, the proper physical measurements for many prosodic variables and even some segmental contrasts are unknown or unclear, at least with respect to their possible contribution to speech intelligibility (Weismer & Martin, 1992). The dissociations between segmental integrity and speech intelligibility shown for speakers with various disorders should therefore not be considered surprising, but rather as a research challenge. Speech intelligibility in persons with speech disorders is a different entity than the speech intelligibility evaluations developed as an index of communication channels. Monsen's (1983) invocation of the speech intelligibility of speakers with hearing impairment as an indeterminate quantity in the absence of very specific information about test detail must be kept in mind for all speech disorders.

35.3.2 Multiple regression models of speech intelligibility

There is an interesting intersection between feature-analytic and transcription measures of speech intelligibility, which reveals a contradiction to the equivocal findings on segmental articulation and speech intelligibility measures. As reviewed above, transcription measures of segmental articulation relate to speech intelligibility in a very inconsistent way, yet when feature-analytic measures or their acoustic underpinnings are used to predict speech intelligibility the results are surprisingly positive. Several studies have used multiple variables to develop regression models of speech intelligibility; selected results for speakers with hearing impairment, dysarthria, and cleft palate are shown in table 35.1. Some studies have used acoustic measures to predict intelligibility (Ansel & Kent, 1992; Metz, Samar, Schiavetti, Sitler, & Whitehead, 1985; Monsen, 1978), others a measure of contrast error rate (or correct transmission) derived from a multiple-choice feature-analytic test (Liu et al., 2000; Weismer

& Martin, 1992; Whitehill & Chau, 2004; Whitehill & Ciocca, 2000). In either case a fairly large group of acoustic or phonetic contrast variables was studied, but a linear combination of only a very small subset accounted for a large proportion of the variance in speech intelligibility scores. In fact, across the studies listed in table 35.1, no more than three variables made significant contributions to the variance in speech intelligibility, and typically *one* variable (the first variable entered into the model) accounted for 50–90 percent of the variance, with the succeeding second and sometimes third variables making more modest contributions to the overall multiple regression solution. Studies using phonetic contrast variables typically produced better prediction of intelligibility scores than those using acoustic variables. This collection of results seems the more remarkable because of variation across studies in disorder type, language, participants, and measures of speech intelligibility; the constant is the wildly successful prediction result. The contradiction to the equivocal results of segmental integrity as a predictor of speech intelligibility is that the phonetic contrast or acoustic variables used in the multiple regression solutions summarized in table 35.1 are reflections of segmental articulation.

Examination of the significant acoustic measures or phonetic contrasts in table 35.1 suggests a variety of segmental, articulatory phenomena that seem to 'explain' intelligibility deficits. The differences across studies in the specific variables that entered into significant multiple regression solutions could, in theory, be explained partially on the basis of different disorder types – that is, each speech disorder requires a unique solution – or of different languages

Table 35.1 Summary of selected studies in which multiple regression models of speech intelligibility have been reported

Study	*S*	*%*	*Significant variables*
Monsen (1978)	HI	73	{t–d VOT; F2 dif. /i/–/u/; nasal/ liquid quality}
Metz et al. (1985)	HI	84	{k–g VOT; sentence duration}
Ansel & Kent (1992)	D	62	{cons. noise duration; F1/F2; vowel duration}
Weismer & Martin (1992)	D	91	{alv. vs. pal. fric.; stop–nasal}
Liu et al. (2000)	D	99	{asp.–unasp cons.; fric.–affric; front–back vowels}
Whitehill & Ciocca (2000)	D	92	{glottal–null; final cons.–null; long–short vowel}
Whitehill & Chau (2004)	ClP	91	{stop–fric; initial–null; affric.–glide}

S = Speaker type (HI = speakers with hearing impairment; D = speakers with dysarthria; ClP = speakers with cleft palate); dif. = difference; cons. = consonant; alv. = alveolar, pal. = palatal; asp. = aspirated, unasp. = unaspirated; fric. = fricative, affric. = affricate.

with their inherently different systems of phonetic contrasts (Mandarin, Cantonese, and English are represented in table 35.1). There is, however, another way to interpret the data in table 35.1, nicely captured by Carney's (1986, p. 52) summary of Monsen's 1978 work: "Monsen's analysis indicated that correct production of these few phonemes per se is not the source of the intelligibility; rather, the presence of these acoustic features suggests that a given speaker has achieved a certain level of articulatory skill."

Weismer and Martin (1992) and Weismer, Jeng, Laures, and Kent (2001) have raised similar concerns about phonetic or acoustic measures and their correlation with speech intelligibility. The extensive intercorrelations *among* the full set of predictor variables in a given study make it difficult to interpret the specific meaning of the few variables that are significant predictors of speech intelligibility (see Weismer & Martin, 1992, tables 3 & 4; also Metz, Samar, Schiavetti, Sitler, & Whitehead, 1985), and the frequent finding of a *single* predictor variable that accounts for so much of the variance in speech intelligibility does not make theoretical sense. For example, in Liu et al.'s (2000) study of phonetic contrasts and speech intelligibility among Mandarin-speaking persons with cerebral palsy and dysarthria, the aspiration–unaspiration contrast accounted for 95 percent of the variance in speech intelligibility scores. Similarly, Metz and colleagues (1985) found that the voice onset time (VOT) difference between /k/ and /g/ accounted for 67 percent of the variance in speech intelligibility for key words in sentence context produced by persons with hearing impairment. It is difficult to imagine a theoretical account of why either of these specific variables would contribute so heavily and independently to intelligibility deficits. More difficult still is a coherent account for the substantial and independent contribution in Metz, Samar, Schiavetti, Sitler, and Whitehead (1985) of the /k/–/g/ VOT difference to speech intelligibility, but *not* the VOT differences for /p/–/b/ or /t/–/d/, which were included in the full set of predictor variables but not selected in the stepwise regression analysis. The underlying speech physiology for the stop voicing distinction in English is common to all places of articulation (Weismer, 2006), so why would the /k/–/g/ VOT difference be chosen independently as a major predictor of speech intelligibility deficits?

Weismer, Jeng, Laures, & Kent (2001), following Monsen (1978) and Carney (1985), argue that significant predictor variables cannot be assumed to be *componential* to speech intelligibility. Rather, the phonetic contrast and acoustic predictor measures seem to be general and interchangeable expressions for severity of articulatory involvement ('articulatory skill', in Carney's terms). Stated otherwise, the set of predictor variables in any given study will all covary with across-speaker variation in severity of speech involvement. The typical experimental approach to determining the explanatory basis of speech intelligibility deficits, in which the study group consists of speakers who vary widely in speech intelligibility, cannot avoid this interpretive ambiguity precisely because of the variation in speaker severity. The only direct approach to identifying the true phonetic (or suprasegmental) components of speech intelligibility is to train selected contrasts within persons who have a speech intelligibility deficit and demonstrate that changes in the 'goodness' of the trained contrast account for increments in intelligibility; untrained control contrasts that do not change across the training must also be employed to make this experiment fully interpretable. An alternate approach to demonstrating true components of speech intelligibility is the use of speech resynthesis to create parametric variations in acoustic characteristics previously shown to be atypical in speech disorders and covariate with across-speaker speech intelligibility. Resynthesis adjustments in the more 'normal' direction should result in speech intelligibility improvements (e.g., see Maassen & Povel, 1984a, 1984b, 1985); adjustments in the opposite direction should make the speech signals less intelligible (Laures & Weismer, 1999).

35.4   Summary

Contemporary studies of speech intelligibility in speech disorders have moved past the use of measures as simple indices of severity and developed tests designed to explain the intelligibility deficit. Following the model of original speech intelligibility tests, 'explanatory' tests have been constructed to reveal the contribution of segmental articulatory characteristics to an intelligibility score. Such a finding would be very similar to the original concept of the articulation index, used to evaluate the intelligibility characteristics of a transmission system. The actual data collected to date, however, point to an intriguing contradiction: when counts or types of segmental articulatory errors are correlated with speech intelligibility deficits, the results are at best equivocal and sometimes frankly contradictory. But when multiple regression models are developed, using phonetic-contrast variables or acoustic measures of those contrasts, a very small number of the variables account for a huge proportion of the variance in intelligibility scores. The multiple regression results, in the present view, are difficult to interpret in theoretical terms and most likely artifacts of the intercorrelations among the predictor variables and their mutual correlation with severity of speaker involvement. More specific studies, involving training of phonetic contrasts and evaluation of speech intelligibility pre- and post-training, are needed to determine the true, underlying components of speech intelligibility in persons with speech disorders. Moreover, it is likely that such studies will reveal a good portion of unexplained variance related to non-segmental factors such as prosody, visual information, and other factors that cannot be captured in simple articulation-oriented test instruments.

REFERENCES

Ansel, B. M. and Kent, R. D. (1992). Acoustic-phonetic contrasts and intelligibility in the dysarthria associated with mixed cerebral palsy. *Journal of Speech and Hearing Research*, 35, 296–308.

Beukelman, D. R. and Yorkston, K. M. (1979). The relationship between information transfer and speech intelligibility of dysarthric speakers. *Journal of Communication Disorders*, 12, 189–96.

Boothroyd, A. (1985). Evaluation of speech production of the hearing impaired: Some benefits of forced-choice testing. *Journal of Speech and Hearing Research*, 28, 185–96.

Bradlow, A. R., Torretta, G. M., and Pisoni, D. B. (1996). Intelligibility of normal speech I: Global and fine-grained acoustic-phonetic talker characteristics. *Speech Communication*, 20, 255–72.

Bunton, K. and Weismer, G. (2001). The relationship between perception and acoustics for a high–low vowel contrast produced by dysarthric speakers. *Journal of Speech, Language, and Hearing Research*, 44, 1215–28.

Bunton, K. and Weismer, G. (2002). Segmental level analysis of laryngeal function in persons with motor speech disorders. *Folia Phoniatrica et Logopaedica*, 54, 223–39.

Carney, A. E. (1986). Understanding speech intelligibility in the hearing impaired. *Topics in Language Disorders*, 6, 47–59.

Egan, J. (1948). Articulation testing methods. *Laryngoscope*, 58, 955–91.

French, N. R. and Steinberg, J. C. (1947). Factors governing the intelligibility of speech sounds. *Journal of the Acoustical Society of America*, 19, 90–119.

Hardin, M. A., Lachenbruch, P. A., and Morris, H. L. (1986). Contribution of selected variables to the prediction of speech proficiency for adolescents with cleft lip and palate. *Cleft Palate Journal*, 23, 10–23.

Hazan, V. and Markham, D. (2004). Acoustic-phonetic correlates of talker intelligibility for adults and children. *Journal of the Acoustical Society of America*, 116, 3108–18.

House, A. S., Williams, C. E., Hecker, M. H. L., and Kryter, K. D. (1965). Articulation-testing methods: Consonantal differentiation with a closed-response set. *Journal of the Acoustical Society of America*, 37, 158–66.

Hustad, K. C. (2006). Estimating the intelligibility of speakers with dysarthria. *Folia Phoniatrica et Logopaedica*, 58, 217–28.

International Phonetic Association (1999). *Handbook of the International Phonetic Association*. Cambridge: Cambridge University Press.

Jeng, J-Y., Weismer, G., and Kent, R. D. (2006). Production and perception of mandarin tone in adults with cerebral palsy. *Clinical Linguistics and Phonetics*, 20, 67–87.

Kent, R. D., Miolo, G., and Bloedel, S. (1994). The intelligibility of children's speech: A review of evaluation procedures. *American Journal of Speech-Language Pathology*, 3, 81–95.

Kent, R. D., Weismer, G., Kent, J. F., and Rosenbek, J. L. (1989). Toward explanatory intelligibility testing in dysarthria. *Journal of Speech and Hearing Disorders*, 54, 482–99.

Klasner, E. R. and Yorkston, K. M. (2005). Speech intelligibility in ALS and HD dysarthria: The everyday listener's perspective. *Journal of Medical Speech-Language Pathology*, 13, 127–39.

Laures, J. and Weismer, G. (1999). The effects of a flattened fundamental frequency on intelligibility at the sentence level. *Journal of Speech, Language, and Hearing Research*, 42, 1148–56.

Licklider, J. C. R. and Miller, G. A. (1951). The perception of speech. In S. S. Stevens (ed.), *Handbook of Experimental Psychology* (pp. 1040–74). New York: John Wiley and Sons.

Liss, J. M., Spitzer, S., Caviness, J. N., and Adler, C. (2002). The effects of familiarization on intelligibility and lexical segmentation in hypokinetic and ataxic dysarthria. *Journal of the Acoustical Society of America*, 112, 3022–30.

Liss, J. M., Spitzer, S., Caviness, J. N., Adler, C., and Edwards, B. (1998). Syllabic strength and lexical boundary decisions in the perception of hypokinetic dysarthric speech. *Journal of the Acoustical Society of America*, 104, 2457–66.

Liss, J. M., Spitzer, S., Caviness, J. N., Adler, C., and Edwards, B. (2000). Lexical boundary error analysis in hypokinetic and ataxic dysarthria. *Journal of the Acoustical Society of America*, 107, 3415–24.

Liu, H-M., Tsao, F-M., and Kuhl, P. K. (2005). The effect of reduced vowel working space on speech intelligibility in Mandarin-speaking young adults with cerebral palsy. *Journal of the Acoustical Society of America*, 117, 3879–89.

Liu, H. M., Tseng, C. H., and Tsao, F. M. (2000). Perceptual and acoustic analysis of speech intelligibility in Mandarin-speaking young adults with cerebral palsy. *Clinical Linguistics and Phonetics*, 14, 447–64.

Luce, P. A. and McLennan, C. T. (2005). Spoken word recognition: The challenge of variation. In D. B. Pisoni and R. E. Remez (eds.), *The Handbook of Speech Perception* (pp. 591–609). Oxford: Blackwell.

Maassen, B. and Povel, D. J. (1984a). The effect of correcting fundamental frequency on the intelligibility of deaf speech and its interaction with temporal aspects. *Journal of the Acoustical Society of America*, 76, 1673–81.

Maassen, B. and Povel, D. J. (1984b). The effect of correcting temporal structure on the intelligibility of deaf speech. *Speech Communication*, 3, 123–35.

Maassen, B. and Povel, D. J. (1985). The effect of segmental and suprasegmental corrections on the intelligibility of deaf speech. *Journal of the Acoustical Society of America*, 78, 877–86.

Metz, D. E., Samar, V. J., Schiavetti, N., Sitler, R. W., and Whitehead, R. L. (1985). Acoustic dimensions of hearing-impaired speakers' intelligibility. *Journal of Speech and Hearing Research*, 28, 345–55.

Miller, G. A. and Nicely, P. E. (1955). An analysis of perceptual confusions among some English consonants. *Journal of the Acoustical Society of America*, 27, 338–52.

Monsen, R. B. (1978). Toward measuring how well hearing-impaired children speak. *Journal of Speech and Hearing Research*, 21, 197–219.

Monsen, R. B. (1981). A usable test for the speech intelligibility of deaf talkers. *American Annals of the Deaf*, 126, 845–52.

Monsen, R. (1983). The oral speech intelligibility of hearing-impaired talkers. *Journal of Speech and Hearing Disorders*, 48, 286–296.

Niemi, J., Koivuselkä-Sallinen, P., and Hänninen, R. (1985). Phoneme errors in Broca's aphasia: Three Finnish cases. *Brain and Language*, 26, 28–48.

Platt, L. J., Andrews, G., Young, M., and Quinn, P. T. (1980). Dysarthria of adult cerebral palsy. I. Intelligibility and articulatory impairment. *Journal of Speech and Hearing Research*, 23, 28–40.

Platt, L. J., Andrews, G., and Howie, P. M. (1980). Dysarthria of adult cerebral palsy. II. Phonemic analysis of articulation errors. *Journal of Speech and Hearing Research*, 23, 41–55.

Rogers, C. L. and Dalby, J. (2005). Forced-choice analysis of segmental production by Chinese-accented English speakers. *Journal of Speech, Language, and Hearing Research*, 48, 306–22.

Schiavetti, N. (1992). Scaling procedures for the measurement of speech intelligibility. In R. D. Kent (ed.), *Intelligibility in Speech Disorders: Theory, Measurement, and Management* (pp. 11–34). Amsterdam: John Benjamins.

Sell, D. (2005). Issues in perceptual speech analysis in cleft palate and related disorders: A review. *International Journal of Language and Communication Disorders*, 40, 103–21.

Sell, D., Grunwell, P., Mildenhall, S., Murphy, T., Cornish, T. C., Williams, A., Bearn, D., Shaw, W. C., Murray, J., and Sandy, J. (2001). The Clinical Standards Advisory Group (CSAG) study. Part 3: Speech outcomes. *Cleft Palate–Craniofacial Journal*, 38, 30–7.

Shriberg, L. D., Flipsen, P., Jr., Kwiatkowski, J., and McSweeny, J. L. (2003). A diagnostic marker for speech delay associated with otitis media with effusion: The intelligibility-speech gap. *Clinical Linguistics and Phonetics*, 17, 507–28.

Smith, C. (1975). Residual hearing and speech production in deaf children. *Journal of Speech and Hearing Research*, 18, 795–811.

Stevens, K. N. (2002). Toward a model of lexical access based on acoustic landmarks and distinctive features. *Journal of the Acoustical Society of America*, 111, 1872–91.

Subtelny, J., Koepp-Baker, H., and Subtelny, J. S. (1961). Palatal function and cleft palate speech. *Journal of Speech and Hearing Disorders*, 26, 213–24.

Subtelny, J. and Subtelny, J. D. (1959). Intelligibility and associated physiological factors of cleft palate speakers. *Journal of Speech and Hearing Research*, 2, 353–60.

Subtelny, J. D., van Hattum, R. J., and Myers, B. B. (1972). Ratings and measures of cleft palate speech. *Cleft Palate Journal*, 9, 18–27.

Tikofsky, R. S. and Tikofsky, R. P. (1964). Intelligibility measures of dysarthric speech. *Journal of Speech and Hearing Research*, 7, 325–33.

Turner, G. S., Tjaden, K., and Weismer, G. (1995). The influence of speaking rate on vowel space and sentence intelligibility in individuals with amyotrophic lateral sclerosis. *Journal of Speech and Hearing Research*, 38, 1001–13.

Weismer, G. (2006). Speech disorders. In M. Traxler and M. Gernsbacher (eds.), *Handbook of Psycholinguistics* (pp. 93–124). Oxford: Blackwell.

Weismer, G., Jeng, J-Y., Laures, J. S., and Kent, R. D. (2001). Acoustic and intelligibility characteristics of sentence production in neurogenic speech disorders. *Folia Phoniatrica et Logopaedica*, 53, 1–18.

Weismer, G. and Martin, R. E. (1992). Acoustic and perceptual approaches to the study of intelligibility. In R. D. Kent (ed.), *Intelligibility in Speech Disorders: Theory, Measurement, and Management* (pp. 67–118). Amsterdam: John Benjamins.

Weston, A. D. and Shriberg, L. D. (1992). Contextual and linguistic correlates of intelligibility in children with developmental phonological disorders. *Journal of Speech and Hearing Research*, 35, 1316–32.

Whitehill, T. L. (2002). Assessing intelligibility in speakers with cleft palate: A critical review of the literature. *Cleft Palate–Craniofacial Journal*, 39, 50–8.

Whitehill, T. L. and Chau, T. H. (2004). Single-word intelligibility in speakers with repaired cleft palate. *Clinical Linguistics and Phonetics*, 18, 341–55.

Whitehill, T. L. and Ciocca, V. (2000). Perceptual-phonetic predictors of single-word intelligibility: A study of Cantonese dysarthria. *Journal of Speeech, Language, and Hearing Research*, 43, 1451–65.

Yavas, M. and Lamprecht, R. (1988). Processes and intelligibility in disordered phonology. *Clinical Linguistics and Phonetics*, 2, 329–45.

Yorkston, K. M. and Beukelman, D. R. (1978). A comparison of techniques for measuring intelligibility of dysarthric speech. *Journal of Communication Disorders*, 11, 499–512.

Yorkston, K. M. and Beukelman, D. R. (1981). *Assessment of Intelligibility of Dysarthric Speech*. Tigard, OR: C. C. Publications.

Yunusova, Y., Weismer, G., Kent, R. D., and Rusche, N. (2006). Breath group intelligibility in dysarthria: Characteristics and underlying correlates. *Journal of Speech, Language, and Hearing Research*, 48, 1294–1310.

Ziegler, W. and Hartmann, E. (1996). Perceptual and acoustic methods in the evaluation of dysarthric speech. In M. J. Ball and M. Duckworth (eds.), *Advances in Clinical Phonetics* (pp. 91–114). Amsterdam: John Benjamins.

36   Connected Speech

SARA HOWARD, BILL WELLS, AND JOHN LOCAL

In attempting to describe the patterns of simplification in informal speech, we are, in a sense, trying to do a ridiculous thing.

(Brown, 1990, p. 58)

36.1   Introduction

Many people with speech difficulties are unintelligible when using longer strings of speech in everyday, spontaneous communication, even though they may be able to produce single words in isolation quite accurately. Despite this common observation, connected speech is not routinely assessed and often is not specifically addressed in intervention.

Using connected speech places a greater load on the speech processing system than does the production of single words. However, the challenge of connected speech is about more than just extra processing load: connected speech is also qualitatively different from single words, in terms of its phonology and therefore its phonetics. Connected speech is more than just a string of individual target segments joined together in series, since each segment is liable to influence the segments that surround it. The precise form that these influences take is determined by the particular language in question, and so the phonology of connected speech is a part of the phonology of the language that the child has to master, just like its systems of vowels and consonants and its phonotactic structures. As adults we display our mastery of the phonology of the language as much by the ways in which we connect words up – our realization of word junctures – as we do by our pronunciation of individual words.

36.2   Connected Speech Processes and Word Junctures

Question: What do you call a mushroom who takes you out for the evening and
pays for all the drinks?
Answer: A [ˈfʌŋgaɪ] to be with.

In spoken English humor, many jokes rely on the listener's subconscious awareness of the tension between the form a lexical item takes when spoken rather
carefully in isolation, and its realization in the company of other words in
connected speech (in the case above, this produces an ambiguity between the
words 'fun guy' and 'fungi'). Such tensions may be said to reflect a set of
simplifying processes which operate on words in larger contexts, and which
have been extensively described in the literature (see, for example, Brown,
1990; Cruttenden, 2001; Nolan & Kerswill, 1990; Shockey, 2003). Connected
speech processes (CSPs) that affect speech production at word boundaries
include assimilation (e.g. RED CAT /rɛd kæt/ → /rɛg kæt/), coalescence (e.g.
MISS YOU /mɪs ju/ → /mɪʃu/), elision (e.g. LAST SUMMER /lɑst ˈsʌmə/ → /lɑs
ˈsʌmə/; IT'S HIM /ɪts ˈhɪm/ but PUT HIM OFF /ˈpʊt ɪm ˈɒf/), and liaison (e.g.,
in a non-rhotic accent, FAR /fɑ/ but FAR AWAY /fɑr əˈweɪ/). Other processes
which contrast words produced in isolation with words in connected speech
include the use of weak forms (e.g. THE /ðə/ or /ðɪ/ rather than /ˈði/; FROM
/frəm/ rather than /ˈfrɒm/) and other vowel reductions connected to the
stress and rhythm patterns of the language in question.
     A significant body of evidence, driven largely by the fact that, as Barry and
Andrews (2001, p. 51) observe, "all languages allow for variation in the time
and effort invested in any given part of an utterance", suggests that similar
phonetic and phonological simplifications in connected speech can be found
across languages and language varieties (see, for example, Barry & Andrews,
2001; Duez, 1995; Engstrand & Krull, 2001; Farnetani, 1997; Ingram, 1989; Kohler,
1990, 2000; Mitterer & Ernestus, 2006; Nicolaidis, 2001). However, it is important
to note that significant differences have also been found between languages.
For example, in English where consonants assimilate at word boundaries, the
direction of this assimilation is typically regressive (i.e. the final consonant of
the first word is influenced by the initial consonant of the following word).
In other languages, however, including German, Portuguese and Swedish, we
see instances of progressive assimilation, where the influence operates in the
opposite direction.
     Cross-linguistic differences provide insights into the important question of
the status of CSPs. One way of characterizing processes such as assimilation
is to regard them as categorical (involving a complete change of segmental
identity) and phonological (a property of the grammar of a specific language).
Alternatively, the same processes can be viewed as gradual (reflecting coarticulatory activity operating on a continuum) and phonetic (a result of the

physical and biomechanical properties of the vocal organs). Farnetani (1997) asks whether this question, at least to some extent, is a methodological artifact reflecting auditory-perceptual versus instrumental approaches to data analysis, the former favoring categorical/phonological interpretation, and the latter supporting coarticulatory/phonetic explanations. Certainly instrumental evidence (in the form of acoustic and electropalatographic investigations) provides strong support for the notion of place and voice assimilation and consonant elision as gradual and variable processes (e.g. Wright & Kerswill, 1989; Barry, 1991; Hardcastle, 1995; Holst, Warren, & Nolan, 1995; Mitterer & Ernestus, 2006; Snoeren, Hallé, & Segui, 2006), although Ellis and Hardcastle (2002), in a study of alveolar-to-velar word-boundary assimilation, identify considerable inter-speaker variation, with some subjects appearing to make continuous, coarticulatory adjustments in these contexts, where others produced what looked much more like categorical changes. Furthermore, the degree to which CSPs occur cross-linguistically may also be governed by grammatical factors. Thus, for example, Rechziegl (2001) compares word-boundary coalescence of /s#j/ to [ʃ] cross-linguistically. We have mentioned above that this is an extremely common process in spoken English: Rechziegl notes that its appearance is quite variable in Dutch, and that in Czech, a strongly inflectional language, grammatical markers at word boundaries appear to exert strong resistance to its occurrence. Bush (2001, p. 256), meanwhile, suggests that the appearance of this process at specific word junctures in spoken English is motivated by lexical collocational frequency: "word-boundary palatalization is more likely between two words if those words occur together in high frequency."

Indeed, there appear to be multiple factors affecting the likely occurrence of CSPs at word boundaries. Shockey (2003) provides a clear summary of phonetic, phonological, prosodic, grammatical, and discourse factors which may all contribute to the likelihood of a particular word-boundary process taking place. Thus, for example, in spoken English, a word-final alveolar (particularly /t/) that forms part of a consonant cluster in an unstressed syllable would be extremely vulnerable to simplification or elision, whereas the same segment appearing as a singleton consonant in initial position in a stressed syllable would be extremely unlikely to be affected by word-boundary speech behaviors. Discourse function and familiarity can also affect a word's realization in connected speech. Fowler and Housum (1987) have suggested that words functioning to provide new information within an utterance are typically more intelligible than words relating to given information, and Bybee (2002) suggests that high-frequency words and phrases are often subject to greater degrees of simplification than low-frequency words, where, presumably, the speaker is maximally facilitating listener comprehension. Indeed, in outlining a usage-based model of language production and change, Bybee (2000, p. 268) cautions that "many cases of what was earlier postulated as structural turn out to be derivable from the way language is used." (See also Sosa and Bybee, chapter 30 in this volume.)

A rather different perspective on the analysis of connected speech has been developed by phonologists working within the tradition of Firthian Prosodic Analysis (Firth, 1948; Kelly & Local, 1989; Ogden & Local, 1994), for whom Junctures (or junctions) have been a particular focus, as they represent one kind of 'prosody'. As a first descriptive step a broad distinction can be made between Open Juncture and Close Juncture, following Sprigg (1957). When a speaker of English produces two words in sequence, there may be features that serve to keep the words distinct (e.g. a silence, audible release of final stop in the coda of first word, or a glottal stop at the onset of the second word if it begins with a vowel, cf. Catford, 1985; Shockey, 2003). Adult speakers may deploy such open juncture for the purposes of emphasis or repair, and it may be more frequent in certain speech activities, e.g. reading aloud. Close juncture on the other hand is characterized by phonetic features that bind adjacent words together. How this can be done depends on the phonological structures that abut at the junction; close juncture types include the connected speech 'processes' outlined above, such as assimilation and elision (two subtypes of consonant – consonant close juncture), and liaison (vowel – vowel close juncture).

36.3   Normal Development

Almost all research on children's phonological development over the past four decades has focused on phonology within the word. As a result, a good deal is known about the emergence of sound types, particularly consonants, often described in terms of processes of simplification (Vihman, 1996, ch. 9). Differences between adult and child productions are accounted for by appeals to the inherent articulatory or perceptual difficulty of certain sound types, cognitive difficulties, and/or the difficulty of producing a sound type when it is subject to contextual influence from other sound types within the target word (e.g. consonant harmony and cluster reduction). While formulations of phonological theory have changed, it is this type of description that has continued to dominate both child phonology research and clinical practice, with spontaneous or connected speech tending to be assessed only in terms of broad perceptual ratings of intelligibility.

This focus on isolated single words, in research and clinical practice, is at odds with the fact that by the end of their second year, typically developing children are starting to produce multi-word utterances, and from then on the use of utterances consisting of a single word is only part of their repertoire (as it is for adults). In fact, the linguistic advance of multi-word speech is predicated upon the phonological advance of producing juncture: the child is challenged to find a phonological solution to word joining.

In principle, then, the study of between-word junctures should be germane to our understanding of early phonological development; in practice, it is conspicuously lacking. This impacts not only on our knowledge of phonological development *per se*, but also on clinical practice with children with speech impairment, for whom between-word junctures are a significant constraint on improved intelligibility. There is a need to understand to what extent the atypical juncture patterns documented in older speech-impaired children reflect normal, early juncture development. Moreover, remedial strategies depend on greater knowledge of how juncture types are deployed and developed in the course of talk-in-interaction.

Various clinically relevant questions can be asked about the development of between word junctures. These are addressed below.

36.3.1   *Do close junctures appear before, after, or at the same time as open junctures?*

Newton and Wells (2002) studied a subset of close junctures in the spontaneous speech of a typically developing boy (CW) learning Southern British English, between the ages of 2;4 and 3;4. One target juncture type studied was: -C#C-, where -C is /d/ or /n/, and where C- is target velar or bilabial, e.g. RED BALLOON, ONE CALLED, i.e. potential sites for alveolar-to-bilabial/velar assimilation in adult English. The earliest recordings showed examples of close juncture (assimilated) forms, but no open juncture forms. As the year progressed, open junctures also appeared, but close junctures (assimilation) were always the majority. This result suggests that this child did not learn to join the two words together phonologically after first learning to combine them grammatically, but that junctural phonology and grammar had emerged simultaneously.

In contrast, Thompson and Howard (2006), in a cross-sectional study investigating the spontaneous speech of six typically developing children from the north of England (three aged from 2;0 to 2;6, and three aged from 3;0 to 3;6), found a clear quantitative shift from a predominance of open junctures for the two-year-olds, to a strong preference for close junctures shown by the three-year-olds. Thompson and Howard tentatively concluded from their data that adult close juncture forms are not all automatic or default, but that children may only learn gradually to negotiate word boundaries.

One related possibility is that adult-like junctures are evident first in the child's stereotypical or formulaic utterances – those multi-word utterances that appear to be learned from the outset as a gestalt and reproduced by the child in that way. As Wray and Perkins (2000, p. 20) observe, "If the same, or similar, groups of elements are being continually encountered and/or produced, it will make good economical sense to store them as separate items" (see also Bybee, 2000). This phonetic mastery of the juncture type may then be extended to those multi-word utterances that represent genuinely novel combinations of independent lexical items, although at this stage we may see significant difference in juncture behaviors between those children who prefer analytic, bottom-up approaches to acquisition – so-called "careful system builders" (Ferguson, 1978) – and children whose more holistic style will favor the production of gestalt forms. Of the latter type of child, Wray (2002, p. 117) remarks, significantly, that "the tendency for gestalt children to speak lengthy utterances that are phonologically indistinct has also made them less popular to study" (see also Peters, 1977). It may also be the case that the patterns of hyperarticulation and hyperelision noted in atypical speech development (see section 36.5 below) are a reflection of analytic versus holistic learning styles.

36.3.2   Do the various subtypes of close and open juncture appear in a developmental sequence?

It is plausible that children will first produce the close junctures that they find 'easiest', just as they appear to produce some individual segments before others. The 'ease' may be articulatory, perceptual or cognitive, and could also be a function of the frequency of the particular juncture in the speech the child hears. Little research has so far addressed this issue. In the study by Newton and Wells (2002), data on CW's development of types of liaison indicated that there was a developmental sequence whereby y- and w-liaison preceded r-liaison. While the former were evident from the onset of multi-word utterances, target r-liaison sites were initially realized by CW as open juncture. Thus r-liaison specifically seems to have been learned as a phonological rule. Newton and Wells argued that from a phonetic perspective this is plausible since, compared to y- and w-liaison, the set of vowels that conditions r-liaison is much more diverse in terms of tongue position. Thompson and Howard (2006) similarly found that r-liaison was only used consistently and appropriately by one of the older children in their study.

A cross-sectional study on the use of adult CSPs by normally developing children from Hereford, in the west of England, was carried out by Newton and Wells (1999). There were 14 children aged 3, and 20 in each of the following age bands: 4, 5, 6 and 7 years. As part of this study the processes of alveolar-to-bilabial and alveolar-to-velar assimilation, final alveolar plosive elision, and /j, w, r/-liaison (e.g., TIDY UP: [taɪdiʲʌp]; SAW A: [sɔˡə]; SHOW US: [ʃəʊʷʌs]), and the use of adult allomorphs of definite and indefinite articles (e.g. AN ORANGE: [ənˈdɹɪndʒ]; THE ORANGE: [ðɪˡˈdɹɪndʒ]) were investigated.

Of the four processes, only one showed a developmental trend: the number of correct allomorphs of the indefinite and definite articles increased progressively through the age bands. The incidence of each of the other processes remained fairly consistent across the age range, at between 70 and 90 percent. This suggests that from a *quantitative* perspective, there is no developmental progression in the frequency of occurrence of adult phonological (as opposed to morphophonological) CSPs, i.e. the frequency of this type of close juncture, as opposed to open juncture, in environments where the CSPs might occur. However, although Newton and Wells (1999) did not explore this issue, it seems more likely that there will be *qualitative* developments in the phonetic realization of these CSP targets. Thompson and Howard's study (2006) of slightly younger children (two- and three-year-olds) suggested, for example, that consonant elision appeared earlier than consonant assimilation in most of the children's speech output.

36.3.3 What phonological factors might influence a child's production of non-adult junctures?

Given the constraints on young children's articulatory capabilities, it is likely that all children produce some junctures that are non-adult in their phonetic form. Some of these have a domain *local* to the juncture. In early recording sessions, for example, CW produced, for target assimilation junctures, tokens such as MAN COME – [mæʔkʌm] (coda consonant elided; glottal stop inserted), and, for target elisions LOST BERTIE – [lɒʔbɜti] (glottal stop for target cluster coda of first word at the juncture). Case studies published in the 1980s have also reported idiosyncratic juncture patterns in normal development. Stemberger (1988) documents instances of nasal assimilation: his daughter Gwendolyn produced GET MORE as [dɛn mou], in variation with [dɛt mou], and Stemberger (1988) and Thompson and Howard (2006) report instances of resyllabification at word junctures (e.g. KNOCK OVER [nɒʔ. 'kəʊvə]). It is possible that the child's failure to realize the target adult juncture in such instances reflects both segmental constraints operating in single-word production, and the task of learning juncture types particular to one's own speech community.

Other non-adult junctures have a long domain. Matthei (1989), for example, reports *onset* (rather than coda) of first word assimilating in place to onset of second word, e.g. his subject E's BIG MOOSE produced as [mɪ mũ]. Bury (2004) notes THEY GO THERE /ðeɪ ɡəʊ ðɛə/ → [ɡaɡə'dɛə], where Robin, at 18 months, appears to assimilate the initial dental fricative of THEY to the onset consonant of GO. Unlike local junctures, these long-domain junctures cannot readily be interpreted as a failed attempt at a target adult juncture. They suggest that, independent of the phonological details of the adult target, binding adjacent words together phonologically may be important for the child, to achieve cohesion of the two elements grammatically, semantically and/or interactionally. Donahue (1986), Stoel-Gammon and Cooper (1984), and Waterson (1978) have all identified speech output in young children which links phonological and grammatical development by various long-domain selection and avoidance strategies. Thus, for example, Donahue (1986, p. 215) reports data from an 18-month-old child who produced two-word utterances such as BIG BOOK and BIG BIRD with clear long-domain harmonies ([bɪb bʊp]; [bɪb bæb]), but "adamantly refused to name or even imitate" syntactically identical structures (e.g. BIG DOG; BIG COOKIE) which did not permit similar harmony patterns.

36.3.4 What other factors might influence a child's use of close and open juncture?

Like adults, children appear to vary between open and close juncture in their realization of the same target sequence of abutting segments. Table 36.1, for example, presents some illustrative data from Robin at CA 18–21 months (Bury, 2004) for the -C#C- juncture between SMOKE and GO. Although we might

Table 36.1

Pattern of realization	Utterance	Gloss
Open juncture	[ˈməʊkʰgɔˈdɛə]	smoke go there
Open juncture	[ˈmɔk .ˈgɔ]	smoke go
Close juncture	[ˈməʊg̊uːˈdɛː]	smoke go there
Close juncture	[ˈmɔkʊˈlɛː]	smoke go there
Close juncture	[ʌˈmɔkᵊˈdɛə]	smoke (?go) there

merely wish to note here that a number of variants coexist in apparent free variation, it may be more illuminating to consider the role of the interactional context in influencing their occurrence. The relationship between talker inter-action and word-boundary behaviors would be a worthwhile topic for future research.

36.4   Methodologies and Assessment

36.4.1   Data collection

As we observed earlier, while children with atypical speech production are often at their least intelligible in spontaneous, multi-word utterances, their speech output skills are nevertheless most often assessed clinically by single-word elicitation tasks such as picture or object naming. Spontaneous speech may be used to give clinicians a 'feel' for the child's general level of intelligibility (Bleile, 2002; Tyler & Tolbert, 2002), but because of the undoubted problems of knowing what the speaker is attempting to say in spontaneous unintelligible speech (Kwiatkowski & Shriberg, 1992), single-word elicited data is most often used for comparing atypical productions of words with normal variants, and assessments of correct versus incorrect phonemes are seen as easier and quicker to define and administer than assessments of general intelligibility (Johnson, Weston, & Bain, 2004) or approaches which aim to identify connected speech behaviors. However, just as Peters (1977) cautioned against the tendency to screen out 'gestalt' children from studies of speech and language development because their speech output was difficult to analyze, so we should also beware of limiting our clinical speech assessments to single words on the grounds of ease and efficiency of analysis: careful and detailed analysis of connected speech, although undoubtedly challenging, may reveal more clinically useful and sig-nificant information about a speaker's output difficulties. Several studies have suggested that children with speech difficulties manifest more difficulties in producing spontaneous speech than in either single-word production or imitation (Faircloth & Faircloth, 1970; Healy & Madison, 1987; Morrison & Shriberg, 1992).

Basically, two approaches to assessment of connected speech have been used: (1) analysis of more or less naturalistic speech samples, and (2) structured testing. The former can be said to have the advantage of an ecological validity not shared by the latter, but, unlike the latter, the use of naturalistic speech samples may seriously limit the occurrence in the data of particular structures and forms of interest. To avoid this problem, Newton (1999) designed a comprehensive set of sentences suitable for repetition by children, targeting the main English CSPs. Normative data from this procedure is presented in Newton and Wells (1999).

Within both approaches, it is possible to carry out quantitative and qualitative analyses. The frequency of occurrence of a CSP relative to the number of target contexts can be calculated, and an individual's score on this measure can be compared to developmental or adult norms (Stackhouse, Vance, Pascoe, & Wells, 2007). Qualitative analysis can be used to investigate the unusual juncture behaviors produced by an individual. This may be done using auditory perceptual analysis alone (Wells, 1994), or supplemented by instrumental analysis such as electropalatography (EPG) (Howard, 2004, 2007; Newton, 1999). Whatever type of analysis is used to record observations of the child's speech in a systematic way, phonological analysis is required to assess the potential impact of the observed juncture behaviors upon the child's intelligibility.

36.4.2   *Phonological interpretation*

As in clinical phonology generally, when interpreting the connected speech patterns of an impaired speaker, we can focus principally on their realization of target forms, i.e. undertake a comparative analysis. This depends on an adequate description of juncture types in the adult language. In the case of English, this is available in a range of sources (e.g. Brown, 1990; Cruttenden, 2001; Lodge, 1984; Shockey, 2003), though the focus of such texts tends to be on 'processes' within a phonemic model. In cases where such CSPs are not found, it is assumed that the citation form is maintained in connected speech, e.g. pronunciation of word-final consonant before a following vowel, although at a phonetic level there are important differences, for example in the pronunciation of a coda plosive before silence as opposed to before an immediately following vowel.

Making a broad distinction between Close and Open Juncture, as described earlier in this chapter, can be a useful initial step towards systematizing and interpreting our observations of juncture behavior (Wells, 1994). This overarching categorization includes the CSPs, which can be thought of as Close Junctures, while their non-application in the same environment would be an instance of Open Juncture. However, the distinction can include other juncture environments too: for example, the occurrence of silence or an epenthetic vowel between a word ending with a consonant and another beginning with a consonant can be interpreted as Open Juncture, whereas the non-release of the coda consonant before an immediately following onset consonant would be

Close Juncture. In relation to adult English phonology, it will be seen that many of the features identified here as characteristic of Close Juncture are associated with non-emphatic utterances in colloquial (not necessarily fast) speech, whereas the open junction features are more often associated with a more formal style and/or emphatic utterances (Brown, 1990; Cruttenden, 2001). Once junctures have been assigned to Close and Open, it may be possible to detect an overall trend in a particular speaker towards the prevalence of one juncture type over the other. Wells and Stackhouse (1997) suggested that the prevalence of Close Juncture could be termed 'hyperelision', while the prevalence of Open Juncture has been termed 'hyperarticulation'.

In the case of a child with speech impairments, juncture realizations can also be compared to those of typically developing children of the same age. As described earlier in this chapter, relatively little information is available about the development of connected speech, compared to what has been reported about consonant and vowel development for English (Grunwell, 1987; Vihman, 1996) and a wide range of other languages (Zhu & Dodd, 2006). While such descriptions are often couched in terms of simplification processes whose domain is the word, drawing on Natural Phonology (Stampe, 1979), the incidence of some of these processes may in part be conditioned by connected speech factors. Such processes include structural simplifications such as Context-Sensitive Voicing – particularly final consonant devoicing, which one might anticipate to be more likely in utterance-final position than before a following word that begins with a vowel. Cluster Reduction is another such process: as the CSP of consonantal elision in adult English has as its domain a coda cluster followed by an onset consonant, one might anticipate that children are more likely to produce radical Cluster Reduction before a word beginning with a consonant. Another structural simplification process, Final Consonant Deletion, was the focus of a single case therapy study described in section 36.6 below.

36.5 Atypical Connected Speech Behaviors in Impaired Speech Production

For individuals with impaired speech production, spontaneous connected speech presents a particular challenge, that of integrating the articulatory and prosodic components of an utterance in order to achieve normal segmental realizations simultaneously with normal patterns of stress, pitch, rate, etc. As Wells (1994, p. 14) notes, "There is . . . a tension for the child between the demands of paradigmatic accuracy, i.e. the need to signal meaning in an intelligible way, and the demands of syntagmatic fluency, i.e. the need to realize phrases and sentences as cohesive wholes." If we concur with Chiat (1989) that the basic building block for speech planning and production is a rhythmic unit, underpinned by respiratory control and organization (Heselwood, Bray, & Crookston, 1995), and that articulatory gestures are constructed around a rhythmic scaffold, we can see how conflicts between articulatory and prosodic control could arise in a speaker with speech production difficulties. For such an individual, these conflicts could potentially impact on articulatory precision (resulting, for example, in segmental misarticulations and/or reductions), on prosody (producing atypical use of stress, rhythm, pause, etc.), or on both (Crystal, 1987). For example, a speaker who favored syntagmatic fluency, and the production of perceptually acceptable prosodic patterns, might accomplish this by extensive use of close juncture patterns at word boundaries, but these might be achieved at the expense of articulatory precision and accuracy in these contexts. Conversely, a child for whom articulatory accuracy is paramount may produce a greater proportion of open junctures at word boundaries, with the beneficial effect on segmental production being counterweighed by the detrimental influence on rhythm and stress patterns. Furthermore, a speaker might, consciously or subconsciously, utilize specific strengths in their speech production abilities in unusual ways in order to compensate for other areas of speech production in which they experience difficulties (Brewster, 1989; Perkins, 2007). All of these factors could have significant effects on a speaker's overall intelligibility.

The relatively few studies which have explored the connected speech behaviors of speakers with impaired speech using detailed phonetic, phonological and prosodic analyses lend support to these predictions. In an early study of the relationship between single-word and connected speech production, Faircloth and Faircloth (1970) selected a number of words which had been misarticulated in the spontaneous speech of an 11-year-old boy with severe speech output difficulties, and elicited the same words from him in isolation. Careful perceptual analysis, based on consensus narrow phonetic transcription, revealed the basis for the boy's increased intelligibility in single-word production compared with connected speech, where the same words variously fell victim to consonant elisions, whole-syllable elisions and significantly reduced segmental accuracy. Many of these features of the boy's connected speech production could be linked to stress and rhythm patterns, with simplifying processes most often occurring in unstressed syllables. As Faircloth and Faircloth (1970, p. 61) note, "The increment in intelligibility [in single word production] appears to be directly related to syllable integrity."

A similar significant mismatch between intelligibility in words spoken in isolation and intelligibility in longer spontaneous utterances is noted in a single case study by Crystal (1987). In attempting to describe and account for linguistic interactions across a number of levels in the speech of a four-and-a-half-year-old boy with a speech and language impairment, Crystal suggests that the most significant feature is the deterioration in prosody and fluency which occurs in syntactically complex structures, with detrimental effects also noted at the level of articulatory accuracy. Significantly, Crystal (1987, p. 18) notes that while there were very few instances of unintelligibility in single-word production, "Several of the more advanced utterances contain words or phrases which are largely or completely unintelligible,

and where the speech is not even transcribable", suggesting that his connected speech has been radically affected by processes associated with
hyperelision.

Wells and Stackhouse (1997) present a case study of an 11-year-old boy,
Richard, whose speech output is characterized by 'hyperelision'. His connected
speech, which non-experts might describe as 'mumbly', and his reduced intelligibility can be linked to a marked tendency to oversimplify word and syllable structures in connected speech production. As well as using elision patterns
found in normal speech production, Richard tends to elide parts of the syllable
rime (nucleus and/or coda) which are not typically elided by most speakers.
On occasions he may elide whole syllables, combining these elisions with the
weak articulation of syllable onsets (e.g. WHEN I GO DOWN FOR MY HOLIDAY IN
POOLE: [wɛ aɪ ɰθ 'daʊ fmaɪ 'hoʊdeɪ n̩ 'pul]). These reduction patterns have
the knock-on effect of destroying the word-boundary contexts where normal
assimilation and elision might take place. These hyperelisions are not random,
but can be closely related to the rhythmic structures of Richard's utterances,
with weak articulation occurring typically in unstressed syllables, and syllable reduction and elision occurring most often in syllables which fall outside
trochaic word templates.

In similar vein, Kelly and Local (1989, pp. 190–202) present data from a girl
aged five, from the north of England, who had been described as having a
'phonological disorder' and who, in spontaneous speech, also appeared to
favor syntagmatic fluency at the expense of articulatory accuracy. By making
use of gemination (consonant lengthening) and glottal closure rather than pro-
nouncing each distinct articulation that made up the sequence, she managed
to retain the rhythmic structure of the target (adult) forms: MUMMY'S WATCH-
ING THEM /'mʌmɪz 'wɒtʃɪn ðəm/ → [m̥ʌm̥e̯ẘw̮ɒ'tɕɪnʲdʲɛmʲ]. A lengthened
labial-velar articulation with close approximation is used instead of the target
/zw/ word juncture sequence. While the rhythm of the target is thus preserved, the primary differentiation in place of articulation is lost, potentially
affecting intelligibility. However, Kelly and Local noted that the *secondary*
articulation, or resonance, does in fact change, from front [ẘ] to back [w̮],
during the course of the labial-velar approximant that spans the word juncture. This shift in resonance reflects the shift from the /z/ of MUMM<u>Y'S</u> to the
/w/ of <u>W</u>ATCHING, indicating that the speaker is aware of the target morphological structure at this juncture, even though she is unable to articulate it
precisely.

In contrast, Wells (1994) and Howard (2007) describe children whose unusual
preference for open junctures at word boundaries disrupts stress patterns
and speech rhythms and results in speech which sounds rather slow, effortful
and disjointed. Zoe, at almost six years old, used idiosyncratic word juncture
behaviors which were context-conditioned and, to a large extent, predictable
(Wells, 1994). She usually achieved close juncture at syllable boundaries within
words, but displayed a strong preference for open junctures at word boundaries. Open juncture in these contexts was realized by a number of phonetic

devices, including sustained glottal closure (e.g. BY THE [baɪʔːtə]), audible release of coda consonants, lack of appropriate assimilation, and between-word pauses (e.g. big car [pɪ̞ːc . kɑ]). The perceptual effect of these behaviors was of jerky, staccato speech, whose slow rate may have related to the rhythmic abnormalities, or may have been a compensatory strategy to maximize intelligibility.

Sam (Howard, 2007), at the age of nine, produced speech, like Zoe, which was characterized by inappropriate use of open juncture at word boundaries. In his case early speech development had been affected by a cleft palate. Sam used glottal onsets at word boundaries where the second item had a vowel onset (e.g. AND ALL ['ʔæŋ. ʔɔʊ) and also inserted glottal plosives at word boundaries where r-liaison would normally be expected to occur (e.g. ARE OPEN ['ʔɑ. ʔəʊpən]). EPG analysis revealed that although he sometimes used appropriate assimilation at word boundaries, on other occasions he avoided highly predictable assimilation both between and within words (e.g. PHONE-BOOK realized as ['fəʊnbʊk]). Sam's connected speech was also characterized by equalisation of stress across syllables, with an avoidance of weak forms and of the expected occurrence of lateral and nasal plosion (thus APPLE ['ʔæ'pʊ]; NEEDLES ['ni'gʊ̥ỹ]), and exaggerated final syllable lengthening, all of which further disrupted the syntagmatic fluency of his speech.

While the above case studies suggest that individual children with connected speech difficulties may be categorized as 'hypereliders' or 'hyperarticulators', this is an oversimplification. Howard (2007) reports on two children who combine hyperelision with hyperarticulation, often within a single utterance. Once again, these tendencies to oversimplify or overarticulate syllables can be related to long-domain patterns of rhythmic organization in their speech production. Tara, who at fourteen still evidenced a strong alveolar backing process in her speech output, had connected speech which was slow in rate, with hyperarticulation. For instance, her production of TABLE NEXT TO HER ['keɪbʊ 'nɛkxk'ku 'hɜ] was syllable-timed, with none of the expected weak-form vowel reduction and with the notable preservation of all of the four consonants in the word-boundary consonant string in NEXT TO. However, she also used hyperelided forms such as the anacrustic HE'S GOT A [ɪɣːaə] in HE'S GOT A 'BOOK.

Holly, a nine-year-old with a developmental dysarthria, also showed both hyper- and hypoelision in her connected speech production. In her case this appeared to link with poor breath control for speech. Her utterances were often characterized by an initial portion which was rapidly articulated, hyperelided and markedly unintelligible, followed by a second portion where her production rate slowed down significantly and where both consonants and vowels were prolonged inappropriately and hyperarticulated, producing the perceptual effect of stress equalization, yet also increasing intelligibility.

That Holly's connected speech difficulties might be traced to problems with respiratory control echoes conclusions drawn by Heselwood, Bray and Crookston (1995). Heselwood and his colleagues present a detailed phonetic, prosodic and acoustic analysis of the speech of Ken, an adult male with a pervasive developmental speech disorder related to Down syndrome. Ken's speech output showed unusual use of word juncture with intelligibility markedly reduced by a tendency to use close juncture at word boundaries, with inappropriate elision of segments and syllables, weak realizations of segments, and accompanying rhythmic disturbances. The authors identify consistent subtle relationships between segmental realizations and rhythmic structures in Ken's speech, which they suggest are the result of more fundamental problems with breath control for speech. The reduced levels of intelligibility in Ken's speech output, like Holly's, can be attributed to neuromuscular difficulties at a basic respiratory level which have knock-on effects throughout speech production.

Specific word juncture devices can also be used to compensate for articulatory constraints, as in the case of Len, who had impaired speech following a partial glossectomy (Perkins, 2007). Perkins notes how Len's utterances comprise an atypically high number of tone units per utterance, with word junctures at tone-unit boundaries having several markers of open juncture (pauses, release of word-final plosives) combined with exaggerated pitch patterns presumably designed to facilitate the listener. Len's connected speech behaviors might be categorized as a component of prosodic deviation, where "a patient may use the prosodic resources of their language to compensate for deficits in other areas" (Brewster, 1989, p. 181).

The case studies reported above describe speakers with pervasive patterns of abnormality in connected speech. For other speakers with atypical speech, connected speech problems are less pervasive. Nevertheless, examination of their utterances reveals that they may have specific problems negotiating word boundaries. Newton (1999) used EPG analysis to explore assimilation and elision in the elicited connected speech production of three boys aged between 11 and 12, each of whom had been diagnosed with a developmental speech impairment. These speakers found coda consonant elision at word boundaries difficult to handle in contrast to their relative success in producing appropriate bilabial and alveolar assimilation of /t/ and /d/. Howard (2004) identified unusual behaviors at similar sites of predicted coda assimilation in the speech of a 13-year-old boy, Danny, with a history of cleft palate. As we have noted, in spoken English regressive assimilation is likely to occur where word-final alveolar stops precede bilabial or velar onsets in initial position in the first syllable of the following word. Auditory perceptual and EPG analysis of Danny's connected speech production in picture description tasks indicated that, in some instances where these conditions prevailed, progressive rather than regressive assimilation took place. This radically disturbs the phonetic and phonological identity of the onset syllable of the second word, which is extremely unusual in English speech production (where information from word onsets plays an important role in word identification) and is likely to be a formidable perceptual hurdle for the listener.

36.6   Intervention

While numerous studies of intervention for phonological and articulatory difficulties have been carried out, very few have incorporated connected speech systematically in the intervention. However, a recent study indicates that this may be a worthwhile approach. Katy, aged 6;5 at the start of the study reported by Pascoe, Stackhouse, and Wells (2005), had severe and persisting speech difficulties. The overall aim of the study was to determine if tailor-made intervention could result in both specific and generalized improvements in speech production. Katy's speech rate was slow with many pauses between words, and many single words emphasized with primary stress. The predominant patterns of phonological simplification found in Katy's speech were: cluster reduction (100%), clusters being typically reduced to one element (e.g. /sp/ and /st/ typically produced as [b] and [d] respectively); final consonant deletion (96%); and prevocalic voicing (40%). All three are structural simplifications that primarily affect the boundaries of words.

It was decided to focus the intervention on Katy's final-consonant deletion pattern. The intervention aimed initially to encourage Katy to produce exemplars of the CVC frame. However, the ultimate aim of the intervention was for Katy to use final consonants in CVC words embedded in sentences, i.e. in connected speech. In order to reach these goals, three phases of therapy were devised as follows:

Phase I: therapy on a specific set of single words
Phase II: therapy on a wider range of single words
Phase III: therapy on connected speech

Items for testing and therapy were chosen to highlight the functional importance of final consonants: when the final consonant is removed, a CVC vs. CV minimal pair is created (e.g. BOAT/BOW). For the intervention study with Katy, words were used in graded phrases to assess final consonant juncture in connected speech. A graded hierarchy of sentences was devised around each of the target single words, moving from a facilitatory context to a more demanding one. For example, in the case of the target word ROPE the facilitatory sentence used as a starting point was THIS ROPE PULLED THE CAR, where the onset consonant of the following word PULLED is the same as the coda consonant of the target word ROPE. The rationale was that children using final consonant deletion should be able to produce the initial [p] in PULLED even if they omit the final [p] in ROPE. In order to achieve an acceptable realization of this final consonant, the child merely has to lengthen the closure phase for the (single) consonant articulation. At the next level the child is required to produce a sentence such as THERE'S ROPE ON THE ROAD, with the target ROPE being followed by a vowel. Finally sentences such as THIS ROPE GOT FRAYED were introduced, requiring change of place of articulation (and voicing) between the final [p] in ROPE and the following consonant [g]. Sentences also varied in terms of the normal adult-like patterns of assimilation that would be expected. For example, in THIS ROPE GOT FRAYED no assimilation between the hetero-organic consonants at the juncture (/p/#/g/) was expected. However, in a sentence like THIS NOTE CAN'T BE READ assimilation of the final /t/ in NOTE, e.g. /'ðɪs nəʊk 'kɑmp bɪ 'rɛd/, would be acceptable.

Although Katy's production of the final consonants of single words produced in isolation improved significantly after Phases I and II, this was not matched by an improvement in her production of the final consonants of the same words when embedded in a sentence. However, the intervention in phase III, described above, was very successful in getting her to use the targeted CVC forms in sentences, something which she had been completely unable to achieve before. This change was not limited to the words in the treatment lists: it extended to untreated words in matched control lists, suggesting that generalized change had been brought about. Gains made with connected speech were maintained in the long term, after a period of no intervention. Thus it seems that improvement in connected speech was only brought about by specifically addressing connected speech in a carefully structured way. Similar children might benefit form this type of specific intervention targeted at connected speech.

36.7   Implications

The description of connected speech features in people with speech difficulties has attracted rather little research interest to date, as has the typical development of these features in children. However, existing research suggests that this may be a fruitful area for clinical phonologists to develop further, as it relates to several key theoretical and clinical areas. Studying connected speech may, for example, offer insights into relationships between phonology and grammar in both normal and impaired speech development, and may particularly complement usage-based, exemplar approaches to speech and language development. Significantly, investigation of connected speech behaviors can throw light on the relationship between segmental phonology and prosody and the ways in which this relationship impacts on intelligibility. This, in turn, could have important implications for the ways we assess and manage impaired speech in the future.

REFERENCES

Barry, M. C. (1991). Temporal modelling of gestures in articulatory assimilation. In *Proceedings of the XIIth International Congress of Phonetic Sciences*, Aix-en-Provence, August 1991, vol. 4 (pp. 14–17).

Barry, W. and Andrews, B. (2001). Cross-language similarities and differences in spontaneous speech patterns. *Journal of the International Phonetic Association*, 30, 51–66.

Bleile, K. (2002). Evaluating articulation and phonological disorders when the clock is running. *American Journal of Speech-Language Pathology*, 11(3), 243–9.

Brewster, K. R. (1989). Assessment of prosody. In K. Grundy (ed.), *Linguistics in Clinical Practice*. London: Taylor & Francis.

Brown, G. (1990). *Listening to Spoken English*. 2nd ed. London: Longman.

Bury, N. (2004). Development of between-word juncture. Unpublished master's dissertation, University of Sheffield.

Bush, N. (2001). Frequency effects and word-boundary palatalization in English. In J. Bybee and P. Hopper (eds.), *Frequency and the Emergence of Linguistic Structure* (pp. 255–80). Amsterdam: John Benjamins.

Bybee, J. (2000). Lexicalisation of sound change and alternating environments. In M. Broe and J. Pierrehumbert (eds.), *Acquisition and the Lexicon*. Papers in Laboratory Phonology, V. (pp. 250–69). Cambridge: Cambridge University Press.

Bybee, J. (2002). Phonological evidence for exemplar storage of multiword sequences. *Studies in Second Language Acquisition*, 24, 215–21.

Catford, J. C. (1985). Rest and open transition in a systemic phonology of English. In J. Benson and W. Greaves (eds.), *Systemic Perspectives on Discourse*. Norwood, NJ: Ablex.

Chiat, S. (1989). The relation between prosodic structure, syllabification and segmental realisation: Evidence from a child with fricative stopping. *Clinical Linguistics and Phonetics*, 3, 223–50.

Cruttenden, A. (2001). *Gimson's Pronunciation of English*. 2nd ed. London: Edward Arnold.

Crystal, D. (1987). Towards a bucket theory of language disability: Taking account of interaction between linguistic levels. *Clinical Linguistics and Phonetics*, 1, 7–22.

Donahue, M. (1986). Phonological constraints on the emergence of two-word utterances. *Journal of Child Language*, 13, 209–18.

Duez, D. (1995). On spontaneous French speech: Aspects of the reduction and contextual assimilation of voiced stops. *Journal of Phonetics*, 23, 407–27.

Ellis, L. and Hardcastle, W. J. (2002). Categorical and gradient properties of assimilation in alveolar to velar sequences: Evidence from EPG and EMA. *Journal of Phonetics*, 30, 373–96.

Engstrand, O. and Krull, D. (2001). Simplification of phonotactic structures in unscripted Swedish. *Journal of the International Phonetic Association*, 31, 41–50.

Faircloth, M. A. and Faircloth, S. R. (1970). An analysis of the articulatory behavior of a speech-defective child in connected speech and in isolated-word responses. *Journal of Speech and Hearing Disorders*, 35, 51–61.

Farnetani, E. (1997). Coarticulation and connected speech processes. In W. J. Hardcastle and J. Laver (eds.), *The Handbook of Phonetic Sciences* (pp. 371–404). Oxford: Blackwell.

Ferguson, C. F. (1978). Learning to pronounce: The earliest stages of phonological development in the child. In F. D. Minifie and L. L. Lloyd (eds.), *Communicative and Cognitive Abilities: Early Behavioral Assessment*. Baltimore, MD: University Park Press.

Firth, J. R. (1948). *Sounds and Prosodies. Transactions of the Philological Society*. Oxford: Blackwell. Reprinted in J. R. Firth (1957), *Papers in Linguistics 1934–1951*. Oxford: Oxford University Press.

Fowler, C. A. and Housum, J. (1987). Talkers' signalling of 'new' and 'old' words in speech and listeners' perception and use of the distinction. *Journal of Memory and Language*, 26, 489–504.

Grunwell, P. (1987). *Clinical Phonology*. 2nd ed. London: Croom Helm.

Hardcastle, W. J. (1995). Assimilations of alveolar stops and nasals in connected speech. In J. Windsor Lewis (ed.), *Studies in English and General Phonetics: Essays in Honour of Professor J. D. O'Connor*. London: Routledge.

Healy, T. J. and Madison, C. L. (1987). Articulation error migration: A comparison of single words and connected speech samples. *Journal of Communication Disorders*, 20, 129–36.

Heselwood, B., Bray, M., and Crookston, I. (1995). Juncture, rhythm and planning in the speech of an adult with Down's Syndrome. *Clinical Linguistics and Phonetics*, 9, 121–38.

Holst, T., Warren, P., and Nolan, F. (1995). Categorising [s], [ʃ] and intermediate electropalatographic patterns: Neural networks and other approaches. *European Journal of Disorders of Communication*, 30, 193–202.

Howard, S. J. (2004). Connected speech processes in developmental speech impairment: observations from an electropalatographic perspective. *Clinical Linguistics and Phonetics*, 18, 405–17.

Howard, S. J. (2007). The interplay between articulation and prosody in children with impaired speech: Observations from electropalatographic and perceptual analysis. *Advances in Speech-Language Pathology*, 9(1), 20–35.

Ingram, J. C. L. (1989). Connected speech processes in Australian English. *Australian Journal of Linguistics*, 9, 21–49.

Johnson, C. A., Weston, A., and Bain, B. A. (2004). An objective and time-efficient method for determining severity of childhood speech delay. *American Journal of Speech-Language Pathology*, 13, 55–65.

Kelly, J. and Local, J. (1989). *Doing Phonology*. Manchester: Manchester University Press.

Kohler, K. (1990). Segmental reduction in German: phonological facts and phonetic explanations. In W. J. Hardcastle and A. Marchal (eds.), *Speech Production and Speech Modelling* (pp. 62–92). Dordrecht: Kluwer.

Kohler, K. (2000). Investigating unscripted speech: implications for phonetics and phonology. *Phonetica*, 57, 85–94.

Kwiatkowski, J. and Shriberg, L. D. (1992). Intelligibility assessment in developmental phonological disorders: Accuracy of caregiver gloss. *Journal of Speech and Hearing Disorders*, 35, 1095–1104.

Lodge, K. R. (1984). *Studies in the Phonology of Colloquial English*. London: Croom Helm.

Matthei, E. H. (1989). Crossing boundaries: More evidence for phonological constraints on early multi-word utterances. *Journal of Child Language*, 16, 41–54.

Mitterer, H. and Ernestus, M. (2006). Listeners recover /t/s that speakers reduce: Evidence from /t/-lenition in Dutch. *Journal of Phonetics*, 34, 73–103.

Morrison, J. A. and Shriberg, L. D. (1992). Articulation testing versus conversational speech sampling. *Journal of Speech and Hearing Research*, 35, 259–73.

Newton, C. (1999). Connected speech processes in phonological development. Unpublished PhD thesis, University College London.

Newton, C. and Wells, B. (1999). The development of between-word processes in the connected speech of children aged between 3 and 7. In B. Maassen and P. Groenen (eds.), *Pathologies of Speech and Language: Advances in Clinical Linguistics and Phonetics* (pp. 67–75). London: Whurr.

Newton, C. and Wells, B. (2002). Between word junctures in early multi-word speech. *Journal of Child Language*, 29, 275–99.

Nicolaidis, K. (2001). An electropalatographic study of Greek spontaneous speech. *Journal of the International Phonetic Association*, 31, 67–85.

Nolan, F. and Kerswill, P. (1990). The description of connected speech processes. In S. Ramsaran (ed.), *Studies in the Pronunciation of English* (pp. 295–316). London: Routledge.

Ogden, R. and Local, J. (1994). Disentangling autosegments from prosodies: A note on the misrepresentation of a research tradition in phonology. *Journal of Linguistics*, 30, 477–98.

Pascoe, M., Stackhouse, J., and Wells, B. (2005). Phonological therapy within a psycholinguistic framework: Promoting change in a child with persisting speech difficulties. *International Journal of Language and Communication Disorders*, 40, 189–220.

Perkins, M. R. (2007). *Pragmatic Impairment*. Cambridge: Cambridge University Press.

Peters, A. M. (1977). Language learning strategies: Does the whole equal the sum of the parts. *Language*, 53, 560–73.

Rechziegl, A. (2001). Consonants in contact: On assimilation and cross-language contrast. In *Proceedings of the IFA Conference* (pp. 103–15). Amsterdam: Institute of Phonetic Sciences, University of Amsterdam.

Shockey, L. (2003). *Sound Patterns of Spoken English*. Oxford: Blackwell.

Snoeren, N., Hallé, P. A., and Segui, J. (2006). A voice for the voiceless: Production and perception of assimilated stops in French. *Journal of Phonetics*, 34, 241–68.

Sprigg, R. K. (1957). Junction in spoken Burmese. In *Studies in Linguistic Analysis* (special volume of the Philological Society) (pp. 104–38). Oxford: Basil Blackwell.

Stackhouse, J., Vance, M., Pascoe, M., and Wells, B. (2007). *Compendium of Auditory and Speech Tasks*. Children's Speech and Literacy Difficulties, 4. Chichester: Wiley.

Stampe, D. (1979). *A Dissertation on Natural Phonology*. New York: Garland.

Stemberger, J. (1988). Between-word processes in child phonology. *Journal of Child Language*, 15, 39–61.

Stoel-Gammon, C. and Cooper, J. A. (1984). Patterns of early lexical and phonological development. *Journal of Child Language*, 11, 247–71.

Thompson, J. and Howard, S. J. (2006). Word juncture behaviours in the speech of preschool children. Poster presented at ICPLA 11: The 11th Meeting of the International Clinical Phonetics and Linguistics Association, Dubrovnik, Croatia, May 31–June 3.

Tyler, A. and Tolbert, L. C. (2002). Speech-language assessment in the clinical setting. *American Journal of Speech-Language Pathology*, 11, 215–20.

Vihman, M. M. (1996). *Phonological Development: The Origins of Language in the Child*. Oxford: Blackwell.

Waterson, N. (1978). Growth of complexity in phonological development. In N. Waterson and C. Snow (eds.), *The Development of Communication*. Chichester: Wiley.

Wells, B. (1994). Junction in developmental speech disorder: A case study. *Clinical Linguistics and Phonetics*, 8, 1–25.

Wells, B. and Stackhouse, J. (1997). Connected speech problems and developmental dyslexia: A case study. Presented at the International Clinical Phonetics and Linguistics Association 6th Annual Conference, Nijmegen, The Netherlands, October 13–15.

Wray, A. (2002). *Formulaic Language and the Lexicon*. Cambridge: Cambridge University Press.

Wray, A. and Perkins, M. R. (2000). The functions of formulaic language: An integrated model. *Language and Communication*, 20, 1–28.

Wright, S. and Kerswill, P. (1989). Electropalatography in the analysis of connected speech processes. *Clinical Linguistics and Phonetics*, 3, 49–57.

Zhu, H. and Dodd, B. (eds.) (2006). *Phonological Development and Disorders in Children: A Multilingual Perspective*. Clevedon: Multilingual Matters.

37 Sociophonetics and Clinical Linguistics

GERRARD DOCHERTY AND GHADA KHATTAB

37.1 Introduction

The term *sociophonetics* refers to the study of those aspects of phonetic realization that vary as a function of a range of social factors, such as age, gender, ethnicity, class, style, and individual identity. In recent years there has been a sharply growing awareness that developing our understanding of how speaker performance is shaped by extra-linguistic factors associated with particular communicative situations is fundamental in building models of speech production, and this interface between the perspectives and paradigms conventionally adopted by sociolinguistic and phonetic research has come to be seen as the domain of sociophonetics (Damico & Ball, chapter 7 in this volume; Foulkes & Docherty, 2006; Hay & Drager, 2007). While the bulk of sociophonetic investigation focuses on speaker performance, there is a growing interest in the way in which the social-indexical information conveyed within the speech signal is accessed and interpreted by listeners, with the result that the scope of sociophonetics now extends uncontroversially to include issues relating to speech processing and perception (e.g. Bent & Pisoni, chapter 24 in this volume; Clopper, 2004; Clopper & Pisoni, 2004a, 2004b; Foulkes, 2005; Hay, Warren, & Drager, 2006).

Likewise, since early perception shapes the child's phonological acquisition and representations, an understanding of sociophonetic variation is fundamental to understanding how children acquire the ability to interpret and generate the social-indexical properties of speech through the various stages of phonological development.

It is also important to consider sociophonetic variation in the context of speakers operating within a multilingual environment. While much work on bilingualism focuses on the interactions between the two or more languages deployed by an individual, much less attention has been paid to how phonetic variability across both languages is harnessed as a means of signaling individual identity in different contexts. One of the aims of this chapter is to highlight this area as one that needs to be factored into clinical speech assessment.

The study of sociophonetic variation is closely associated with theories of phonological change and, as part of this, with studies of geographically determined accent variation and of the phenomena which are observed when accents come into contact or when a shift in social structures leads to greater or less differentiation in the social-indexical properties of language performance.[1] A good example of this is the work which has been taking place over the past two decades on the process of dialect leveling in the UK (e.g. Dyer, 2002; Kerswill, 2001, 2003; Torgersen & Kerswill, 2004; Watt, 2002), where it appears that greater social and spatial mobility and increased fuzziness of social hierarchies has led to a decrease in the use of some strongly regionally marked phonological variants and a rapid spread of innovative forms across speakers located in widely distributed urban centres (Britain, forthcoming; Kerswill, 1996a; Kerswill & Williams, 2000; Watt & Milroy, 1999; Williams & Kerswill, 1999). However, for the purposes of this chapter, we do not plan to focus on variation which is spatially differentiated in this way (that is, we are not going to compare different 'accents' or consider how they have changed over time); rather, our objective is to focus on the factors which can give rise to variation within the same community and to consider the implications of these for clinical phonological assessment.

37.2   The Nature of Sociophonetic Variability

The study of sociophonetic variability has been heavily influenced by methodologies arising from sociolinguistic research. A key aspect of this is the adoption of the linguistic variable as the fundamental object of study (Milroy & Gordon, 2003). Linguistic variables can be identified at different levels of analysis (phonological, discourse, lexical, syntactic, morphological), but in each case they are defined as being a locus of socially correlated variation in speaker performance. Note that an aspect of speech performance that could constitute a linguistic variable in one variety of a language may not apply in another variety, and, likewise, different variables may be relevant across languages. Once a linguistic variable has been identified as a focus for analysis, the analysis proceeds by scoring the relative frequencies of the range of variants which are found for all of the occurrences of a particular variable within a corpus of speech.

So, for example, in a study of sociophonetic variation in Newcastle upon Tyne, Watt (2002) investigated the variation encountered in the realization of the vowel nuclei encountered in words of the GOAT lexical set (e.g. *go, load, slow*).[2] Watt's results can be seen in figure 37.1. Watt's study tracked the relative frequencies of the four variants ([oː, ʊə, oʊ, ɵ]) that were found to be associated with this variable across the performance of 32 speakers distributed equally across groups defined by social class, sex, and age. While the monophothongal [oː] form was the variant which occurred by far the most frequently (72 percent across the total sample of 1464 tokens), the distribution of variants was

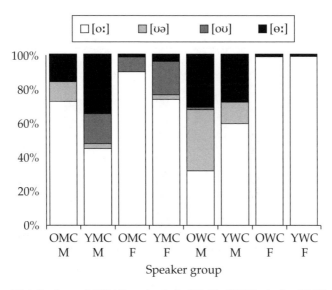

Figure 37.1 Distribution of GOAT variants in Watt's (2002) study. OMC = old middle-class; YMC = young middle-class; OWC = old working-class; YWC = young working-class; F = female; M = male.

not even across different categories of speaker. As shown in figure 37.1, two groups (young middle-class males and older working-class males) used [o:] much less frequently (45% and 32% respectively) but had relatively high usage of the [ə] and [ʊə] variants; looking across different social classes and ages, Watt's results suggested that male speakers were significantly more likely to produce variants which are localized (i.e. more characteristic of the Newcastle vernacular) than variants which are present across a wide extent of the north of England. Furthermore, Watt discovered a good deal of congruence in the patterns which emerged across a number of vowels (for example, across the FACE and NURSE lexical sets) within the performance of Newcastle speakers, suggesting that, in general, his observations were reflecting a fairly generalized characteristic of the social-indexicality conveyed by variation in vowel production in Newcastle.

As well as exemplifying the methodology which is typically applied within sociophonetic studies, Watt's work illustrates the fact that differences observed across speakers are usually not categorical; i.e., sociophonetic differentiation does not typically come about by virtue of one group of speakers adopting a particular variant 100 percent of the time while another group adopts a different variant in 100 percent of tokens. More typically, investigators find non-categorical distributions in which the speakers are differentiated by the relative frequency with which particular variants occur, but tokens of more than one variant and often of a number of variants are found in the performance of all speaker groups.

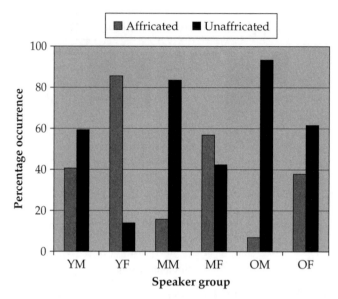

Figure 37.2   Frequency of occurrence of affricated and unaffricated variants of (ch) in Jarabo-Larenzo's (1998) data from Santa Cruz de Tenerife.

Sociophonetic variation of this sort has been most thoroughly investigated in relation to vowel production, but in recent years there has been an increasing focus on consonantal variation revealing very similar types of patterns of variation. For example, figure 37.2 shows for speakers of Spanish in Santa Cruz de Tenerife (Jarabo-Lorenzo, 1998) the distribution of two variants of the (ch) variable ([tʃ] and [ʃ]) as a function of speakers' age and sex, as scored from lexical items such as *chico* (boy) realized as [tʃiko] or [ʃiko].

As can be seen, while tokens of both variants are found across all speaker groups, there is a clear differentiation in the relative frequencies of the affricated and fricated forms as a function of speaker sex, with the fricated forms being much more strongly associated with male speakers than with female speakers (although there is something of an interaction with age as can be seen from the fact that the older female speakers also seem to produce predominantly fricated forms).

Many other consonantal variables have been investigated within recent sociophonetic studies (see Foulkes & Docherty, 2007, for an overview with regard to British English); and there is now ample evidence regarding the diverse ways in which variation in consonantal realization can be associated with speakers' social characteristics and orientation.

Perhaps not surprisingly, social-indexical marking in speech performance is not the exclusive domain of segmental units, and an increasing body of evidence demonstrates the roles of prosody and voice quality as carriers of social-indexicality. Stuart-Smith (1999) found variation in voice quality and vocal timbre in speakers from Glasgow as a function of age, sex, and (most of all) social class. Other investigators have suggested that the social-indexical role of creaky voice quality is different across USA and UK varieties of English, being predominantly a marker of young female speakers in the former while being more of a marker of maleness in the latter (Henton & Bladon, 1988). A different dimension of social marking has been explored in work on the role of prosodic and intonational characteristics in the judgments made by listeners about 'gay-sounding' male speech (Levon, 2006; Munson, McDonald, DeBoe, & White, 2006; Smyth, Jacobs, & Rogers, 2003). Despite the fact that perceived intonational variability does not always correlate with more objective acoustic measures of mean F0 and its variance, 'gay-sounding' voices are often perceived to have higher pitch and more exaggerated variation in the intonation. Thus, it appears that no aspect of speech production is ruled out of being harnessed for social-indexical purposes, and it is all the more surprising that it is only in recent years that the full range of variation of this sort has started to be subject to detailed phonetic investigation.

37.3   Focusing on Individuals

One of the outcomes of this increased focus on social-indexical variation is a growing realization that the social factors which have typically been considered in studies of this sort (e.g. age, gender, class) are a less than satisfactory basis on which to build a full understanding of social-indexicality within speech. There are two key issues here. One is that these social categories are themselves quite complex and subject to different interpretations (for example, age can be handled on a simple chronological basis, but equally, as suggested by Eckert, 1996, and Llamas, 2006, there is a case for handling it in terms of 'life stage', since this may be a more direct influence on age-related language patterns). A second issue is that the social categories are perhaps best thought of as "analysts' categories" (Milroy & Gordon, 2003, p. 116) since there is nothing intrinsic to those social variables that leads speakers to perform in a particular way (for example, being a young, working-class male from Newcastle does not in itself determine that such an individual would have a certain percentage of [oː] tokens in the GOAT lexical set). Rather it appears that what investigators are tapping into with their observations is a much more complex process whereby individuals deploy their linguistic (including phonological) resources to position themselves within the communities with whom they interact (much as they do along many other dimensions of human behavior). We can see evidence of this in the style-shifting that speakers undertake in different contexts, driven in some cases by an implicit accommodation to or divergence from an interlocutor (Giles, 1984; Giles, Coupland, & Coupland, 1991), but in others by an individual's beliefs about the impact of particular linguistic behavior within a particular situation (see for example, Sangster's (2002) work on phonological variation amongst students at Oxford who had originated from Liverpool, which explores the explicit motivation that some individuals had for either retaining or diminishing aspects of their Liverpool variety).

It is self-evident that the observations that arise from studies of social-indexical variation in speech which are based on traditional social categories are really an amalgam of the behavior of the individual participants within the study. With this in mind, it is important to emphasize that the linguistic behavior of the *individual* is the most relevant level to focus on if we are to develop explanatory accounts of social-indexicality in speech. Fundamentally, sociophonetic variation appears to be best understood as a key element in the formation and projection of individual identity (or identities) across the range of interactions maintained by a speaker. This appears to be a dimension of speech production which develops only gradually during early childhood (Foulkes & Docherty, 2006), but which is probably heavily influenced by growing awareness of gender identity, by encountering peer groups at the onset of schooling, and perhaps most of all by the process of adolescence (Eckert 1996; Kerswill, 1996b).

Even though the sociophonetic properties relating to individual speaker identity tend to stabilize in adulthood, many adult speakers will anecdotally report that they are conscious of phonological style-shifting in different contexts (indeed the first author of this chapter, who lived in Scotland until the age of seven before moving to the north of England, is variably rhotic, but much more so when in interaction with rhotic speakers from Scotland).

37.4   Interpreting Sociophonetic Variability

As might be expected, the ability to execute what is often very fine-grained tuning of speech performance in the interest of identity projection is mirrored by the fact that individuals are extremely adept at *interpreting* this dimension of the speech signals that they are exposed to. While listeners often find it difficult to articulate what it is in the physical manifestation of speech that drives their evaluations, anecdotal evidence and personal experience suggests that listeners readily make a wide range of judgments about their interlocutors based on properties of their speech. Research into the perception and interpretation of social-indexical properties of speech is far less well advanced than the work on speaker performance. One line of research, commonly referred to as 'perceptual dialectology', has focused on the extent to which listeners are able to identify the regional provenance of speakers (see, for example, Clopper, 2004; Preston & Long, 2002; Thomas, 2002 as good sources of background on this). Another has begun to explore how listeners' implicit knowledge (built up over time and through experience) of how a particular category of speaker typically performs, e.g. males vs. females (Strand, 1999), Americans vs. Canadians (Niedzielski, 1999), and Australians vs. New Zealanders (Hay, Nolan, & Drager, 2006), impacts on a range of speech perception tasks, thus demonstrating the likely integration of the social-indexical channel into speech processing.

In reviewing the impact of sociophonetic variation on speech communication, it is important to highlight that over time in most communities, ideologies evolve arising from conventional beliefs about the social meaning of particular phonetic forms (Lippi-Green, 1997; Milroy, 2006). For example, within the UK, while the use of a glottal-stop variant of word-medial /t/ (in words like 'water' or 'bottle') is known to be a rapidly spreading feature of the speech performance of younger speakers across geographically diverse urban centers, a full account of this pattern of variation should reflect the fact that these variants are at the same time highly stigmatized for many members of the same community (most prominently for older speakers) and highly acceptable to many other members of the same community (typically the younger speakers). Socially constructed beliefs center on factors such as perceived prestige, or the alleged aesthetic qualities of a particular variant (or accent as a whole; consider the case of the Birmingham variety of English in the UK, which is much-maligned in the popular media and about which many individuals from outside, and even within, that region will readily express negative opinions), or around other collective stereotypical judgments (e.g. what characteristics are typically thought to correlate with an individual's sexual orientation – see Smyth, Jacobs, and Rogers (2003) – or with particular ethnic groups). These beliefs further shape and reinforce individuals' behavior and lead to the situation where some forms are highly salient (with the potential to be evaluated positively or negatively), whereas others are abundantly present but with far lower overt awareness on the part of speakers and listeners.

While a recent sharp growth in the attention being paid by investigators to sociophonetic variation has rapidly increased our understanding of the dimensions of social-indexicality within speech, there are still some fundamental questions regarding how speakers handle this type of variation in the act of producing or processing an utterance (see Docherty, 2007; Foulkes & Docherty, 2006, for overviews). With regard to speech production, we lack a full account of how this social-marking dimension of speech is interwoven with the lexical-contrastive dimension; most work on speech production modeling to date has focused on the latter, and, while a lot of work in experimental phonetics has looked on certain types of variability such as coarticulation, prosodic modulation, and rate (e.g. Cho & McQueen, 2005; Hardcastle & Hewlett, 1999; Tsao, Weismer, & Iqbal, 2006), little progress has been made in building a sociophonetic dimension into such models. A similar picture applies to speech processing; from the point of view of perception, we need to know much more about listeners' sensitivity to different aspects of variation and how this maps on to the ideologies which exist around particular aspects of variation. We also need to develop a much greater understanding of how children factor sociophonetic variation into the process of mastering the sound patterns of their native language(s), and, as indicated above, how this relates to their social-identity development more generally. This applies also to people who are learning a language as an L2.

37.5   Sociophonetic Variability in Multilingual Contexts

Few bilingual studies have considered the sociophonetic dimensions of phonological acquisition (cf. Agnihotri, 1979; Verma & Firth, 1995), or their impact on the cognitive representation of two languages. This may be due to the fact that, until recently, linguists interested in early bilingualism have mainly focused on whether bilingual children start with one phonological system for both of their languages or differentiate their systems from the start (e.g. De Houwer, 1995; Genesee, 1989; Leopold, 1970; Paradis, 2001). Since the emphasis has often been on the issue of separation rather than the phonetic detail and potential variation within each system, researchers have mainly been interested in the child's ability to acquire aspects of the phonology that are important for lexical contrast. The targets for each language are often based on the standard dialect, and little attempt is made to look at social-indexical sound features that identify the child as belonging to a particular community, age, gender, social class, etc. The targets are also generally assumed to be invariable (i.e., often only one realization is expected for each target sound under investigation).

While more and more studies on monolingual acquisition are pointing to the importance of looking at variation in the input that the child receives (e.g. Docherty, Foulkes, Tillotson, & Watt, 2006; Foulkes, Docherty, & Watt, 2005; Roberts, 1997), variable targets are even more pertinent to any discussion of bilingual input, as the child's linguistic input may consist of standard, non-standard, and non-native varieties for two languages. In many minority communities, first-generation immigrants often learn the host language as adults and speak it with a foreign accent, while it is assumed that their offspring will acquire a native-like accent due to a more naturalistic context and increasing peer influence, and that they will eventually 'catch up' with their monolingual peers. Chambers (2002, p. 121) refers to this phenomenon as the 'Ethan experience', after the son of eastern European immigrants to Toronto. Ethan's parents were advanced speakers of English with a pronounced foreign accent, but Ethan learned English with a native-like accent by 'filtering out' the foreign accent features that were present in his parents' input. While it is true that many children of immigrants end up sounding more like their monolingual peers than their parents, the possibility that they possess multiple representations for the same lexical, phonological and/or phonetic phenomena which they can call upon according to context cannot be discounted. Evidence for this position comes from comparing the English spoken by bilinguals in the presence of their monolingual peers with that addressed to their parents or other bilinguals or second language learners.

For instance, Khattab (2007) found that English-Arabic bilinguals growing up in Yorkshire acquire native-accent features that are more typical of their immediate than their wider community, and in certain contexts they may also produce L2 features that are typical of their parents' speech. For instance, while the bilinguals' production paralleled their monolingual friends' use of northern realizations for BATH, and the fronted [əː] realization for the GOAT vowel, which is undergoing change (e.g. Watt & Tillotson, 2001), their realization of START, FACE and STRUT was more typical of the standard-like [ɑː], [eɪ], and [ʌ] realizations that were found in their circle of monolingual friends and families, despite evidence for the use of [aː], [ɛː], and [ʊ] respectively in the wider community (Grabe & Nolan, 2001). The bilinguals' parents produced foreign-accented variants that were typical of L1 interference, e.g. [ɛ] for BATH, [eː] for FACE, [oː] for GOAT, syllable-final clear [l]s, taps or trills for /r/s and a rhotic accent. However, the bilingual children also produced these features when communicating with their parents and code-switching to English from an Arabic base. A detailed analysis of the use of these features showed a strong influence of the base language (Arabic) but also a tendency for the children to accommodate to their parents' English accent. The features found in the code-switched data reflect the bilinguals' wider linguistic repertoire and suggest that the foreign-accent features that are present in their parents' speech are not ignored or filtered out. Instead, these are learned and stored as knowledge that is only activated in particular social contexts and that has particular social-indexical value. Bilinguals may also choose to use features of their L1 when producing their L2 as a way of preserving their ethnic identity through the L2 accent (Verma & Firth, 1995).

Khattab's study underlines the importance of awareness of the variable native targets in a particular community to establishing what is acceptable in a bilingual speaker's production. The study also underlines the importance of collecting data from controls who have close links with the bilinguals, since these are essential for the identification of the bilinguals' targets, especially in cases where English is being learned mainly outside the home and peer influence becomes more pervasive.

The notion of various degrees of activation depending on the context is not new to the discussion of bilingual competence, but has often been limited to language choice. For instance, it has been shown that the bilingual's choice of language in a particular conversational setting is influenced by factors like topic, interlocutor(s), and social context (Grosjean, 2001; Hamers & Blanc, 2000). Knowledge of these choices constitutes part of the sociolinguistic repertoire which children acquire. Sociophonetic research suggests that the bilingual's choices may not only be limited to which language to use with whom, but may also extend to which particular phonetic variants to use, depending on the linguistic context and the accent of the interlocutor. The ability shown by children to accommodate their speech to their interlocutor is part of the development of sociolinguistic competence that has been reported in monolingual situations (e.g. Chambers, 1973; Street & Cappella, 1989), and in cases of contact between different varieties of English (e.g. Rampton, 1995).

37.6   Sociophonetic Variability and Clinical Assessment

We now consider some of the implications of the presence of abundant social-indexical variation in speech for clinical assessment of speech production, focusing on three issues: (1) establishing a baseline against which to score a speaker's performance in the presence of abundant variability in typical speech production, (2) the approach to sociophonetic variation in the context of assessing a multilingual speaker, and (3) the extent to which ideologies relating to sociophonetic variation could influence clinical assessment.

37.6.1   *Establishing a baseline*

A key tension which arises from the findings of sociophonetic research is how they impact on the application of assessment tools that require a fixed frame of reference of some sort against which to score an individual's speech performance (either with or without standardization against a population sample). There are at least two important dimensions that can be highlighted. First, phonological assessment tools based around a 'standard' of some sort are clearly problematic because even regional 'standards' are unlikely to be representative of the speech performance of many speakers from that region. For example, within the UK context, it is possible to conceive of assessments being adapted to a Scottish standard or a North of England standard in order to deal with some of the differentiation from a Southern English standard, but what we know of sociophonetic variation suggests that such regional adaptations would struggle to capture the range of variation encountered *within* a single population; i.e., while regional adaptations would go some way to tackling some of the more obvious aspects of regional variation, they would not address the fact that within a single region individual speech patterns are heavily shaped by social factors such as those reviewed above. In light of this, it is striking that the vast majority of off-the-shelf tests do not make any attempt to deal even with coarse-grained regional variation, and in many cases steer away from this problem focusing exclusively or primarily on consonants, for example, the South Tyneside Assessment of Phonology, or STAP (Armstrong & Ainley, 1988), and the Diagnostic Evaluation of Articulation and Phonology, (DEAP – Dodd, Zhu, Crosbie, Holm, & Ozanne, 2002).

A second problematic issue raised by sociophonetic work with respect to assessment against some type of 'standard' is the need for assessment tools to be able to deal with the token-to-token variation in phonetic realization which sociophonetic work suggests will be readily encountered in the speech performance of speakers, whether they are children or adolescents following typical patterns of development, or in the performance of adults.

We can exemplify this by referring to the findings of a recent study (Docherty, Foulkes, Tillotson, & Watt, 2006; Foulkes, Docherty, & Watt, 2005) that set out to investigate the emergence of sociophonetic variation in children, alongside other aspects of their acquisition of native-language sound-patterning. Focusing on a cross-sectional sample of 39 children from a 'working-class' speech community in Newcastle upon Tyne, aged 2;0, 2;6, 3;0, 3;6, and 4;0, this study analyzed the realization of /t/ in a number of different contexts in utterances produced by children recorded interacting with their mothers in a play situation. The analysis focused on the extent to which the children were reproducing the patterns of phonetic realization which previous research on inter-adult speech in the same community had shown to be social-indexically structured. One such pattern was the use of a pre-aspirated variant in the realization of /t/ in word-final prepausal position (e.g. 'bet' realized as [bɛʰt]), which in inter-adult speech was shown to be predominantly a feature of female speech performance.

Figure 37.3 shows, for the children in the Newcastle study, the percentage usage of pre-aspirated variants in the 1,396 tokens of word-final prepausal /t/ that were analyzed. It can readily be seen that the pre-aspirated variant is amply present across the sample of speakers as a whole (on average 38 percent of all /t/ tokens were produced with this variant). While the children's performance did not in general reflect the social-indexical structuring of the usage of pre-aspirated /t/ in the adult community (with the exception of the 3;6 speakers), the results nevertheless suggest that any attempt to state what is age-typical in respect of the realization of /t/ in this environment for this

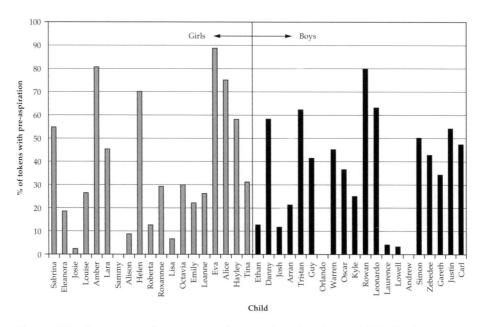

Figure 37.3 Frequency of occurrence of pre-aspirated variants of (t) in Docherty et al.'s (2006) data from Newcastle children.

variety of English cannot neglect the pre-aspirated forms (i.e. in considering what is 'normal' for children who are learning this variety, an expectation which referred only to a canonical [t] realization would not be appropriate). A further striking aspect of this data is the varying degrees of inconsistency both within and between speakers. While three speakers attain levels of >80% in usage of the pre-aspirated variant, others evince no usage of it all, while for the majority of speakers pre-aspirated [ʰt] is one of a number of variants which they produce for /t/ in this context (the principal others being a canonical released [t] and a glottalized variant). This suggests that there are some who are quite consistent in respect of the degree of their use of this particular variant, and others who are much less so.

Space does not permit a further exploration of these findings or of the findings for /t/ in other environments, but similar patterns of variability were observed for /t/ in other environments, although pre-aspirated tokens do not figure highly as they are largely encountered in prepausal environments.

While the Newcastle study reports on variants which are a reflection of the sociophonetic variability within the child's immediate speech community, there are of course many reports of variability in the speech of typically developing children arising from other factors such as motor control and articulatory coordination (see, for example, Whiteside, Henry and Dobbin's (2003) study of VOT variability as a function of age in children ranging from age 5 to 13; Smith, Kenney, and Hussain's (1996) study of duration and temporal variability in children's productions; or Yildirim, Narayanan, Byrd, and Khurana's (2003) study of vowel variability in the production of preschoolers). The presence of these sources of variability in the performance of typically developing children points to a need for phonological assessment tools to avoid two particular pitfalls: forcing the clinician to base a judgment of typical/atypical performance on a single token of a particular target sound in a particular context, and requiring a decision with respect to typicality by reference to a 'standard' which provides only a single 'correct' target for each particular context. The risk is that where this can't be achieved, children may be scored as performing atypically when in fact they are within the range of normal variability for a particular target, or, conversely, as performing typically when they are outside that range.

In light of the above, it is noteworthy that the presence of variability such as that discussed above has started to be acknowledged in the design of phonological assessment tools. For example, the DEAP (Dodd, Zhu, Crosbie, Holm, & Ozanne, 2002) specifically sets out to rate the degree of consistency shown by a speaker over three repetitions of single-word responses to 25 picture stimuli. While the primary motivation for this is Dodd's previous work (1995) suggesting that inconsistency above a certain threshold is a strong diagnostic indicator, this approach clearly embodies a view that typical speech production is not free of token-to-token variability. However, by adopting this approach, the DEAP places additional demands on the clinician in respect of understanding the nature of typical variability within the client's speech community. When scoring the inconsistency test, if the within-word inconsistency rate crosses the threshold of 40 percent which Dodd, Zhu, Crosbie, Holm, and Ozanne (2002) identify as the diagnostic threshold, the clinician is advised to reassess the inconsistencies which have been identified and to exclude from the percentage calculation those that are 'developmentally age-appropriate'. But how would a clinician handle the Newcastle children's pre-aspirated variants discussed above? They do not fall into the category of a typical developmental process, and yet since they are simply reflecting variability in the speech community which the child is part of, they clearly should not be classified as *a*typical. This suggests that the laudable move to incorporate into clinical assessment what we know about typical patterns of variability in speech needs to be mediated by an awareness of the parameters of variation within the client's immediate speech community. Interestingly, while the DEAP does not bring these together in respect of the inconsistency analysis, it does to some extent in respect of its approach to error analysis, where clinicians are urged not to class as an 'error' tokens which are present within the regional accent concerned. As we have tried to indicate above, it is not simply regional accent features that will be relevant in this case, but also the social-indexical variation present within the client's speech community.

37.6.2   *Working with multilingual speakers*

Bilingual assessments are scarce, and a long way from being able to account for sociophonetic variability in one or more of the bilingual/multilingual's languages. In some cases there are more urgent issues to deal with, like finding out what other language(s) and/or dialects the client speaks (Stow, 2004; Stow & Pert, 2006), due to the scarcity of data on languages other than English (cf. McLeod, 2007). For instance, in the case of the Pakistani heritage languages spoken in the UK, the prestige that is attached to Urdu may lead clients to claim it as their mother tongue when they might actually be Mirpuri speakers. The lack of standardized tests on languages other than English may also mean that the assessment in these languages is more informal and, if code switching is the norm in the bilingual's community, then the data elicited with the help of the bilingual SLTA (speech and language therapy assistant) are bound to contain many instances of code switching. While in many studies of normal bilingual development it has become standard to account for language mode by using different interlocutors for each language session, this is not always possible in a clinical context where the clinician might speak only one of the languages of the bilingual client. While bilingual assistants may be trained to elicit data from the bilingual's L1, the SLT (speech and language therapist; US SLP (speech-language pathologist)) is often present and the context is rarely conducive to a 'monolingual' state. Any bilingual assessment will need to take into consideration the fact that speakers might be exposed to several varieties of a particular language or to closely related languages and that their production might contain phonological (amongst other) features from more than one of these varieties, especially if code switching is common in their community.

There are hardly any standardized tests that can deal with code switching in terms of scoring (cf. Stow & Pert, 1998a, 1998b), and many SLTs still view code switching as a sign of lack of competence in one of the bilingual's languages. This may be true in the very early stages of the bilingual's development. While normally developing bilinguals may reach a state of competence in both of their languages that would allow them to function in a near-monolingual mode, many bilingual children who are referred for SLT may be in the early stages of acquiring one of their languages or experiencing delay in one of these languages and may therefore still be relying on the other to communicate. However, in immigrant communities where bilingualism is the norm, the amount of code switching may actually increase as the children grow older and become more competent in both of their languages (Pert & Letts, 2006). This is because fluent code switching preserves the grammatical, syntactic and morphological rules of both languages. Code switching in this context should therefore be expected as the norm for the bilingual's daily interactions, but most clinical assessments are too rigid in terms of their scoring systems to accommodate bilingual discourse and what counts as an 'acceptable' or 'correct' answer.

In cases of balanced bilingualism, bilingual behavior seems to suggest that bilinguals can control language activation: competent bilinguals have been shown to behave in a 'monolingual' manner when speaking to other monolingual speakers by producing separate phonetic realizations of particular phonological variables that are similar in their languages (Bullock & Gerfen, 2004; Bullock, Toribio, Davis, & Botero, 2005). When code-switching, however, speakers may 'carry over' phonetic properties from the base language onto the 'guest' language. This could be due either to internal factors like language base influence (termed 'linguistic convergence' by Bullock, Toribio, Davis, & Botero, 2005) or to external factors like the bilingual's accommodation to their interlocutor. These signs of interaction between the bilingual's languages should not be interpreted as interference, since they tend to occur mainly in bilingual contexts. This is not to suggest that competent bilinguals are immune from interference between their languages. In fact, psycholinguistic experiments suggest that both of the bilingual's languages are often activated even if the context requires the use of only one language (Roelofs & Verhoef, 2006), and that selection is often delayed till the phonetic level (as opposed to the lexical, morphological, or phonological level).

Roelofs and Verhoef (2006) also suggest that the bilingual may have shared representations for phonologically 'similar' material, e.g. similar phonemes, and that this similarity triggers phonetic activation from both languages, leading to the 'wrong' one (the phonetic realization that belongs to the other language) being used at times. Evidence for bilinguals treating phonological material from their languages as 'similar' could be taken from their use of phonetic realizations that are typical of one language in the production of the other language. For instance, English-Arabic bilinguals can develop different realizations for /r/ for each of their languages, but occasionally produce taps in English and approximants in Arabic, or even combine patterns from both languages by producing retroflex taps (Khattab, 2002). The bilingual's developing phonetic repertoire may therefore be wider than the combined repertoires of two mono-lingual children. SLTs need to be aware of these 'atypical' realizations, which may not be indicative of a disorder but which may be a necessary step in the bilingual's development as they formulate hypotheses about their languages. Similar observations have been made by Holm and Dodd (1999) for their Cantonese-English bilinguals, who showed 'error' patterns which the authors argue should be considered normal developmental stages in the development of Cantonese-English bilinguals, even if they were atypical for monolinguals.

37.6.3 *Ideology and assessment*

As a further illustration of the importance of building a sociophonetic dimen-sion into clinical assessment, we consider the status of labial and/or labiodental variants of /r/ in speakers of British English. Historically, the realization of /r/ as a labiodental approximant [ʋ] (also labeled by Lindsey and Hirson, 1999, as a "hypolingual /r/") was widely interpreted as a developmental misarticula-tion which for some speakers would persist beyond the age at which it could be classified (in, for example, Dodd and colleagues' terms) as developmental-age-appropriate.[3] Thus labiodental realizations of /r/ constitute the large part of Ward's (1936, pp. 30ff.) discussion of "defective R sounds". Likewise, Cruttenden's 2001 revision of *Gimson's Pronunciation of English* indicates that labiodental /r/ is "regarded as a speech defect" (p. 207). For most of the last century, it would not be unusual for UK-based SLTs to assess and treat clients presenting with a labiodental /r/. However, for contemporary young speakers of UK varieties of English, the situation is very different, with labiodental /r/ now significantly more prevalent, but crucially now not being interpreted as a 'speech defect' or indeed being a feature which speakers and listeners show much awareness of at all. The nature of this change is documented in Foulkes and Docherty (2000), and is perhaps best exemplified in Trudgill's account of phonological variation in Norwich (Trudgill, 1974, 1988, 1999), the original report of which (Trudgill, 1974) revealed only a handful of 'idiosyncratic' speakers using [ʋ]. However, Trudgill's 1988 study found that a third of the speaker sample born between 1959 and 1973 made use of [ʋ] variants of /r/.

  With labial /r/ we see an example of where, for reasons which are yet to be fully deduced, the social evaluation of a particular pattern of realization has evolved (in this case rather rapidly), so that what was once stigmatized and treated as a speech defect warranting intervention by a speech and language therapist now passes virtually unnoticed (although one might hypothesize that many older individuals would still be inclined to interpret labial /r/ as a 'problem'). This gives rise to an interesting follow-on question: What is the role of the social evaluation prevalent within a particular speech community with respect to what is considered to be atypical or 'disordered' speech? On the one hand, there are clearly many cases where social evaluation has presumably no part to play – fronting of /k/ to [t], for example, which results in the collapse of a very significant consonantal contrast in English and potentially severe problems of intelligibility, whatever the individual's variety of English. On the other hand, there is a range of 'misarticulations', the impact of which is differentially interpreted by both speakers and listeners. For example, for many speakers, a degree of lisping of /s/ is a feature that they would wish to change in their own performance (or that parents may wish to change in their children's speech), whereas other speakers may feel less motivated to change because it has simply become part of their own phonetic 'signature'. We can see a similar situation in the case of a rather different phonetic parameter, voice quality. It is well known (Laver, 1980) that it is difficult to define the 'normal voice' (resulting in the use of the term *modal* voice to attempt to define a baseline against which *amodal* voices can be compared), meaning that the definition of what is 'normal' needs to be established for each individual speaker, with the expectation that what is acceptably normal for one speaker could be unacceptably abnormal for another. Furthermore, as shown by Stuart-Smith's (1999) work in Glasgow referred to above, it is likely that these judgments are shaped not solely by how individuals perceive normality in respect of their habitual voice quality, but also by constructed societal beliefs about what constitutes a 'normal' and/or 'appealing' voice quality (so it might be hypothesized that the harsh voice quality which is relatively widespread amongst working-class males in Glasgow would be on the margins of what is considered normal by other social groups within that same city). The key point here is that a clinician's interpretation of what is normal or not for an individual speaker in respect of voice quality needs to be mediated by an understanding that voice (like other phonetic parameters referred to above) is one of the aspects of speech production which are closely tied to an individual's identity.

37.7   Practical Solutions?

While research into the sociophonetic properties of speech is progressively providing us with a more rounded account of their function within speech communication, painting an apparently ever more complex picture in the process, work on determining how these properties should be dealt with in clinical assessment is some way behind. Clearly, clinicians can refer to standard texts which provide accounts of particular varieties of a language (e.g., for English, see Foulkes & Docherty, 1999, and Schneider, 2007; or journals like *English World-Wide*), but these tend to represent a snapshot in time and do not necessarily cover in sufficient detail all of the parameters of variability relevant for the assessment of a particular individual. A more productive approach would be the development of tools to allow sociophonetic variation to be factored into a clinical assessment. For example, while, as pointed out above, assessment of vowel production has a relatively low profile in routine clinical assessment, it is likely that Wells's lexical sets analysis could be applied quite straightforwardly as a means of determining not only the predominant vocalic features of an individual's accent but also the main dimensions along which the speaker varies. It would seem reasonable to suggest that a similar approach could be taken to the assessment of consonants: since, typically, consonant assessments are based on a sample of words which provide exemplars of all consonants in most if not all environments in which they can occur, it would not be difficult to tag those consonant/environment conjunctions that are known to be most likely to give rise to sociophonetic variation across different varieties of English, so that the clinician can pay particular attention to the variability which might be encountered with those particular items.

There would probably also be much to gain by bringing to bear a greater focus on stylistic variation in clinical phonological assessment, as assessing speaker performance across different styles is likely to give greater insight into the range of variants that a speaker is able to generate and the extent to which they can be deployed in a way that reflects the stylistic variation present within that speaker's community. While, for some time now, a comparison of single-word performance with that on longer stretches of speech has been widely used in assessing speech performance in speakers with atypical speech motor control (e.g. Kent & Kent, 2000; Kent, Kent, Rosenbek, Vorperian, & Weismer, 1997), in other areas (most notably the assessment of developmentally atypical phonology) the predominant approach is to base an assessment on the production of words in isolation (cf. Howard, 2007; Howard, Local and Wells, chapter 36 in this volume). There is clearly a cost in time arising from incorporation of a wider range of styles, but if this enables a more complete assessment of an individual's sound patterning to emerge, then it is arguably valuable for that additional time to be invested.

Likewise, when dealing with bilingual or multilingual clients, studies by Stow and Pert (1998a, 1998b) and Pert and Letts (2003) are leading the way in documenting the normal patterns of discourse of speakers of the Pakistani heritage languages in the UK and in creating assessments for languages other than English as well as bilingual phonological assessments. More bilingual phonological assessments are needed that can accommodate code switching and take into account the variable phonetic and phonological patterns of bilingual speech that depend on issues like language activation and the demands of the situation.

Hand in hand with developing tools which would enable greater account to be taken of sociophonetic variability in clinical assessment, it is crucial that the issues discussed within this chapter are given a significant profile within the education and training of clinicians. While it is probably many years now since any program for training speech and language therapists advocated a prescriptive approach to the assessment of speech production, it is important that, in learning how to assess clients, trainee clinicians learn to guard against subconscious appeals to a 'standard' as somehow representing the 'target' against which an individual's performance should be evaluated, and situations in which their clinical judgments could be influenced by their own implicit ideologies relating to phonological variation (as described in section

37.7.3 above). This is perhaps all the more important in contexts (such as that which currently holds in the UK, for example) where the social and ethnic make-up of the SLT profession is far from representative of that of society as a whole (Thanki, 2002), and where there is evidence of certain ethnic groups leading the way in inducing language/accent change (Torgersen, Kerswill, & Fox, 2006). Many approaches to addressing this could be taken, but it would seem important to build this awareness fundamentally into the values under-pinning any SLT program so that the basic message is reinforced by all of those involved in its delivery at every opportunity (as opposed, for example, to seeing this issue simply as a point to be handled via the course in socio-linguistics or phonetics).

37.8   Prospects

Looking into the future, the handling of sociophonetic variation in clinical assess-ment very much depends on how phonology itself is conceived of both within a clinical setting and beyond. While the historically dominant view of phono-logical representation as specifying the invariant underlying building blocks of lexical items (subject to different types of 'rules' which provide a mapping to speech production targets) is likely to continue to be strongly present in the work of linguists and clinicians, this approach is increasingly being challenged by a 'usage-based' model (Bybee, 2001, 2002; Pierrehumbert, 2003; Sosa & Bybee, chapter 30 in this volume) which sees phonological knowledge as dynamic and non-invariant, strongly driven by experience, and embodying not only the sound-referent associations relevant to lexical meaning but also all of the other significant associations experienced by individuals (e.g. those relating to indi-viduals, situations, contexts, as discussed here). This overall approach is not uncontested (not least because it raises very significant theoretical issues re-garding, for example, the nature of the lexicon), and has many issues that need to be elaborated in much greater detail (see discussion in Foulkes & Docherty, 2006; Pierrehumbert, 2000, 2006), but to the extent that it is a valid approach, it clearly paints a very different view of the nature of phonological representa-tion and therefore of the object of a clinical phonological assessment. It is a view that has not yet had much influence on the practice of clinicians, but ultim-ately it is one that might allow for a more rounded account to be formulated in clinical assessment of the sorts of variation described in this chapter.

ACKNOWLEDGMENT

We would like to thank Paul Foulkes and the volume editors for their very helpful comments on a draft of this chapter.

NOTES

1   The term 'social-indexical' is applied here to those properties of speech which are correlated with relevant social dimensions of a speech community either at the level of groups of speakers or in relation to individuals.
2   As a means of facilitating the analysis of vowel variables, Wells (1982) introduced the notion of standard 'lexical sets' to refer to groups of English words that share the same vowel pronunciation across two or more varieties. Since the vowel that is associated to a particular lexical set may vary across different dialects, the vowel differences between these dialects can be conveniently expressed in terms of these lexical sets.
3   But it should be noted that, developmentally, [w] is more common than [ʋ], so it is not obvious that this is a persisting developmental pattern.

REFERENCES

Agnihotri, R. K. (1979). Processes of assimilation: A sociolinguistic study of Sikh children in Leeds. Unpublished PhD thesis, University of York.

Armstrong, S. and Ainley, M. (1988). *South Tyneside Assessment of Syntactic Structures*. Ponteland, UK: STASS Publications.

Britain, D. (forthcoming). One foot in the grave? Dialect death, dialect contact and dialect birth in England. *International Journal of the Sociology of Language*.

Bullock, B. and Gerfen, C. (2004). Phonological convergence in a contracting language variety. *Bilingualism, Language, and Cognition*, 7(2), 1–10.

Bullock, B., Toribio, J. A., Davis, K. A., and Botero, C. G. (2005). Phonetic convergence in bilingual Puerto Rican Spanish. In B. Schmeiser, V. Chand, A. Kelleher, and A. Rodriguez (eds.), *Proceedings of the West Coast Conference on Formal Linguistics 23*. Somerville, MA: Cascadilla Press.

Bybee, J. (2001). *Phonology and Language Use*. Cambridge Studies in Linguistics, 94. Cambridge: Cambridge University Press.

Bybee, J. (2002). Phonological evidence for exemplar storage of multiword sequences. *Studies in Second Language Acquisition*, 24, 215–21.

Chambers, J. K. (1973). Canadian raising. *Canadian Journal of Linguistics*, 18, 113–35.

Chambers, J. K. (2002). Dynamics of dialect convergence. *Journal of Sociolinguistics*, 6, 117–30.

Cho, T. and McQueen, J. M. (2005). Prosodic influences on consonant production in Dutch: Effects of prosodic boundaries, phrasal accent and lexical stress. *Journal of Phonetics*, 33, 121–57.

Clopper, C. G. (2004). Linguistic experience and the perceptual classification of dialect variation. Doctoral dissertation, Indiana University.

Clopper, C. G. and Pisoni, D. B. (2004a). Effects of talker variability on perceptual learning of dialects. *Language and Speech*, 47, 207–39.

Clopper, C. G. and Pisoni, D. B. (2004b). Homebodies and army brats: Some effects of early linguistic experience and residential history on dialect categorization. *Language Variation and Change*, 16, 31–48.

De Houwer, A. (1995). Bilingual language acquisition. In P. Fletcher and B. MacWhinney (eds.), *Handbook of Child Language* (pp. 219–50). Oxford: Blackwell.

Docherty, G. J. (2007). Speech in its natural environment: Accounting for social factors in phonetic variability. In J. Cole and J.-I. Hualde (eds.), *Papers in Laboratory Phonology, IX* (pp. 1–36). Berlin: Mouton.

Docherty, G. J., Foulkes, P., Tillotson, J., and Watt, D. J. L. (2006). On the scope of phonological learning: issues arising from socially structured variation. In L. Goldstein, D. H. Whalen, and C. T. Best (eds.), *Laboratory Phonology 8* (pp. 393–421). Berlin: Mouton de Gruyter.

Dodd, B. (1995). *Differential Diagnosis and Treatment of Children with Speech Disorder*. London: Whurr Publishers.

Dodd, B., Zhu, H., Crosbie, S., Holm, A., and Ozanne, A. (2002). *Diagnostic Evaluation of Articulation and Phonology*. London: Psychological Corporation.

Dyer, J. (2002). 'We all speak the same round here': dialect leveling in a Scottish-English community. *Journal of Sociolinguistics*, 6, 99–116.

Eckert, P. (1996). Age as a sociolinguistic variable. In Florian Coulmas (ed.), *The Handbook of Sociolinguistics*. Oxford: Blackwell.

Foulkes, P. (2005). Sociophonetics. In K. Brown (ed.), *Encyclopedia of Language and Linguistics*. 2nd ed. (pp. 495–500). Amsterdam: Elsevier Press.

Foulkes, P. and Docherty, G. J. (eds.) (1999). *Urban Voices: Accent Studies in the British Isles*. London: Edward Arnold.

Foulkes, P. and Docherty, G. J. (2000). Another chapter in the story of /r/: 'Labiodental' variants in British English. *Journal of Sociolinguistics*, 4, 30–59.

Foulkes, P. and Docherty, G. J. (2006). The social life of phonetics and phonology. *Journal of Phonetics*, 34(4), 409–38.

Foulkes, P. and Docherty, G. J. (2007). Phonological variation in England. In D. Britain (ed.), *Language in the British Isles*, 2nd ed. Cambridge: Cambridge University Press.

Foulkes, P., Docherty, G. J., and Watt, D. J. L. (2005). Phonological variation in child directed speech. *Language*, 81, 177–206.

Genesee, F. (1989). Early bilingual development: One language or two? *Journal of Child Language*, 6, 161–79.

Giles, H. (ed.) (1984). The dynamics of speech accommodation. *International Journal of the Sociology of Language*, 46, 1–155.

Giles, H., Coupland, N., and Coupland, J. (eds.) (1991). *The Contexts of Accommodation: Dimensions in Applied Sociolinguistics*. New York: Cambridge University Press.

Gimson, A. C. (2001). *Gimson's Pronunciation of English*. 6th ed., revised by A. Cruttenden. London: Edward Arnold.

Grabe, E. and Nolan, F. (2001). *English Intonation in the British Isles: The IViE Corpus*. CD-ROMs produced as part of ESRC grant R000237145.

Grosjean, F. (2001). The bilingual's language modes. In J. L. Nicol (ed.), *One Mind, Two Languages* (pp. 1–22). Oxford: Blackwell.

Hamers, J. F. and Blanc, M. H. A. (2000). *Bilinguality and Bilingualism*. 2nd ed. Cambridge: Cambridge University Press.

Hardcastle, W. J. and Hewlett, N. (eds.) (1999). *Coarticulation: Theory, Data and Techniques*. Cambridge: Cambridge University Press.

Hay, J. and Drager, K. (2007). Sociophonetics. *Annual Review of Anthropology*, 36, 89–103.

Hay, J., Nolan, A., and Drager, K. (2006) From fush to feesh: Exemplar priming in speech perception. *Linguistic Review*, 23, 351–79.

Hay, J., Warren, P., and Drager, K. (2006) Factors influencing speech perception in the context of a merger-in-progress. *Journal of Phonetics*, 34(4), 458–84.

Henton, C. and Bladon, A. (1988). Creak as a sociophonetic marker. In L. M. Hyman and C. N. Li (eds.), *Language, Speech and Mind: Studies in Honour of Victoria A. Fromkin* (pp. 3–29). London: Routledge.

Holm, A. and Dodd, B. (1999). A longitudinal study of the phonological development of two Cantonese-English bilingual children. *Applied Psycholinguistics*, 20, 349–76.

Howard, S. J. (2007). The interplay between articulation and prosody in children with impaired speech: observations from electropalatography and perceptual analysis. *Advances in Speech-Language Pathology*, 9(1), 20–35.

Jarabo-Lorenzo, F. (1998). Sociolinguistic variation and change in the Spanish of Santa Cruz de Tenerife. Unpublished PhD dissertation, University of Newcastle upon Tyne.

Kent, R. D. and Kent, J. F. (2000). Task-based profiles of the dysarthrias. *Folia Phoniatrica and Logopaedica*, 52, 48–53.

Kent, R. D., Kent, J. F., Rosenbek, J. C., Vorperian, H. K., and Weismer, G. (1997). A speaking task analysis of the dysarthria in cerebellar disease. *Folia Phoniatrica and Logopaedica*, 49, 63–82.

Kerswill, P. (1996a). Milton Keynes and dialect levelling in south-eastern British English. In D. Graddol, J. Swann, and D. Leith (eds.), *English: History, Diversity and Change* (pp. 292–300). London: Routledge.

Kerswill, P. (1996b). Children, adolescents and language change. *Language Variation and Change*, 8, 177–202.

Kerswill, P. (2001). Mobility, meritocracy and dialect levelling: The fading (and phasing) out of Received Pronunciation. In P. Rajamäe and K. Vogelberg (eds.), *British Studies in the New Millennium: The Challenge of the Grassroots*. Tartu: University of Tartu, pp. 45–58.

Kerswill, P. (2003). Dialect levelling and geographical diffusion in British English. In D. Britain and J. Cheshire (eds.), *Social Dialectology: In Honour of Peter Trudgill*, pp. 223–43. Amsterdam: Benjamins.

Kerswill, P. and Williams, A. (2000). Mobility and social class in dialect levelling: Evidence from new and old towns in England. In Klaus Mattheier (ed.), *Dialect and Migration in a Changing Europe* (pp. 1–13). Frankfurt: Peter Lang.

Khattab, G. (2002). /l/ production in English-Arabic bilingual speakers. *International Journal of Bilingualism*, 6, 335–54.

Khattab, G. (2007). Variation in vowel production by English-Arabic bilinguals. In J. Cole and J. I. Hualde (ed.), *Papers in Laboratory Phonology IX* (pp. 383–410). Berlin: Mouton de Gruyter.

Laver, J. (1980). *The Phonetic Description of Voice Quality*. Cambridge: Cambridge University Press.

Leopold, W. F. (1970). *Speech Development of a Bilingual Child: A Linguist's Record*, vol. 2. New York: AMS Press.

Levon, E. (2006). Hearing 'gay': Prosody, interpretation and the affective judgments of men's speech. *American Speech*, 81, 56–78.

Lindsey, G. and Hirson, A. (1999). Variable robustness of nonstandard /r/ in English: Evidence from accent disguise. *Forensic Linguistics: The International Journal of Speech, Language and the Law*, 6(2), 278–88.

Lippi-Green, R. (1997). *English with an Accent: Language, Ideology, and Discrimination in the United States*. London and New York: Routledge.

Llamas, M. C. (2006). Age. In M. C. Llamas, L. Mullany, and P. Stockwell (eds.), *The Routledge Companion to Sociolinguistics* (pp. 69–76). London: Routledge.

McLeod, S. (ed.) (2007). *The International Guide to Speech Acquisition*. Clifton Park, NY: Thomson Delmar Learning.

Milroy, J. (2006). Language ideologies. In M. C. Llamas, L. Mullany, and P. Stockwell (eds.), *The Routledge Companion to Sociolinguistics* (pp. 133–9). London: Routledge.

Milroy, L. and Gordon, M. (2003). *Sociolinguistics: Method and Interpretation*. Language in Society, 34. Malden, MA: Blackwell.

Munson, B., McDonald, E., DeBoe, N., and White, A. (2006). Acoustic and perceptual bases of judgments of women and men's sexual orientation from read speech. *Journal of Phonetics*, 34, 202–40.

Niedzielski, N. A. (1999). The effect of social information on the perception of socio-linguistic variables. *Journal of Social Psychology*, 18(1), 62–85.

Paradis, J. (2001). Do bilingual two-year-olds have separate phonological systems? *International Journal of Bilingualism*, 5(1), 19–38.

Pert, S. and Letts, C. (2003). Developing an expressive language assessment for children in Rochdale with a Pakistani heritage background. *Child Language Teaching and Therapy*, 19(3), 267–89.

Pert, S. and Letts, C. (2006). Codeswitching in Mirpuri speaking Pakistani heritage preschool children: Bilingual language acquisition. *International Journal of Bilingualism*, 10(3), 349–74.

Pierrehumbert, J. (2000). The phonetic grounding of phonology. *Bulletin de la Communication Parlée*, 5, 7–23.

Pierrehumbert, J. (2003). Phonetic diversity, statistical learning, and acquisition of phonology. *Language and Speech*, 46(2–3), 115–54.

Pierrehumbert, J. (2006). The next toolkit. *Journal of Phonetics*, 34(6), 516–30.

Preston, D. and Long. D. (eds.) (2002). *Handbook of Perceptual Dialectology*, vol. 2. Amsterdam: John Benjamins.

Rampton, B. (1995). *Crossing: Language and Ethnicity among Adolescents*. London: Longman.

Roberts, J. (1997). Hitting a moving target: Acquisition of sound change in progress by Philadelphia children. *Language Variation and Change*, 9, 249–66.

Roelofs, A. and Verhoef, K. (2006). Modeling the control of phonological encoding in bilingual speakers. *Bilingualism: Language and Cognition*, 9, 167–76.

Sangster, C. (2002). Inter- and intra-speaker variation in Liverpool English: A socio-phonetic study. Unpublished DPhil dissertation, University of Oxford.

Schneider, E. (2007). *Postcolonial English: Varieties around the World*. Cambridge: Cambridge University Press.

Smith, B. L., Kenney, M. K., and Hussain, S. (1996). A longitudinal investigation of duration and temporal variability in children's speech production. *Journal of the Acoustical Society of America*, 99, 2344–9.

Smyth, R., Jacobs, G., and Rogers, H. (2003). Male voices and perceived sexual orientation: An experimental and theoretical approach. *Language and Society*, 32, 329–50.

Stow, C. (2004). Meeting the bilingual challenge. *RCSLT Bulletin*, 623, 14–15.

Stow, C. and Pert, S. (1998a). *The Rochdale Assessment of Mirpuri Phonology with Punjabi and Urdu* (RAMP). Rochdale: Pert.

Stow, C. and Pert, S. (1998b). The development of a bilingual phonology assessment. *International Journal of Language and Communication Disorders*, 33 (Supplement), 338–43.

Stow, C. and Pert, S. (2006). Phonological acquisition in bilingual Pakistani heritage children in England. In Z. Hua and B. Dodd (eds.), *Phonological Development and*

Disorders in Children: A Multilingual Perspective (pp. 326–45). Clevedon: Multilingual Matters.

Strand, E. A. (1999). Uncovering the role of gender stereotypes in speech perception. *Journal of Language and Social Psychology*, 18(1), 86–99.

Street, R. L. and Cappella, J. N. (1989). Social and linguistic factors influencing adaptation in children's speech. *Journal of Psycholinguistic Research*, 18(5), 497–519.

Stuart-Smith, J. (1999). Glasgow: Accent and voice quality. In Foulkes and Docherty (1999) (pp. 201–22).

Thanki, M. (2002). White women only: The challenge for change. *Royal College for Speech and Language Therapy (RCSLT) Diversity Strategy Report*. London: RCSLT.

Thomas, E. R. (2002). Sociophonetic applications of speech perception experiments. *American Speech*, 77, 115–47.

Torgersen, E. and Kerswill, P. (2004). Internal and external motivation in phonetic change: Dialect levelling outcomes for an English vowel shift. *Journal of Sociolinguistics*, 8, 24–53.

Torgersen, E., Kerswill, P., and Fox, S. (2006). Ethnicity as a source of changes in the London vowel system. In Frans Hinskens (ed.), *Language Variation: European Perspectives* (pp. 249–63). Amsterdam: John Benjamins.

Trudgill, P. (1974). *The Social Differentiation of English in Norwich*. Cambridge: Cambridge University Press.

Trudgill, P. (1988). Norwich revisited: Recent linguistic changes in an English urban dialect. *English World-Wide*, 9, 1–33.

Trudgill, P. (1999). *The Dialects of England*. 2nd ed. Oxford: Blackwell.

Tsao, T-C., Weismer, G., and Iqbal, K. (2006). The effect of intertalker speech rate variation on acoustic vowel space. *Journal of the Acoustical Society of America*, 119, 1074–82.

Verma, M. and Firth, S. (1995). Old sounds and new sounds: Bilinguals learning ESL. In M. Verma, K. P. Corrigan, and S. Firth (eds.), *Working with Bilingual Children* (pp. 128–42). Clevedon: Multilingual Matters.

Ward, I. C. (1936). *Defects of Speech: Their Nature and Their Cause*. 3rd ed. London: J. M. Dent and Co.

Watt, D. (2002). 'I don't speak with a Geordie accent, I speak, like, the Northern accent': Contact-induced levelling in the Tyneside vowel system. *Journal of Sociolinguistics*, 6, 44–63.

Watt, D. and Milroy, L. (1999). Patterns of variation and change in three Newcastle vowels: Is this dialect levelling? In Foulkes and Docherty (1999) (pp. 25–46).

Watt, D. and Tillotson, J. (2001). A spectrographic analysis of vowel fronting in Bradford English. *English World-Wide*, 22(2), 269–302.

Wells, J. C. (1982). *Accents of English* (3 vols.). Cambridge: Cambridge University Press.

Whiteside, S. P., Henry, L., and Dobbin, R. (2003). Patterns of variability in voice onset time: A developmental study of motor speech skills. *Neuroscience Letters*, 347, 29–32.

Williams, A. and Kerswill, P. (1999). Dialect levelling: Change and continuity in Milton Keynes, Reading and Hull. In Foulkes and Docherty (1999) (pp. 141–62).

Yildirim, S., Narayanan, S., Byrd, B., and Khurana, S. (2003). Acoustic analysis of preschool children's speech. In M. J. Solé, D. Recasens, and J. Romero (eds.), *Proceedings of the 15th International Congress of Phonetic Sciences*, Barcelona, August (pp. 949–52). Rundle Mall, Adelaide: Causal Productions.

38 Cross-Linguistic Phonological Acquisition

DAVID INGRAM

38.1 Introduction

A complete understanding of phonological acquisition in children will not be achieved until in-depth studies are available on how children acquire the wide range of phonological systems that characterize human language. This challenging enterprise is complicated by the large number of languages that exist, the need to determine the full range of ways that languages differ phonologically, and the manner in which phonological properties interact with grammatical properties. Estimates of the number of languages vary, but the numbers are typically in the thousands. Linguistic studies have made great strides in the last one hundred years in understanding the structure of language, but many languages have not been studied in depth, and many aspects of language structure are far from being completely understood.

Table 38.1 presents a summary of the major aspects that need to be considered in developing a phonological typology of languages. As shown, languages will differ in their prosodic systems, syllable structure, consonantal and vocalic systems, phonotactics, and interactions with morphology and syntax. Phonologists are actively studying each of these areas to add to our understanding of their universal and language-specific properties, but many gaps exist in our current knowledge.

In addition to developing accurate phonological characterizations of languages, research into phonological acquisition deals with both theoretical and practical issues. Theoretical issues involve the assumptions that need to be made about the nature of phonological acquisition in general. At one extreme, research can take a strong theoretical stand, e.g. assuming a particular theory such as Optimality Theory (OT), and view phonological data from that perspective (cf. Ball & Kent, 1997). At the other end, research can be more descriptively driven, collecting data and determining patterns of acquisition with minimal theoretical speculation. For example, research could be initiated on a language such as Igbo (an African language of the Niger–Congo family) to

Table 38.1 Properties of a phonological typology of languages

1. *Prosody*	systems of stress, tone, and pitch accent; stress vs. syllable timing
2. *Syllable structure*	nature of onsets, codas, consonant clusters, reduplication, and mora structure
3. *Vowels*	systems of vowels, e.g. number of vowels, existence of vowel length, nasalization, tense vs. lax vowels, and degrees of frontness; vowel harmony systems.
4. *Consonants*	types of consonants in relation to place, voice and manner; states of the larynx; common vs. rare sounds (e.g. 'ř' in Czech).
5. *Phonotactics*	constraints on consonant and vowel co-occurrences (e.g. final devoicing in German)
6. *Grammatical interactions*	morphological and syntactic conditioning (e.g. English plural)

provide data on the patterns of its acquisition, without posing specific theoretical questions. Here, I will make some basic yet conservative theoretical assumptions about how phonological acquisition takes place, while providing preliminary cross-linguistic data.

Besides selecting a theory of phonology, research also needs to work within a theory of phonological acquisition. Issues in phonological acquisition concern assumptions about the extent to which children form linguistic systems comparable to those of adult speakers. At one end we have maturational accounts that propose children are not like adults, and that they follow a path of discontinuous development. This would occur, for instance, if the early words produced by children were constrained by the maturation of the articulators, so that less complex syllables and sounds are acquired before more complex ones (e.g. MacNeilage & Davis, 2000; Locke, 1983). Such theories have important implications for the study of both typical children (monolingual and bilingual) and children showing a phonological delay or disorder. If such theories are accurate, then children across languages should look very similar to one another, regardless of their typicality. Alternatively, children could begin phonological acquisition with the basic cognitive and articulatory skills to begin the establishment of a phonological system, albeit a simple one, that is constructed with the same phonological units that characterize adult language. This is a long-standing position (Jakobson, 1968) that still has its proponents today (Ingram, 1989).

It would be impossible to cover all these aspects of cross-linguistic acquisition in a single article, because of both the scope of the enterprise and a lack of research on many of them. The present chapter will approach the topic by concentrating on two descriptive aspects as they relate to two theoretical questions.

The descriptive part presents data from selected languages concerning differences in consonantal acquisition, and whole-word complexity, across languages. These data are discussed in relation to these theoretical questions: (1) Is early phonological acquisition universal or influenced by the linguistic environment? (2) Is an impairment in early word production the result of an articulatory or a phonological impairment? It will be concluded that children show noticeable cross-linguistic differences in phonological acquisition, and that these differences demonstrate early phonological organization of the input. Further, the limited data that exist indicate that children with phonological impairments show the same ambient characteristics as their peers who are typically developing. These results provide evidence that phonological impairment is indeed phonological, not just the result of articulatory limitations. These three results together provide strong evidence for the early use of phonological organization.

38.2   Determinants of Early Phonological Acquisition

38.2.1   *Early consonantal inventories*

A question fundamental to the understanding of phonological acquisition is: When do children begin phonological organization of the target language? The Russian linguist Roman Jakobson, in his classic work (Jakobson, 1968), proposed that it begins with children's very first words, but that properties of the ambient language emerge soon after. The first words have phonological characteristics in the sense that there are basic linguistic contrasts made through the use of universal distinctive features. A number of researchers (e.g. Locke, 1983, MacNeilage & Davis, 2000) have challenged this perspective, arguing that the limited range of early speech sounds is due to limitation of the articulatory system. From this perspective, phonology does not begin until later, e.g. around the acquisition of the fiftieth word (Locke, 1983).

One way to examine this question is through cross-linguistic research. If children are constrained by the maturation of the articulatory system, then we should see similar patterns in word production across languages. If, however, children are more advanced in their articulatory development, and ready for phonological organization of the input, we should expect cross-linguistic variation. This question was examined in Pye, Ingram, and List (1987) through a very simple methodology of examining the early consonantal inventories of children acquiring different languages. In their study, the languages studied were English and K'iche' (a Guatemalan language). Their results indicated that the two inventories were in fact distinct.

Here, I will review the results in Pye, Ingram, and List (1987) and add other data as well, to demonstrate that children in different linguistic environments produce different consonantal inventories from very early on in their word acquisition. That presentation will be followed by a discussion of possible explanations of these results.

Starting with English, studies have shown that children show variability in their early consonant acquisition, but that grouped data indicate a general system shown in (1) (Ingram, 1981; Stoel-Gammon, 1991). (The data throughout this section will be based on word-initial consonant acquisition.)

(1)   Early consonantal system of English-speaking children

    m   n   y
    b   d   g
    p   t   k
    f   s   h
    w   j

English children show three places of articulation (labial, coronal, velar), four classes (nasals, stops, fricatives, glides), and early use of a voice contrast between stops. The question then becomes whether or not children in other linguistic environments will show similar categories, subject of course to the distinctions being found in their ambient language.

Below is the consonantal system reported by Pye and colleagues for five K'iche' children.

(2)   Early consonantal system of K'iche'-speaking children

    m   n
    p   t tʃ k
                    x
    w   l

There are certain similarities between this system and the English one. They share four classes of consonants, and three places of articulation. One difference, the lack of a voice contrast within stops, can be explained by the fact that K'iche' does not have such a difference. Other differences, however, cannot be accounted for in this fashion. First, the K'iche' inventory has two consonants that occur in English, /l/ and /tʃ/, but these consonants are not found in the English early inventory. Also, these two consonants not only appear in early K'iche', but they are the two most frequently occurring consonants. Another noticeable difference is seen within the fricatives. While K'iche' has an /s/, it does not occur early. Instead, K'iche' children show the use of an early velar fricative /x/ not found in English. Pye and colleagues conclude that the data support the view that the ambient language influences early phonological acquisition. Their more specific proposal for this influence will be returned to later.

I have found similar differences in the early consonantal inventories of every language for which I have been able to obtain data. (3) gives the early consonant system of French children. This is based on my analyses of diary data found in Deville (1890, 1891), Roussey (1899, 1900), and Vinson (1915).

(3)   Early consonantal system of French-speaking children

```
m  n
b  d
p  t
f  s
   l
```

Like the K'iche' system, this shows some similarities to the English inventory. There are three similar classes (nasals, stops, fricatives), similar consonants for these three classes, and an early voice distinction. There are also two notice- able differences. One is the early occurrence of /l/, an observation also made for the K'iche' inventory. Second, there is a lack of early velar stops, even though French has them. Given the small number of children being analyzed, it is possible that these sounds might be part of early French if a wider range of children were studied. Independent evidence for the lack of velars, however, is found in de Boysson-Bardies and Vihman (1991). They studied the early consonants in the babbling and first 25 words of children acquiring French, English, Japanese, and Swedish. Table 38.2 gives the distribution of labial, dental and velar consonants for the first 25 words acquired. The data indicate that that French children produced the lowest rate of velars (9%), versus rates ranging from 20% to 26% for the other languages.

Another example of consonantal differences across languages is Cantonese. (4) gives the consonant system for early Cantonese, based on data in So and Dodd (1995). The data are for 26 children between the ages of 2;0 and 2;6, for those word-initial consonants that were used by 90 percent of the subjects.

(4)   Early consonantal system of Cantonese-speaking children

```
m  n  ŋ
p  t  k
w  j
      h
```

As with the other languages, the data are as interesting for what is missing as for which sounds occur. Cantonese has both an /f/ and an /s/, but neither

Table 38.2   The percentage of occurrence of labial, dental, and velar consonants in the early words for four languages (de Boysson-Bardies & Vihman, 1991)

Language	Labials (%)	Dentals (%)	Velars (%)
French	52	39	9
English	40	40	20
Japanese	22	51	26
Swedish	20	58	23

meets the So and Dodd criteria for acquisition until 4;0 and 4;6 collectively (ages when both boys and girls have acquired them). Cantonese has a contrast between aspirated and unaspirated stops (the closest thing to the voice vs. voiceless difference in English and French), and this distinction is not acquired until age 4;0. Also, Cantonese has an /l/, but it does not appear early as it does in French and K'iche'.

Lastly, (5) presents the early consonantal system for five Spanish-speaking children from 2;2 to 2;11, reported in Loatman (2001).

(5)   Early consonantal system of Spanish-speaking children

      m   n

      b   g

      p   t   k

             tʃ

       l

         j

The Spanish data show the early occurrence of both /l/ and /tʃ/ as has been noted for K'iche'. There is also an early voice contrast, though /d/ does not appear in the early system. Spanish has three fricatives, /f/, /s/, and /x/, but none of these met the criterion for inclusion in the early inventory.

Data such as these provide a strong case that children across language environments do not begin acquisition with the same consonants. What then, is the explanation behind these differences? Pye, Ingram, and List (1987) explored this question by looking at the distribution of the English and K'iche' inventories across the words in each language that the children were acquiring. They found significant correlations with the frequency of occurrence of the individual consonants and the number of word types they occurred in. Stated differently, the more words a consonant occurred in, the more likely it was that the children would acquire it. This relationship is one that has been referred to as *functional load* (cf. Meyerstein, 1970). The functional load of any particular phoneme refers to its importance within the phonological system. While the specifics of determining functional loads for individual phonemes are complex, simple examples can demonstrate the general point. Take for example, English /s/ versus /ʒ/. The /s/ phoneme is very frequent in English, and is found to be an early acquisition. The phoneme /ʒ/, however, is restricted to the coda position and is not in many English words; it is thus a late acquisition. In discussing functional load, it is also important to emphasize that functional load concerns type frequency, not token frequency. For example, the English phoneme /ð/ is low in functional load in the sense that it primarily occurs in a small number of function words, such as the article 'the' and pronouns such as 'this', 'that'. It is high in token frequency, however, since those function words in which it occurs are used frequently in the language. The phoneme /ð/, however, is a late acquisition for English children, either due to its low functional load or articulatory difficulty. The latter options can be teased out by studying a language such as Greek, where /ð/ has a higher functional load than in English. Unfortunately, the data on Greek acquisition are limited, but there is some indication that it is an earlier acquisition in Greek than it is in English (Petinou, n.d.).

Recently, Stokes and Surendran (2005) have explored more systematically the interaction of the three candidates for accounting for the acquisition of speech sounds, these being articulatory complexity, functional load, and ambient (i.e. token) frequency. They developed a procedure to measure each, and applied the measures to the early phonologies of children acquiring English, Cantonese and Dutch. Regression analyses were performed on the influence of each factor on the emergence of consonants, and the accuracy of consonant production. The results showed that the factors had different effects both across languages and on the two aspects of consonant emergence and accuracy. Functional load had a strong influence on the emergence of consonants in English, though their accuracy was more predicted by articulatory complexity. The token frequency of consonants was a strong predictor for the emergence of consonants in Cantonese, and also for the accuracy of production for Dutch. While a very preliminary study, it showed that the three factors may play very different roles depending on the language being investigated.

38.2.2   *Whole-word complexity and proximity*

While the study of phonological acquisition has mostly focused on segmental development, recent research has expanded to syllables and whole-word properties. Ingram (2002) has suggested two aspects of whole words to incorporate into phonological analyses, whole-word complexity, and proximity. Whole-word complexity refers to the extent to which one word can be said to be more complex than another. A thorough measure of complexity will need to consider syllabic and segmental complexity, and some way to weigh the two. Ingram (2002) proposed a simpler measure, one for providing a relatively fast and simple way to establish an initial impression, referred to as the *phonological mean length of utterance*, or pMLU. The pMLU is a basic count of the number of sounds in a word, and the number of consonants. Each vowel receives one point, and each consonant two points, under the assumption that consonants, particularly when combined into consonant clusters, add more complexity to a word than vowels. An English word like 'bee' will receive a score of 3, while a word like 'between' would score 10. The mean of these counts across a child's vocabulary can give some idea of whether or not a child is acquiring simpler or more complex words, and it can be used to assess the complexity of words on articulation tests. The calculation of the pMLU of a child's productions is done slightly differently, where consonants are scored with one point, and only receive a second point if they are produced correctly. The child who produces 'truck' as [gak] will receive four points: three points for the three segments, and one more point for the correct /k/. The scoring of *proximity* involves comparing the child's pMLU to that of the adult targets, by dividing the latter into the former. The child who produces all its words correctly (technically, all consonants correctly and some effort for each vowel) will have a score of 1.0 or 100%. In the example above for 'truck', the proximity would be .57, by dividing 7 (the pMLU of the target word) into 4 (the pMLU of the child's word). Ingram (2002) reported proximity scores for English children acquiring their first 25 words of around 64 percent.

The study of whole-word measures is still at a very early stage, and much more needs to be done concerning the specific rules for their calculation and appropriate sample sizes. There has been, however, preliminary research applying the measures cross-linguistically, and also to phonological disorders and bilingualism, areas to be covered later. The measurement of pMLU cross-linguistically has been reported in Ingram (2002) for English, Cantonese and Spanish, in Saaristo-Helin, Savinainen-Makkonen, and Kunnari (2006) for Finnish, and in Taelman, Durieux, and Gillis (2005) for Dutch. I also have some preliminary data on pMLU for French children, and new data on Spanish since Ingram (2002) in Hase (2005). Table 38.3 provides a summary of the data for pMLU in each of these languages, and also proximity when available.

Obviously, an accurate comparison of whole-word measures across languages will require controlled comparisons matching children on age and vocabulary size. Even without such data, the comparisons in table 38.3 suggest that children differ on these measures cross-linguistically, at least in the early stages of phonological development. The Cantonese child showed relatively low pMLU scores and high proximity, suggesting that she was having little trouble acquiring Cantonese phonology. The Finnish children have higher pMLUs for the first 25 words than the English children, and also higher proximity, suggesting that longer words with relatively simple syllable structure do not impede phonological acquisition. The Spanish children were older than the Finnish

Table 38.3 A comparison of pMLU and proximity for six languages

Language	Ages/samples/children	pMLU	Proximity
English	0;11 to 1;10/first 25 words/5 children	3.2	.64.
	1;3 to 2;3/longitudinal/Jennika	3.6 to 5.1	.67 to .74
	1;4 to 1;8/longitudinal/Kristen	4.2 to 5.6	.65 to .86
Cantonese	1;7//Wai	4.8	.93
Dutch	1;4 to 1;10//7 children	4.4	not given
	1;11 to 2;4//6 children	5.4	not given
	2;6 to 2;11//4 children	6.0	not given
Finnish	1;5 to 2;0/first 25 words/17 children	5.1	.78
French	1;5 to 1;11/first 250 words/Fernande	3.5 to 3.8	.62 to .68
Spanish	2;6//5 children	6.3	.82
	2;7//7 children	6.4	.84
	3;0//8 children	7.0	.92

children, but showed a similar pattern, with a relatively high proximity. The English and Dutch data indicate that the phonologies of these languages are harder to acquire, since the pMLUs are lower and proximity is lower also (at least for the available English data). The French child showed a low pMLU and low proximity comparable to the English children during the first 50 words. The two English children with longitudinal data showed a gradual increase in both, but the French child maintained those lower measures across the first 250 words. Of course, such small samples need to be treated with great caution, but the preliminary data are suggestive of cross-linguistic differences.

38.3   The Nature of Phonological Impairment

Traditionally, children who showed atypical or delayed speech were assumed to have a speech problem, that is, an inability to move the articulators appropriately to produce words correctly. In the late 1960s, researchers conducted phonological analyses on children with impaired speech, and found that their patterns required a phonological, not just an articulatory, explanation (Ingram, 1976). For example, a child who produced an /s/ as a [t] could nonetheless produce an [s] as a substitute for a /ʃ/. This is the classic Jakobsonian argument that speech development is phonological, not just articulatory. Word acquisition requires the child to form phonological representations of words, and to be capable of mapping those representations into speech forms.

Cross-linguistic phonological acquisition provides an excellent test case to explore the articulatory versus phonological nature of speech impairments. If, in fact, the primary characteristic of a speech disorder is an inability to make sounds, then children with speech problems should look similar across linguistic environments. On the other hand, if these children are nonetheless making an effort to establish a phonological system along the lines of their language peers, then their word productions should look more similar to those of typical children in their language environment than to children with speech problems in a different linguistic environment.

The determination of consonant inventories, as done earlier, can be used to study the nature of a child's phonological impairment. The methodology is basically to determine inventories for children with typical development, and compare them with those of children with speech impairments. Relatively little cross-linguistic research of this kind has been done, since such research would involve studies that plan such comparisons with careful matching of the children. Nonetheless, some data exist where one set comprises studies on normal phonological acquisition, and another set involves studies on phonological impairment. These data can then be compared on an ad hoc basis to get an initial impression on how the two sets of data compare. If there is a trend in the sets of comparisons, such trends can at least be suggestive of whether children with impairments compare more closely to their same-language peers, or to children with phonological impairments in other languages. Here, data will be presented for comparison for English, Italian, Swedish, Turkish, and Greek.

Ingram (1981) matched 15 typically developing children (1;5 to 2;2, median age 1;9) to 15 children with phonological impairments (3;11 to 8;0, median age 5;3), according to their Articulation Scores (AS). The AS is a measure that weighs the number of consonants a child is using by their frequency of use. (6) gives the consonant inventories of each group, with the number of children who used each consonant. Data are only provided for consonants that occurred in at least one-third of the samples.

(6)   Consonantal systems of English-speaking children

	Typical			Atypical	
m (14)	n (11)		m (13)	n (6)	
b (15)	d (15)	g (8)	b (15)	d (15)	g (5)
p (7)	t (9)	k (9)	p (9)	t (15)	k (9)
f (5)	s (5)		f (7)	s (5)	
w (11)		h (9)	w (12)		h (10)

Except for some small numerical differences, the two inventories are the same. With just one language being compared, however, it is not possible to conclude either that the similarities are due to a language effect or that they are due to articulatory complexity.

Evidence for a language effect in phonological impairment increases when other languages are considered. Bortolini, Ingram, and Dykstra (1993) compared nine Italian children with typical language (2;2 to 2;11) with nine Italian children identified as having a phonological impairment (4;9 to 7;1). Analyses of their word-initial consonant inventories gave the results shown in (7). The most frequent consonants are marked with an asterisk (*), and less frequent ones are within parentheses.

(7)   Consonantal systems of Italian-speaking children

Typical				Atypical			
b*	d*		g	b*	d		(g)
p*	t*		k*	p*	t*		k*
f*	s*	tʃ*		f*	s	(tʃ)	
v*	z			v			

The first thing to note is that the Italian data from typical children provide further support for cross-linguistic differences. The early acquisition of /tʃ/ is found, and also the early and frequent use of /v/, a fricative acquired very late by English children. The inventory for the atypical children looks very similar to both the inventory for atypical English children in (6) and the Italian children. It is more similar to the Italian children, however, in the occurrence of /v/ and /tʃ/. Elsewhere, Ingram (1988) has reported the early acquisition of /v/ in languages other than English. The fact that the Italian children with a phonological impairment still produce a /v/, presumably due to its import- ance in the ambient language, is support for the hypothesis that their impair- ment is not overriding their developing a phonological system for the more important phonemes in the language.

Data on the phonological systems of Swedish are found in Nettelbladt (1983) and Magnusson (1983). Nettelbladt conducted detailed analyses on 10 children with delayed phonological development (4;4 to 7;11), and collected longitudinal data on one typical child, Tor, at four ages, 1;8, 2;0, 2;2 and 2;5. Magnusson reported phonological data on 32 children between 3;9 and 6;6 who were classified as language-impaired. It is not clear whether these data should be considered typical or not, but the comparison of these data to the Nettelbladt children suggests that their phonologies were delayed. (8) gives the consonantal inventories for these subjects, with the following selection crit- eria: for Nettelbladt's children with impairment, those consonants used by at least five children; for Magnusson, the 10 consonants with the highest per- centages of correct use (as reported in Locke, 1983, table 2.7); and consonants produced correctly by Tor at 2;2.

(8)   Consonantal systems of Swedish-speaking children

Atypical (Nettelbladt)				*Atypical* (Magnusson)			*Tor*		
m	n			m	n		m	n	
p	t			p	t		p	t	
b				b	d		b	d	
f	s/θ		h	f	s	h	f	θ	h
v		j		v				l	

The phonemes /v/ and /j/ are phonetically fricatives, but described by Nettel- bladt as functionally glides. There are also dialectal variations between the use of [s] and [θ], so these two sounds have been treated as phonemic variants. The three sets of data are similar. Of particular interest is the production of /v/ by both groups of impaired children, despite its later acquisition by the typical children. The early use of /v/ was also found in the Italian data above. The phoneme /j/ did not meet the criterion for inclusion for the Magnusson children, but it was just below the cutoff. Tor is clearly acquiring both these sounds later. He does have an /l/, which is not found in the atypical group. Only one of Nettelbladt's ten subjects showed its acquisition.

The next two sets of data on Turkish and Greek are among the relatively rare cases where a single researcher has compared typical phonological acquisition with that of children with a phonological impairment. Topbaş (1996) reported the phonological development of 10 Turkish children classified as speech-disordered, aged five to seven. The study included consonantal inventories for each of the ten children. (9) gives the inventories for those consonants in two charts, one with consonants used by at least eight of the children, the other of consonants used by at least six children. These inventories can be compared to the data in Topbaş (1992), where developmental data from the ages of 1;0 to 3;0 are given for 22 typically developing Turkish children.

(9)   Consonantal systems of Turkish-speaking children

	Atypical (80% of children)				*Atypical* (60% of children)			
m	n			m	n		
p	t	tʃ		p	t	tʃ	k
b	d			b	d		
					s	ʃ	
	l				l		
	j				j		

	Typical (1st 9 consonants)				*Typical* (1st 12 consonants)			
m	n			m	n		
p	t	tʃ	k	p	t	tʃ	k
b	d			b	d	dʒ	g
						ʃ	
	j				j		

The nine consonant inventories share seven of the consonants, and the 12 consonant inventories share 10. One particularly interesting difference is that the /l/ phoneme appears in both sets of the inventories for the atypical children, but it is not in either of those for typical children. This is evidence against the suggestion, based on the previous data on Swedish, that /l/ may be a difficult sound.

Lastly, preliminary data are available from Greek children in Petinou (n.d.). Petinou examined the phonetic inventories of four typically developing children and four children classified as having a specific expressive language delay (SELD). The mean age of the SELD group was 26 months, suggesting these were a group of late talkers. No ages were given for the group of normally developing children (ND). Petinou concluded that the SELD children used fewer consonants than the ND children. This is not surprising given the differences in vocabulary size. The ND children had an average vocabulary of 171 words compared to only 27 words for the SELD children (with a standard deviation of 13). Of interest here is the actual nature of the consonants used. The ND children used the full range of Greek consonants. The SELD children, however, only used nine consonants. These consonants are given in (10) (data were reported for only three children).

(10)   Consonantal systems of Greek-speaking children

Atypical			Typical				
m	n		m	n			ŋ
b	d		b	d	dʒ		g
p	t	k	p	t	tʃ		k
			f	θ	s	ʃ	ɣ
	ð̃		v	ð	z	ʒ	x
	l			l			
				r			

Greek has an extensive fricative system with 10 consonants. The system for atypical children contains just one fricative, /D/. If phonological delay were the result of impaired articulatory ability alone, this would be one of the last fricatives to be acquired, according to analysis based on English data and the relatively limited distribution of this sound cross-linguistically. As discussed earlier, this sound has a high functional load in Greek, and its occurrence in the very limited inventory of three children suggests that the environment is playing a role in its use. There is also the early appearance of /l/, which was just seen in the Turkish data.

In summary, comparisons of consonantal inventories in English, Italian, Swedish, Turkish, and Greek show children with atypical acquisition having inventories more like those of their language peers than those of children with other languages. Such data provide strong support for the position that phonological impairment shows similar environmental effects to typical acquisition.

38.4   Future Directions

Cross-linguistic research is critical in the effort to understand phonological acquisition in typically developing children, and children with phonological impairments. It provides strong support for the view that children are capable of phonological organization at the time of the first words, and that difficulties in speech acquisition have a phonological component. Research into these questions, however, is still at a very early stage. Many aspects of the questions identified in table 38.1, as well as other theoretical questions, have been little researched to date. One area with a great need for more research is that of prosodic development. Languages differ in their timing, stress patterns, and intonation, and the ways in which children acquire these differences need to be better understood (e.g. Dupoux & Peperkamp, 2002). Another area is that of bilingual phonological acquisition. It has become clear in recent years that bilingual children show an early separation of their phonological systems, but that the systems can influence each other in several possible ways (Kesharvarz & Ingram, 2003). The examination of these possibilities will require the study of a wide range of bilingual situations. Bunta, Davidovich, and Ingram (2005) have shown in their study of an English-Hungarian bilingual child that the child's pMLU may vary between the languages, but not the proximity. This finding suggests that it may be more important for children to approximate the phonological properties of the target language than to add more complex sounds. Virtually no research exists that applies the whole-word measures discussed earlier to typical and atypical populations cross-linguistically. The kinds of results reviewed here, however, show that cross-linguistic studies are vital for the advancement of our knowledge of phonological acquisition.

REFERENCES

Ball, M. J. and Kent, R. D. (1997). *The New Phonologies: Developments in Clinical Linguistics.* San Diego, CA: Singular Press.

Bortolini, U., Ingram, D., and Dykstra, K. (1993). The acquisition of the feature [voice] in normal and phonologically delayed Italian children. Paper presented at the *Symposium of Research in Child Language Disorders*, University of Wisconsin-Madison, May 21–2.

Bunta, F., Davidovich, I., and Ingram, D. (2005). The relationship between the phonological complexity of a bilingual child's words and those of the target languages. *International Journal of Bilingualism*, 10, 71–88.

De Boysson-Bardies, B. and Vihman, M. (1991). Adaptation to language: Evidence from babbling and first words. *Language*, 67, 297–319.

Deville, G. (1890). Notes sur le développement du langage. *Revue de Linguistique et de Philologue Comparée*, 23, 330–43.

Deville, G. (1891). Notes sur le développement du langage. *Revue de Linguistique et de Philologue Comparée*, 24, 10–42, 128–43, 242–57, 300–20.

Dupoux, E. and Peperkamp, S. (2002). Fossil markers of language development: Phonological deafnesses in adult speech processing. In B. Laks and J. Durand (eds.), *Phonetics, Phonology, and Cognition* (pp. 168–90). Oxford: Oxford University Press.

Hase, M. (2005). A comparison of two phonological assessment tools for monolingual Spanish-speaking children. Master's thesis, Arizona State University.

Ingram, D. (1976). *Phonological Disability in Children.* London: Edward Arnold.

Ingram, D. (1981). *Procedures for the Phonological Analysis of Children's Language.* Baltimore, MD: University Park Press.

Ingram, D. (1988). The acquisition of word initial [v]. *Language and Speech*, 31, 77–85.

Ingram, D. (1989). *First Language Acquisition.* Cambridge: Cambridge University Press.

Ingram, D. (2002). The measurement of whole word productions. *Journal of Child Language*, 29, 713–33.

Jakobson, R. (1968) (trans. A. R. Keiler). *Child Language, Aphasia, and Phonological Universals*. The Hague: Mouton. Originally published as *Kindersprache, Aphasie, und allgemeine Lautgesetze*. Uppsala: Almqvist and Wiksell, 1941.

Kesharvarz, M. and Ingram, D. (2003). The early phonological development of a Farsi-English bilingual child. *International Journal of Bilingualism*, 6, 255–69.

Loatman, C. (2001). Phonological patterns of two-year-old monolingual Mexican-American Spanish speakers. Master's thesis, Arizona State University.

Locke, J. L. (1983). *Phonological Acquisition and Change*. New York: Academic Press.

MacNeilage, P. F. and Davis, B. L. (2000). On the origin of internal structure of word forms. *Science*, 288, 527–31.

Magnusson, E. (1983). *The Phonology of Language Disordered Children: Production, Perception, and Awareness*. Travaux de l'institut de linguistique de Lund, XVII. Lund: CWK Gleerup.

Meyerstein, R. S. (1970). *Functional Load: Descriptive Limitations, Alternatives of Assessment and Extensions of Application*. The Hague: Mouton.

Nettelbladt, U. (1983). *Developmental studies of dysphonology in children*. Travaux de l'institut de linguistique de Lund, XIX. Lund: CWK Gleerup.

Petinou, K. (n.d.). Phonological patterns in two groups of Cypriot Greek-speaking children. Unpublished study.

Pye, C., Ingram, D., and List, H. (1987). A comparison of initial consonant acquisition in English and Quiché. In K. E. Nelson and A. van Kleeck (eds.), *Children's Language* (pp. 175–90). Hillsdale, NJ: Erlbaum.

Roussey, C. (1899). Notes sur l'apprentissage de la parole chez un enfant. *La Parole*, 1, 790–880.

Roussey, C. (1900). Notes sur l'apprentissage de la parole chez un enfant. *La Parole*, 2, 23–40, 86–97.

Saaristo-Helin, K., Savinainen-Makkonen, T., and Kunnari, S. (2006). The phonological mean length of utterance: Methodological challenges from a crosslinguistic perspective. *Journal of Child Language*, 33, 179–90.

So, L. and Dodd, B. (1995). The acquisition of phonology by Cantonese-speaking children. *Journal of Child Language*, 22, 473–95.

Stoel-Gammon, C. (1991). Normal and disordered phonology in two-year olds. *Topics in Language Disorders*, 11(4), 21–32.

Stokes, S. F. and Surendran, D. (2005). Articulatory complexity, ambient frequency, and functional load as predictors of consonant development in children. *Journal of Speech, Language, and Hearing Research*, 48, 577–91.

Taelman, H., Durieux, G., and Gillis, S. (2005). Notes on Ingram's whole-word measures for phonological acquisition. *Journal of Child Language*, 32, 391–405.

Topbaş, S. (1992). A pilot study of phonological acquisition by Turkish children and its implications for phonological disorders. Paper presented to the 6th International Conference on Turkish Linguistics, Eskisehir, Turkey.

Topbaş, S. (1996). Phonological analysis in speech disordered children in Turkish. Paper presented to the VIIth International Congress for the Study of Child Language, Istanbul.

Vinson, J. (1915). Observations sur le développement du langage chez l'enfant. *Revue Linguistique*, 49, 1–39.

Author Index

Subject Index